Periodontal Disease: A Clinical Approach

Periodontal Disease: A Clinical Approach

Edited by **Regina Stuart**

hayle medical

New York

Published by Hayle Medical,
30 West, 37th Street, Suite 612,
New York, NY 10018, USA
www.haylemedical.com

Periodontal Disease: A Clinical Approach
Edited by Regina Stuart

International Standard Book Number: 978-1-63241-318-5 (Hardback)

Printed in China.

Contents

Preface

A clinical approach towards periodontal disease has been described in this up-to-date book. The aim of this book is to cater to modern practitioners as well as students and educators in the field of periodontology. An elucidation of the contemporary concepts illustrating the complex interactions of multiple genotypes, microbial fingerprint and host modulations has been presented in this book. Furthermore, an analysis of the clinical outcome of the disease's progression, as influenced by the epigenetic factors, has been provided. This elucidative book also provides in-depth explanations of the rising concepts on periodontitis as a bilateral modulating factor and as a risk factor for several systemic diseases.

This book is a result of research of several months to collate the most relevant data in the field.

When I was approached with the idea of this book and the proposal to edit it, I was overwhelmed. It gave me an opportunity to reach out to all those who share a common interest with me in this field. I had 3 main parameters for editing this text:

1. Accuracy - The data and information provided in this book should be up-to-date and valuable to the readers.

2. Structure - The data must be presented in a structured format for easy understanding and better grasping of the readers.

3. Universal Approach - This book not only targets students but also experts and innovators in the field, thus my aim was to present topics which are of use to all.

Thus, it took me a couple of months to finish the editing of this book.

I would like to make a special mention of my publisher who considered me worthy of this opportunity and also supported me throughout the editing process. I would also like to thank the editing team at the back-end who extended their help whenever required.

Editor

Part 1

Aetiology of Periodontal Diseases

1

The Microbial Aetiology of Periodontal Diseases

Charlene W.J. Africa
University of the Western Cape
South Africa

1. Introduction

The study of the aetiology of periodontal diseases has continued for decades with much progress shown in the last two decades. Having moved through periods of "whole" plaque (with emphasis on mass) being attributed to the disease process, to "specific" species being implicated, we have finally returned to examining the oral microbiota as an ecological niche involving not only a selected few species but looking at plaque as a whole where all the players are invited to participate with their roles no longer individually defined but viewed as a team effort with recognition of their individual strengths and contributions. Recent findings using advanced technology, are confirming findings viewed by electron microscopy nearly half a century ago, but we now have the knowledge and expertise to interpret those findings with deeper understanding. This chapter will attempt to examine the microbial succession within the plaque biofilm from health to disease, bearing in mind the susceptibility of the host, the microbial heterogeneity and the expression of virulence by the putative pathogens.

2. Theories proposed by early pioneers

Microbial plaque has been implicated as the primary aetiologic factor in chronic inflammatory periodontal disease (CIPD, Listgarten, 1988). Studies of experimental gingivitis in man and in animal models have confirmed that a positive correlation exists between plaque accumulation and CIPD, and that plaque control reverses the inflammatory process (Lindhe *et al.*, 1973; Löe *et al.*, 1965; Page & Schroeder, 1976, 1982 Theilade *et al.*, 1966). It has also become evident, at least in relation to chronic gingivitis, that plaque mass rather than quality is the main correlate with disease severity (Abdellatif & Burt, 1987; Ramfjord *et al.*, 1968). It was initially postulated that CIPD occurred as the result of an overgrowth of indigenous plaque microorganisms (Gibbons *et al.*, 1963; Löe *et al.*, 1965; Socransky *et al.*, 1963; Theilade *et al.*, 1966). But, since many of the organisms observed in periodontal health were also observed at diseased sites (Slots, 1977), the results indicated that shifts in microbial populations rather than specific pathogens would play a role in initiating disease. Failure to demonstrate an overt pathogen gave rise to the non-specific plaque hypothesis (NSPH, Loesche, 1976), which generally assumes that all plaque is capable of causing disease. If the plaque mass is increased, irritants produced by the plaque microbes are increased until gingival inflammation ensues.

However, the NSPH failed to explain why certain individuals with longstanding plaque and gingivitis do not develop periodontitis, while others, with minimal plaque, had lower resistance to disease. Comparisons of health and diseased sites, demonstrated an increase in Gram-negative organisms in the latter (Hemmens & Harrison, 1942; Rosebury *et al.*, 1950; Scultz-Haudt *et al.*, 1954). By 1977, the focus had shifted from supra to subgingival plaque and since sampling and cultural methods had improved, more sophisticated studies were possible in relation to the microbial aetiology of CIPD. It was shown that subgingival plaque composition differs, not only between subjects, but also between sites within the same mouth (Listgarten & Hellden, 1978; Socransky *et al.*, 1992). The culture of plaque samples from single diseased sites lead to the association of certain bacterial species with various forms of CIPD (Listgarten, 1992; Socransky & Haffajee, 1992,).

While the NSPH focuses on quantitative changes, the specific plaque hypothesis (SPH) focuses on qualitative changes. Evidence for the specific plaque hypothesis has been derived from studies of subgingival microflora associated with health and disease, from evaluations of the pathogenic potential of various members of the periodontal microbiota as well as selective suppression of the microflora by chemotherapy using both human and animal models. These criteria have been used in association studies, since no single pathogen has been isolated which fulfils the criteria for Koch's postulates, namely, that a specific organism should be isolated in pure culture in all lesions of the disease and a similar disease produced in animals when inoculated with the causative organism, resulting in the recovery of that same organism from the lesions of the infected animals. These postulates have proved inadequate for CIPD since cultural studies of CIPD have revealed over 700 bacterial species, many of which are extremely difficult to cultivate, creating problems with animal inoculations. Another factor is that the disease produced in experimental studies with animals need not necessarily be the same disease observed in humans (Socransky, 1979), nor does a bacterium which is known to be pathogenic always cause disease in selected hosts even though they may be of the same species (Socransky & Haffajee 1992). It is therefore impracticable to compare virulence in different host species, even though the same pathogen is used. Alternatives for Koch's postulates were suggested by Socransky (1979), namely, that there be association of the organism with disease followed by elimination after treatment, and that host response, animal pathogenicity and mechanisms of pathogenicity are considered.

Association of a given organism with disease is demonstrated by an increase in the proportion of that organism at the site of infection and a decrease or absence in health and after treatment. The marked differences between plaques seen in health and disease, and the establishment in the subgingival plaque of species such as *Porphyromonas gingivalis* and *Aggregatibacter actinomycetemcomitans* (Aa), which are seldom, if ever, detected in health or gingivitis, led to the hypothesis that severe periodontitis was caused by exogenous microorganisms (Genco *et al.*, 1988). However, this hypothesis failed to define a specific means of host entry or colonisation. Nor was the acquisition or mode of transmission adequately explained. Although treatment resulted in suppression or elimination of these species, the authors failed to include the effect of treatment on many of the indigenous species as well. Acceptance of an exogenous infection hypothesis was considered by many as an over-simplification of a very complex situation. Re-evaluation of the different hypotheses indicated that they all contained contradictions. Overlaps often occurred regarding suspected "periodontopathogens" in active and inactive sites. This negated both the SPH and the NSPH. Eradication of "exogenous pathogens" resulted in a microbial shift from a disease-related to a health-associated microbiota, incorporating both the SPH and the NSPH. To confuse the issue even further, miscroscopic (Africa *et al.*, 1985a; Reddy *et al.*, 1986) and cultural studies (Africa, unpublished data) of plaque from two groups of subjects with heavy plaque accumulations, showing no clinical evidence of associated loss of attachment, demonstrated disease-associated microbial species. High percentages of spirochaetes and motile rods were indicated in these darkfield studies, while the cultural studies demonstrated the presence of *Porphyromonas gingivalis* and *Prevotella intermedia* amongst their predominant cultivable species. However, distinct differences in the cultivable microflora accompanying these species were observed when the periodontitis group was compared with the two periodontitis-resistant groups. This would indicate that the host response, along with microbial interactions within the plaque microbiota, determined disease progression and that neither the SPH nor the NSPH *per se* could be applied in this case. Theilade (1986) proposed an acceptance of a compromise between the two, in order to accommodate the microbial succession from health to disease, when attempting to establish the association of specific species with CIPD.

The inability to explain why some individuals developed disease and others not, created difficulties in comparing data, especially since inter-individual as well as intra-individual variability was often demonstrated. With more than 700 microbial species inhabiting the periodontal pocket, many of which are uncultivable and/or difficult to identify, contradictions often occur regarding the association of specific species with a particular disease entity.

These research outcomes are complicated by differences in sampling and detection methods and inaccuracies in the classification and diagnosis of disease. Added to that, is the fact that animal models of disease are often used for *in vivo* investigations of monomicrobial infections. The disease is therefore induced and differs from natural pathogens in humans (Arnett and Viney, 2007) where the disease process is initiated by the normal microbiota overcoming the tolerance threshold of the host, resulting in a polymicrobial infection (Gemmell *et al.*, 2002; Kesavalu *et al.*, 1997).

Because a precise definition of disease activity has not been clearly established, earlier studies of the microbial aetiology of CIPD have failed to implicate any single plaque bacterial species as the definitive causative species. Many of the subgingival flora could not be classified by existing taxonomic schema at the time, with the result that oral microbiologists often forced their isolates into existing species descriptions, a process which was not only incorrect but which confused and hampered the process of implicating specific aetiological agents in periodontal disease. The bacteria discussed in the subsequent sections can only be implicated by association with disease and have not been proven as single pathogens fulfilling the criteria of Koch's postulates. The flora of sites sampled at a particular time may not relate to that present at a time of an episode of disease activity or quiescence. Results may reflect previous episodes of disease activity and may have no bearing on the current level of disease activity (Listgarten, 1992; Socransky & Haffajee, 1992).

3. The ecological plaque hypothesis

The finding of suspected pathogens in mouths free of disease could either be due to avirulent clonal types of the microbial species or due to low levels of bacterial species in an insusceptible or "carrier" host. With the advent of molecular biology, our understanding has been greatly improved and our approach to identifying the putative pathogens has gone full circle. We are once again looking at bacterial succession and ecological changes but with improved knowledge where, with the assistance of modern technology, we are viewing bacterial plaque as a "biofilm" of microbes possessing the chromosomal and extra chromosomal genetic properties necessary to initiate disease in a susceptible host. In order to initiate disease, a potential pathogen has to colonise a susceptible host with an appropriate infectious dose in an environment conducive to optimal bacterial interactions which will favour the expression of its virulence properties (Socransky & Haffajee, 1992). This environmental activity results in patterns of bacterial succession favouring the ecological plaque hypothesis (Marsh, 1991). The ecological plaque hypothesis suggests that periodontal disease is an opportunistic endogenous infection brought about by an ecological shift in the plaque biofilm from a predominantly Gram-positive facultatively anaerobic microflora to a Gram-negative obligate anaerobic or micro-aerophilic flora, resulting from host-microbial and microbe-microbe interactions, creating an anaerobic environment which favours their growth (Konopka, 2006). Thus any bacterial species may be pathogenic since ecological changes in the environment may dictate the pathogenicity and virulence mechanisms for that particular organism (Marsh, 1991, 1994, 1998). Disease may thus be prevented by interruption of the environmental factors responsible for the ecological shifts as well as elimination of the putative pathogen.

4. The oral cavity as a microbial ecosystem

The oral cavity is home to a multitude of microbes colonising a variety of surfaces, namely the tooth, tonsils, tongue, hard and soft pellets, buccal cavity, lips and associated gingival tissue. (Kolenbrander & Landon, 1993; Paster *et al.*, 2001; Rosan & Lamont, 2000; Whittaker *et al.*, 1996). With specific microbial species demonstrating tropism for specific tissues (Aas *et al.*, 2005; Gibbons, 1996; Mager *et al.*, 2003; Van Houte *et al.*, 1970), all of which interact with each other as well as with the oral environment, the oral cavity meets the criteria for the definition of a microbial ecosystem (Konopka, 2006; Marsh, 1992; Raes & Bork, 2008).

Factors which determine the oral microflora include environmental factors (temperature, oxygen tension, pH, availability of nutrients), host factors (host tissues and fluids, genetics, diet) and microbial factors (adherence, retention and coaggregation, microbial intra- and interspecies interactions, clonal heterogeneity, virulence mechanisms) thus creating a dynamic and complex ecosystem (Kuramitsu *et al.*, 2007; Kolenbrander, 2006; Marsh, 2005; Overman, 2000; Rosan & Lamont, 2000; Sissons *et al.*, 2007; Socransky & Haffajee, 2002; Ten Carte, 2006).

Dental plaque is a dynamic biofilm formed by the ordered succession of > 700 bacterial species. The recognition of dental plaque as an oral biofilm has now become widely accepted. (Aas *et al.*,2005; Bowden, 2000; Filoche *et al.*, 2010; Haffajee *et al.* ,2008; Jenkinson & Lamont, 2005; Marsh, 1991, 2003, 2006; Marsh & Percival, 2006; Socransky & Haffajee, 2005). In health these endogenous species live in symbiosis with the host , but changes in the oral microbial ecology due to nutritional and atmospheric gradients, synergistic and/or antagonistic interactions between microbial species, may alter the balance of the host and render an organism pathogenic (Carlsson, 1997; Kolenbrander, 2000; Lamont & Jenkinson, 1998; Marsh, 1999, Newman, 1988; Pratten & Wilson 1999, Quireynen *et al.* 1995, 2001, Rosan & Lamont, 2000; Sbordone & Bortolaia, 2003; Socransky & Haffejee, 1992, 1995; Socransky *et al.*, 1998). Most periodontopathogens are commensals in the oral cavity and express their virulence only in a susceptible host or when changes occur in their ecosystem. Microbial species exhibit different properties when they form communities in the plaque biofilm and work together rather than in isolation. With synergy prevailing over antagonism, they respond to changes in the environment as a single unit rather than as individual species (Caldwell *et al.,* 1997). Formation of the plaque biofilm and a discussion of ecological succession in the development of CIPD, is essential in understanding the changes which occur in the periodontium during the progression from health to disease. Ecological succession is the process whereby a microbial population (e.g. plaque microbiota) undergoes a continuous series of changes in composition as different species colonise and become established at the expense of others. The microbial population present at any given time will determine the subsequent successional changes.

4.1 Formation of the plaque biofilm

The tooth surface is a non-shedding surface which allows for the colonisation of microbial species and the establishment of a plaque biofilm. If a tooth surface is professionally cleaned, a deposit called the acquired pellicle develops within 15-30 minutes. It is a thin, clear cuticle composed of mainly glycoproteins and its source is generally considered to be precipitations of mucoids from saliva, containing molecules which are recognised by bacterial adhesins during the initial selective adsorption of Gram-positive cocci (streptococci) to the surface of the acquired pellicle.

Saliva not only provides substrates for bacterial growth by the secretion of proteins and glycoproteins (endogenous nutrients) but also serves as a mode of transport for carbohydrates and peptides (exogenous nutrients) of dietary origin (Homer *et al.,* 1996; Palmer *et al.,* 2001; Scannapieco, 1994). When a microorganism adsorbs to the acquired pellicle, growth and multiplication will occur, accompanied by accumulation of bacterial products. Attachment of microorganisms is further enhanced by the production of dextrans by the streptococci and by the ability of bacterial cells to coaggregate (Kolenbrander, 2000). Differences in microbial growth rates cause population shifts to occur quickly once the initial microbial population has been established.

The cleansing activities of the mouth such as saliva, abrasion and swallowing are limited to the colonisation of supragingival plaque only. The subgingival plaque, due to the anatomy of the gingival sulcus, is undisturbed by the cleansing activites of the mouth and because a relatively stagnant environment is formed, harbours many more motile bacteria than supragingival plaque. Because the oxidation-reduction potential (Eh) of the gingival sulcus is very low (Loesche, 1988), the subgingival environment would favour the growth of a more anaerobic microflora than would be found in supragingival areas where the environment selects for the growth of aerobic and facultative microflora. The indigenous anaerobic microflora includes members of the genera *Actinomyces, Bacteroides, Bifidobacterium, Campylobacter, Capnocytophaga, Fusobacterium, Leptotrichia, Peptococcus, Peptostreptococcus, Propionibacterium, Veillonella* and many motile organisms such as *Selenomonas,* a few spirochaetes and vibrios. Many of these species co-exist with facultative and capnophilic bacteria in periodontal health and disease.

4.2 Bacterial interactions during biofilm development

Pathogens do not exist in isolation in the oral cavity but as part of a microbial community which may display synergistic or antagonistic interactions. Microbial diversity is spatially structured, not only by geographic location, but also by environment (O'Malley, 2008).

Early plaque is composed of mainly Gram-positive cocci which are gradually replaced by more filamentous Gram-positive forms and finally, an abundance of Gram-negative forms which were not found initially (Kolenbrander *et al.*, 1985 ; Haffajee & Socransky, 1988). Gram-negative colonisation of the gingival sulcus occurs only after the lawn of Gram-positive organisms has been established, since Gram-negative organisms cannot adhere directly to the tooth surface (Slots, 1977). An increase in the thickness of the plaque biofilm results in the creation of nutritional and atmospheric gradients which alter the environment, reducing oxygen levels and allowing for the growth of anaerobes (Bradshaw *et al.*, 1998; Cook *et al.*, 1998; Lamont & Jenkinson, 1998). Coaggregation enables the colonisation of organisms that do not have receptor sites. Their colonisation is therefore facilitated by the colonisation of a synergistic species. Coaggregation can be defined as intrageneric, intergeneric or multigeneric cell-to-cell recognition (Kolenbrander, 1989) in a biofilm community and was reported to occur between viable as well as dead cells, providing evidence that interactions are mediated by existing specific surface molecules rather than cells responding actively to each other (Kolenbrander, 1993). An important factor of plaque biofilm formation is the spatial relationship of the community members (Dawes 2008; Mager *et al.* 2003; Mineoka *et al.*, 2008). The proximity of phenotypes allows for their interactions and influences their ability to survive within the biofilm.

Among the early studies of spatial relationships in plaque biofilm formation are the studies by Nyvad and colleagues (Nyvad, 1993; Nyvad & Fejerskov, 1987a; Nyvad & Fejerskov, 1987b; Nyvad & Killian, 1987). Using a stent that holds enamel pieces (commonly used in supragingival oral film investigations), they placed it in the oral cavity and monitored the formation of plaque biofilms. Among the first species to colonise were streptococci and actinomyces, including *Streptococcus sanguinis, Streptococcus oralis, Streptococcus mitis, Streptococcus salivarius* and *Actinomyces viscosus.* Plaque biovars were seen to develop at exactly the same rate from individual to individual, reaching a plateau around 12 hours after stent insertion (Nyvad & Kilian, 1987). Electron microscopy confirmed a change in species composition over the next 12 hours with both Gram-positive and Gram-negative bacteria appearing, providing evidence for direct interaction between species in the biofilm (Nyvad & Fejerskov, 1987b).

Further studies confirmed the importance of cell-to-cell recognition in early plaque development and examination of undisturbed plaque. Palmer *et al,(*2003) used antibodies to detect adhesins or their complimentary receptors on bacteria known to coaggregate. They examined the reactions using immunofluorescence and confocal microscopy and found that many of the cells which reacted with the adhesin antibody were adjacent to cells reactive with the receptor antibody. Diaz *et al., (*2006) used ribosome-directed fluorescence in situ hybridisation (FISH) to examine spatial relationships and produced similar results.

Electron microscopy has demonstrated that where 2 or more species coaggregate with a common partner using the same mechanism, they are likely to compete for receptor sites e.g. "corncob" formations, where coccoid cells such as streptococci attach to a long rod such as *Fusobacterium nucleatum* (Jones, 1972; Listgarten *et al.*, 1973) or *S. sanguinis* and *Corynebacterium matruchotii* (Bowden, 1999; Palmer, 2001; Socransky *et al.*, 1998; Wilson, 1999). Another example is the " test-tube brush" arrangement formed by *Eubacterium yurii* (Margaret & Krywolap, 1986). If 2 or more bacteria coaggregate with a common partner using different mechanisms of adhesion, the common partner acts as the coaggregation bridge for the coaggregation of the other 2 species e.g. *Prevotella loescheii* PK 1295 provides the bridge linking *Streptococcus oralis 34* to *Actinomyces israelii* PK 14 (Weiss *et al.*, 1987).

Intergeneric coaggregations occur with *Fusobacterium* and other bacteria such as *Aggregatibacter actinomycetemcomitans* (Rosen *et al.*, 2003), *Tannerella forsythia* (Sharma *et al.*, 2005), and oral *Treponema* (Kolenbrander, 1995). Intrageneric coaggregations occur among different strains of oral fusobacteria (Kolenbrander, 1995), *P. gingivalis* (Lamont *et al.*, 1992), oral streptococci, and *Actinomyces* (Kolenbrander *et al.*, 1989). Coaggregation bonds between *P. gingivalis* and oral streptococci or *Actinomyces naeslundi* are rendered resistant to removal if *P. gingivalis* adheres directly *to Streptococcus gordonii* (Brooks *et al.*, 1997; Cook et al., 1998; Demuth *et al.*, 2001, Rosan & Lamont, 2000; Quirynen *et al.*, 1995).
The production of metabolic products by plaque bacteria may promote or inhibit the growth of other species (Kolenbrander, 2000; Quirynen *et al.*, 1995, 2001). Examples of cross-feeding include but are not limited to, the production of lactic acid by *Streptococcus* and *Actinomyces*, needed for the metabolism of *Veillonella* which, in turn, produce menadione which favours the growth of *Porphyromonas* and *Prevotella*. *Fusobactrium* produces fatty acids needed for the growth and metabolism of *Treponema* and in synergy with *P. gingivalis*, produces metabolic products needed for the growth of *Mogibacterium (Eubacterium) timidum* (Miyakawa & Nakazawa, 2010). Other beneficial microbial interactions include the prevention of colonisation of a pathogenic species by using receptors which may be needed for the attachment of latecomers (Rosen *et al.*, 2003) or by the production of substances which affect the growth of, or prevent the production or expression of, virulence factors by the pathogen (Socransky & Haffajee, 1992).

4.3 Quorum sensing

Another mechanism by which bacteria are able to communicate is via quorum sensing molecules. Quorum sensing has been described in both Gram-positive and Gram-negative bacteria. It has been defined by Miller (2001) as "the regulation of gene expression in response to fluctuations in cell population density".As they grow, quorum sensing bacteria produce to the external environment a series of molecules called autoinducers. The autoinducers accumulate as the bacterial population increases and once they reach a certain threshold, different sets of target genes are activated, thus allowing the bacteria to survive environmental changes. Cell-cell communication may occur between and within bacterial species (Miller, 2001) and controls various functions reflecting the needs of a specific bacterial species to inhabit a particular niche such as the production of virulence factors, or by the transmission and acquisition of the generic information needed to produce virulence factors from other species in the biofilm development (Passador *et al.*, 1993; Reading *et al.*, 2006). Several strains of *P. intermedia, T. forsythia, F. nucleatum* and *P. gingivalis* were found to produce quorum sensing signal molecules (Frias *et al.*, 2001; Sharma *et al.*, 2005).

4.4 Host susceptibility and inter-individual variation

It was previously understood that plaque control was effective in preventing and treating periodontal diseases. Now it is clear that the plaque biofilm alone is not enough to initiate or control the disease process. A susceptible host is needed and the susceptibility is genetically determined with individuals responding differently to various stimuli (Relman, 2008; Tombelli & Tatakis, 2003).
The severity of periodontal diseases differs amongst populations of different race (Douglas *et al.*, 1983), in different areas of the same country, (Teixeira *et al.*, 2006; Viera *et al*, 2009,) as well as in different countries (Cortelli *et al.*, 2005; Gajardo *et al.*, 2005; Haffajee *et al.*, 2004;

Sanz *et al.*, 2000; Rylev & Kilian, 2008). Asian and African popoulations have on average more severe periodontal disease than Europeans and Americans (Glickman, 1972; Baelum *et al.*, 1986; Botero *et al*, 2007). While this may largely be due to differences in oral hygiene habits, customs and traditions, confounding factors may affect the immune response which, in turn, will affect the level of disease activity (Table 1).

As previously mentioned, not all individuals are susceptible to periodontitis and the literature shows that some individuals present with gingivitis which appears to remain contained. A much quoted study of the plantation workers in Sri Lanka (Löe, 1986), who practised no oral hygiene and had no access to professional dental care, demonstrated that some, but not all, developed periodontitis, while others remained with minimal disease. Studies by Africa *et al.*, (1985a) and Reddy *et al.*(1986) reported on a periodontitis resistant population in South Africa . Although one of the first studies to report on increased prevalence of suspected periodontopathogens in the absence of periodontitis, thus suggesting a variability in host susceptibility to periodontitis as well as 'carriers" of avirulent strains, no genetic studies were done to confirm this.

Plaque biofilm formation has been described as a highly ordered sequential attachment of specific species over time, a process found to occur at the same rate for everyone (Palmer 2003). However, the architecture and function is person-specific and even though the same bacterial species may often be found in the same site of many different individuals, each individual may have a unique microbial fingerprint (Dethlefsen *et al.*, 2007), which dictates the outcome of disease progression and response to treatment (Filoche *et al.*, 2007, 2008; Haffajee *et al.*, 2006; Preza *et al.*, 2008; Sissons *et al.*, 2007; Teles *et al.*, 2006). Not only do different persons harbour different oral microbiota, but different sites within the same mouth as well as different sites of the same tooth in the same mouth also differ in microbial composition due to environmental differences (Dawes *et al.*, 2008; Haffajee *et al.*, 2006, 2009; Mager *et al.*, 2003; Mineoka *et al.*, 2008).

The bacterial challenge presented by the bacteria of the plaque biofilm activates the host inflammatory response which is also influenced by the factors listed in Table 1. The severity of periodontal disease is modified by the expression of three elements of the host response, namely, interleukin-1 (IL-1), prostaglandin-E_2 (PGE_2) and matrix metalloproteinases (MMPs) that destroy both collagen and bone. Increased production of IL-1 appears to be hereditary with specific IL-1 gene variation associated with response to the bacterial challenge (Assuma *et al.*, 1988; Cavanaugh *et al.*, 1998; Gemmell *et al.*, 1998; Ishihara *et al.*, 1997; McGee *et al.*, 1998; Okuda *et al.*, 1998; Roberts *et al.*, 1997).

Factor	Selected References
Smoking	Bergström *et al.*, 2000; Calsina *et al.*, 2002; Feldman *et al.*, 1983; Haber, 1994; Haber *et al.*, 1993; Stam, 1986;
Genetics	Engebretson *et al.*, 1999; Genco, 1998; Gore *et al.*, 1998; Grossi *et al.*, 1998; McDevitt *et al.*, 2000; Mark *et a*l., 2000; Michalowicz *et al.*, 2000; Lang *et al.*, 2000; Shirodaria *et al.*, 2000;
Diabetes	Genco, 1988; Grossi *et al.*, 1998
Hormones	Marcuschamer *et al.*, 2009
Stress	Armitage 1999; Bascones & Figuero 2006; Flemming, 1999; Genco, 1998; Newman, 1998.
Age	Genco, 1998; Horning *et al*, 1992

Table 1. Factors which may influence host susceptibility.

4.5 Gene expression

As mentioned above, host susceptibility may be genetically determined; so also, can many important virulence traits be ascribed to heterogeneity among subspecies of bacteria. Some strains are associated with health or "carrier" states while others are associated with disease. In order to confirm this, researchers have embarked on demonstrating multiple clonal types within the periodontopathogens and reported on their different virulence properties.

Gene expression is regulated in response to changes in the environment with either up- or down-regulation of the production of virulence factors (Finlay & Falkov, 1989; Maurelli *et al.*, 1989; Miller *et al.*, 1989), or when the organism comes into direct contact with partner community bacteria (Sharma, 2010) thus acquiring their virulence through cell-cell interactions (Araki *et al.*, 2004; Brook *et al.*, 1984; Kuriyama et al, 2010; Van Dalen *et al.*, 1998).

The persistence of clones appears to vary for different species, with many clones simultaneously inhabiting the oral cavity at different periods. Genomic polymorphisms within bacterial strains along with the response of the host will determine the disease situation and progression in the individual patient (Hohwy *et al.*, 2001; Kononen *et al.*, 1994; Tambo *et al.*, 2010). Early colonising species showing wide clonal diversity (reflected in antigenic variety) elicit natural immunity which benefits the host, while frequent turnover of clones within a particular host may allow the species to overcome the host response and exert its pathogenicity (Smith, 1988).

Multiple genotypes have been demonstrated in *Prevotella* (Yanagiswa *et al.*, 2006), *P. gingivalis* (Amano *et al.*, 2000; Nakagawa *et al.*, 2000), *F. nucleatum* (George *et al.*, 1997; Haraldsson *et al.*, 2004; Thurnheer *et al.*, 1999), *T. denticola* and other spirochaetes (Choi *et al.*, 1994; Reviere *et al.*, 1995), and Aa (Preus *et al.*, 1987a,b). Cross-sectional and longitudinal studies of *T. forsythia* in periodontal disease (Hamlet *et al.*, 2002, 2008) found the prtH genotype to be significantly raised in subjects with disease and lowered in subjects showing no attachment loss. It is generally accepted that species involved in infection will display a high degree of genetic similarity (Perez-Chaparo *et al.*, 2008). In the case of *P. gingivalis*, many different individuals may be colonised by a single genotype, but their clonal types may differ. Based on their nucleotide sequences, *P. gingivalis fima* gene has been classified into 5 genotypes (I-V). Types I and V are most prevalent in healthy adults (Amano *et al.*, 2000), with type I showing the most significant association (Amano *et al.*, 1999a; Nakagawa *et al.*, 2000). Anamo *et al.*(1999, 2000) reported Type II to be significantly associated with periodontitis, followed by type IV while the converse was found by Griffen *et al.*(1999), using ribosomal intergenic spacer region (ISR) heteroduplex typing, and Teixeira *et al.* (2009). These differences may be attributed to differences in techniques used and/or study population. Another explanation may be that virulent alles may be distributed at several genetic loci throughout the clones with only certain combinations producing a strain which may be associated with disease (Loos *et al.*, 1993). More than 100 genes were reported to be missing from the genome of a non-invasive strain of *P. gingivalis* (Dolgilevich *et al.*, 2011). Types III and IV of *P. gingivalis* are believed to be virulent, showing reduced ability to adhere to host proteins, while non-encapsulated strains of type I are recognised as avirulent and showed better adhesion to salivary proteins (Nakagawa *et al.*, 2000).

A key virulence factor of Aa is the powerful leucotoxin which is able to disrupt and destroy cells of the immune system. Aa serotypes c and b have been associated with health and disease respectively (Asikainen *et al.*, 1991). The leucotoxic clone JP2 is associated with serotype b and is characterised by enhanced leucotoxin expression associated with the 530bp deletion in the promoter region of the *ltx* operon. It is speculated that the clone might have a distinct host tropism being found mostly in adolescents in Mediterranean regions of Africa (e.g. Morocco) and West Africa from where it was transferred to the Americas during the slave trade. Although frequently found in subjects with aggressive periodontitis, clonal types other than JP2 have been associated with disease and carrier states. Recent evidence of aggressive periodontitis amongst adolescents in Morocco who do not have the JP2 clone (Rylev *et al.* 2011), and the finding of the JP2 clone in a Caucasian mother and daughter in Sweden who have no disease (Claesson *et al.* (2011), indicate that carriers do exist in Caucasians and that other serotypes may be associated with disease in African populations. Table 2 shows some examples of different serotypes in different population groups.

Ethnicity	%Aa isolates	Serotype distribution					
		a	b	c	d	e	NT
Chinese (Mombelli *et al.*, 1998)	61.6	15	0	38.3	0	8.3	0
Chinese (Mombelli *et a*l., 1999)	62.7	18	7.7	57.7	0	7.1	9.4
Vietnamese Finish (Holtta 1994)	78 13	36 6	27 6	63 0	0 0	0 0	0 0
Turkey (Dogan *et al.*, 2003)	66	0	0	34	0	0	34
Germans Koreans (Kim *et al.*, 2009)	27 22	20 0	33 0	25 61.9	0 19	0 0	0 0
Spanish (Blasi, 2009)	72.5	37.5	20	15	0	0	0
Brazilian (Roman-Torres *et al*, 2010)	80	31.8	<10	52.9	0	0	0

Table 2. Distribution of serotypes in different ethnic groups (NT = non typeable).

Serotypes a and b are prevalent in Europeans while serotype c is prevalent in Asian and Mediterranean groups (Table 2 and Sakellari *et al.*, 2011). Cortelli *et al.*, (2005) recommended that serotype b be used as a diagnostic marker for aggressive periodontitis since they found a high prevalence of the JP2 clone in a Brazilian population. These findings have been contradicted by other studies on Brazilians which showed very low, if any, serotype b strains (Vieira et al., 2009; Roman-Torres *et al.*, 2010). Yet another study showed similar frequencies of serotypes b and c but associated serotype b with health and c with disease (Teixeira *et al.*, (2006). The contradictions in these results may be due to the fact that Brazil has a multi-ethnic population of predominantly African and Mediterranean origin, while the native Brazilians, descending from almost extinct ethnic groups who live in cultural isolation with no mixing with other ethnic groups (Vieira *et al.*, 2009), have not been exposed to the toxic strains of Aa.

5. Plaque bacteria associated with health and periodontal disease

5.1 Plaque in health

The tooth surface harbours a microbial population which not only lives in harmony with host tissues, but also serves a protective function by occupying an ecological niche which would otherwise be colonised by potentially pathogenic bacteria. Bacterial species belonging to the genera *Streptococcus* and *Actinomyces* rapidly colonise bacteria-free surfaces, thus explaining their prevalence in dentitions which are well maintained (Listgarten, 1988). The relatively aerobic environment of the healthy gingival sulcus tends to preclude the growth of obligate anaerobes and the predominant flora includes members of the genera *Actinomyces, Atopobium, Eubacterium, Micromonas, Peptococcus, Staphylococcus, Streptococcus, Veillonella* while phylotypes Bacteroidetes and Deferribacteres have also been reported. Vibrios and spirochaetes are present in low numbers if at all (Dalwai *et al.*, 2006; Grossi *et al.*, 1994; Kumar *et al.*, 2003; Listgarten & Helldén, 1978; Loesche, 1980; Marsh, 1994; Rosan & Lamont, 2000).

Direct darkfield and phase contrast microscopic counts from healthy sites also indicate that spirochaetes (1-3%) and motile rods (1-6%) are present in low numbers, while coccoid cells (62-79%) predominate (Lindhe *et al.*, 1980; Addy *et al.*, 1983; Africa *et al.*, 1985b; Adler *et al.*, 1995; Stelzel *et al.*, 2000). Studies of healthy sites following treatment also show similar low counts of these forms due to their reduction or complete elimination, with a concomitant increase in cocci (Listgarten et al 1978; Loesche et al 1987; Africa *et al.*, 1985b; Adler *et al.*, 1995; Stelzel *et al.*, 2000).

In the section that follows, the association of microbial species with periodontal diseases will be discussed according to the classification outlined in the World Workshop Proceedings (Armitage, 1999) and will be restricted to a selection of the species most frequently associated with periodontal diseases.

5.2 Plaque in gingivitis

The new classification of periodontal diseases recognises that gingivitis is more prevalent than periodontitis and has thus included in the classification of "gingival diseases" all the previous sub-classifications of periodontitis related to endocrine and host immune disturbances, associations with therapeutic agents and malnutrition. In addition, plaque induced gingivitis has been classified separately from non-plaque induced gingivitis involving other aetiologic agents such as *Treponema pallidum, Neisseria gonorrhoeae,* streptococci, herpesviruses, and *Candida* which may also present in the oral cavity (Armitage, 1999). A detailed description of the classification is outside of the scope of this chapter and readers are advised to read the chapter on disease classification for details.

For ease of reading and association, this section will describe the microbiota under the broad headings of gingivitis, chronic periodontitis and aggressive periodontitis only, since many of the species overlap in the subclassifications of the three disease entities and may all be contained within the broad listing of putative pathogens in Table 3.

If the plaque biofilm remains undisturbed, demonstrable inflammation of the gingiva will occur in 2-4 days due to the production of various noxious bacterial metabolites such as endotoxins, mucopeptides, lipoteichoic acids, metabolic end-products and proteolytic agents, which may penetrate the gingival tissues. In addition, the increased production of gingival fluid contains growth-promoting factors for a wide range of bacteria. The initial phase of gingivitis is characterised by predominantly Gram-positive cocci, followed by fusiform bacilli after 2-4 days. Neutrophil transmigration through junctional and pocket epithelium is enhanced, accompanied by perivascular collagen destruction. Thinning and ultimate ulceration of the cuff epithelium may occur, followed by infiltration of lymphocytes and other mononuclear cells. Further loss of collagen from the marginal gingiva will occur, accompanied by an increase in vibrios and spirochaetes (Table 3) with a predominantly polymorphonuclear (PMN) leucocyte and plasma cell infiltrate apparent in the connective tissue. Bleeding on probing may occur and a relatively shallow gingival pocket may be evident. At this stage, chronic gingivitis can either be induced or eliminated by plaque control.

Bacterial species	**Gingivitis**	**Chronic periodontitis**	**Aggressive periodontitis**	
			Localised	**Generalised**
Aggregatibacter actinomycetemcomitans (Aa)		+	+	+
Campylobacter rectus	+	+		+
Capnocytophaga	+		+	+
Cryptobacterium curtum		+		
Eikenella corrodens	+	+	+	+
Enterobacteriaceae		+	+	
Eubacterium saphenum		+		
Fusobacterium nucleatum	+	+	+	
Micromonas (Peptostreptococcus) micros		+	+	
Mogibacterium (Eubacterium) timidum		+		
Peptostreptococcus anaerobius	+	+		
Pophyromonas endodontalis		+		
Porphyromonas gingivalis	+	+		+
Prevotella intermedia	+	+	+	+
Slackia (Eubacterium) exigua		+		
Tannerella forsythia		+		+
Treponema amylovorum		+		+
Treponema denticola	+	+		+
Treponema lecithinolyticum				+
Treponema maltophilum		+		
Treponema medium	+	+		
Treponema pectinovorum	+	+		+
Treponema socranskii	+	+		+
Treponema vincentii	+	+		+
Veillonella parvula	+			

Table 3. Bacterial species most frequently detected in periodontal diseases.

5.3 Plaque in chronic periodontitis

Previously referred to as adult periodontitis, this disease affects many teeth with no evidence of rapid progression. The onset appears to be after 30 years, but the condition may also be found in children and adolescents. Amounts of microbial deposits are usually associated with the severity of disease. Although chronic periodontitis can occur in a localised and a generalised form, both forms appear to be identical in their aetiology and pathogenesis. The microbial pattern varies, with reports of unusual species appearing in the literature. The species listed in Table 3, date post 1999 only, following the reclassification of periodontal diseases, since studies before 1999 might now fall within a different disease category under the new classification and create confusion.

When periodontal disease becomes active or destructive, the numbers of the bacteria in the unattached zone increases and Gram-negative organisms, particularly the motile organisms, predominate. If this condition is allowed to persist, the periodontal tissues are rapidly destroyed. Direct microscopy studies using both darkfield and phase contrast have revealed significant differences between subgingival microbial floras of healthy and diseased subjects. Listgarten & Helldén (1978) demonstrated that in chronic periodontitis-affected subjects, spirochaetes constituted 37.7% and motile rods 12.7% of the total microscopic count, with coccoid cells as low as 22.3%. These microbiological changes may signal an increase in periodontal disease activity. Many cycles of exacerbation and remission may continue till the alveolar bone is destroyed and the teeth lost (Socransky *et al.*, 1984).

Table 3 lists some of the species most frequently associated with periodontal diseases (Botero *et al.*, 2007; Casarin *et al.*, 2010; Dogan *et* al., 2003, Gajardo *et al.*, 2005; Kumar *et al.*, 2003; Teixeira *et al.*, 2006; Riep *et al.*, 2009). Species associated with chronic periodontitis are predominantly Gram-negative with few Gram-positive anaerobes. Spirochaetes predominate along with *P. gingivalis* and *T. forsythia*. Bacterial antagonism and synergism are indicated with Aa seldom reported along with *P. gingivalis* , while species like *F. nucleatum, P. intermedia* and other species of the "orange complex" (Socransky *et al.*,(1998) are necessary for the colonisation of the "red complex" consortium. Subjects with high proportions of *P. gingivalis* were found to have few or no *P. intermedia* and *vice versa* (Loesche *et al.*, 1985, Africa, unpublished data). Recent studies would indicate that this inhibition has been overcome, probably due to interactions of emerging species or due to clonal diversity within the two species, resulting in a mutual tolerance.

Recently, our attention has been drawn to the colonisation of the asaccharolytic anaerobic Gram-positive rods (AAGPRs) which have been associated with periodontitis (Miyakawa & Nakagawa, 2010). Although some of these species have been reported in the past, their role in disease has not received much attention. While they have an inability to form biofilms when cultured individually, they appear to be dependent on *P. gingivalis* and *F. nucleatum* for their colonisation of, and establishment in, the plaque biofilm. Their irregular finding in plaque cultural studies may be due to their fastidious growth requirements and difficulties in their colony recognition. Some of the AAGPR species may form part of the viable but not cultivable (VNC) species in the oral cavity, playing a role in prolonging and stabilising of biofilms formed by *P. gingivalis.* Because they are able to inhibit cytokine production by human gingival fibroblasts stimulated by other bacteria, it is possible that they may prolong inflammation, causing chronic disease (Miyakawa & Nakagawa, 2010).

The role of Enterobacteriaceae in chronic periodontitis is not clear and they are thought to indicate superinfection. It is speculated that they are opportunists which thrive after periodontal treatment. The drugs of choice for treating periodontal disease include amoxicillin, doxycycline, tetracycline and metronidazole. The Enterobacteriaceae show resistance to these drugs and may therefore persist after administration of therapy (Botero *et al.*, 2007). More studies are needed to explain their presence in the plaque biofilm and to elucidate their role in infection.

Herpes viruses may contribute to the pathogenesis of chronic and aggressive periodontitis (Table 4). There is speculation that Epstein-Barr virus-1 (EBV-1) and cytomegalovirus (CMV) may be involved in synergistic mechanisms with Aa, *P. gingivalis* and *T. forsythia* (Chalabi *et al.*, 2010; Dawson et al., 2009; Imbronito *et al.*, 2008; Slots 2010, Fritschi *et al.*, 2008).

Microbe	Chronic Periodontitis	Localised Aggressive Periodontitis	Generalised Aggressive Periodontitis
Herpes simplex virus-1	+	-	+
Cytomegalovirus	+	-	
Epstein-Barr virus	+	-	+
Dialister pneumosintes	+	-	-
Prevotella denticola	+	-	-
Staphylococcus aureus	-	-	+

Table 4. Species less frequently reported but also implicated in periodontal diseases.

5.4 Aggressive periodontitis

This form of periodontitis is less common than chronic periodontitis and mostly affects young patients. Localised and general forms of the disease differ in aetiology and pathogenesis. Localised aggressive periodontitis (LAP) mostly restricted to the first molars and incisors, is characterised by rapid loss of attachment and bone destruction in otherwise clinically healthy individuals while generalised aggressive periodontitis (GAP) presents a clinical picture similar to LAP but the bone loss is generalised. Aggressive periodontitis was previously called localised and generalised juvenile periodontitis. Plaque films are thinner than in chronic periodontitis and age is no longer a criterion for diagnosis (Armitage, 1999).

Comparison of the microbiology of chronic periodontitis with aggressive periodontitis shows major overlaps , with very few species showing unique specificity for either condition (Table 3). The organisms most strongly associated with LAP and GAP are Aa and *P. gingivalis* respectively. The prevalence of Aa in LAP and GAP is often contradictory with some reporting it only in LAP and others reporting it in both LAP and GAP. However, the prevalence appears to be higher in LAP. A positive correlation was found between a highly toxigenic group of Aa and deep pockets, young age and mean attachment loss (Cortelli *et al.*, 2005). Aa was found to be present in very low numbers in a Colombian population (Botero *et al.*, 2007) when compared with Asian populations (Yang *et al.*, 2005; Leung *et al.*, 2005) and a Brazilian population (Cortelli *et al.*, 2005). The Colombian population harboured *E. corrodens, P. gingivalis* and *T. forsythia* along with Enterobacteriaceae. The latter may be associated with halitosis in humans (Goldberg et al., 1997). As with chronic periodontitis, very few studies make a distinction between LAP and GAP. Most studies report on "aggressive periodontitis" (Botero *et al.*, 2007; Cortelli *et al.*, 2005; Sakellari *et al.*, 2004) which, in the context of this chapter is interpreted as GAP.

6. Virulence mechanisms of plaque bacteria

Although the terms pathogenicity and virulence relate to the ability of a microorganism to produce disease, pathogenicity refers to the species and virulence refers to degrees of pathogenicity of strains within species. Microbial virulence is investigated by comparing the properties of virulent and avirulent strains. *In vitro* studies of enzymes, antigens, metabolic and biological properties indicate virulence markers which may be responsible for inhibiting host defence mechanisms or tissue damage. These results could often be misleading since many bacteria from infected animals have been shown to differ chemically and biologically from tissue grown *in vitro*. This could be explained by differences in growth conditions and phenotypic changes. However, there are some bacterial virulence determinants which were originally examined *in vivo* and then reproduced *in vitro* by approximate changes in cultural conditions (Smith, 1976). In order for bacteria to be considered pathogenic, they should be examined for their ability to colonise the appropriate site and initiate infection, multiply within the host's tissues, resist and overcome the host's defences and cause damage to the host's tissues. This section is limited to the discussion of selected microbial species and is based purely on association studies and the demonstration *in vitro* of their pathogenic potential but bearing in mind that true virulence is expressed in a susceptible host, rather than *in vitro*, where nutritional and other environmental conditions differ. Tables 5-8 list the important virulence factors of four of the species most frequently associated with periodontal diseases namely, *T. denticola, P. gingivalis,* Aa and *T. forsythia* respectively.

6.1 Adhesion and colonisation

Many of the suspected periodontopathogens have surface structures necessary for attachment, including fimbriae, capsules and lipopolysaccharides.

6.1.1 Fimbriae

The interaction between bacterial fimbriae and host factors could be an important component of the disease process.

Fimbriae are extracellular appendages which facilitate the adhesion of a Gram-negative organism to a surface. Aa possesses fimbriae and amorphous material which assist in adhesion (Fives-Taylor *et al.,* 1999). Protein sequence homology of *P. gingivalis* fimbriae polymers of repeating fimbrillin monomer subunits with a molecular weight of about 43kDa (Yoshimura *et al.*, 1984; Lee *et al.*, 1991) show no homology with the fimbriae of other Gram-negative bacteria. The *fim*A gene of *P. gingivalis* appears to be involved in most of the adhesive mechanisms of the organism. *P. gingivalis* fimbriae also facilitate coaggregation with other plaque organisms such as *T. denticola*, oral streptococci, fusobacteria, actinomyces and oral epithelial cells, amongst others. Other reported functions of fimbriae include chemotaxis and cytokine induction (Goulbourne & Ellen, 1991; Hashimoto *et al.,* 2003; Ishihara et al 1997; Rosen *et al.*, 2008; Yao *et al.*, 1996).

6.1.2 Capsules and surface layers (S-layers)

The outer layer of bacteria is often referred to as a capsule (uniform consistency) or a slime layer (ill- defined and loosely formed). Because it is this outer layer that is in direct contact with the environment, it is largely responsible for the ultimate survival of the producer bacterial cell.

The composition of capsular polysaccharide may vary among strains and may be composed of either carbohydrate or protein, depending on the conditions under which they were grown (Hofstad, 1992). *In vitro* studies have demonstrated a capsule on *P. gingivalis* (Listgarten & Lai, 1979; Woo *et al.*, 1979), fusobacteria and peptostreptococci (Brook and Walker, 1985, 1986). Besides having adhesive properties, capsules are known to provide immunologic specificity and protection against phagocytosis.

T. forsythia lacks fimbriae and possesses a surface layer of glycoproteins. These serve as ligands for lectin-like receptors on other bacteria e.g. *F. nucleatum* (Murray *et al.*, 1988), epithelial cell adherence and invasion (Tanner *et al.*, 1996; Sakakibara *et al.*, 2007) and as an external protective layer (Sleytr & Messner, 1988), highly regulated to respond to environmental changes (Kato *et al.*, 2002). S-layers have also been reported for *C. rectus* (Haapasalo *et al.*, 1990), *Prevotella buccae* (Kornman & Holt, 1981) and *Eubacterium yunii* (Kerosuo *et al.*, 1988).

The oral spirochaetes possess an outer sheath or slime layer which envelopes the complete cell. In *T. denticola*, this layer is composed of 50% protein and 31% total lipid, of which 95% and 11% are phospholipid and carbohydrate respectively (Masuda & Kawata, 1982; Weinberg & Holt, 1990). The adhesive properties of *T. denticola* to hydroxyapatite (Cimansoni *et al.*, 1987), human gingival epithelial cells (Olsen, 1984; Reijntjens *et al.*, 1986), fibroblasts (Weinberg & Holt, 1990), fibronectin (Dawson & Ellen, 1990; Haapasalo *et al.*, 1992) fibrinogen and laminin (Haapasalo *et al.*, 1992) as well as erythrocytes (Mikx & Keulers, 1992), have been demonstrated. The putative *T. denticola* adhesin was characterised as being a surface-bound 53 kDa protein (Cockayne *et al.*, 1989; Umemoto *et al.*, 1989; Haapasalo *et al.*, 1992), while Weinberg & Holt (1990) described outer sheath surface proteins of 64 kDa and 54-58 kDa depending on the strain examined. These proteins were considered to be major degradation components of high molecular mass oligomers (Haapasalo *et al.*, 1992). *T. denticola* major sheath protein (Msp) is thought to be responsible for its binding *to F. nucleatum, Streptococcus crista, P. gingivalis* and *T. forsythia* (Kolenbrander *et al.*, 2000).

6.1.3 Haemagglutinins

Haemagglutinins are known virulence factors for a number of bacteria of which *P. gingivalis* produces 5 haemagglutinating molecules. Their role in colonisation is to mediate the binding of bacteria to human cell receptors. Our understanding of the complexities of the genetics and functions of the haemagglutinin process has been greatly informed by the cloning of the first haemagglutinin gene (*hag*A) from *P. gingivalis* (Progulske-Fox *et al.*, 1989). Because *P. gingivalis* requires haem for growth, the binding to erythrocytes may also serve as a nutrient source (Progulske-Fox *et al.*, 1989). Co-expression of genes associated with haemagglutination and proteolytic activity of *P. gingivalis*, suggest that they function in complexes on the cell surface (Shah *et al.*, 1992). Haemagglutinating activity has also been described for *T. forsythia* (Tables 5- 8).

6.2 Impairing host immune systems

For adhesion to lead to colonisation, bacteria must be able to resist the host defence mechanisms such as phagocytosis and the protective antimicrobial factors which would otherwise destroy them. The innate immune system is the host's first line of defence against bacterial infection. Immunomodulation by bacteria allows for their survival and subsequent invasion.

6.2.1 Interfering with PMN function

The ability of *T. denticola* to suppress the production of β-defensin 3 by human gingival epithelial cells (Table 5) has been reported (Shin *et al.,* 2010). By preventing binding of such antimicrobial peptides, *Treponema* can evade the host defences and survive. Neutrophil chemotaxis and phagocytic activity may be impaired by *Treponema* Msp interactions, leading to reorganisation of host cells.

Aa produces a leukotoxin that alters cell membranes of PMNs and monocytes and interferes with antibody production (Table 7) thus ensuring its own survival (Fives-Taylor et al., 1999). The leukotoxin is encoded by a ltx operon consisting of four known genes, namely, ltxA, ltxB, ltxC and ltxD, which appear to be present in all strains of Aa with varied levels of expression with the JP2 ltx promoter being associated with high levels of leukotoxin expression.

Virulence mechanism	References
Adhesion and colonisation	
Haemagglutinin	Grenier, 1991
Major sheath protein (Msp)	Batista de silva et al., 2004; Kaplan *et al.,* 2009; Kolenbrander *et al.,* 1995, Rosen *et al.,* 2008, Yao *et al.,* 1996
Outer sheath (S-layer), outer sheath vesicles (OSV)	Kuchn & Kesty, 2005
Impairment of host defences	
Methyl mercaptan	Johnson *et al.,* 1992; Lancero *et al.,* 1996
Lipoproteins	Dashper *et al,* 2011
Suppression of β-defensin production	Shin *et al.,* 2010
Internalisation by epithelial cells	Colombo *et al.,* 2007
Tissue invasion / bone resorption	
Motility	Li *et al.,* 1999; Kataoka *et al.,* 1997
Metabolic end products	Chu *et al.,* 2002; Fiehn, 1989; Fukamachi *et al.,* 2005; Kuramitsu *et al.,* 2007; Yoshimura *et al.,* 2000
Phosphatases	Ishihara *et al.,* 1995; Laughon *et al.,* 1982;
Trypsin-like protease	Loesche *et al.,* 1987; Ohta *et al.,* 1986
Tissue degrading enzymes	Fiehn 1986b; Mikx, 1991; Uitto *et al.,* 1986

Table 5. Virulence factors of *T. denticola.*

Spirochaetes, including *T. denticola,* have been reported to inhibit lysosome release (Taichman *et al.,* 1982) thereby inhibiting PMN degranulation and other immune reactions to spirochaetes and other plaque microrganisms in the periodontal pocket (Hurlen *et al.,* 1984). Besides interfering with PMN function, spirochaetes are also able to suppress proliferation of fibroblasts (Boehringer *et al.,* 1984), endothelial cells (Taichman *et al.,* 1984) and lymphocyte responsiveness (Taichman *et al.,* 1982; Shenker *et al.,* 1984). The ability of bacteria to overcome the host defence mechanisms may also place the host at risk for opportunistic infections and could be relevant to the progression of periodontitis.

Virulence mechanism	References
Adhesion and colonisation Haemin Fimbriae Outer membrane proteins	Holt & Bramanti, 1991 Dickinson *et al.*, 1988; Lamont & Jenkinson, 1998
Impairment of host defences Induction of cytokines Ability to subvert host intracellular events and localise intracellularly Proteases	Frandsen *et al.*, 1987; Hanazawa *et al.*, 1992; Murakami *et al.*, 2002; Schifferie *et al.*, 1993; Shapira *et al.*, 1997
Tissue invasion / bone resorption Hyaluronidase, heparin Chondroitin sulphatase Phopholypase A Acid and alkaline phosphatases	Bulkacz *et al.*, 1981; Capestany *et al.*, 2004; Frank, 1980; Frank & Vogel, 1978; Holt & Bramanti, 1991; Kawata *et al.*, 1994; Lindemann *et al.*, 1988; Sismey-Durrant & Hopps, 1991;

Table 6. Virulence factors of *P. gingivalis.*

Oppa, a *T. denticola* lipoprotein has been proposed to act as an adhesin for the purpose of covering the surface of *T. denticola* with host proteins in order to avoid, or at least delay, immune recognition (Dashper *et al.*, 2011), while surface proteins of *T. forsythia* activate host cells to release pro-inflammatory cytokines and induce cellular apoptosis (Hasebe *et al.*, 2004).

6.2.2 Endotoxins

True endotoxins are derived only from Gram-negative bacteria and normally exist within the bacterium as integral components of the bacterial cell wall in the form of unique glycolipid, lipopolysaccharide (LPS). Endotoxin can be released from cells during active growth as well as by cell lysis. Normal macrophages are not cytotoxic but following exposure to LPS, can selectively release lysosomal enzymes. So also can PMNs and lymphocytes (Koga et al., 1985). Most of the LPS-related injury in tissues seems to be due to constituents of PMN lysosomes which, not only may digest connective tissue components, but also increase vascular permeability and activate other mediators of inflammation (kinins). LPS is thought to be able to induce B-lymphocyte differentiation, resulting in the production of immunoglobulin-synthesising cells, mainly IgG and IgM. It can also reduce adhesion of periodontal ligament fibroblasts and stimulate bone resorption *in vitro* (Koga *et al.*, 1985; Wilson *et al.*, 1986). Toll-like receptors (TLRs) bind to host epithelial cells and macrophages which sense LPS, thereby preventing triggering of intracellular signalling systems which lead to the production of inflammatory mediators and the migration of macrophages and PMNs to the site of infection (Dauphinee & Karsan, 2006).

Treponemes lack the genes encoding the enzymes for LPS synthesis. The treponemal outer sheath contains lipooligosaccharides (LOS) with a diacylglycerol lipid anchor and hexose-hexosamine-hexose core. Fragments in the lipid anchor resemble a glycolipid membrane anchor found in Gram-positive lipoteichoic acid (Dashper *et al.*, 2010). The function of LOS

is similar to LPS, stimulating the expression of MMPs and fibroblasts thereby inducing the production of a variety of inflammatory mediators which could exacerbate the disease process (Choi *et al.*, 2003).
Induction of cytokine production from macrophages has been demonstrated with LPS in *Bacteroides, Prevotella,* and *Porphyromonas* (Fujiwara *et al.*, 1990; Yoshimura *et al.*, 1997). Because of the immunologic and physiologic effects that LPS has on the host-parasite relationship in periodontal disease, it should be considered as highly significant.

Virulence mechanism	References
Adhesion and colonisation Fimbriae Vesicles Amorphous material	Fives-Taylor et al., 1994
Impairment of host defences Chemotaxis inhibitor Resistance to phagocytosis Capsular polysaccharide Surface antigens Inhibition of fibroblast cytokines Leukotoxin	Ebersole *et al.*, 1996; Fives-Taylor & Meyer, 1999; Mangan *et al.*, 1991; Nakashima *et al.*, 1997; Wilson & Henderson, 1995
Tissue invasion / bone resorption Lipopolysaccharide (LPS) Haemolysin Proteinases Phospholipase C Extracellular vesicles Collagenase Acid and alkaline phosphatases Epithelial toxin	Kimizuku *et al.*, 1996; Lai *et al.*, 1981; Mayrand *et al.*, 1996; Saglie et al., 1988; Wang *et al.*, 2001; Wilson & Henderson, 1995; Zambon, 1983

Table 7. Virulence factors of *Aggregatibacter actinomycetemcomitans* (Aa).

6.2.3 Protease production

Porphyromonas, Prevotella and *Capnocytophaga* produce proteases against IgA and IgG (Grenier *et al.*, 1989). Although all their virulence mechanisms have not been studied in great detail, bacterial species that produce these proteases are associated with invasion of mucous membranes where IgA may be found (Hofstad, 1992). *Prevotella* and *P. gingivalis* (Table 6) each produce different antigenic forms of IgAI protease (Frandsen *et al.*, 1987).

6.3 Colonisation and multiplication in vivo

Having established themselves, the bacteria must be able to multiply within the host. Factors such as temperature, nutrients and atmospheric conditions should be supplied by the tissues or through bacterial interactions. In the gingival crevice, there is much evidence for symbiosis amongst plaque bacteria.

Virulence mechanism	References
Adhesion and colonisation Haemagglutinin S-layer Leucin rich proteins BspA Glucosidases	 Murakami *et al.* 2002 Sabet *et al.*, 2003 Sakakibara *et al.*, 2007 Sharma *et al.*, 1998, 2010
Impairment of host defences Proteolytic enzymes corrupt host immunity Surface lipoproteins induce apoptosis	 Holt & Bramanti 1991 Hasebe *et al.*, 2004
Tissue invasion / bone resorption Trypsin-like protease α-D-glucosidase and N-acetyl-β-glucosaminidase PrtH proteinase (forsythe detachment factor) Methylglyoxal product	 Grenier, 1995 Hughes et al., 2003 Maiden et al., 2004 Saito et al., 1997

Table 8. Virulence factors of *T. Forsythia.*

6.3.1 Synergistic virulence expression

Many virulence genes in plaque bacteria are only expressed when the bacterial species comes into contact with the host or with other partner community bacteria, e.g. the virulence properties of *P. gingivalis* are enhanced by interaction with *F. nucleatum* (Frias *et al.*, 2001; Kinder & Holt, 1989; Kolenbrander & Andersen, 1987), *T. denticola* (Grenier, 1992; Ikegami *et al.*, 2004), and *T. forsythia* (Yao *et al.*, 1996).

T. denticola and *P. gingivalis* display a symbiotic relationship in degrading proteins, utilisation of nutrients and growth promotion (Grenier, 1992; Grenier & Mayrand, 2001; Hollman & van der Hoeven, 1999; Kigure *et al.*, 1995; Nilius *et al.*, 1993; Yoneda *et al.*, 2001).

Interactions between *T. forsythia* and other bacteria such as members of the "red complex" result in synergistic mechanisms in alveolar bone loss and immune-inflammatory responses in rats (Kesavalu *et al.*, 2007). This bacterial consortium has frequently been associated with the clinical progression of chronic and aggressive periodontitis (Holt & Ebersole, 2005; Lamont & Jenkinson, 1998; Socransky *et al.*, 1998). Because of its motility, *T. denticola* is able to respond chemotactically to environmental stimuli. It appears that *T. forsythia* may be a necessary precursor for the colonisation of *T. denticola* and *P. gingivalis*, since these species were rarely found in subgingival plaque without *T. forsythia* (Dashper *et al.*, 2011). Studies of subcutaneous abscess showed that inoculation with *P. gingivalis* resulted in more severe, ulcerative lesions than monoinfection with *T. denticola, T. pectinovorum* or *T. vincentii* (Kesavalu *et al.*, 1997, 2007). Low doses of *P. gingivalis* co-infected with *T. denticola* significantly enhanced tissue damage, showing that *P. gingivalis* was needed for invasion and tissue damage to occur.

6.3.2 Toxin-antitoxin systems

Toxin-antitoxin systems (TA) are composed of a stable toxin and a labile antitoxin which retard essential cell components and counteract the effects of the toxin respectively. They play a major role in biofilm formation in that they are involved in programmed cell death and reversible bacteriostasis (Kim *et al.*, 2009; Makarova *et al.*, 2009). *T. denticola* contains 33 predicted TA systems which, when they show an increase in expression, may demonstrate a role for them in biofilm persistence and resistance to environmental assaults (Jayaraman, 2008; Lewis, 2000).

6.4 Damage of the host's tissues

An increase in microorganisms results in high concentrations of endotoxin, mucopeptides, lipoteichoic acids, metabolic products and proteolytic activity in the subgingival area.

6.4.1 Outer membrane vesicles

Gram-negative bacteria produce outer membrane vesicles (OMV) previously thought to be random blebbing of the outer sheath resulting in the formation of spherical vesicles 50-100nm in diameter (Devoe & Gilchrist, 1977; Grenier & Mayrand, 1987b). We now know that their formation is a highly regulated response to strengthen the bacterium during environmental changes. Such blebs have been identified in *P. gingivalis* (Grenier & Mayrand, 1987b), Aa (Kato et al., 2002) and *Treponema. T. denticola* outer sheath vesicles have been reported to penetrate tissues more readily than the bacterium itself (Cimansoni & McBride, 1987).

6.4.2 Leucin-rich repeat proteins

Leucin-rich repeat proteins (LRR) are found in many eukaryotic and prokaryotic cells with a variety of cellular locations and functions. They belong to the CTD family of proteins involved in protein-protein interactions and signal transduction. Genes encoding LRR proteins have been identified in *P. gingivalis, T. denticola, P. intermedia* and *F. nucleatum. T. denticola* LrrA protein plays a role in coaggregation with *T. forsythia* but not *P. gingivalis* or *F. nucleatum*. lrrA also mediates binding to epithelial cells (Ikegami *et al.*, 2004, Rosen *et al.*, 2008). Six Lrr proteins are predicted in the *T. denticola* genome. Two Lrr proteins have been characterised from *P. gingivalis*. The InlJ protein of *P. gingivalis* (Capestany *et a*l., 2006) is secreted and attached to the surface of the cell. It is important in coaggregation and biofilm development as well as for epithelial cell invasion. OMV of *P. gingivalis* promote the BspA-mediated invasion of epithelial cells by *T. forsythia* (Inagaki *et al.*, 2006, Lewis *et al.*, 2008). *T. forsythia* BspA protein is also associated with alveolar bone loss (Capestany *et al.*, 2006; Dashper *et al.*, 2009; Inagaki *et al.*, 2006; Sharma *et al.*, 1995, 2005). To date, one Lrr protein has been characterised and another five predicted. *P. intermedia* BspA protein (Lewis *et al.*, 2008) is associated with bacterial adherence and invasion, and triggers the release of bone-resorping proinflammatory cytokines from monocytes (Hajishenghallis *et al.*, 2002).

6.4.3 Enzymes

Many Gram-negative bacteria contain proteolytic and hydrolytic enzymes in their periplasmic space and in addition, they produce extracellular enzymes. Plaque bacterial enzymes are many, with a resultant variety in capacity to damage the host tissues or modulate the behaviour of other strains; for example, they alter bacterial attachment and interfere with host defence systems by inactivating important proteinase inhibitors.

Spirochaetes are able to damage periodontal tissue directly by the production of surface components such as endotoxins and histolytic enzymes. Indirect damage may result from the initiation of excessive inflammation or tissue reaction in response to toxins, products of tissue breakdown, or specific hypersensitivity of the protective host inflammatory response to bacterial plaque antigens (Holt & Bramanti, 1991; Kontani *et al.*, 1996; Kuramitsu *et al.*, 1995; Potempa & Pike, 2009; Travis *et al.*, 1997).

Certain plaque bacteria such as *Capnocytophaga, T. forsythia, T. denticola, T. vincentii* and *P. gingivalis* produce collagenolytic proteases referred to as trypsin-like enzyme (Laughon *et al.*, 1982; Yoshimura *et al.*, 1984). This enzyme is able to break down intrinsic protease inhibitors such as α-antitrypsin and could therefore interfere with the control of normal proteolytic processes on human mucosal surfaces (Travis *et al.*, 1997). Trypsin-like enzymes also activate latent tissue collagenase (Uitto *et al.*, 1986). The *P. gingivalis* trypsin-like enzyme differs from the *T. denticola* enzyme (Yoshimura *et al.*, 1984) in that it is a true protease capable of degrading albumin, azocoll and gelatin and is stimulated by reducing agents such as dithiothreitol. Both enzymes are cell-bound and released by cell lysis (Loesche *et al.*, 1987).

Mucopolysaccharidases (e.g. hyaluronidase and chondroitin sulphatase) are able to exert their effects by diffusing into the tissues and breaking down the intercellular acidic mucopolysaccharides of the epithelium without there being any direct bacterial penetration of the host tissues (Fiehn 1986b, Reijntjens *et al.*, 1986). Hyaluronidases are produced by the gingival tissues as well as by oral spirochaetes and *P. gingivalis* and are present in most salivas but increased in subjects with poor oral hygiene and periodontal disease (Holt & Bramanti, 1991). Both *P. gingivalis* and *T. denticola* demonstrate chondroitin sulphatase activity (Fiehn, 1986b; Holt & Bramanti, 1991).

Collagenolytic activity also requires gelatinase and other proteases (Uitto, 1987). Gelatinase may originate from both the plaque bacteria and human leucocytes and is potent in degrading basement membrane collagen (Uitto, 1987). Elastase participates in collagen degradation by solubilising the polymeric collagen fibres into individual tropocollagen molecules. Spirochaetes are known gelatinase and elastase producers (Uitto *et al.*, 1986). The ability of spirochaetes to degrade basement membrane collagen could well be related to their ability to penetrate host tissues (Ellen & Galimanas, 2005; Kigure *et al.*, 1995). Dentilisin is a protease located on the surface of the cell which contributes to disease by disrupting intercellular adhesion proteins (Choi *et al.*, 2003) allowing for *T. denticola* to penetrate epithelial cell layers.

The *T. forsythia* genome encodes several glycosidases which can hydrolyse terminal glycosidic linkages in oligosaccharides and proteoglycans from saliva, gingival crevicular fluid and periodontal tissue, thus promoting disease progression. They can also be involved in adherence, colonisation and cross-feeding of community bacteria (Sharma, 2010). Bacterial glycosidases may expose host cell-surface sugars which bind to haemagglutinins identified in *T. forsythia* (Murakami *et al.*, 2002). Glycosidase activity was sometimes observed with *T. denticola* (Mikx, 1991) but not with *T. vincentii* nor *T. pectinovorum* (Fiehn, 1986b; Mikx, 1991).

P. gingivalis and oral spirochaetes show esterase activity (Lamont & Jenkinson, 1998; Mikx, 1991). In conjunction with phospholipase, esterases may play a role in tissue destruction. Phospholipase may provide prostaglandin precursors and help initiate prostaglandin-mediated bone resorption (Bulkacz *et al.*, 1981).

A neutral phosphatase gene has been cloned and expressed from *T. denticola* (Ishihara & Kuramitsu, 1995). Bacterial acid and alkaline phosphatases cause alveolar bone breakdown, and have been demonstrated in small spirochaetes (Fiehn, 1986) and *P. gingivalis* (Frank & Voegal 1978, Slots, 1991), while peptidases contribute to the pathogenesis of periodontal disease by directly penetrating and degrading basement membrane collagen (Fiehn 1986b, Grenier *et al.*, 1990).

The outer envelope of Gram-negative bacteria consists of 2 layers, namely, the outer membrane and the peptidoglycan layer. The purpose of the peptidoglycan layer is to maintain cell shape. Cell lysis will therefore not only yield membrane fragments but fragments of peptidoglycan as well which interact with host tissue, resulting in a range of biological activities, including activation of complement and immunosuppression. Peptidoglycan is also considered to be involved in stimulating bone resorption (Nissengard *et al.*, 1988) and may therefore constitute an important virulence factor in periodontal disease.

6.4.4 Metabolic end-products

A variety of potentially cytotoxic metabolites are synthesised by oral bacteria including hydrogen sulphide, low molecular weight organic acids and ammonia. Hydrogen sulphide is a metabolic end product of cysteine fermentation and is cytotoxic for epithelial cells and gingival fibroblasts (Beauchamp *et al.*, 1984), exerting both pro-and anti-inflammatory mediators which may disturb host defences (Chen *et al.*, 2010). Both T. *denticola* and *P. gingivalis* produce hydrogen sulphide. *T. denticola* produces hydrogen sulphide from glutathione and thus glutathione metabolism plays an important role in pathogenicity mediated by *T. denticola* (Chu *et al.*, 2002).

Volatile sulphur compounds may increase the permeability of the oral mucosa and reduce collagen and non-collagenous protein synthesiss. Methyl mercaptan, a volatile sulphur compound produced by *T. denticola* and *P. gingivalis* and derived from methionine, is known to reduce protein synthesis by human gingival fibroblasts, as well as inhibit cell migration in periodontal ligament cells (Johnson *et al.*, 1992; Lancero *et al.*, 1996).

T. forsythia releases metabolites which favour the growth of *P. gingivalis* which in turn, degrades host proteins releasing nutrients such as peptides and amino acids for *T. forsythia*. The synergy between these two species and with *T. denticola*, provide evidence for their combined virulence expression in periodontal disease.

Virulence is multifactorial, being influenced by microbial interactions (which often differ *in vivo* and *in vitro*) as well as host susceptibility. Molecular biology has contributed greatly to our understanding of virulence and disease progression but many questions still remain unanswered.

7. Conclusion

Certain subgingival plaque morphtypes predominate in different forms of periodontal disease and shifts in microbial proportions probably relate to health and disease. There is no proof of a causal relationship between the organisms described above and periodontal disease. One can only suggest an association. Because the oral microbiota contains around 700 species of microrganisms, it has been accepted that periodontal disease is a polymicrobial infection, with shifts in the proportions of some species relating to different forms of periodontal disease.

Identification and monitoring of specific bacteria could aid in management and treatment by determining the causative species, monitoring of treatment and deciding on recall intervals. Most methods currently employed in microbiological assessment have major shortcomings. Inconsistencies between cultural microbiological data from cases with similar clinical features are often encountered. These inconsistencies may be attributed to differences in detection methods as well as to different stages of the disease process. Differences in data from different research centres could indicate not only technical problems, but also problems related to the classification of a given site as active or inactive. However, major advances have occurred during the past decade and continued efforts are being made to facilitate and standardise the microbiological diagnosis of periodontal diseases. Although this chapter describes a role for many species with different forms of periodontal disease, the interaction and role of bacterial products is vast and complex. Therefore the association of a given organism with disease (even though it may be constantly present) could be considered as being the result rather than the cause of disease. However, in examining association studies, spirochaetes cannot be ignored since they have been considered amongst the most highly suspect of the plaque microbiota, being consistently observed in different forms of periodontal disease and demonstrating significant pathogenic potential.

The increased prevalence of Aa, *T. denticola, P. gingivalis* and *T. forsythia* in different forms of periodontal disease has earned them the recognition as diagnostic markers in the disease process. However, they should not be considered with the exclusion of other important contributers such as *F. nucleatum*. New and unusual species are emerging which may, in time, prove to be the real initiators of the disease process with the above species having to relinquish their position at the top of the list of suspected periodontopathogens. Many contradictions occur and while some advocate the use of microbial biomarkers, others find them misleading and suggest that microbiota should be examined for both pathogenic and protective flora and results interpreted as they pertain to the susceptibility of the host (Quirynen *et al.*, 2001; Riep, 2007).

Treatment must be effected with the bacterial communities of the biofilm in mind and should concentrate on preventing biofilm formation, interfering with the process of bacterial succession and elimination of specific organisms in the biofilm. The recent isolation of an Aa serotype b bacteriophage, which is able to lyse bacteria within a biofilm, holds some promise in this area (Castillo-Ruiz *et al.*, 2011). Until this can be put to practice, professional plaque control coupled with individual oral hygiene practices will continue to serve in maintaining a healthy oral ecosystem.

8. Acknowledgement

This material is based upon work supported financially by the National Research Foundation, South Africa.

9. Disclaimer

Any opinion, findings and conclusions or recommendations expressed in this material are those of the author and therefore the NRF does not accept any liability in regard thereto.

10. References

Aas, J.A., Paster,B.J., Stokes, L.N., Olsen, I. & Dewhirst, P.E. (2005). Defining the bacterial flora of the oral cavity, *J Clin Microbiol* 43: 5721-5732.

Abdellatif, H.M. & Burt, B.A. (1987) An epidemiological investigation into the relative importance of age and oral hygiene status as determinants of periodontitis, *J Dent Res* 66: 13-18.

Addy, M., Newman, H., Langeroudi, M.& Gho, J.G.L. (1983). Darkfiled microscopy of the microflora of plaque, *Br Dent J* 155: 269-273.

Adler, A., Oberholzer, R., Ebner, J.P., Guindy, J., Meyer, J., & Rateltschak, K.(1995). Subgingival plaque due to gingivitis and inactive periodontitis sites in the adult periodontitis patient, *Odontol Stomatol* 105 (2): 155-158.

Africa, C.W., Parker, J.R. & Reddy, J.(1985a). Bacteriological studies of a periodontitis-resistant population. I. Darkfield Microscopical studies, *J Periodont Res* 20: 1-7.

Africa, C.W., Parker, J.R. & Reddy, J. (1985b). Darkfield microscopy of the flora of subgingival plaque of patients with severe periodontitis and its use in therapeutic assessment, *J* Dent *Ass S.A.* 39: 5-9.

Albandar, J.M.& Tinoco, E.M. (2002). Global epidemiology of periodontal diseases in children and young persons, *Periodontol 2000* 29: 153-176.

Albrect, G., Freeman, S. & Higginbotham, N.(1998) Complexity and human health: The case for a trans-disciplinary paradigm, *Cult Med Psychiatry* 22: 55-92.

Allenspach-Petrzilka, G.E. & Guggenheim , B. (1983). Bacterial invasion of the periodontium; an important factor in the pathogenesis of periodontitis, *J Clin Periodontol* 10: 609-617.

Amano, A., Nakagawa, I., Okahashi, N.& Hamada, N., (2004) Variations of *Porphyromonas gingivalis* Fimbriae in relation to microbial pathogenesis, *J Penodontal Res* 39:136-142.

Amano, A., Nakagawa, I., Kataoka, K., Morisaki, I.& Hamada, S. (1999a). Distribution of *Porphyromonas gingivalis* strains with *fim* A genotypes in periodontitis patients, *J Clin Microbial* 37: 1426-1430.

Amano, A., Kuboniwa, M., Nakagawa, I., Akiyama, S., Morisaki, I.& Hamada, S. (2000) Prevalence f specific Genotypes of *Porphyromonas gingivalis fim* A and periodontal health status, *J Dent Res* 79(9): 1664-1668.

Araki, H., Kuriama, T., Nakagawa, K & Narasawa T. (2004). The microbial synergy *of Peptostreptococcus micros* and *Prevotella intermedia* in a murine absess model, *Oral Microbiol Immunol* 19 (3): 177-181.

Armitage, G.C. (1999). Development of a classification system for periodontal diseases and conditions, *Ann Periodontal* 4(1): 1-6.

Armitage, G.C. (2010). Comparison of the microbiological features of chronic and aggressive periodontitis, *Periodontol 2000* 53: 70-88.

Arnett, H.A. & Viney, J.L. (2007). Considerations for the sensible use of rodent models of inflammatory disease in predicting efficacy of new biological therapeutics in the clinic, *Adv Drug Deliv Rev* 59: 1084-1092.

Asikainen, S., Lai, C.H., Alaluusua, S. & Slots J. (1991). Distribution *of Actinobacillus actinomycetemcomitans* serotypes in periodontal health and disease, *Oral Microbiol Immunol* 6(2): 115-118.

Assuma, R., Oates, T., Cochran, D., Amat, S. & Graves D.T. (1998). Interleukin-1 and tumour necrosis factor antagonists inhibit the inflammatory response and bone loss in experimental periodontitis, *J Immunol* 160: 403-409.

Baelum, V., Fejerskov, O. & Karring, T. (1986). Oral hygiene, gingivitis and periodontal breakdown in adult Tanzanians. *J Perio Res* 21: 221-232.

Batista da Silva A., Lee,W., Bajenova, F., McCulloch, C. & Ellen, R. (2004). The major outer sheath protein of *Treponema denticola* inhibits the binding step of collagen phagocytosis in fibroblasts, *Cell Microbial* 6: 485-498.

Barthold ,P.M., Gully, N.J., Zilm, P.S. & Rogers, A.H. (1991). Identification of components in *Fusobacterium nucleatum* chemostat culture supernatants that are potent inhibitors of human gingival fibroblast proliferation, *J Periodontal Res* 26: 314-322.

Barua, P.K., Dyer, D.W. & Neiders, ME. (1990). Effect of iron limitation *on Bacteroides gingivalis, Oral Microbial Immunol* 5: 263-268.

Bascones Martinez, A. & Figuero Ruiz, E. (2006). Periodontal diseases as bacterial infection, *AV Periodon Implantol* 17 (3): 111-118.

Beauchamps, R.O.Jr., Bus, J.S., Popp, J.A., Boreiko, C.J. & Andjelkovich, D.A. (1984). A critical review of the literature on hydrogen sulphide toxicity, *Crit Rev Toxicol* 13: 25-97.

Beck, J.D. (1990). Identification of risk factors. *In* Bader J.D., *Risk Assessment In Dentistry.* Chapel Hill: University of North Carolina pp 8-13

Bergstrom, J., Eliasson, S. & Dock, J. (2000). A 10 year perspective study of tobacco smoking and periodontal health, *J Periodontal* 71(8): 1338-1347.

Bick, P., Betts Carpenter, A., Holderman, H.V., Muller, G.A.,Ranny, R.R., Pulcanis & Tew, T.G. (1981). Polyclonal B cell activation induced by extracts of Gram-negative bacteria isolated from periodontally diseased sites, *Infect Immun* 34: 43-49.

Bik, E.M., Armitage, G.C., Looner, P., Emerson, J., Morigodin, E.F., Nelson, K.E.,Gill, S.R., Fraser-Liggett, C.M. & Relman, D.A. (2010). Bacterial diversity in the oral cavity of 10 healthy individuals, *Isme J* 4(8): 962-974.

Blasi, A. (2009). Characterisation and serotype distribution of *Aggregatibacter actinomycetemcomitans* detected in a population of periodontitis patients in Spain, Thesis, *University Degli Studi di Napoli Federico II*

Blomhof, L., Otteskog, P. & Soder, P. (1980). Various lipopolysaccharides reduce adhesion of periodontal ligament fibroblasts, *Scand J Dent Res* 88: 10-14.

Boehringer, H., Taichman, N.S. & Shenker, B. (1984). Suppression of fibroblast proliferation by oral spirochaetes, *Infect Immun* 45: 155-159.

Botero, J.E., Contreras ,A., Lafaurie ,G., Jaramillo, A., Betancourt ,M. & Arce ,R.M.(2007). Occurrence of Periodontopathic and Super-infecting bacteria in chronic and aggressive periodontitis subjects in a Colombian population, *J Periodontol* 78: 696-704.

Bowden, G.H. (1999). Controlled environment model for accumulation of biofilms of oral bacteria, *Methods Enzymol* 310: 216-224.

Bradshaw, D.J., Marsh, P.D., Watson, D.K.. & Allison C. (1998). Role of *Fusobacterium nucleatum* and coaggregation in anaerobe survival in planktonic and biofilm oral microbial communities during aeration, *Infect Immun* 66: 4729-4732.

Bramanti, T.E. & Holt, S.C. (1990). Iron-regulated outer membrane proteins in the bacterium, *Bacteroides gingivalis, Biochem Biophys Res Comm* 166: 1146-1154.

Brogan, J.M., Lally, E.T., Poulsen, K., Demuth D.R. (1994). Regulation *of Actinobacillus actinomycetemcomitans* leukotoxin expression: analysis of the promoter regions of leukotoxic and minmaly leukotoxin strains, *Infect Immun* 62(2): 501-508.

Brook, I., & Walker, R.I. (1985). The role of encapsulation in the pathogenesis of anaerobic Gram-positive cocci, *Canad J Microbiol* 31: 176-180.

Brook, I., & Walker, R.I.(1986) The relationship between *Fusobacterium* species and other flora in mixed infection, *J Med Microbiol* 21: 93-100.

Brooks, W., Dermuth, D.R., Gi,l S. & Lamont, R.J. (1997). Identification of a *Streptococcus gordonii SspB* domain that mediates adhesion to *Porphyromonas gingivalis, Infect Immun* 65: 3753-3758.

Bulkacz, I., Erbland, J.F. & MacGregor , J. (1981). Phospholipase A activity in supernatants from cultures of *B. melaninogenicus, Biochem Biophys Acta* 664: 148-155.

Caldwell, D.E., Atuku, E., Wilkie, D.C., Wivcharuk, K.P., Karthikeyan, S., Korber, D.R., Schmid, D.F. & Wolfaard G.M. 1997). Germ theory versus community theory in understanding and controlling the proliferation of biofilms, *Adv Dent Res* 11: 4-13.

Calsina, G, Ramon, J.M. & Echeverria, J.J. (2002). Effects of smoking on periodontal tissues, *J Clin Periodontol* 29:771-776.

Carlsson, J. (1997). Bacterial metabolism in dental biofilms, *Adv Dent Res* 11: 75-80.

Capestany, C.A., Kuboniwa, M., Jung, I-Y., Park ,Y., Tribble, G.D. & Lamont R.J. (2006). Role of *Porphyromonas gingivalis* In IJ protein in homotypic and heterotypic biofilm development, *Infect Immun* 74: 3002-3005.

Carlsson, J. (1997). Bacterial Metabolism in dental biofilms, *Adv Dent Res* 11: 75-80.

Carrasi, A., Abatis, S., Santarelli, G. & Vogel, G. (1989). Periodontitis in a patient with chronic neutropenia, *J Periodontol* 60: 352-357.

Carranza, F.A., Saglie, R., Newman, M.G. & Valentin, P.L. (1983). Scanning and transmission electron microscopy of tissue-invading micro-organisms in localised juvenile periodontitis, *J Periodontol* 54: 598-617.

Casarin, R.C.V., Del Pelosa Ribeiro, E.,Mariano, F.S., Nociti, F.H. Casati, M.Z. & Goncalves, R.B. (2010). Levels of *Aggregatibacter actinomycetemcomitans, Porphyromonas gingivalis,*inflammatory cytokines and species-species immunoglobulin G in generalised, aggressive and chronic periodontitis, *J Periodontol Res* 45(6): 635-642.

Castillo-Ruiz, M., Vines, E.D., Montt, C., Fernandez, J., Degado, J.M., Hormazaba I.J.C. & Bittner, M. (2011). Isolation of a novel *Aggegatibacter actinomycetemcomitans* serotype b bacteriophage capable of lysing bacteria within a biofilm, *Appl Environ Microbiol* 77(9): 3157-3159.

Cavanaugh, J.A., Callen, D.F., Wilson, S.R., et al (1998). Analysis of Australian Crohn's disease pedigrees refines the localisation for susceptibility to inflammatory bowel disease on chromosome 16, *Ann Human Genet* 62:291-298.

Chalabi, M., Rezaie, F., Moghim, S., Mogharehabed, A., Rezaei, M. & Mehraban, B. (2010). Periodontitis bacteria and herpesviruses in chronic periodontitis, *Mol Oral Microbial* 25(3): 236-240.

Chen, C., Makinen, K.K., Makinen, P.L. , Ohta, K. & Loesche, W.J. (1988). Structure of a Benzoylarginine peptidase from *Treponema denticola* ASLM. *J Dent Res* 67: 395 Abst 2255.

Chen, W., Kajiya ,M., Giro, G., Ouhara, K. Mackler, H.E., Mawardi, H. *et al.* (2010). Bacteria-derived hydrogen sulphide promotes Interleukin -8 production from epithelial cells, *Biochem Biophys Res Commun* 391: 645-650.

Cheng, K.J. & Costerton, J.W. (1973). Localisation of alkaline phosphatase in three Gram-negative rumen bacteria, *J Bacteriol* 116: 424-440.

Choi, B.K., Paster, B.J., Dewhirst, F.E. & Gobel, U.B. (1994). Diversity of cultivable and uncultivable oral spirochaetes from a patient with severe destructive periodontitis, *Infect Immun* 62: 1889-1895.

Choi, B.K., Lee, H.J., Kang, J.H., Jeong, G.J., Min, C.K. & Yoo Y.J. (2003). Induction of osteoclastogenesis and matrix metalloproteinasis expression by the LOS of *Treponema denticola, Infect Immun* 71: 226-233.

Chu, L., Dong, Z., Xu, X., Cochran, D.L. & Ebersole J.L. (2002). Role of glutathione metabolism of *Treponema denticola* in bacterial growth and virulence expression, *Infect Immun* 70:1113-1120

Chu, L., Lai, Y., Eddy, S., Yang, S., Song, L. *et al.* (2008). A 52-kDa leucyl aminopeptidase from *Treponema denticola* is a cysteinylglycinase that mediates the second step of glutathione metabolism, *J Biol Chem* 283: 19351-19358.

Cimasoni, G., Song, M. & McBride (1987). Effect of crevicular fluid and lysosomal enzymes on the adherence of streptococci and *Bacteroides* to hydroxyapatite, *Infect Immun* 55:1484-1489.

Claesson,R, Lagevall, M., Hoglund-Aberg, C., Johansson, A. & Haubek, D. (2011). Detection of the highly leukotoxic JP2 clone of *Aggregatibacter actinomycetemcomitans* in members of a Caucasian family living in Sweden, *J Clin Periodontol* 38 (2):115-121.

Cockayane, A., Sanger, R. & Ivic, A. (1989). Antigenic and structural analysis of *Treponema denticola, J Gen Microbiol* 135: 3209-3218.

Cook, G.S., Costerton, J.W. & Lamont, R.J. (1998). Biofilm formation by *Porphyromonas gingivalis* and *Streptococcus gordonii, J Periodontal Res* 33 (6): 323-327.

Colombo, A., da Silva, C. & Haffajee, A. (2007). Identification of intracellular oral species within human crevicular epithelial cells from subjects with chronic periodontitis by fluorescence *in situ* hybridisation, *J Periodontal Res* 42: 236-243.

Cortelli, J.R., Cortelli, S.C., Jordan, S., Haraszthy, V.I. & Zambon J.J. (2005). Prevalence of periodontal pathogens in Brazilians with aggressive or chronic periodontitis,*J Clin Periodontol* 32(8): 860-866.

Cosgarea ,R., Baumer, A., Pretzi ,B., Zehaczek, S. & Ti-Sun K. (2010). Comparison of 2 different microbiological test kits for detection of periodontal pathogens, *Acta Odontol Scand* 68(2):115-121.

Courtois, G.J., Cobb, C.M. & Killoy, W.J. (1983). Acute necrotising ulcerative gingivitis, A transmission eclectron microscope study, *J Periodontol* 54: 671-679.

Daep, C.A., James ,D.M., Lamont, R.J. & Desmuth ,D.R . (2006). Structural characterization of peptide - mediated inhibition of *Porphyromonas gingivalis* biofilm formation, *Infect Immun* 74(10): 5756-5762.

Dalwai, F., Spratt, B.J., Pratten, J. (2006) Modeling shifts in microbial populations in health and disease, *Appl Enviroment Microbiol* 72: 3678-3684.

Darby, I.B., Hodge, P.J., Riggio, M.P. & Kinane ,D.F. (2000). Microbial comparison of smoker and non-smoker adult and early-onset periodontitis patients by polymerase chain reaction, *J Clin Periodontol* 27: 417-424.

Dashper, S.G., Ang, C.S., Veith, P.D., Mitchell, H.I., Lo, A.W., Seers, C.A. *et al.* (2009). Response of *Porphyromonas gingivalis* to home limitation in continuous culture, *J Bacteriol* 9:1044-1055.

Dashper, S.G., Seers, C.A., Tan, K.H. & Reynolds, E.C. (2011). Virulence factors of the oral spirochaete *Treponema denticola, J Dent Res* 90: 691-703.

Dauphinee, S.M. & Karsan, A. (2006) Lipopolysaccharide signalling in endothelial cells, *Lab Invest* 86: 9-22.

Davey, M.E. (2006). Techniques for the growth of *Porphyromonas gingivalis* biofilms, *Periodontol 2000* 42: 27-35.

Dawes, C. (2008). Salivary flow patterns and the health of hard and soft oral tissue, *J. Am Dent Assoc* 139: 185-245.

Dawson, J.L. &Ellen, R.P. (1990). Tip-oriented adherence of *Treponema denticola* to fibronectin, *Infect Immun* 58: 3924-3925.

Dawson, D.R., Wang,C. Danaher, R.J., Lin, Y., Kryscio, R.J., Jacob, R.J. & Miller, C.S. (2009). Real-time PCR to determine the prevalence and copy member of EBV amd CMV DNA in subgingival plaque at individual healthy ahd periodontal disease sites, *J Periodontol* 80(7): 1133-1140.

Demuth, D.R., Irvine, D.C., Costerton, J.W., Cook, G.S. & Lamont R.J. (2001). Discrete protein determinant directs the species - specific adherence of *Porphyromonas gingivalis* to oral streptococci, *Infect Immun* 69: 5736-5741.

Dethlefsen, L., Mc Fall-Ngai, M. & Relman, D.A. (2007). An ecological and evolutionary perspective on human-microbe mutualism and disease. *Nature* 449: 811-818.

Devoe I.W., Gilchrist J.E. (1973). Release of endotoxin in the form of cell wall blebs during *in vitro* growth of *Neisseria meningitidis* , *J Exp Med* 138: 1156-1167.

Diaz, I., Chalmers, N.I., Rickard, A.H., Kong, C., Milburn, C.L., Palmer, R.J. Jr., Kolenbrander, P.E. (2006). Molecular characterization of subject-specific oral microflora during initial colonisation of enamel, *Appl Environ Microbiol* 72: 2837-2848.

Dickinson, D.P., Kubiniec, H., Yoshimura, F. & Genco R.J. (1991). Molecular cloning and sequencing of the gene encoding the protein from *Porphyromonas (Bacteroides) gingivalis.,Biochem Biophys Res Commun.* 175: 713-719.

Dogan, B., Antinhelmo, J., Cetiner, D. et al. (2003). Subgingival microflora in Turkish patients with periodontitis, *J Periodontol* 74: 803-814.

Dolgilevich, S., Rafferty, B., Luchinskaya, D. & Kozarov, E.(2011). Genomic comparison of invasive and rare non-invasive strains reveals *Porphyromonas* genetic polymorphisms, *J Oral Micro* 3: 5764.

Dorn, B.R., Burks, J.N., Seifert, K.N. & Progulske-Fox, A. Invasion of endothelial and epithelial cells by strains of *Porphyromonas gingivalis, FEMS Microbiol Let* 187: 139-144.

Douglass, C.W., Jette, A.M., Fox, C.H., et al. (1993). Oral health status of the elderly, in *New Engl. J Gerodontol* 48:39-46.

Downes, J., Munson, M.A., Spratt, D.A., Kononen, E., Tarkka, E., Jousimies-Somer, H., & Wade ,W.G. (2001). Characterisation of *Eubacterium*-like strains isolated from oral infections, *J Med Microbiol* 50: 947-951.

Dziarski, R. (1978). Immunosuppressive effect of *Staphylococcus aureus* on antibody response in mice, *Int Arch Allergy Appl Immunol* 57: 304-311.

Dzink, J., Socransky, S.S. & Haffajee, A. (1988). The predominant cultivable microflora of active and inactive lesions of destructive periodontal disease, *J Clin Periodontol* 15: 316-323.

Ebersole, J.L, Hall, E.E. & Steffen, M.J. (1996). Antigenic diversity in the periodontopathogen, *Actinobacillus actinomycetemcomitans Immunol Invest* 25: 203-214.

Eckles, T.A., Reinhardyer, J.K., Tussing, G.J., Szydlowski , W.M. & Du Bois, L.M. (1980). Intracrevicular application of tetracycline in white petroleum for the treatment of periodontal disease, *J Clin Perio* 17: 454-462.

Elamin, A.M., Skaug, N., Ali, R.W., Bakken, V. & Albander, J.M. (2010). Ethnic disparities in the prevalence of periodontitis among high school students in Sudan, *J Periodontol* 81(6): 891-896.

Ellen, R. & Galimanas, V.B. (2005). Spirochaetes at the forefront of periodontal infections,*Periodontol 2000* 38: 13-32.

Engebretson, S.P. *et al* (1999). The influence of interleukin gene polymorphism on expression of interleukin -l Beta and TNFA-Alfa in periodontal tissue and gingival crevicular fluid, *J Periodontol* 70(6): 567-573.

Eisenstein, B.I. (1990). New Molecular techniques for microbial epidemiology and the diagnosis of infectious diseases, *J Inf Dis* 161: 595-602.

Eriksen, H.M. & Dimitrov, V. (2003). Ecology of oral health: a complexity perspective, *Euro J Oral Sciences* 111(4): 285-293.

Farquharson, S.I., Germaine, G.R. & Gray, G.R. (2000). Isolation and characterisation of the cell-surface polysaccharides of *Porphyromonas gingivalis* ATCC 53978, *Oral Microbiol Immunol* 15:151-157.

Faveri, M., Mayer, M.P., Feres, M., de Fiqueredo, L.C., Dewhirst, F.E. & Paster, B.J. (2008). Microbiological diversity of generalised aggressive periodontitis by 16Sr RNA clone analysis, *Oral Microbiol Immunol* 23(2):112-118.

Feldman, R.S., Bravacos, J.S. & Close (1983). Association between smoking different tobacco products and periodontal disease indexes, *J Periodontol* 54: 481-487.

Fiehn, N-E. (1986a). Nutrient and environment growth factors for eight small-sized oral spirochaetes, *Scand J Dent Res* 94: 208-218.

Fiehn, N-E. (1986b). Enzyme activities from eight small-sized oral spirochaetes, *Scand J Dent Res* 94: 132-140.

Fiehn, N-E. (1989). Small-sized oral spirochaetes and periodontal disease, *Acta Path Microbiol Immunol Scand suppl* 97: (7).

Fiehn, N-E. & Westergaard, J. (1984). Cultivation on solid media of spirochaetes in subgingival plaque from advanced marginal periodontitis in humans, *Scand J Dent Res* 92: 426-435.

Filoche, S., Wong, L. & Sissons C.H. (2010). Oral biofilms : Emerging concepts in Microbial ecology, *J Dent Res* 89(1): 8-18.

Finlay, B.B. & Falkow, S. (1989). Common themes in microbial pathogenicity, *Microbiol Rev*53: 210-230.

Fives-Taylor, P.M., Meyer, D.H., Mintz, K.P. & Brissette, C. (1999). Virulence factors of *Aggregatibacter actinomycetemcomitans, Periodontol 2000* 20: 136-167.

Flemming, T.F. (1999). Periodontitis, *Ann Periodontol* 4: 32-38.

Frandsen, E.V.G., Reinholdt, J. & Kilian, N. (1987). Enzymatic and antigenic characterisation of immunoglobulin Al proteases from *Bacteroides* and *Capnocytophaga* species, *Infect Immun* 55: 631-638.

Frank, R.M. (1980). Bacterial penetration in the apical pocket wall of advanced periodontitis in humans, *J Periodont Res* 15: 563-573.

Frank, R.M. & Vogel, J.C. (1978). Bacterial bone resorption in advanced cases of human periodontitis, *J Perio Res* 13: 251-261.

Frias, J., Olle, E. & Alsina M. (2001). Periodontal pathogens produce quorum sensing signal molecules, In*fect Immun* 69(5): 3431-3434.

Fritschi, Z., Kiszely, A. & Persson G.R. (2008). *Staphylococcus aureus* and other bacteria in untreated periodontitis, *J Dent Res* 87(6): 589-593.

Fukamachi, H., Nakano, Y., Okano, S., Shibata, Y., Abiko, Y. & Yamashita, Y.(2005). High production of methyl mercaptan by L-methionine- alpha-deamino-gamma-mercapto-methane lyase from *Treponema denticola, Biochem Biophys Res Commun* 331: 127-131.

Fujise, O., Hamachi, T., Inouc, K., Miura, M. & Maeda, K. (2002). Microbiological markers for prediction and assessment of treatment outcome following non-surgical periodontal therapy, *J Periodontol* 73(11): 1253-1259.

Fujiwara, T., Ogawa, T., Sohue, S. & Hamada, S. (1990). Chemical immunological and antigenic characterisations of Lipopolysaccharides from *Bacteroides gingivalis* strains, *J Gen Microbiol* 136: 319-326.

Furuichi, Y., Ramberg, P., Krok, L. & Lindhe, J. (1997). Short-term effects of triclosan on healing following subgingival scaling, *J Clin Periodontol* 24(10): 777-782.

Gaetti-Jardim, E.Jr. & Avila-Campos, M.J. (1999). Haemagglutination and haemolysis by oral *Fusobacterium nucleatum, New Microbiol* 22: 63-67.

Gajardo, M., Silva, N. & Gomez, L. (2005). Prevalence of periodontopathic bacteria in aggressive periodontitis patients in a Chilean population, *J Periodontol* 76(2): 289-294.

Garrison, S.W. & Nicols, F.C. (1989). Lipopolysaccharide elicited secretory responses in monocytes; altered release of prostaglandin E2 but not Interleukin- l beta in patients with adult periodontitis, *J Periodont Res* 24: 88-95.

Gemmell, E. & Seymor, G.J. (1998). Cytokine profiles of cells extracted from humans with periodontal diseases, *J Dent Res* 77: 16-26. (1988). The origin of periodontal infections, *Adv Dent Res* 2: 245-259.

Genco, R.J., Zambon, J.J. & Christersson, L.A. (1988). The origin of periodontal infections, *Adv Dent Res* 2: 245-259

George, K.S., Reynolds, M.A. & Falkler W.A. Jr. (1997). Arbitrarily primed polymerase chain reaction fingerprinting and clonal analysis of oral *Fusobacterium nucleatum* isolates, *Oral Microbiol Immunol* 12: 219-226.

Gibbons, R.J., Hay, D.,Cisor, J.O. & Clark W.B. (1988). Adsorbed salivary proline-rich protein-l and statherin : receptors for type l fimbriae of A*ctinomyces viscosus* TI4V/Jl on apatitic surfaces, *Infect Immun* 56: 2990-2993.

Gibbons, R.J., Hay, D.I. & Schlesinger, D.H. (1991). Delineation of a segment of adsorbed salivary acidic proline-rich proteins which promotes adhesion of *Streptococcus gordonii* to apatitic surfaces, *Infect Immun* 59: 2948-2954.

Gibbons, R.J., Socransky, S.S., Sawyer, S., Kapsimales, B. & MacDonald, J.B. (1963). The microbiota of the gingival crevice area of man II, The predominant cultivable microorganisms, *Arch Oral Biol* 8: 281-289.

Glickman, I. (1972). in *Clinical Periodontology*. Saunders , Philadelphia , 4th edition.

Goldberg, S., Cardash, H., Browning, H. III., Sahly, H. & Rosenberg, M. (1997). Isolation of Enterobacteriaceae from the mouth and potential association with malodour, *J Dent Res* 76: 1770-1775.

Goodson, J.M., Tanner, A.C., Haffajee ,A.D.,Somberger, G.C. & Socransky, S.S. (1982). Patterns of progression and regression of advanced destructive periodontal disease, *J Clin Periodontol* 9:472-481.

Gore, E.A., Sanders, J.J., Pandey, J.P., Palesch, Y. & Galbraith, G.M.P.(1998). Interleukin – 1-Beta + 3953 allele 2: association with disease status in adult periodontitis, *J Clin Peridontol* 25: 781-785.

Goulbourne, P.A. & Ellen, R.P. (1991). Evidence that *Porphyromonas* (*Bacteroides*) *gingivalis* fimbriae function in adhesion to *Actinomyces viscosus, J Bact* 173: 5266-5274.

Greenblatt, J., Boackle, R.J. & Schwab, J.H. (1978). Activation of the alternate complement pathway by peptidoglycan from streptococcal cell wall, *Infect Immun* 19: 296-303.

Grenier, D. (1992). Demonstration of bimodal coaggregation reaction between *Porphyromonas gingivalis* and *Treponema denticola, Oral Microbiol Immunol* 7: 280-284.

Grenier, D. (1995) .Characterisation of the trypsin-like activity of *Bacteroides forsythus, Microbiol* 141: 921-926.

Grenier, D. & Mayrand D. (1987a). Selected characteristics of pathogenic and non-pathogenic strains of *Bacteroides gingivalis, J Clin Microbiol* 25: 738-740.

Grenier, D. & Mayrand, D. (1987b). Functional characterisation of extracellular vesicles produced by *Bacteroides gingivalis, Infect Immun* 55: 111-117.

Grenier, D. & Mayrand, D. (2001). Cleavage of human immunoglobulin G by *Treponema denticola, Anaerobe* 7: 1-4.

Grenier, D., Mayrand, D. & McBride, B.C. (1989). Further studies on the degradation of immunoglobulins by black-pigmented *Bacteroides, Oral Microbiol Immunol* 4: 12-18.

Grenier,D., Uitto, V.J. & McBride, B.C. (1990). Cellular location of a *Treponema denticola* chymotrypsin-like protease and importance of the protease in migration through the basement membrane, *Infect Immun* 58: 347-351.

Griffen, A.L., Lyons, S.R., Becker, M.R., Moeschberger, M. L &, Leys, E.J. (1999). *Porphyromonas gingivalis* strain variability and periodontitis, *J Clin Microbiol* 37: 4028-4033.

Grossi, S.G. & Genco ,R.J. (1998). Periodontal Disease and diabetes mellitus: a two-way relationship, *Ann Periodontol* 3(1): 51-61.

Guentsch, A., Kramesberger, M., Sroka, A., Pfister, W., Potempa, J. & Eick, S. (2011). Comparison of gingival crevicular fluid sampling methods in patients with severe, chronic periodontitis, *J Periodontol Jan 14 n.d.*

Haapasalo, M., Kerosuo, E. & Lounatmaa, K. (1990). Hydrophobicities of human polymorphonuclear leucocytes and oral *Bacteroides* and *Porphyromonas spp., Wolinella recta* and *Eubacterium yurii* with special reference to bacterial surface structures, *Scand J Dent Res* 98: 472-480.

Haapasalo, M., Miler, K.H., Uitto, V-J., Keung Leung , W. & McBride, B.C. (1992). Characterisation, cloning and binding properties of the major 53 kDa *Treponema denticola* surface antigen, *Infect Immun* 60: 2058-2065.

Haber, J. (1994). Smoking is a major risk factor for periodontitis, *Curr Opin Periodontol* 12: 8.

Haber, J., Wattles, J., Crowle,y M., Mandel,l R., Joshipura, K.& Kent, R.L. (1998). Evidence for cigarette smoking as a major risk factor for periodontitis, *J Periodontol* 64: 16-23.

Haffajee, A.D., Bogren, A., Hasturk, H., Feres, M., Lopez, N.J. and Socransky, S.S. (2004). Subgingival microbiota of chronic periodontitis subjects from different geographic locations, *J Clin Periodontol* 31: 996-1002.

Haffaje,e A.D. & Socransky, S.S. (1994). Microbial aetiological agents of destructive periodontal disease, *Periodontol 2000* 5: 78-111.

Haffajee, A.D., Socransky, S.S. & Goodson, J.M. (1992). Subgingival temperature: I Relation to baseline clinical parameters, *J Clin Periodontol* 19: 417-422.

Haffajee, A.D., Socransky, S.S.,Patel, M.R. & Song X. (2008). Microbial complexes in subgingival plaque, *Oral Microbial Immunol* 23: 196-205.

Haffajee, A., Socransky, S.S., Smith, C. & Dibart, S. (1991). Relation of baseline microbial parameters to future periodontal attachment loss, *J Clin Periodontol* 18: 744-750.

Haffajee, A.D., Teles, R.P., Patel, M.R., Song, X., Yaskell, T. & Socransky S.S. (2009). Factors affecting human supragingival biofilm composition II Tooth position, *J Periodontal Res* 44: 520-528.

Haffajee, A.D., Teles, R.P. & Socransky S.S. (2006). The effect of periodontal therapy on the composition of the subgingival microbiota. *Periodontol 2000* 42: 219-258.

Hajishengallis, G., Martin, M., Sojar, H.T., Sharma, A., Schifferie, R.E., De Nardin, E., Russell, M.W. & Genco R.J. (2002). Dependence of bacterial protein adhesins on Toll-like receptors for proinflammatory cytokine induction, *Clin Diagn Lab Immunol* 9: 403-407.

Hamlet, S.M., Taiyeb-Ali, T.B., Cullinan, M.P., Westerman, B., Palmer, J.E., & Seymour G.J.(2007).*Tannerella forsythensis prt* H genotype and association with periodontal status, *J Periodontol* 78: 344-350.

Han, Y.W., Shi, W., Huang, G.T., Kinde,r H.S., Park, N.H. & Kuramitsu, H *et al.* (2000). Interactions between periodontal bacteria and human oral epithelial cells: *Fusobacterium nucleatum* adheres to and invades epithelial cells, *Infect Immun* 68: 3140-3146.

Hanazawa, S., Murakami, Y., Takeshita, A., Kitami, H., Chita, K., Amano, S. & Kitano, S. (1992). *Porphyromonas gingivalis* fimbriae induce expression of the neutrophil chemotactic factor kc gene of mouse peritoneal macrophages: role of protein kinase c, *Infect Immun* 60:1544-1549.

Hannig, C., Hannig,M., Rehmer, O., Braun, O., Hellwig, E.& Al-Ahmad A. (2007). Fluorescence microscopic visualisation and quantification of initial bacterial colonization on enamel *in situ*, *Arch Oral Biol* 52: 1048-1056.

Haraldsson, G., Holbrook, W.P. & Kononen E. (2004). Clonal similarity of salivary and nasopharyngeal *Fusobacterium nucleatum* in infants with acute otitis media experience, *J Med Microbiol* 53: 161-165.

Hasebe, A.,Yoshimura ,A., Into, T., Kataoka, H., Tanak,a S., Arakawa, S., Ishikura, H., Golenbock, D.T., Sugaya, T., Tsuchida, N., Kawanami, M., Har,a Y. & Shibata, K. (2004). Biological activities of *Bacteroides forsythus* lipoproteins and their possible pathological roles in periodontal diseas,. *Infect Immun* 72: 1318-1325.

Hashimoto, M., Ogawa, S., Asai, Y., Takai, Y., Ogawa, T. (2003). Binding of *Porphyromonas gingivalis* fimbriae to *Treponema denticola* dentilisin, *FEMS Microbiology Letters* 226 : 267-271.

Hausmann, E. & Kaufman, E. (1969). Collagenase activity in a particulate fraction from *B. melaninogenicus, Biochem Biophys Acta* 194: 612-615.

Hemmens, E.S. & Harrison, R.W. (1942). Studies on the anaerobic bacterial flora of suppurative periodontitis, *J Infec Dis* 70: 131-146.

Hill, G.B., Ayers, M.O. & Kohan, A.P. (1987). Characteristics and sites of infection of *Eubacterium nodatum, E.timidium, E. brachy* and other assacharolytic eubacteria, *J Clin Microbiol* 25: 1540-1545.

Hofstad, T. (1992). Virulence factors in anaerobic bacteria, *Euro J Clin Microbiol Infect Dis* 11 (11): 1044-1048.

Hohwy, J., Reinhold,t J. & Kilian M. (2001). Population dynamics of *Streptococcus mitis* in its natural habitat, *Infect Immun* 69: 6055-6063.

Hollman, R., Van der Hoeven, H.J. (1999). Inability of intact cells of *Treponema denticola* to degrade human serum proteins IgA, IgG and albumin, *J Clin Periodontol* 26: 477-479.

Holt, S.C. &Bramanti, T.E. (1991). Factors in virulence expression and their role in periodontal disease pathogenesis, *Crit Rev Oral Biol Med* 2: 177-281.

Holt, S.C & Ebersole, J.L. (1991). The surface of selected periodontopathic bacteria: possible role in virulence, In *Periodontal disease, Pathogens and host immune responses* (Ed) Hamada, S., Holt, S.C. & McGhee, J.R., Quintessence Publishing company, Tokyo. pp 79-98.

Holtta,P.,Alaluusua,S.,Saarela, M. & Asikainen,S. (1994). Isolation frequency and serotype distribution of mutans streptococci and *Actinobacillus actinomycetemcomitans* and clinical periodontal status in Finish and Vietnamese children, *Scand J Dent Res* 102(2): 113-119.

Homer, K. A., Kelley, S., Hawkes, J., Beighton, D. & Grootveld, M.C. (1996). Metabolism of glycoprotein-derived sialic acid and N-acetylglucosamine by *Streptococcus oralis. Microbiol* 142:1221-1230.

Horning, G.M., Hatch, C. & Cohen, M.E. (1992). Risk indicators for periodontitis in a military treatment population, *J Periodontol* 63: 297-302.

Hughes, C.V., Malki, G., Loo,C., Tanner, A.C. & Ganeshkumar, N. (2003). Cloning and expression of α-D-glucosidase and N-acetyl-β-glucosaminidase from the periodontalpathogen, *Tannerella forsythensis, Oral Microbiol Immunol* 18:309-312.

Hurlen, B., Olsen, J., Lingaas, E. & Midtredt, T. (1984). Neutrophil phagocytosis of *Treponema denticola* as indicated by extracellular release of lactoferrin, *Acta Pathol Microbiol Scand Sect B;* 92: 171-173.

Iino, Y. & Hopps, R.M. (1984). The bone-resorbing activities in tissue culture of lipopolysaccharides from the bacteria *Actinobacillus actinomycetemcomitans, Bacteroides gingivalis and Capnocytophaga ochracea* isolated from human mouths, *Arch Oral Biol* 29: 59-63.

Ikegami ,A., Honma, K., Sharma, A & Kuramitsu, H.K. (2004). Multiple functions of the leucine-rich repeat protein LrrA of *Treponema denticola, Infect Immun* 72: 4619-4627.

Imbronito, A.V., Okuda, O.S., de Freitas, N.M., Lotufo, R.F.M. & Nunes F.O. (2008). Detection of Herpesviruses and periodontal pathogens in subgingival plaque of patients with chronic periodontitis, generalised aggressive periodontitis or gingivitis, *J Periodontol* 79(12): 2313-2321.

Inagaki, S., Onishi, S., Kuramitsu, H.K. & Sharma, A. (2006). *Porphyromonas gingivalis* vesicles enhance attachment and the leucine- rich repeat BspA protein is required for invasion of epithelial cells by *Tannerella forsythia, Infect Immun* 74: 5023-5028.

Ishihara, K. & Kuramitsu, H. K. (1995). Cloning and Expression of a Neutral Phosphatase Gene from *Treponema denticola Infect Immun* 63,(4): 1147–1152.

Ishihara, Y. *et al.* (1997). Gingival crevicular interleukin - I and interleukin- 1 receptor antagonist levels in periodontally, healthy and diseased sites, *J Periodont Res* 32: 524-529.

Ishihara,K., Miura, T., Kuramitsu, H.K & Okuda, K. (1996). Characterisation of the *Treponema denticola pn*P gene encoding a prolyl-phenylalanine-specific protease (dentilisin), *Infect Immun* 64:5178-5186.

Jarayaman, R. (2008). Bacterial persistence. Some new insights into an old phenomenon, *J Biosci* 13: 795-805.

Jenkinson, H.F.& Lamont, R.J. (2005). Oral Microbial communities in sickness and in health,*Trends Microbial* 13: 589-595.

Johnson, P.W., Ng, W. & Tonzetich J.(1992). Modulation of human fibroblast cell metabolism by methyl mercaptan, *J Periodontol Res* 27: 476-483.

Jones ,S.J. (1972). A special relationship between spherical and filamentous microorganisms in mature human dental plaque, *Arch Oral Biol* 17: 613-616.

Kamma, J.J., Nakou, M., Gmur, R. & Baehni, P.G. Microbiological profiles of early onset /aggressive periodontitis patients, *Oral Microbiol Immunol* 19 (5): 314-321.

Kaplan, C.W., Lux, R., Haake, S.K. & Shi, W. (2009). The *Fusobacterium nucleatum* outer membrane protein RadD is an arginine inhibitable adhesin required for inter-species adherence and the structured architecture of multispecies biofilm *Mol Microbiol*, 71: 35–47.

Kashket, S., Moudin, M.F., Haffajee, A.D. & Kashket E.R. (2003). Accumulation of methylglycosal in the gingival crevicular fluid of chronic periodontitis patients. *J Clin Periodontol* 30: 364-367.

Kataoka, M., Li, H., Arakawa, S. & Kurumitsu,H. (1997). Characterisation of a methyl-accepting chemotaxis protein gene, *dmc*A from the oral spirochaete, *Treponema denticola, Infect Immun* 65:4011-4016.

Kato, S., Kowashi, Y.,& Demuth, D.R. (2002). Outer membrane-like vesicles secreted by *Actinobacillus actinomycetemcomitans* are enriched in leukotoxin, *Microb Pathog* 32: 1-13.

Kawamoto,D., Ando, E., Longo, P., Nunes, C.,Wikstrom, M & Mayer, M. (2009). Genetic diversity and toxic activity of *Aggregatibacter actinomycetemcomitans* isolates, *Oral Microbiol Immunol* 24(6): 493-501.

Kawata, Y.S., Hanazawa, S, Amano, S., Murakami, Y., Marsumoto, T., Nishida, K. & Kitano, S. (1994). *Porphyromonas gingivalis* fimbriae stimulate bone resorption *in vitro, Infect Immun* 62: 3012-3016.

Kerosud, E., Haapasalo, M., Lounatmaa, K., Ranta, H. & Ranta K. (1988). Ultrastructure of a novel anaerobic Gram-positive non-sporing rod from dental root canal. *Scand J Dent Res* 96: 50-55.

Kesavalu, J., Salhishkumar, S., Balthavatchalu, V., Mathews, C., Davison, D., Steffan, M. & Ebersole J. (2007). Rat Model of polymicrobial infection. Immunity, and alveolar resorption in periodontal disease, *Infect Immun* 75: 1704-1712.

Kigure, T., Saito, A., Seida, K., Yamada, S., Ishihara, K. & Okuda, K. (1995). Distribution of *Porphyromonas gingivalis and Treponema denticola* in human subgingival plaque at different periodontal pocket depths examined by immunohistochemical methods, *J Periodontal Res* 30: 332-341.

Kilian, M., Frandsen, E.V., Haubek, D. & Poulsen K. (2006). The etiology of periodontal disease revisited by population genetic analysis, *Periodontol 2000* 42: 158-179.

Kim, S., Chu, L. & Holt, S. (1996). Isolation and characterisation of a hemin-binding cell envelope protein from *Porphromonas gingivalis, Microb Pathog* 21: 65-70.

Kim, T-S., Frank, P., Eickholz, P., Eick, S. & Kim C.K. (2009). Serotypes of *Aggregatibacter actinomycetemcomitans* in patients with different ethnic backgrounds, *J Periodontol* 80: 2020-2027.

Kim, Y., Wang, X., Ma, Q., Zhang, X.S. & Wood T.K. (2009). Toxin-anti toxin systems in *Escherichia coli* influence biofilm formations through YjgK (*Tab* A) and fimbriae, *J Bacteriol* 191: 1258-1267.

Kinder, S.A. & Holt ,S. (1989). Characterisation of coaggregation between *Bacteroides gingivalis* T22 and *Fusobacterium nucleatum* T18, *Infect Immun* 57: 3425-3433.

Koch, R. (1884). Erste Conferenz zur Eroterung der Cholerafrage *Berliner Klinische Wochenschrift* 30: 20-49.

Koga, T., Nishihara, T., Fujiwara, T., Nisizawa, T., Okahashi, N., Noguchi, T. & Hamada, S. (1985). Biochemical and immunological properties of lipopolysaccharide from *Bacteroides gingivalis* and comparison with lipopolysaccharide from *Escherichia coli, Infect Immun* 47: 638-647.

Kolenbrander, P.E. (1989). Surface recognition among oral bacteria: multi –generic coaggregations and their mediators, *Crit Rev Microbial* 17: 137-159.

Kolenbrander, P.E. Coaggregation: adherence in the human and microbial ecosystem. *In:Microbial Cell-Cell Interactions* (Divorkin M.) American Society for Microbiology, Washington D.C.pp 303-329. nd.

Kolenbrander, P.E. (2000). Oral Microbial Comumunities: biofilms, interactions and genetic systems, *Annu Rev Microbiol* 54: 413-437.

Kolenbrander, P.E., & Andersen, R.N. (1989). Inhibition of coaggregation between *Fusobacterium nucleatum* and *Porphyromonas gingivalis* by lactose and related sugars, *Infect Immun* 57: 3204-3209.

Kolenbrander ,P.E., Andersen, R.N., Blehert, D.S., England, P.G., Fostar, J.S.& Palmer, R.J. Jr. (2002). Communication among oral bacteria, *Microbiol Mol Biol Rev* 66: 486-505.

Kolenbrander, P.E., Andersen, R.N. & Holderman L.V. (1985). Coaggregation of oral *Bacteroides* species with other bacteria: central role in coaggregation bridges and competitions, *Infect Immun* 48: 741-746.

Kolenbrander, P.E., Andersen R.N. & Holderman L.V. (1990). Intrageneric coaggregation among strains of human oral bacteria : potential role in primary colonisation of thetooth surface, *Applied Environmen Microbiol* 56: 3890-3894.

Kolenbrander, P.E. & Landon J. (1993). Adhere today, here tomorrow: oral bacterial adherence, *J Bacteriol* 175: 3247-3252.

Kolenbrander, P.E., Palmer, R. J. Jr., Richard, A.H., Jakubovics, N.S., Chalmers ,N.I. & Diaz P.I. (2006). Bacterial interactions and successions during plaque development, *Periodontol 2000* 42: 47-79.

Kolenbrander, P.E., Parrish, K.D., Andersen, R.N. & Greenberg E.P. (1995). Intergeneric coaggregation of oral *Treponema* spp. with *Fusobacterium* spp. and intrageneric coaggregation among *Fusobacterium* spp., *Infect Immun* 63(12): 4584-4588.

Kononen, E.,Asikainen, S., Saarela, M., Karjalainen, J. & Jousimies –Somer H.(1994). The oral Gram-anaerobic microflora in young children: longitudinal changes from edentulous to dentate mouth, *Oral Microbiol Immunol* 9: 136-141.

Kononen, E., Kanervo, A., Salminen, K. & Jousimies-Somer H.(1999). Beta-lactamase production and antimicrobial susceptibility of oral heterogenous *Fusobacterium nucleatum* populations in young children, *Antimicrob Agents Chemother* 43: 1270-1273.

Konopka, A. (2006). Microbial ecology: searching for principles, *Microbe* l: 175-179.

Kontani, M., Ono, H., Shibata, Y., Okamura, Y., Tanaka, T., Fujiwara, T., Kimura, S. & Hamada, S. (1996). Cystein protease of *Porphyromonas gingivalis* 381 enhances binding of fimbriae to cultured human fibroblasts and matrix proteins, *Infect Immun* 64: 756-762.

Kornman, K.S., Crane, A., Wang, H.Y., de Giovine, F.S., Newman M.G., Pirk, F.W., Wilson, T.G.,Jr, Higginbottom, F.L., Duff, G.W. (1997). The interleukin-1 genotype as a severity factor in adult periodontal disease, *J Clin Periodontol* 24(1):72-77.

Kornman, K.S. & Holt S.C. (1981). Physiological and ultrastructural characterisation of a new *Bacteroides* species (*Bacteroides capillus)* isolated with severe localised periodontitis, *J Periodont Res* 16: 542-555.

Kritschevsky, B. & Seguin, P. (1924). The unity of spirochetosis of the mouth, *Dent Cosmos* 66: 511-520, 622-631.

Kuehn, M. J. & Kesty, N. C. (2005). Bacterial outer membrane vesicles and the host-pathogen interaction. *Genes Dev* 19: 2645-2655.

Kumar, P.S., Griffen, A.L., Barton, J.A., Paste,r B.J., Moeschberger, M.L. & Leys E.J. (2003). New bacterial species associated with chronic periodontitis, *J Dent res* 82(5): 338-344.

Kuramitsu, H.K.,He, X., Lux, R., Andersen, M.H. & Shi W.(2007). Interspecies interactions within oral microbial communities, *Microbiol Mol Biol Rev* 71: 653-670.

Kuramitsu, H.K., Yoneda ,M. & Madden T. (1995). Proteases and collagenases of *Porphyromonas gingivalis, Adv Dent Res* 9: 37-40.

Laine, M.A. (2002). Effect of pregnancy on periodontal and dental healt,. *Acta Odontol Scand* 60:257-264.

Lakio, L., Kuula, H., Dogan, B. & Asikainen, s. (2002). *Actinobacillus actinomycetemcomitans* proportion of subgingival bacterial flora in relation to its clonal type, *E J Oral Sci* 110(3): 212-217.

Lamont, R.J., Hersey, S.G. & Rosan, B. (1992). Characterisation of the adherence of *Porphyromonas gingivalis* to oral streptococci, *Oral Microbiol Immunol* 7: 193-197.

Lamont, R.J., Hsiao, G.W. & Gill S. (1994). Identification of a molecule of *Porphyromonas gingivalis* that binds to *Streptococcus gordonii, Microb Pathog* 17: 355-360.

Lamont, R.J. & Jenkinson, H.F. (2000). Subgingival colonisation by *Porphyromonas gingivalis. Oral Microbiol Immunol* 15: 341-349.

Lamont, R.J. & Jenkinson H.F. (1998). Life belowthe gumline: Pathogenic mechanisms of *Porphyromonas gingivalis, Microbiol Mol Biol Rev* 62: 1244-1263.

Lang, N., Bartold, P.M., Cullinan, M., Jeffcoat, M., Mombelli, A., Kurakam,i S., Page, R., Papapanou, P., Tonetti ,M. & Van Dyke, T. (1999). Consensus report: aggressive periodontitis, *Ann Periodontol* 4: 53.

Lancero, H., Niu ,J., &Johnson, P.W. (1996). Exposure of periodontal ligament cells to methyl mercaptan reduces intracellular pH and inhibits cell migration, *J Dent Res* 75: 1994-2002.

Lang, N.P., Tonetti, M.S., Suter, J., Sorrell, J., Duff, G.W. & Korman K.S. (2000). Effect of interleukin – l gene polymorphisms on gingival inflammation assessed by bleeding on probing in a periodontal maintenance population, *J Periodontal Res* 35(2): 102-107.

Laughon, B.E., Syed, S.A. & Loesche, W.J. (1982). API-ZYM system for the identification of *Bacteroides* species, *Capnocytophaga* species and spirochaetes of oral origin, *J Clin Microbiol 15:* 97-102.

Lee, J-Y., Sojar, H.T., Bedi, G.S. & Genco, R.J. (1991). *Porphyromonas (Bacteroides) gingivalis* fimbrillin: size, amino-terminal sequence, and antigenic heterogeneity, *Infect Immun* 59:383-389.

Leung, W.K., Ngai, V.K., Yau, J.Y., Cheung, B.P., Tsang, P.W. & Corbet E.F. (2005). Characterisation of *Actinobacillus actinomycetemcomitans* isolated from young Chinese aggressive periodontitis patients, *J Periodontal Res* 40: 258-268.

Lewis, K. (2000). Programmed death in bacteria, *Microbial Mol Bio Rev* 64: 503-514.

Lewis, J.P., Lye,r D., He, H., Miyazaki ,H., Yeudall, A. & Anaya, C. (2008). Identification and characterisation of adhesins from *Prevotella intermedia* 17, *J Dent Res* 87: (Spec Iss A): 0997.

Li,H., Arakawa, S., Deng, O & Kuramitsu,H. (1999). Characterisation of a novel methyl-accepting chemotaxis gene,*dmc*B from the oral spirochaete, *Treponema denticola, Infect Immun* 67:694-699.

Liljenberg, B. & Lindhe, J. (1980). Juvenile periodontitis , some microbiological, histopathological and clinical characteristics, *J Clin Periodontol* 7: 48.

Lindhe, J, Hampp, S-E & Loe, H. (1973). Experimental periodontitis in the Beagle dog, *J Periodont Res* 8: 1-10.

Lindemann, R.A.,Economou, S. & Rothermel, H. (1988). Production of IL-1 and TNF by human peripheral monocytes activated by periodontal bacteria and extracted lipopolysaccharide, *J Dent Res* 67: 1131-1135.

Listgarten, M.A. (1965). Electron microscopic observations on the bacterial flora of acute necrotising ulcerative gingivitis, *J Periodontol* 136: 328-339.

Listgarten,M.A. (1976). Structure of the microbial flora associated with periodontal health and disease in man, a light and electron microscope study, *J Periodontol* 47: 1-17.

Listgarten, M.A. (1988). The role of dental plaque in gingivitis and periodontitis, *J Clin Periodontol* 15: 485-487.

Listgarten, M.A. (1992). Microbiological testing in the diagnosis of periodontal disease, *J Periodontol* 63: 332-337.

Listgarten, M.A. & Hellden, L. (1978). Relative distribution of bacteria at clinically and periodontally diseased sites in humans, *J Clin Periodontol* 5: 115-132.

Listgarten, M.A. & Lai C.H. (1979). Comparative ultrastructure of *Bacteroides melaninogenicus* subspecies. *J Periodont Res* 14: 332-340.

Listgarten, M.A., Mayo, H. & Amsterdam M. (1973). Ultrastructure of the attachment device between coccal and filamentous microorganisms in "corn cob" formation of dental plaque, *Arch Oral Biol* 18: 651-656.

Loe, H., Anerud, A., Boysen, H. & Morrison, E. (1986). Natural history of periodontal disease in man: rapid, moderate and no loss of attachment of Sri Lankan labourers 14-46 years of age, *J Clin Periodontol* 13: 431-440.

Loe, H & Silness ,J. (1963). Periodontal disease in pregnancy l. Prevalence and severity, *Acta Odontol Scand* 21: 533-551.

Loe, H., Theilade, E. & Jensen, S.B. (1965). Experimental gingivitis in man, *J Periodontol* 36: 177-187.

Loesche, W.J. (1969). Oxygen sensitivity of various anaerobic bacteria, *Appl Microbiol* 18: 723-727.

Loesche, W.J. (1976). Chemotherapy of dental plaque infections, *Oral Sci Rev* 9: 65-107.

Loesche, W.J. (1988) The spirochaetes, In Newman, M.G. and Nisengard, R. (Eds), *Oral Microbiology and Immunology* W.B. Saunders Co., U.S.A.

Loesche, W., Grossman, N.S. (2001). Periodontal Disease as a specific, albeit chronic , infection: Diagnosis and Treatment, *Clin Microbiol Rev* (Oct): 727-752.

Loesche, W.J., Syed, S.A., Schmidt, E. & Morrison, E.C. (1987). Trypsin-like activity in subgingival plaque, A diagnostic marker for spirochaetes and periodontal disease ?, *J Periodontol* 58: 266-273.

Loos, B. G., Dyer, D. W., Whittam, T. S. & Selander, R. K. (1993). Genetic structure of populations of *Porphyromonas gingivalis* associated with periodontitis and other oral infections. *Infect Immun* 61: 204–212.

Lopez, N.J., Mellado, J.C. & Leighton G.X. (1996). Occurrence of *Actinobacillus actinomycetemcomitans* , *Porphyromonas gingivalis* and *Prevotella intermedia* in juvenile periodontitis, *J Clin Periodontol* 23: 101-105.

Lundstrom, A., Johansson, L.A. & Hampp, S.E. (1984). Effect of combined systemic antimicrobial therapy and mechanical plaque control in patients with recurrent periodontal disease, *J Clin Periodontol* 11: 321.

MacFarlane, T.W., Jenkins, W.M.M., Gilmour, W.H., McCourtie, J. & McKenzie, D. (1988). A longitudinal study of untreated periodontitis, II Microbiological findings, *J Clin Periodontol* 15: 331-337.

McDevitt, M. J., Wang, H. Y., Knobelman, C., Newman M.G., di Giovine, F. S., Timmis, J., Duff, G.W. & Kornman, K. S. (2000). Interleukin-1 genetic association with periodontitis in clinical practice, *J Periodontol* 71(2):156-163.

McGee, J.M., Tucci ,M.A., Edmundson, T.P., Serio, C.L. &Johnson R.B. (1998). The relationship between concentrations of pro-inflammatory cytokines within gingival and the adjacent sulcular depth, *J Periodontol* 69: 865-871.

McKee, A.S., McDermid ,A.S., Baskervill,e A., Dowsett, A.B. & Ellwood, D.C. (1986). Effect of hemin on the physiology and virulence of *Bacteroides gingivalis* W50. *Infect Immun* 52: 349-355.

McKee, A.S., McDermid, A.S., Wai,t R., Baskerville, A. & Marsh, P.D. (1988). Isolation of clonal variants of *Bacteroides gingivalis* W50 with a reduced virulence, *J Med Microbiol* 27: 59-64.

Maeda, K., Nagata, H., Kuboniwa, M., Kataoka ,K., Nishida, N., Tanaka, M. & Shizukuishi.(2004). Characterisation of the binding of *Streptococcus oralis* glyceraldehyde -3-phosphate dehydrogenase to *Porphyromonas gingivalis* major fimbriae, *Infect Immun* 72: 5475-5477.

Mager, D.L., Ximenez-Fyvie, L.A., Haffajee, A.D. & Socransky S.S. (2003). Distribution of selected bacterial species on intraoral surfaces, *J Clin Periodontol* 30: 644-654.

Magnusson, I., Lindhe, J., Yoneyama, T. & Liljenberg, B. (1984). Recolonisation of a subgingival microbiota following scaling in deep pockets, *J Clin Periodontol 11:* 193-207.

Maiden, M.F.J., Pham, C. & Kashket, S. (2004). Glucose toxicity effect and accumulation of methylglyoxal by the periodontal pathogen *Bacteroides forsythus, Anaerobe* 10:27-32.

Makarova, K.S. , Wolf, Y.I. & Koonin, E.V. (2009). Comprehensive comparative-genomic analysis of type 2 toxin-antitoxin systems and related mobile stress response systems in prokaryotes, *Biol Direct*, 3(4):19.

Makinen, K.K., Syed, S.A., Makinen, P-L. & Loesche, W.J. (1986). Benzoylarginine peptidase and immunopeptidase profiles of *Treponema denticola* strains isolated from the human periodontal pocket, *Curr Microbiol* 14: 85-89.

Makinen, K.K., Syed, S.A., Loesche, W.J. & Makinen, P-L. (1988). Proteolytic profile of *Treponema vincetii* ATCC 35580 with special reference to collagenolytic and argenine aminopeptidase activity, *Oral Microbiol Immunol* 3: 121-128.

Mangan, D.F. et al (1991). Lethal effects of *Actinobacillus actinomycetemcomitans* leukotoxin on human T lymphocytes. *Infect Immun* 59(9): 3267-3272.

Manor, A., Lebendiger, M., Shiffer, A. & Tovel,H. (1984). Bacterial invasion of periodontal tissues in advanced periodontitis in humans, *J Periodontol* 55: 567-573.

Marcuschamer, E., Hawley,C.E., Speckman, I. Romero R.M. & Molina, J.N. (2009). A lifetime of normal events and their impact on periodontal health, *Perinatol Reprod Hum* 23(2):53-64.

Margaret, B.J. & Krywolap G.N. (1986). *Eubacterium yurii* subsp. *yurii* sp. nov; test tube brush bacteria from subgingival dental plaque, *Int J Systemat Bacteriol* 36: 145-149.

Mark, L.L *et al.* (2000). Effect of the interleukin- 1 genotype on monocyte interleukin- 1 beta expression in subjects with adult periodontitis, *J Periodontal Res* 35(3): 172-177.

Marsh, P.D. (1999). Microbiologic aspects of dental plaque and dental caries, *Dent Clin North Am* 43: 599-614.

Marsh, P.D. (2003). Are dental diseases examples of ecological catastrophes? *Microbiol 149:* 279-294.

Marsh, P.D. (2005). Dental plaque: biological significance of a biofilm community life-style, *J Clin Periodontol* 32(6): 7-15.

Marsh, P.D. (2006). Dental plaque as a biofilm and a microbial community – implications for health and disease, *BMC Oral Health* 6(1): 14.

Marsh, P.D.& Percival R.S. (2006). The oral microflora – friend or for ? Can we decide? *Int Dent J* 56(4): 233-239.

Mashimo, P., Yamamoto, Y., Slots, J., Park, B.H. & Genco, R.J. (1983). The periodontal microflora of juvenile diabetics: culture, immunofluorescence and serum antibody studies, *J* Periodontol 54: 420-430.
Masuda, K. & Kawata, T. (1982). Isolation, properties and reassembly of outer sheath carrying a polygonal array from an oral treponeme, *J Bacteriol* 150: 1405-1413.
Maurelli, A.T. (1989). Temperature regulation of virulence genes in pathogenic bacteria: a general strategy for human pathogens, *Microbial Pathogenesis* 7: 1-10.
Mayrand, D. & Holt, S.C. (1988). Biology of asaccharolytic black-pigmented *Bacteroides* species, *Microbiol Rev* 52: 134-152.
Mayuko, O. (2006). Quantitative analysis of periodontal pathogens in aggressive periodontitis patients in a Japanese population, *J of the Stomtological Society Japan.* 73(1): 70-78.
Mergenhagen, S.E., Hampp, E.G. & Scherp, H.W. (1961). Preparation and biological activities of endotoxin from oral bacteria, *Infect Dis* 108: 304-310.
Michalowicz, B.S. et al. (2000). Evidence of a substantial genetic basis for risk of adult eriodontitis, *J Periodontol* 71: 1699-1707.
Mikx,F.H.M. (1991). Comparison of peptidase , glucosidase and esterase activities of oral and non-oral *Treponema* species, *J Gen Micro* 137: 63-68.
Mikx, F.H.M. & deJong, M.H. (1987). Keratinolytic activity of cutaneous and oral bacteria, *Infect Immun 55:* 621-625.
Mikx, F.H.M., & Keulers. (1992). Haemagglutination activity of *Treponema denticola* grown in serum-free medium in continuous culture, *Infect Immun* 60: 1761-1766.
Mikx, F.H.M, Malta, J.C. &van Campen, G.J. (1990). Spirochaetes in early lesions of necrotizing ulcerative gingivitis experimentally induced in beagles, *Oral Microbiol Immunol* 5: 86-89.
Mikx, F.H.M. and van Campen, G.J. (1982). Microscopial evaluation of the microflora in relation to necrotizing ulcerative gingivitis in the beagle dog, *J Perio Res* 17: 576-584.
Millar, S.J., Goldstein, E.G., Levine, M.J. & Hausmann, E. (1986). Lipoprotein: a Gram-negative cell wall component that stimulates bone resorption, *J Periodont Res* 21: 56-59.
Miller, M.B. & Bassler ,B.L. (2001). Quorum sensing in bacteria, *Annu Rev Microbiol* 55: 165-199.
Miller, J.F., Mekalanos, J.J. & Falkow, S.F. (1989). Co-ordinate regulation and sensory transduction of bacterial virulence, *Science* 243: 916-922.
Mineoka, T., Awano, S., Rikimaru ,T., Kurata, H., Yoshida, A. & Ansai T. et al. (2008). Site-specific development of periodontal disease is associated with increased levels of *Porphyromonas gingivalis, Treponema denticola* and *Tannerella forsythia* in subgingival plaque, *J Periodontol* 79: 670-676.
Miyakawa, H. & Nakazawa ,F. (2010). Role of asaccharolytic anaerobic Gram-positive rods on periodontitis. Review (New Strategy of Study for Oral Microbiology!) *J Oral Biosci* 52(3):240-244.
Mombelli, A., Gmur, R., Frey, J., Meyer, J., Zee, K.Y., Tam, J.O.W., Lo, E.C.M., Di Rienzo, J., Lang, N. & Corbet, E.F. (1998). *Actinobacillus actinomycetemcomitans* and *Porphyromonas gingivalis* in young Chinese adults, *Oral Microbiol Immunol* 13(4): 231-237.

Mombelli, A., Gmur, R., Lang, N.P., Corbewt, E. & Frey, J. (1999). *Actinobacillus actinomycetemcomitans* in Chinese adults: serotype distribution and analysis of the leukotoxin gene promoter locus, *J Clin Periodontol* 26(8): 505-510.

Moore, L.V.H., Moore, W.E.C., Cato, E.P., Smibert, R.M., Burmeister, J.A. & Best, A.M. (1987). The bacteriology of human gingivitis, *J Dent Res* 66: 989-995.

Moore, W.E.C., Holdeman, L.V., Cato, E.P., Smibert, R.M., Burmeister, J.A. & Ranney, R.R. (1983). Bacteriology of moderate (chronic) periodontitis in mature adult humans, *Infect Immun* 42: 510-513.

Moore, W.E.C. & Moore, L.V.H. (2000). The bacteria of periodontal diseases, *Periodontol* 51: 66-77.

Moter, A., Riep, B., Haban, V., Heuner, K., Siebert, G., Berning, M., Wyss, C., Ehmke, B., Flemming, T. & Gobel, U. (2006).Molecular epidemiology of oral treponema in patients with periodontitis and in periodontitis-resistant subjects, *J Clin Microbiol* 44(9):3078-3085.

Mousques, T., Listgarten, M.A. & Phillips, R.W. (1980). Effect of scaling and root planning on the composition of the human subgingival microflora, *J Periodont Res* 15: 144-151.

Mullally, B.H., Dace, B., Shelburne, C.E., Wolff, L.F.,& Coulter W.A. (2000). Prevalence of periodontal pathogens in localised and generalised forms of early -onset periodontitis, *J Periodontal Res* 35: 232-241.

Muller, H-P. & Flores de Jacoby, L. (1985). The composition of the subgingival microflora of young adults suffering from juvenile periodontitis, *J Clin Periodontol* 12: 113-123.

Muller, H-P., Muller, R.F. & Lange, D.E. (1990). Morphological compositions of subgingiva microbiota in *Actinobacillus actinomycetemcomitans* -associated periodontitis, *J Clin Periodontol* 17: 549-556.

Murakami, Y.,Higuchi, N., Nakamura, H., Yoshimura, F. & Oppenheim, F.G. (2002). *Bacteroides forsythus* haemagglutinin is inhibited by N-actylneuramenyllactose, *Oral Microbiol Immunol* 17:125-128.

Murray, P.A., Kern, D.G.,& Winkler, J.R.(1988). Identification of a galactose binding lectin on *Fusobacterium nucleatum, Infect Immun* 56: 1314-1339.

Nair, B.C., Mayberry, W.R., Dziak, R., Chen, P.B., Levine, M.J. & Hausmann, E. (1983). Biological effects of a purified lipopolysaccharide from *Bacteroides gingivalis, J Periodont Res* 18: 40-49.

Nakagawa, I., Amano, A., Kimura,R.K., Nakamura, T., Kawabata, S., & Hamada, S. (2000). Distribution and molecular characterisation of *Porphyromonas gingivalis* carrying a new type of *fim* A gene, *J Clin Microbiol* 38: 1901-1914.

Nakashima, K., Schenkein, H.A., Califano, J.V. & Tew, J.G. (1997). Heterogeneity of antibodies reactive with the dominant antigen of *Actinobacillus actinomycetemcomitans, Infect. Immun* 65(9): 3794-3798.

Neides, M.E., Chen, P.B., Suido, H., Reynolds, H.S., & Zambon J.J. (1989). Heterogeneity of virulence among strains of *Bacteroides gingivalis, J Peridont Res* 24: 192-198.

Newman, H.N. (1976). The apical border of plaque in chronic inflammatory periodontal disease, *Br Dent J* 141: 105-113.

Newman, H.N.(1998). Periodontal therapeutics -a viable option? *Int Dent J* 48: 173-179.

Nisengard, R.J., Newman, M.G. & Zambon, J.J. (1988). Periodontal disease, In: *Oral Microbiology and Immunology* (Ed) Newman, M.G. & Nisengard, W.B. Saunders Pub., Harcourt Brace Jovanocich Inc. pp 411-437.

Noiri ,Y. & Ebisu, S. (2000). Identification of periodontal disease - associated bacteria in the "plaque- free zone", *J Periodontol* 71: 1319-1326.

Noiri, Y., Li, L.,& Ebisu, S.(2001). The localisation of periodontal disease - associated bacteria in human periodontal pockets, *J Dent Res* 80: 1930-1934.

Noiri, Y., Ozaki, K., Nakae ,H., Matsuo, T. & Ebisu S. (1997). An immunohistochemical study on the localization of *Porphyromonas gingivalis, Campylobacter rectus* and *Actinomyces viscosus* in human periodontal pockets, *J Periodontal Res* 32: 598-607.

Nyfors, S., Kononen, E., Syrjanen, R., Komulainen, E.,& Jouismies - Somer, H. (2003). Emergence of penicillin resistance among *Fusobacterium nucleatum* populations of commensal oral flora during early childhood, *J Antimicrob Chemother* 51: 107-112.

Nyvad, B. (1993). Microbial colonization of human tooth surfaces, *Apmis* 101: 7-45.

Nyvad, B. & Fejerskov, O. (1987a). Scanning electron microscopy of early microbial colonization of human enamel and root surfaces *in vivo, Scand J Dent Res* 95: 287-296.

Nyvad, B. & Fejerskov, O. (1987b). Transmission electron microscopy of early microbial colonization of human enamel and root surfaces *in vivo. Scand J Dent Res* 95: 297-307.

Nyvad, B. & Kilian, M. (1987). Microbiology of the early colonization of human enamel and root surfaces *in vivo., Scand j Dent Res* 95: 369-380.

Offenbacher, S. (1996). Periodontal diseases: pathogenesis, *Ann Periodontol* 8: 21-78.

Offenbacher, S., Barros, S.P., Singer, R.E., Moss, K., Williams, R.C., & Beck J.D. (2007). Periodontal disease at the Biofilm - Gingival Interface, *J Periodontol* 78(10): 1911-1925.

Offenbacher, S., Odle, B. & van Dyke, T. (1985). The microbial morphotypes associated with periodontal health and adult periodontitis; composition and distribution, *J Clin Periodontol* 12: 736-749.

Ohta, K., Makinen, K.K. & Loesche, W.J. (1986). Purification and characterisation of an enzyme produced by *Treponema denticola* capable of hydrolysing synthetic trypsin substrates, *Infect Immun* 53: 213-220.

Okuda, K., Naito, Y., Ohta, K., kukumoto, Y., Kimura, Y., Ishikawa, I., Kinoshita, S. & Takazoe, I.(1984). Bacteriological study of periodontal lesions in 2 sisters with juvenile periodontitis and their mother, *Infect Immun* 45: 118-121.

Olsen, I. (1984). Attachment of *Treponema denticola* to cultured human epithelial cells, *Scand J Dent Res* 92: 55-63.

O'Malley, M.A. (2008). Everything is everywhere: but the envi ronment selects ubiquitous distribution and ecological determinism in microbial biogeography, *Stud Hist Philos Biol Biomed Sci* 39: 314-325.

Omar, A.A., Newman, H.N., Bulman, J. & Osborn, J. (1990). Darkground microscopy of subgingival plaque from the top to the bottom of the periodontal pocket, *J Clin Periodontol* 17: 364-370.

Ono, Okuda, K. & Takazoe, I. (1987) Purification and characterisation of a thiol-protease from *Bacteroides gingivalis* strain 381, *Oral Microbiol Immunol* 2: 77-81.

Overman, P.R. (2000). Biofilm: a new view of plaque, *J Contmp Dent Pract* 1: 18-29.

Page, R.C., & Kornman, K.S. (1997). The pathogenesis of periodontitis. *Periodontology 2000* 14: 112-157.

Page, R.C.& Schroeder, H.E. (1982). Periodontitis in man and other animals, A comparative review, Karger Basil, New York.

Palmer, R.J., Diaz, P.I., & Kolenbrander ,P. (2006). Rapid succession within the *Veillonella* population of a developing human oral biofilm *in situ, J Bacteriol* 188: 4117-4124.

Palmer, R.J. (Jr.) Gordon, S.M., Cisar, J.O. & Kolenbrander, P.E. (2003). Co-aggregation - mediated interactions of streptococci and actinomyces detected in initial human dental plaque, *J Bacteriol* 185: 3400-3409.

Palmer, R.J., Jr. Wu, R., Gordon, S., Bloomquist, C.G., Liljemark, W.F., Kilian, M., & Kolenbrander, P.E. (2001). Retrieval of biofilms from the oral cavity, *Methods Enzymol* 337: 393-403.

Pan, Y.P., Li ,Y., & Caufield, P.W. (2001). Phenotypic and genotypic diversity of *Streptococcus sanguis* in infants, *Oral Microbiol Immun* 16: 235-242.

Park, Y., Simionato, M.R., Sekiya, K., Murakami ,Y., James, D.M., Chen ,W., Hackett, M., Yoshimura, F., Desmuth, D.R. & Lamont R.J. (2005). Short fimbriae of *Porphyromonas gingivalis* and their role in co-adhesion with *Streptococcus gordonii, Infect Immun* 73: 3983-3989.

Passador, L., Cook, J.M., Gambello, M.J., Rust, L., & Iglewski, B.H. (1993). Expression of *Pseudomonas aeruginosa* virulence genes requires cell-to-cell communication, *Science* 260: 1127–1130.

Paster, B.J., Beches, S.K., Galvirin, J.I., Ericson, R.E. Lai, C.N., Levanos, V.A., Sahasralbudie, A. & Dewhirst F.E. (2001). Bacterial diversity in subgingival plaque, *J Bacteriol* 183: 3770-3783.

Perez-Chaparro, P.J., Gracieux, P., Lafaurie, G.I., Donnio, P.Y., Bonnaure-Mallet, M. (2008). Genotypic characterization of *Porphyromonas gingivalis* isolated from sub-gingival plaque and blood samples in positive bacteraemia subjects with periodontitis, *J Clin Periodontol.* 35:748–753.

Perry, M.B., Maclean, I.M., Brissen, J.R. & Wilson, M. (1996). Structures of the antigenic O-polysaccharides of Lipopolysaccharides produced by *Actinobacillus actinomycetemcomitans* Serotypes a,c,d,e, *Eur J Biochem* 242: 682-688.

Perry, M.B., Maclean, I., Gmur, R.,& Wilson, M. (1996). Characterisation of the O-polysaccharide structure of Lipopolysaccharide from *Actinobacillus actinomycetemcomitans* Serotype b. *Infect Immun* 61: 1215-1219.

Plancak, D., Jorgic - Srdjak, K., Curilovic, Z. (2001). New classification of Periodontal Diseases, *Acta Stomat Croat* 35: 89-93.

Potempa, J., & Pike, R. (2009). Corruption of innate immunity by bacterial proteases, *J Innate Immun* 1: 70-87.

Preus, H.R., Olsen, I.,& Namork, E. (1987). Association between bacteriophage- infected *Actinobacillus actinomycetemcomitans* and rapid periodontal destruction, *J Clin Periodontol* 14: 245-247.

Preus, H.R., Olsen, I., & Namork E. (1987). The presence of phage-injected *Actinobacillus actinomycetemcomitans* in juvenile periodontitis patients, 14: 605-609.

Preza, D., Olsen, I., Aas JA et al (2008). Bacterial profiles of root caries in elderly patients, *J Clin Microbiol* 46: 2015–2021.

Progulske-Fox, A., Tumwasorn, S., & Holt S.C. (1989). The expression and function of a *Bacteroides gingivalis* haemagglutinin gene in *Escherichia coli, Oral Microbial Immunol* 4: 121-131.

Quirynen, M.,& Bollen, C.M. (1995). The influence of surface roughness and surface–free energy on supra- and subgingival plaque formation in man. A review of the literature, *J Clin Periodontol* 22: 1-14.

Quirynen, M., De Soete, M., Dierick ,K.,& van Steenberger, D.(2001). The intra-oral translocation of periodontopathogens jeopardises the outcome of periodontal therapy. A review of the literature, *J Clin Periodontol* 28: 499-507.

Ramfjord, S.P., Emslie, K.D., Greene, J.C., Held, A.J. & Waerhaug, J. (1968). Epidemiological studies of periodontal diseases, *Am J Publ Health* 58: 1713-1722.

Rams, T.E. ,& Slots, J. (1992). Antibiotics in periodontal therapy: an update. *Compendium* 13:1130-1134.

Reading, N.C., & Sperandio, V. (2006). Quorum sensing: the many languages of bacteria. *FEMS Microbiol Lett* 254(1): 1-11.

Reddy, J., Africa, C.W. & Parker, J.R. (1986). Darkfield Microscopy of subgingival plaque of an urban black population with poor oral hygiene, *J Clin Periodontol* 13: 578-582.

Reijntjens, F.M.J., Mikx, F.H.M., Wolters Lutgerhorst, J.M.L. & Maltha, J.C. (1986). Adherence of oral treponemes and their effect on morphological damage and detachment of epithelial cells *in vitro, Infect Immun* 51: 642-647.

Relman, D. A. (2008). "Till death do us part": coming to terms with symbiotic relationships. *Nat. Rev.* 6: 721-724.

Riep,B., Edesi-Neu B.L.,Claessen, F.Skarabis, H., Ehmke,B. et al.(2009). Are putative periodontal pathogens reliable diagnostic markers? *J Clin Microbiol* 47(6): 1705-1711.

Riggio, M.P., Macfarlane, T.W., Mackenzie, D., Lennon, A., Smith,A.J. & Kinan,e D. (1996). Comparison of polymerase chain reaction and culture methods for detection of *Actinobacillus actinomycetemcomitans* and *Porphyromonas gingivalis* in subgingival plaque samples, *J Periodontal Res* 31: 496-501.

Riviere, G.R., Smith, K.S., Carranza, N., Tzagaroulcki, E., Kay ,S. I. & Dick, M. (1995). Subgingival distribution of *Treponema denticla, Treponema socranskii,* and pathogen-related oral spirochaetes: prevalence and relationship to periodontal status of sampled sites, *J Periodontol* 66: 829-837.

Riviere, G.R., Wagner, M.A., Baker-Zander, S., Weisz, K.S.., Adams, D.F. & Simonson, L. (1991a). Identification of spirochaetes related to *Treponema pallidum* in necrotizing ulcerative gingivitis and chronic periodontitis, *N Eng J Med* 325: 539-543.

Riviere, G.R., Weisz, K.S., Adams, D.F. & Thomas, D.D. (1991b). Pathogen-related oral spirochaetes from dental plaque are invasive, *Infect Immun* 59: 3377-3380.

Roberts,F.A., Richarson, G.J.& Michalek, S.M.(1997). Effects of *Porphyromonas gingivalis* and *Escherichia coli* lipopolysaccharide on mononuclear phagocytes, *Infect Immun* 65:3248-3254.

Roman-Torres, C.V.G., Aquerio, D.R., Cortelli, S. C., Franco, G.C.N., dos Santos, J.G., Corraini, P., Holzhausen, M., Dintz, M.G., Gomez, R.s. & Cortelli, J.R. (2010). Prevalence and distribution of serotype-specific genotypes of Aa in chronic periodontitis in Brazilian subjects, *Arch Oral Biol* 55(3): 242-245.

Rosan, B. & Lamon,t R.J. (2000). Dental plaque formation . *Microbes Infect* 2: 1599-1607.

Rosebury, T., MacDonald, J.B. & Calrk, A.R. (1950). A bacteriological survey of gingival scrapings from periodontal infections by direct examination, guinea pig inoculation and anaerobic cultivation, *J Dent Res* 29: 718-731.

Rosen, G., Nisimov, I., Helcer, M. & Sela, M.N. (2003). *Actinobacillus actinomycetemcomitans* serotype b *Lipopolysaccharides* mediates coaggregation with *Fusobacterium nucleatum. Infect Immun* 71(6): 3652-2656.

Rylev ,M., Bek-Thomsen, M., Reinholdt, J., Ennibi, O.K. & Kilian, M. (2011). Microbiological and Immunological characteristics of young Moroccan patients with aggressive periodontitis with and without detectable *Actinobacillus actinomycetemcomitans* JP2 infection, *Molecular Oral Microbiol* 26(1):35-51.

Rylev, M & Kilian, M. (2008). Prevalence and distribution of principal periodontal pathogens worldwide, *J Clin periodontal* 35(8): 3465-3615.

Sabet,M., Lee,S .W., Nauman, R.K., Sims, T.& Um, H. S. (2003). The surface s-layer is a virulence factor of *Bacteroides forsythus, Microbiol* 149: 3617-3627.

Saglie, F.R., Carranza, F.A., Newman, M.G., Cheng, l. & Lewin, K.J. (1982). Identification of tissue-invading bacteria in human periodontal disease, *J Periodont Res* 17: 452-455.

Saglie,F.R., Marfony,A.& Camargo, P. (1988). Intragingival occurrence of *Actinobacillus actinomycetemcomitans and Bacteroides gingivalis* in active destructive periodontallesions, *J Periodontol* 59:259-265.

Saito, Y., Fujii, R., Nakagawa, K., Kuramitsu, H.K., Okuda, K. & Ishihara, K. (2008). Stimulation of *Fusobacterium nucleatum* biofilm formation *by Porphyromonas gingivalis, Oral Microbiol Immunol* 23:1-6.

Saito, T., Ishihara, K., Kato, T., & Okuda, K. (1997). Cloning, expression, and sequencing of a protease gene from *Bacteroides forsythus* ATCC 43037 in *Escherichia coli. Infect Immun* 65:4888-4891.

Sakakibara, J., Nagano, K., Murakami, Y., Higuchi, N., Nakamura, H., Shimozato, K. & Yoshimura, F. (2007). Loss of adherence ability to human gingival epithelial cells in S-layer protein-deficient mutants of *Tanerella forsythensis, Microbiol* 153:866-876.

Sakellari, D., Katsikari, A., Slini, T., Ioannidi,s I., Konstamtinidis, A. & Arsenakis, M. (2011). Prevalence and distribution of *Aggregatibacter actinomycetemcomitans* serotypes and the JP2 clone in a Greek population. *JClin Periodontol* 38: 108-114.

Sanz, M., van Winkelhoff, A.J., Herrer,a D., Lemijn - Kippuw, N., Simon, R.& Winkel, E. (2000). Differences in the compostion of the subgingival microbiota of two periodontitis populations of different geographic origin. A comparison between Spain and the Netherlands, *Eur J Oral Sci* 108: 383-392.

Sarel-Carrinaga, R.M., Pires, J.R., Sogumo, P.M., Salmon, C.R., Peres, R.C.R. & Spolidono D.M.P. (2009). A familial case of aggressive periodontitis! Clinical, microbiolocal and genetic findings, *Rensta de Odontologia da UNESP.* 38(3): 175-183.

Sbordone, L. & Bortolaia, C. (2003). Oral microbial biofilms and plaque-related diseases: microbialcommunities and their shifts from oral health to disease, *Clin Oral Invest* 7:181-188.

Sbordone, L., Di Genio, M. & Bortolaia, C. (2000). Bacterial virulence in the aetiology of periodontal diseases, *Minerva Stomatol* 49:485-500.

Scannapieco, F. A. (1994). Saliva-bacterium interactions in oral microbial ecology. *Crit Rev Oral Biol Med* 5: 203–248.

Schei, O., Waerhaug, J., Lovdal, A & Arno, A (1959). Alveolar bone loss as related to oral hygiene and age , *J Periodontal* 30: 7-16.

Schifferie, R.E., Wilson, M.E., Levine, M.J. & Genco, R.J. (1993). Activation of serum complement by polysaccharide-containing antigens of *Porphyromonas gingivalis, J Periodont Res* 28: 248-254.

Selvig, K.A., Hofstad, T. & Kristoffersen, T. (1971). Electron microscopic demonstration of bacterial lipopolysaccharides in dental plaque matrix, *Scand* J Dent Res 79: 409-421.

Shah, H.N., Seddon, S.V. & Garbia, S.E. (1989). Studies on the virulence properties and metabolism and pleiotropic mutants of *Porphyromonas gingivalis* W50, *Oral Microbiol Immunol* 4:19-23.

Shapira, L., Sylvia, V.L., Halabi, A.,Soskolne, A., Van Dyke, T.E., Dean, D., Boyan, B. & Swartz, Z.(1997). Bacterial lipopolysaccharide induces earlyand late activation of protein kinase C in inflammatory macrophages by selective activation of PKC, *Biochem Biophys Res Commun* 240:629-634.

Sharma, A. (2010). Virulence mechanisms of *Tannerella forsythia., Periodontol 2000.* 54: 106-116.

Sharma, A., Inagaki, S., Sigurdson, W. & Kuramitsu, H.K. (2005). Synergy between *Tannerella forsythia* and *Fusobacterium nucleatum* in biofilm formation, *Oral Microbiol Immunol* 20(1): 39-42.

Shenker, B,J., Listgarten, M.A. & Taichman, N.S. (1984). Suppression of human lymphocyte responses by oral spirochaetes; a monocyte dependent phenomenon, *J Immunol B* 132: 2039-2045.

Shin,J.E., Kim, J.S., Oh, J-E., Min, B-M. & Choi, Y. (2010). *Treponema denticola* Suppresses Expression of Human β-Defensin-3 in Gingival Epithelial Cells through Inhibition of the Toll-Like Receptor 2 Axis Infection and Immunity, 78(2): 672-679

Shirodaria, S., Smith, J., McKay, I.J., Kennech, C.N. & Hughes, F.J. (2000). Polymorphisms in the Interleukin -lA gene are correlated with levels of interleukin -lx protein in gingival crevicular fluid of teeth with severe periodontal disease, *J Dent Res* 79(11): 1864-1869.

Siboo,R., Chan, E.C.S & Cheng, S-L. (1988). The production of phospholipase C by oral spirochaetes, *J Dent Res* 67: 202 Abs 719.

Sismey-Durrant, H. Hopps, R.M.(1991). Effect of lipopolysaccharide *from Porphyromonas gingivalis* on prostaglandin E2and IL-1β release from rat peritoneal and human gingival fibroblasts *in vitro, Oral Microbiol Immunol* 6: 378-380.

Sissons , C.H., Anderson, S.A., Wong, L., Coleman, M.J. & White, D.C. (2007). Microbiota of plaque microcosm biofilms: effect of three times daily sucrose pulses in different simulated oral environments, *Caries Res* 41: 413-422.

Sleytr, U.B. & Messner, P. (1983). Crystalline surface layers in procaryotes, *J Bacteriol 170:* 2891-2897.

Slots, J. (1977). Microflora in the healthy gingival sulcus in man, *Scand Dent Res* 85: 247-254.

Slots, J. (1981). Enzyme characterisation of some oral and non-oral Gram-negative bacteria with API-ZYM system, *J Clin Microbiol* 14: 288.

Slots, J. (2010). Human viruses in periodontitis, *Periodontal 2000* 53(1): 89-110.

Slots, J., Emrich, L., Genco, R.J. & Rosling, B.G. (1985). Relationship between some subgingival bacteria and periodontal pocket depth and gain or loss of periodontal attachment after treatment of adult periodontitis, *J Clin Periodontol* 12: 540-552.

Slots, J. & Genco, R.J. (1984) Black pigmented *Bacteroides* species, *Capnocytophaga* species and *Actinobacillus actinomycetemcomitans* in human disease: virulence factors in colonisation, survival and tissue destruction, *J Dent Res* 63: 412-421.

Smalley, J.W., Birss, A.J., Kay, H.M., McKee, A.S. & Marsh, P. (1989). The distribution of trypsin - like enzyme activity in cultures of a virulent and avirulent strain of *Bacteroides gingivalis* W50, *Oral Microbiol Immunol* 4: 178-181.

Smibert, R.M. & Burmeister, J.A. (1983). *Treponema pectinovorum* sp. nov. isolated from humans with periodontitis, *Int J Syst Bacteriol* 33: 852-856.

Smith, D.J., King, W.F., Gilbert, J.V. & Taubman , M.A. (1998). Structural integrity of infant salivary immunoglobulin A (I gA) in IgAl protease –rich environments, *Oral Microbiol Immunol* 13: 89-96.

Socransky, S.S. (1984). Microbiology of plaque, *Compend Contin Educ Dent Suppl* 5: S53-S56.

Socransky S.S. & Haffajee, A.D. (1992). The bacterial aetiology of destructive periodontal disease: current concepts, *J Periodontol* 63(4): 322-331.

Socransky, S. S. & Haffajee, A.D. (2002). Dental biofilms: difficult therapeutic targets, *Periodontol 2000* 28:12-55.

Socransky, S.S. & Hafajee, A.D. (2005). Periodontal microbial ecology, *Periodontol 2000* 38:135-187.

Socransky, S.S., Hafajee, A.D., Dzink, J.L. & Hillman, J.D.(1988). Association between microbial species in subgingival plaque samples, *Oral Microbiol Immunol* 3:1-7.

Socransky, S.S., Hafajee, A.D. & Cugini, M.A. (1998). Microbial complexes in subgingival plaque, *J Clin Periodontol* 25:134-144.

Socransky, S.S., Hafajee, A.D., Goodson, J.M. & Lindhe, J. (1984). New concepts of destructive periodontal disease, *J Clin Periodontol* 11(1):21-32.

Socransky, S.S., Loesche, W.J., Hubersak, C. & McDonald, J.B. (1964). Dependency of *Treponema microdentium* on other oral organisms for isobutyrate, polyamines and a controlled oxidation reduction potential, *J Bacteriol* 88: 200-209.

Sohar, H.T. & Genco, R.J. (2005). Identification of glyceraldehyde-3-phosphate dehydrogenase of epithelial cells as a second molecule that binds to *Porphyromonas gingivalis* fimbriae, FEMS *Immunol Med Microbiol* 45:25-30.

Stam, J.W. (1986). Epidemiology of gingivitis, *J Clin Periodontol* 13:360-366.

Stelzel, M. & Flores-de-Jacoby, L. (2000). Topical metronoidazole application as an adjunct to scaling and root planning, *J Clin Periodontol* 27(6):447-452.

Sunde, P.T., Olsen, I., Gobel, U.B., Theegarten, D., Winter, S., Debelian, G.J., Tronstad, L & Motor, A. (2003). Flourescence *in situ* hybridusation (FISH) for direct visualisation of bacteria in peri-apical lesions of asymptomatic no-filled teeth, *Microbiol* 149:1095-1102.

Susser, M. (1996). Choosing a future for epidemiology. II. From block boxes to Chinese boxes and eco-epidemiology, *Am J Pub Health* 86:674-677.

Sveen, K. & Skaug, N. (1980). Bone resorption stimulated by Lipopolysaccharides from *Bacteroides, Fusobacterium* and *Veillonella* and by lipid A and polysaccharide parts of *Fusobacterium* lipopolysaccharides, *Scand J Dent Res* 88: 535-542.

Takeuchi, Y., Umeda, M., Ishizuka, M., Huang, Y & Ishikawa, I. (2003). Prevalence of periodontopathic bacteria in aggressive periodontitis patients in a Japanese population, *J Periodontol* 74(10):1460-1469.

Taichman, N.S., Bohringer, H.R., Lai, C.H., Shenker, B.J.,Tsa, C.C., Berthold, P.H., Listgarten, M.A. & Shapiro, I.S. (1982). Pathobiology of oral spirocaetes in periodontal disease, *J Periodont Res* 17: 449-451.

Tambo, T., Kunyama, T., karaswa, T., Nakagawa, K., Yamamoto, E. & Williams, D.W. (2010). Genetic heterogeneity of *Prevotella* strains involved in dentoalveolar abscess, *Arch Clin Microbiol* 1 (4): n.p.

Tan, K.S., Woo, C.H., Ong, G & Song, K.P. (2001). Prevalence of *Actinobacillus actinomycetemcomitans* in an adult ethnic Chinese population, *J Clin Periodontol* 28(9): 886-890.

Tanner, A.C.R., Listgarten, M.A., Ebersole, J.L. & Strzempko, M.N. (1986). *Bacteroides forsythus* sp.nov. a slow-growing fusiform *Bacteroides* species from the human oral cavity, *Int J Systemat Bacteriol* 36:213-221.

Teixeira, R.E., Mendes, E.N., de Carvalho, M., Nicoli, J.R., de Macedo Farias, L.& Magalhaes, P.P. (2006). *Actinobacillus actinomycetemcomitans* serotype specific genotypes and periodontal status in Brazilian subjects, *Can J Microbiol* 52: 182-188.

Teixeira, S.R.L.,Mattarazo, O.F., feres, M., Fugueredo, L.C., de Faveri, M., Simionato, M. & Mayer, M.P.A. (2009). Quantification of *P. gingivalis* and FimA genotypes in smoker-chronic periodontitis, *J Clin Periodontol* 36(6): 482-487.

Teles RP, Haffajee AD, Socransky SS. Microbiological goals of periodontal therapy. *Periodontol 2000* 2006: 42: 180–218.

Ten carte, J. M. (2006). Biofilms, a new approach to the microbiology of dental plaque, *Odontol* 94:1-9.

Theilade, E. (1986). The non-specific theory in microbial aetiology of inflammatory periodontal diseases, *J Clin Periodontol* 13: 905-911.

Theilade, E., Wright, W. H., Borglum-Jensen, S. &Loe, H. (1966). Experimental gingivitis in man II, A longitudinal clinical and bacteriological investigation, *J Periodont Res* 1: 1-13.

Thiha, K., Takeuchi, Y., Umeda, M., Huang, Y., Ohnishi, M. & Ishiwara, I. (2007). Identification of periodontopathic bacteria in gingival tissue of Japanese periodontitis patients, *Oral Microbiol Immunol* 22(3): 201-207.

Thomas, D., Navab, M., Haake, D.A., Fogelman, A.M., Miller,J.N. & Lovett, M.A. (1988). *Treponema pallidum* invades intercellular junctions of endothelial cell monolayers, *Proc Nat l Acad Sci USA* 85: 3608-3612.

Thurnheer, T., Guggenheim, B., Gruica, B. & Gmur, R. (1999). Infinite serovar and ribotype heterogeneity among oral *Fusobacterium nucleatum* strains, *Anaerobe* 5: 79-92.

Tonzetich, J. & McBride, B. L. (1981). Characterisation of volatile sulphur production by pathogenic and non-pathogenic strains of oral *Bacteroides, Arch Oral Biol* 26: 963-969.

Travis, J., Pik, R., Imamura, T. & Potempa, J. (1997). *Porphyromonas gingivalis* proteinases as virulence factors in the development of periodontitis, *J Periodontal Res* 32:120-125.

Travis, J & Salvesen, G.S. (1983). Human plasma proteinase inhibitors, *A rev Biochem* 52:655-709.

Trombelli, L. & Tatakis, D.N. (2003). Periodontal diseases: current and future indications for local antimicrobial therapy, *Oral Dis* 9:11-15.

Trope,M., Rosenberg, E. & Tronstad, L. (1992). Darkfield microscopic spirochaete count in the differentiation of endodontic and periodontal abscesses, *J Endodon* 18(2): 82-86.

Uematsu, H. & Hoshino, E.(1992). Predominant obligate anaerobes in human periodontal pockets, *J Periodont Res* 27:15-19.

Uitto, V-J. (1983). Degradation of basement membrane collagen by proteinases from human gingiva, leukocytes and bacterial plaque, *J Periodontol* 54: 740-745.

Uitto, V-J. (1987). Human gingival proteases, l: extraction and preliminary characterisation of trypsin-like and elastase-like enzymes, *J Periodont Res* 22: 58-63.

Uitto,V-J., Chan, E.C.S. & Chin Quee, T. (1986). Initial characterisation of neutral proteinases from oral spirochaetes, *J Periodont Res* 21: 95-100.

Umemoto, T., Namikawa, I., Suido & Asai, S. (1989). A major antigen on the outer envelope of a human oral spirochaete, *Treponema denticola, Infect Immun* 57: 2470-2474.

Van Dalen, P., Van Winkelhoff, A., & Van Steenbergen, T. (1998). Prevalence of *Peptostreptococcus micros* morphotypes in patients with adult periodontitis, *Oral Microbiol Immunol* 13: 62-64.

Van dyke, T.E., Duncan, E.L., Cutler, C.W., Kalmer, J.R.& Arnold, R.R. (1988). Mechanisms and consequences of neutrophil interaction with the subgingival microbiota, In: *PeriodontologyToday*, Int Congr Zurich, Karger, Basel,pp 209-217.

Van Palenstein-Helderman, W.H. & Hoogeveen, C.J. (1976). Bacterial enzymes and viable counts in crevices of non-inflamed and inflamed gingiva, *J Periodont Res* 11: 25-34.

Van Steenbergen, T.J., Delemarre, F.G., Namavar, F & De Graaf, J. (1987). Differences in virulence within the species *Bacteroides gingivalis, Antonie van Leeuwenhoek* 53; 233-244.

Vieira, E.M.M., Rasian, S.A., Wahasugui,T.C., Avila-Campos, M. et al.(2009). Occurrence of *Aggregatibacter actinomycetemcomitans* in Brazilian Indians fromUmutina reservations, Matogrosso, Brazil, *J App Oral Sci* 17(5):440-445.

Vrahopoulos, T.P., Barber, P.M.& Newman, H.N. (1992). The apical border plaque in chronic adult periodontitis, An ultrastructural study, II: Adhesion, matrix and carbohydrate metabolism, *J Periodontol* 63: 253-261.

Wang,L., Azuma, Y., & Khinohara, O. (2001). Effect of *Actinobacillus actinomycetemcomitans* protease on the proliferation of gingival epithelial cells, *Oral Diseas* 7(4): 233-237.

Wecke, J., Kersten, T., Madela, K., Motor, A., Gobel, U., Friedman, a & Bernimoulin, J.P. (2000). A novel technique for monitoring the development of bacterial biofilms in human periodontal pockets, FEMS *Microbiol Lett* 191; 95-101.

Weinberg, A. & Holt, S.C. (1990). Interaction of *Treponema denticola* TD-4, GM-l and M325 with human gingival fibroblasts, *Infect Immun* 58: 1720-1729.

Weinberg, A., Nitzan, D.W., Shyter, A. & Sela, M.N. (1986). Inflammatory cells and bacteria in pericoronal exudates from acute pericoronitis, *Int J Oral Maxillofac Surg* 15: 606-613.

Weiss, E.I., Kolanbrander, P.E., London, J., Hand, A.R. &Andersen, R.N. (1987). Fimbria-associated proteins of *Bacteroides loescheii* PK1295 mediate intergeneric coaggregations, *J Bacteriol* 169:4215-4222.

Whittaker, C.J., Klier, C.M. & Kolenbrander, P.E. (1996). Mechanisms of adhesion by oral bacteria, *Annu Rev Microbiol* 50: 513-552.

Willis, S.G., Smith, K.S., Durin, V.L., Gapter, L.A., Riviere, K.H. & Riviere, G.R. (1999). Identification of seven *Treponema* species in health and disease-associated dental plaque by nested-PCR, *J Clin Microbiol* 37 (3): 867-869.

Wilson, M. (1999). Use of constant depth film fermenter in studies of biofilms of oral bacteria, *Methods Enzymol* 310: 264-279.

Wilson, M& Hendersen, B. (1995). Virulence factors of *Actinobacillus actinomycetemcomitans* relevant to the pathogenesis of inflammatory periodontal disease, FEMS *Microbiol Rev* 17(4):365-379.

Wilson, M., Meghji, S. & Harvey, W. (1986). Inhibition of bone collagen synthesis *in vitro* by lipopolysaccharide from *Actinobacillus actinomycetemcomitans* , *IRCS Med Sci* 14:536-537.

Woo, D.D.L., Holt, S. & Leadbetter, E.R. (1979). Ultrastructure of *Bacteroides* species, *B. asaccharolyticus, B. fragilis, B. melaninogenicus* subspecies *melaninogenicus, B. melaninogenicus* subspecies *intermedius, J Infect Dis* 139: 534-546.

Wyss, C., Choi, B.K., Schupbach, P., Guggenheim, B. & Gobel, U.B. (1997). *Treponema amylovorum* sp. nov. , a saccharolytic spirochaete of medium size isolated from an advanced human periodontal lesion, *Int J Syst Bacteriol* 47: 842-845.

Xajigeorgiou, C., Sakellari, D., Slini, T, Baka, A. & Konstantinidis, A. (2006). Clinical and microbiological effects of different antimicrobials on generalised aggressive periodontitis, *J Clin Periodontol* 33 (4): 254-264.

Xie, H., Gibbons, R.J. & Hay, D.I. (1991). Adhesive properties of strains of *Fusobacterium nucleatum* ss *nucleatum vincentii* and polymorphism, *Oral Microbiol Immunol* 6: 257-263.

Yacoubi, A., Djamila, B., Makhrelouf, L. & Bensoltane, A. (2010). Microbiological study of periodontitis in the west of Algeria, *World J Med Sciences* 5(1):7-12.

Yamaji, Y., Kubota,T., Sasuguri, K., Sato, S., Suzuki, Y., Kumada, H & Umemoto, T. (1995). Inflammatory cytokine gene expression in human periodontal ligament fibroblasts stimulated with bacterial lipopolysaccharide, *Infect Immun* 63:3576-3581.

Yanagisawa, M., Kuriyama, T., Williams, D.W., Nakagawa, K. & Karasawa, T. (2006). Proteinase activity of *Prevotella* species associated with oral purulent infection, *Curr Microbiol* 52:375-378.

Yang, H.W., Huang, Y.F., Chan, Y. & Chou, M.Y. (2005). Relationship of *Actinobacillus actinomycetemcomitans* serotypes to periodontal condition: prevalence and proportions in subgingival plaque, *Eur J Oral Sci* 113: 28-33.

Yao, E.S., Lamont, R.J., Leu, S.P. & Weinberg, A. (1996). Interbacterial binding among pathogenic and commensal oral bacterial species, *Oral Microbial Immunol* 11: 35-41.

Yilmaz, O., Young, P.A., Lamont, R. J. & Kenny, G. E. (2003). Gingival epithelial cell signalling and cytoskeletal responses to *Porphyromonas gingivalis* invasion, *Microbiol* 149: 2417-2426.

Yoneda, M., Hirofuji, T., Anan, H., Matsumoto, A., Hamachi, T., Nakayama, K. *et al.* (2001). Mixed infection of *Porphyromonas gingivalis* and *Bacteroides forsythus* in a murine abscess model: involvement of gingipains in a synergistic effect, *J Periodontal Res* 36:237-243.

Yoshimura, F., Nishikata, M., Suzuki, T., Hoover, C & Newbrun , E. (1984). Characterisation of a trypsin-like protease from the bacterium *Bacteroides gingivalis* isolated from human dental plaque, *Arch Oral Biol* 29: 559-564.

Yoshimura, F., Takahashi, K., Nodasake, Y & Suzuki, T. (1984). Purification and characterisation of a novel type of fimbriae from the oral *anaerobe Bacteroides gingivalis, J Bacteriol* 160:949-957.

Zambon, J.J. (1983). Recent research on the role of dental plaque microorganisms; Aa in the aetiology of localised juvenile periodontitis, *Bull Eighth Dist Dent Soc* 17(3):16-17.

Zambon, J.J. (1985). *Aggregatibacter actinomycetemcomitans* in human periodontal disease, *J Clin Periodontol* 12(1):1-20.

Zambon, J.J. (1996). Periodontal diseases: microbial factors, *Ann Periodontol* 1(1): 879-925.

Zijnge, V., Meljar, H., Lie, M-A., Tromp, J.A.H., Deyener, J.E., Harmsen, J.M. &Abbas, F.(2010). The recolonisation hypothesis in a full mouth or multiple lesion treatment protocol: a blinded randomised clinical trial, *J Clin Periodontol* 37(6):518-525.

2

Microbiological Diagnosis for Periodontal Diseases

Akihiro Yoshida and Toshihiro Ansai
Division of Community Oral Health Science, Kyushu Dental College
Japan

1. Introduction

Periodontitis, an infectious disease caused by bacteria, brings about destructive changes leading to loss of bone and connective tissue attachment (Williams, 1990). Several oral bacteria are considered to be possible pathogens in periodontitis (Darveau et al., 1997). In particular, the black-pigmented, Gram-negative anaerobic rods *Porphyromonas gingivalis* and *Tannerella forsythia* have been implicated as major pathogens in the etiology of this disease. These two species are frequently isolated together, implying the existence of an ecological relationship between these organisms (Darveau et al., 1997). *Treponema denticola*, a helical oral spirochete, has also been considered as a major pathogen in periodontitis (Darveau et al., 1997). Mixed infection with these three bacteria in periodontal sites is correlated strongly with the severity of adult periodontitis (Socransky & Haffajee, 1998). Socransky named this combination the "red complex" and found that these bacteria were most crucial for the progression of this disease (Socransky & Haffajee, 1998). Thus, the detection of these organisms provides essential information about the severity of periodontitis. *Aggregatibacter actinomycetemcomitans* is suspected to be the most probable causal factor for aggressive periodontitis in adolescents (Darveau et al., 1997).

Although we cannot completely rule out the possibility of exogenous infection, periodontitis is thought to be primarily an endogenous infection caused by oral bacteria. Various systems for the detection of oral pathogens have been reported, but most are qualitative (Yoshida et al., 2005a; Yoshida et al., 2005b). Because periodontal pathogens exist not only in infected pockets but also in the healthy sulcus, qualitative detection is not suitable for the diagnosis of periodontitis. For this purpose, we have developed a quantitative detection system that uses real-time polymerase chain reaction (PCR) methodology (Yoshida et al., 2003a; Yoshida et al., 2003b).

The best time for the detection of oral bacteria remains unclear. When during the periodontal treatment process should a diagnostic system be used? Can a quantitative detection system be used for the initial diagnosis of periodontitis? Furthermore, periodontitis is influenced by multiple factors such as genetic, environmental, and lifestyle-related factors that complicate the determination of a microbial cut-off value for disease onset. The use of microbiological detection for the initial diagnosis of periodontitis is thus likely to be of limited value. Nevertheless, microbiological diagnosis is meaningful in evaluating the effects of periodontal therapy. During periodontal therapy, factors associated with the etiology of periodontitis, other than microbiological factors, are relatively stable, whereas the number of bacteria is variable. Previously, we found a positive relationship between pocket depth and *P. gingivalis* and *T. denticola* counts and percentages, and the cell numbers were significantly lower after initial periodontal treatment compared with before treatment, which included scaling, tooth-brushing instruction, and professional mechanical tooth cleaning (Kawada et al., 2004; Yoshida et al., 2004).

A microbiological diagnosis involving bacterial detection can be useful for periodontal treatment. However, before considering these applications, the purpose of bacterial examinations in the course of treatment and the etiology of periodontitis must be understood. In this chapter, we describe the factors associated with the diagnosis of periodontitis and discuss the role of microbiological diagnosis in periodontal treatment.

2. Periodontal disease as an infectious disease

Previous investigations have revealed that periodontal disease is an infectious disease caused by oral bacteria and that it has complex associations with immunological, genetic, and environmental factors (Williams, 1990). It also is associated closely with dental plaque, which has been recognized as a biofilm contributing to representative oral diseases such as dental caries and periodontal disease (Keyes & Likins, 1946). The features of periodontitis as an infectious disease are listed in Table 1.

1.	Endogenous infection by normal oral microbiological flora
2.	Mixed infection by various normal oral microbiological flora
3.	*Porphyromonas gingivalis, Tannerella forsythia, Treponema denticola,* and *Aggregatibacter actinomycetemcomitans* as possible causative bacteria
4.	Biofilm-associated infectious disease caused by subgingival microflora

Table 1. Features of periodontitis as an infectious disease.

2.1 Etiology of periodontal disease

Numerous bacterial products are released in the crevice fluid in the periodontal pockets. This fluid contains histiolytic enzymes, endo- and exotoxins, and nontoxic materials that interfere with cell function. Of these, collagenase and other proteases released by bacteria in the periodontal pockets are related to the features of periodontitis, such as the extensive destruction of collagen and the connective-tissue matrix (Kuramitsu, 1998). Bacterial lipopolysaccharide can also induce bone destruction (Miyata et al., 1997). Low-molecular-weight metabolites released by oral bacteria such as sulfides are considered to be cytotoxic molecules in the periodontium (Socransky, 1990). On the other hand, some bacteria can inactivate a specific antibody, which enables them to prevent their own death by phagocytosis. *A. actinomycetemcomitans* produces a leukotoxin that specifically kills human leukocytes (McArthur et al., 1981). Thus, some bacteria can inhibit the normal immune-defense system of the host. The bacterial etiological agent is pathogenic because of its capacity to induce response mechanisms that destroy periodontal tissue. Bacterial substances can thus directly and indirectly destroy periodontal tissues, and it is difficult to distinguish "good" from "bad" bacteria because one bacterial species may behave both beneficially and destructively in humans. However, some bacteria are considered to be periodontopathic due to the production of etiological agents; the monitoring of these pathogens is important in periodontal treatment.

2.2 Infection mechanism of periodontal disease

Periodontal disease is characterized by inflammation caused by periodontopathic bacteria in the subgingival plaque. In general, periodontal infection is thought to be endogenous. In contrast to an exogenous infection, endogenous periodontal infection involves the internal proliferation of the normal bacterial flora in the oral environment. This significantly influences the potential use of microbiological examinations in the diagnosis of periodontal disease, as will be described later. Periodontopathic bacteria proliferate in periodontal environments such as the sulcus and induce inflammation around the periodontium. Both vertical transmission (e.g., between child and mother) and horizontal transmission (e.g., between husband and wife) of periodontopathic bacteria are commonly observed (Kobayashi et al., 2008).

Periodontitis usually involves infection with a combination of oral bacteria, and several specific bacterial species are suspected as contributors to this disease. *Porphyromonas gingivalis*, a Gram-negative anaerobic rod, is thought to be a major pathogen in adult and aggressive periodontitis. *Tannerella forsythia*, another Gram-negative anaerobic rod, and *Treponema denticola*, an oral spirochete, are associated with adult periodontitis, whereas *A. actinomycetemcomitans*, a Gram-negative anaerobic rod, is related to aggressive periodontitis. Socransky reported that a "red complex" of three bacteria, *P. gingivalis*, *T. forsythia*, *T. denticola*, is associated with the severity of periodontitis (Socransky & Haffajee, 1998). Oral bacterial examinations to monitor periodontal status generally focus on these three bacteria.

2.3 Bacterial examination of periodontal disease

To date, many detection methods for bacteria in periodontal disease have been reported (Suzuki et al., 2004a; Suzuki et al., 2004b; Yoshida et al., 2003a; Yoshida et al., 2003b). Representative methods for the microbiological examination of periodontal disease are shown in Table 2. The selection of a suitable examination method requires the definition of clear objectives for the results. For example, in order to confirm the horizontal or vertical transmission of a specific periodontal pathogen or to select appropriate antibiotics, the presence of target bacteria must be determined.

Bacterial examination methods that detect the presence of bacteria, but not the amount, are termed qualitative examinations. Owing to the endogenous nature of periodontal infection, periodontal bacteria often exist in both healthy gingival sulcus and diseased periodontal pockets, making qualitative methods unsuitable for the diagnosis of periodontal disease. We propose that the most important application of microbiological examination in periodontal disease is in monitoring changes in bacterial numbers after periodontal treatment compared with before treatment, providing an assessment of the effectiveness of periodontal treatment. For this purpose, quantitative bacterial examinations are required.

Method	Principle	Advantages	Disadvantages	Comments
Culturing	Culturing of oral specimens on a medium	Detection of viable bacteria. Antibiotic sensitivity.	Unculturable bacteria. Requires bacteriology skill.	Important for antibiotic selection.
Enzymatic	Measurement of enzymatic activities produced by oral bacteria	Rapid and low-cost method.	Cannot identify bacterial species.	Commercial kits are available.
Immunological	Detection of specific bacteria using antibodies	Available for specific bacteria.	Cannot discriminate between living and dead cells.	Requires special techniques.
Conventional PCR	Detection of bacteria by DNA amplification	High sensitivity, qualitative analysis.	Same as above. Quantitative detection is not available.	Requires a thermal cycler.
Real-time PCR	Detection of bacteria by DNA amplification	High sensitivity, quantification.	Cannot discriminate between living and dead cells.	Requires a thermal cycler.
Loop-mediated isothermal amplification (LAMP)	Isothermal DNA amplification	High sensitivity, isothermal amplification, visual detection.	Same as conventional PCR.	Developed by Eiken Chemical Co., Ltd.

Table 2. Representative microbiological examination methods in dental practice.

3. Microbiological examination methods for periodontal disease

In selecting the appropriate microbiological examination method, the objectives and purposes of the analysis must be defined, as specimen collection procedures vary according to the goals of the assessment. Clinical specimens to be analyzed for a patient's periodontopathic bacterial levels should be collected from the saliva or tongue coat. Saliva samples should be diluted with phosphate-buffered saline (PBS), and salivary components and debris must be removed by centrifugation before the sample is analyzed. Tongue-coat samples are collected from the tongue dorsum and suspended in PBS, and debris is then removed by centrifugation. For the analysis of bacteria in specific periodontal pockets, subgingival plaque or crevicular fluid samples are suitable. To collect subgingival plaque, a paper point is inserted into the periodontal pocket and then transferred to a tube containing PBS; the subgingival plaque is suspended, and debris is removed by centrifugation (Fig. 1). Properly prepared samples can then be analyzed by qualitative and quantitative methods.

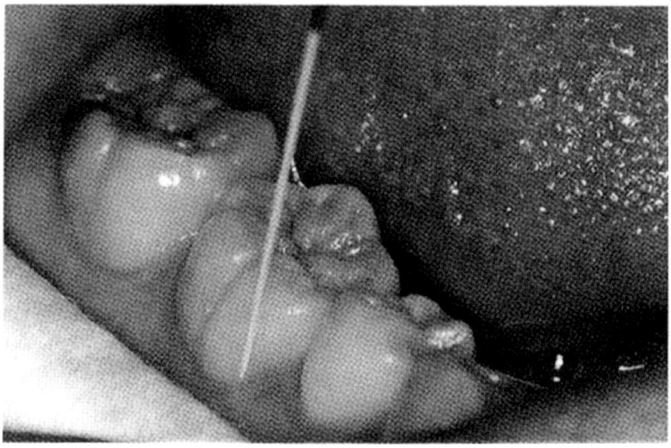

Fig. 1. Sampling of the subgingival plaque using by paperpoint.

3.1 Qualitative examination of periodontal disease

Both enzymatic and PCR-based methods are often used for the qualitative examination of periodontal bacteria. Enzymatic methods do not require special technology or equipment, are relatively inexpensive, and are commercially available as kits (Schmidt et al., 1988). However, because enzymatic methods identify only a group of bacteria associated with periodontitis and not specific bacteria, these analyses are not helpful in the selection of antibiotics.

We previously developed a detection system for hydrogen sulfide (H_2S), a causative agent for oral malodor produced by bacteria, especially periodontopathic bacteria (Yoshida et al., 2009). This type of detection system can be used to evaluate treatment efficiency even when specific bacteria cannot be identified, providing that the treatment objectives and detection targets are the same. Hydrogen sulfide produced by oral bacteria reacts with bismuth chloride to form bismuth sulfide as a black precipitate, as described by the following reaction:

$$3H_2S + 2\,BiCl_3 \rightarrow Bi_2S_3\downarrow + 6\,HCl$$

Hydrogen sulfide-producing bacteria can be detected by measuring the absorbance of the black precipitate. As shown in Fig. 2, these precipitates are detectable in small subgingival plaque samples from periodontal pockets, obtained using paper points. This system for the comprehensive detection of hydrogen sulfide-producing bacteria can be used to evaluate the elimination of these organisms.

On the other hand, PCR techniques are relatively sensitive and can be used with species-specific primers to identify specific bacteria (Yoshida et al., 2005b). A major disadvantage of PCR techniques is that they cannot discriminate between viable and dead bacteria, because PCR methods use chromosomal DNA as a template. This makes PCR techniques unsuitable for sensitivity tests guiding the selection of antibiotics. A modification of the PCR method, loop-mediated isothermal amplification (LAMP), was developed by Eiken Chemical Co., Ltd. (Japan). LAMP reactions are performed under isothermal conditions, in contrast to the thermal cycling necessary for PCR. In addition to this advantage, LAMP technology has a rapid analysis time of about 1 h and requires no special detection equipment, as the results can be observed by the naked eye (Fig. 3). Using this technology, we have developed a method for the rapid detection of the "red complex" of *P. gingivalis, T. forsythia,* and *T. denticola,* which is closely related to the severity of periodontitis (Yoshida et al., 2005a). Osawa et al. have developed a LAMP-based detection system for *A. actinomycetemcomitans,* one of the causative bacteria for aggressive periodontitis (Osawa et al., 2007). LAMP technology is currently one of the most rapid bacterial diagnostic methods (Kato et al., 2007; Nagashima et al., 2007).

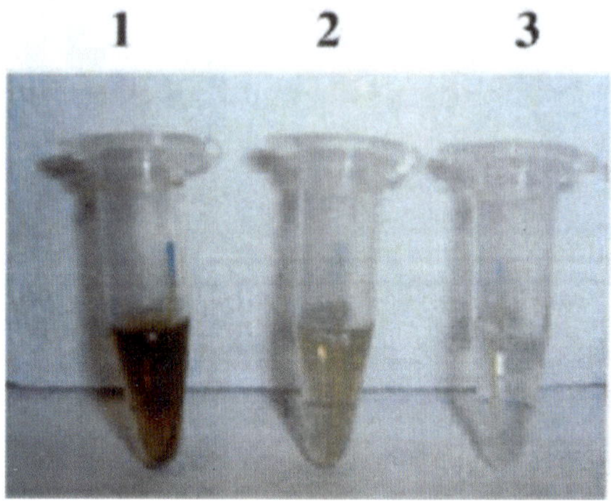

Fig. 2. Visualization of hydrogen sulfide production by precipitation of bismuth trichloride. 1. *Poryphyromonas gingivalis* ATCC 33277 culture; 2. Subgingival fluid sample (*P. gingivalis* positive); 3. Subgingival fluid sample (*P. gingivalis* negative)

3.2 Quantitative examination of periodontal disease

Recently, real-time PCR has become a popular method for the quantitative detection of periodontal bacteria (Suzuki et al., 2004a; Suzuki et al., 2005). Originally used for the measurement of DNA copy numbers, this technique has also been applied to the quantification of bacteria (Yoshida et al., 2003a; Yoshida et al., 2003b). One advantage of this technique is its wide dynamic range of bacterial detection, making it suitable for the determination of oral bacteria, which occur in various and variable amounts. We have developed a detection system based on real-time PCR for the quantification of periodontopathic bacteria, including *P. gingivalis, A. actinomycetemcomitans, T. denticola,T. forsythia,* and *Prevotella* species, in oral specimens such as saliva and subgingival plaque (Kato et al., 2005; Suzuki et al., 2004a; Nagashima et al., 2005; Yoshida et al., 2003a). Using this system to quantify *P. gingivalis* and *T. denticola* in subgingival plaque samples taken from periodontitis patients, we demonstrated a correlation between the numbers of these organisms and periodontal pocket depth (Kawada et al., 2004; Yoshida et al., 2004). The number of *P. gingivalis* bacteria increased ten-fold with every millimeter increase of pocket depth (Fig. 4).
Furthermore, the number of this organism decreased significantly after scaling and root planning (Kawada et al., 2004). Thus, this method can be used to quantitatively evaluate the number of periodontopathic bacteria at periodontal sites, making it applicable for the evaluation of therapeutic efficacy. Although the specific equipment and chemical

requirements of real-time PCR technology may limit its use, several laboratories have recently begun to offer real-time PCR analytical services for the quantification of periodontopathic pathogens, expanding access to this type of analysis.

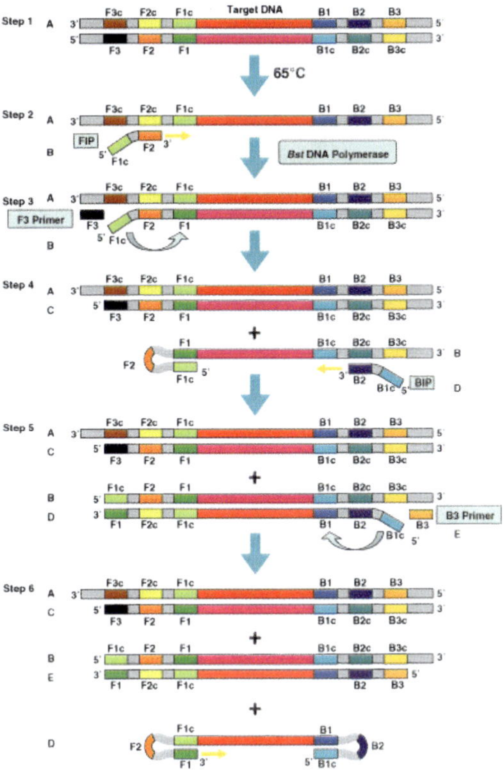

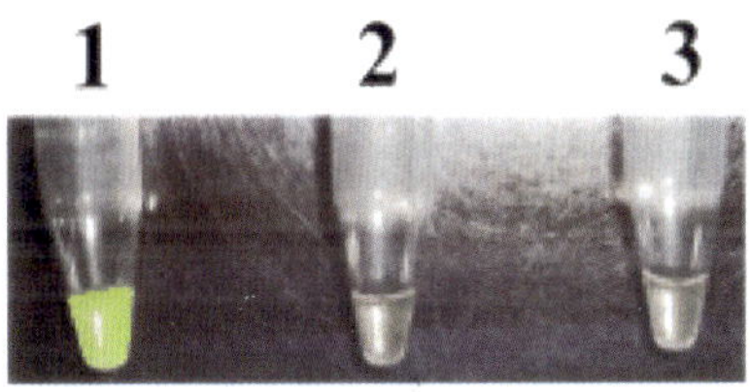

(a) Principles of LAMP technology; (b) Visualization of *P. gingivalis* in subgingival plaque

Fig. 3. Principles of LAMP technology (a) and visualization of *Porphyromonas gingivalis* in subgingival plaque (b). 1. *P. gingivalis* positive subgingival plaque; 2. *P. gingivalis* negative subgingival plaque; 3. Negative control (without DNA)

We also have provided technical support for GC Corporation Co., Ltd. (Japan), which provides services for the quantitative analysis for periodontopathic bacteria (Fig. 5).

One disadvantage of this technology is that because PCR uses DNA as a template, it quantifies both viable and dead bacteria, which usually results in overestimated cell numbers. To discriminate between living and dead bacteria, we have used propidium monoazide, which selectively penetrates the membranes of dead cells and combines with the DNA, thereby inhibiting its amplification by PCR. Masakiyo et al. evaluated the LED-based fluorescence microscopy which distinguishes between live and dead bacteria for oral bacteria (Masakiyo et al., 2010). Future investigations of the relationship between bacterial cell viability and the severity of periodontitis would further clarify the etiology of periodontitis.

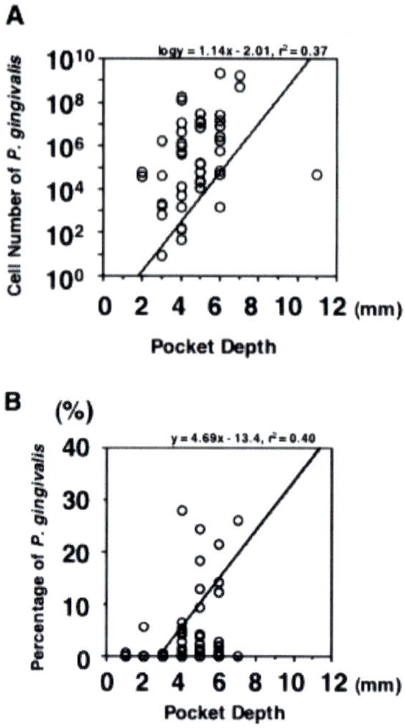

Fig. 4. The correlation between the amount of *P. gingivalis* and pocket depth. A. The correlation between the cell number and pocket depth. B. The correlation between the percentages and pocket depth.

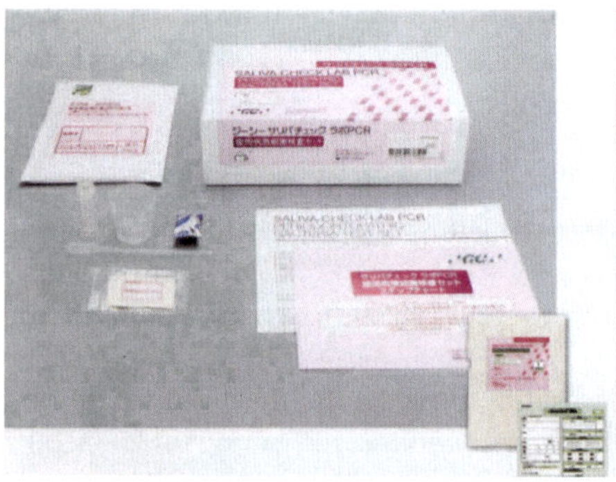

Fig. 5. The commercial kit of real-time PCR assay for periodontopathic bacteria.

4. Microbiological examinations for the purpose of diagnosis

Although quantitative detection methods may be necessary for evaluating therapeutic efficacy, as described above, qualitative methods may be sufficient and even preferable for diagnostic purposes. For example, qualitative culturing methods are more practical than molecular methods for evaluating antibiotic sensitivity. After antibiotic sensitivity has been established, quantitative methods, ideal one that incorporates a way of discriminating between viable and dead cells, can be used to evaluate the therapeutic efficiency of the antibiotics.

The specific periodontal characteristics of a patient should also be considered when choosing a microbiological method for diagnosis. In patients with a specific periodontal locus, subgingival plaque samples would provide the most relevant information. To identify the population of periodontopathic bacteria present in the oral cavity of a patient, saliva or tongue-coat samples would be appropriate.

5. Microbiological examinations for the purpose of antibiotic selection

Periodontal tissue debridement and root planing are the initial therapeutic approaches for periodontal disease. However, mechanical periodontal debridement can have poor therapeutic efficacy in some cases, owing to the invasion of periodontopathic bacteria into the periodontal tissue. In such cases, antibiotic therapy is often effective (Slots et al., 2004). Antibiotics can be chosen based on the specific pathogens identified by microbiological examination. *Porphyromonas gingivalis, A. actinomycetemcomitans, T. forsythia,* and *T. denticola* are common target bacteria. Table 3 shows the recommended antibiotics according to bacterial type.

	Red complex: *Porphyromonas gingivalis, Tannerella forsythia, Treponema denticola*	*Aggregatibacter actinomycetemcomitans*	Orange complex: *Prevotella intermedia, Fusobacterium nucleatum*
Pathogenicity	High	High	Moderately high
Amoxicillin	-	+	-
Clindamycin	+	-	+
Doxycycline	+	+	+
Minocycline	+	+	+
Azithromycin	-	+	-
Ciprofloxacin	-	+	-
Metronidazole	+	-	+
Amoxicillin + Metronidazole	+	+	+

Table 3. Periodontopathic bacteria and recommended antibiotics (Shaddox & Waller, 2009).

However, this table presents only theoretical or *in vitro* data, and antibiotics selected based on these data may not be effective. Bacteria present in biofilm often obtain antibiotic-resistance genes through horizontal gene transfer, and periodontopathic bacteria may thus acquire novel antibiotic-resistance genes in addition to those they naturally possess, nullifying theoretical antibiotic data. To assess the effectiveness of antibiotics for an individual case of periodontitis, bacterial culturing and the construction of an antibiogram are useful methods for obtaining patient-specific antibiotic data.

6. Conclusions

In this chapter, the concept, selection, and procedure of microbiological examination have been described. Although not required in all cases, the importance of microbiological examinations in the diagnosis and treatment of periodontal disease cannot be ignored in some cases. When a patient's treatment history, present periodontal condition, and information required for diagnosis and treatment (e.g., bacterial species identification, antibiotic selection) are considered, a suitable microbiological examination method and timing can be determined.

Although many of the examination methods described in this chapter are difficult to perform in a private clinical setting, most can be performed in cooperation with commercial laboratories. We are currently focusing on the research and development of a periodontal microbiological examination that satisfies the accuracy, ease of handling, speed, and cost requirements of private clinics.

7. References

Darveau, R.P., Tanner, A. & Page, R.C. (1997). The microbial challenge in periodontitis.*Periodontology 2000*, Vol.14(No. 1): 12-32.

Kato, H., Yoshida, A., Awano, S., Ansai, T. & Takehara, T. (2005). Quantitative detection of volatile sulfur compound- producing microorganisms in oral specimens using real-time PCR. *Oral Diseases*, Vol.11 (No.11, Suppl 1):67-71.

Kato, H., Yoshida, A., Ansai, T., Watari, H., Notomi, T. & Takehara, T. (2007). Loop-mediated isothermal amplification method for the rapid detection of *Enterococcus faecalis* in infected root canals. *Oral Microbiology and Immunology*, Vol. 22(No.2):131-135.

Kawada, M., Yoshida, A., Suzuki, N., Nakano, Y., Saito, T., Oho, T. & Koga, T. (2004). Prevalence of *Porphyromonas gingivalis* in relation to periodontal status assessed by real-time PCR. *Oral Microbiology and Immunology*, Vol.19(No.5):289-292.

Keyes, P.H. & Likins, R.C. (1946). Plaque formation, periodontal disease, and dental caries in Syrian hamsters. *Journal of Dental Research*, Vol. 25:166.

Kobayashi, N., Ishihara, K., Sugihara, N., Kusumoto, M., Yakushiji, M. & Okuda, K. (2008). Colonization pattern of periodontal bacteria in Japanese children and their mothers. *Journal of Periodontal Research*, Vol.43 (No.2):156-161.

Kuramitsu, H.K. (1998). Proteases of *Porphyromonas gingivalis*: what don't they do? *Oral Microbiology and Immunology*, Vol.13 (No.5):263-270.

Masakiyo, Y., Yoshida, A., Takahashi, Y., Shintani, Y., Awano, S., Ansai, T., Sawayama, S., Shimakita, T. & Takehara, T. (2010). Rapid LED-based fluorescence microscopy distinguishes between live and dead bacteria in oral clinical samples. *Biomedical Research*, Vol.31(No.1):21-26.

McArthur, W.P., Tsai, C.C., Baehni, P.C., Genco, R.J. & Taichman, N.S. (1981). Leukotoxic effects of *Actinobacillus actinomycetemcomitans* modulation by serum components. *Journal of Periodontal Research*, Vol.16 (No.2):159-170.

Miyata, Y., Takeda, H., Kitano, S., Hanazawa, S. (1997). *Porphyromonas gingivalis* lipopolysaccharide-stimulated bone resorption via CD14 is inhibited by broad-spectrum antibiotics. *Infection and Immunity*, Vol.65 (No.9):3513-3519.

Nagashima, S., Yoshida, A., Suzuki, N., Ansai, T. & Takehara, T. (2005). Use of the genomic subtractive hybridization technique to develop a real-time PCR assay for quantitative detection of *Prevotella* spp. in oral biofilm samples. *Journal of Clinical Microbiology*, Vol.43(No.6):2948-2951.

Nagashima, S., Yoshida, A., Ansai, T., Watari, H., Notomi, T., Maki, K. & Takehara T. (2007). Rapid detection of the cariogenic pathogens *Streptococcus mutans* and *Streptococcus sobrinus* using loop-mediated isothermal amplification. *Oral Microbiology and Immunology*, Vol.22(No.6):361-368.

Osawa, R., Yoshida, A., Masakiyo, Y., Nagashima, S., Ansai, T., Watari, H., Notomi, T. & Takehara, T. (2007). Rapid detection of *Actinobacillus actinomycetemcomitans* using a loop-mediated isothermal amplification method. *Oral Microbiology and Immunology*, Vol.22(No.4):252-259.

Schmidt, E.F., Bretz, W.A., Hutchinson, R.A. & Loesche, W.J. (1988). Correlation of the hydrolysis of benzoyl-arginine naphthylamide (BANA) by plaque with clinical parameters and subgingival levels of spirochetes in periodontal patients. *Journal of Dental Research*, Vol.67(No.12):1505-1509.

Shaddox, L.M. & Walker, C. (2009). Microbial testing in periodontics: value, limitations and future directions. *Periodontology 2000*. Vol.50(No.1):25-38.

Slots, J., Research, Science and Therapy Committee. (2004). Systemic antibiotics in periodontics. *Journal of Periodontology*, Vol.75(No.11): 1553-1565.

Socransky, S.S. (1970). Relationship of bacteria to the etiology of periodontal disease. *Journal of Dental Research*, Vol.49(No.2):203-222.

Socransky, S.S., Haffajee, A.D., Cugini, M.A., Smith, C. & Kent, R.L. Jr. (1998). Microbial complexes in subgingival plaque. *Journal of Clinical Microbiology*, Vol.25(No.2):134-144.

Suzuki, N., Nakano, Y., Yoshida, A., Yamashita, Y. & Kiyoura, Y. (2004a). Real-time TaqMan PCR for quantifying oral bacteria during biofilm formation. *Journal of Clinical Microbiology*, Vol.42(No.8):3827-3830.

Suzuki, N., Yoshida, A., Saito, T., Kawada, M. & Nakano, Y. (2004b). Quantitative microbiological study of subgingival plaque by real-time PCR shows correlation between levels of *Tannerella forsythensis* and *Fusobacterium* spp. *Journal of Clinical Microbiology*, Vol.42(No.5):2255-2257.

Suzuki, N., Yoshida, A. & Nakano, Y. (2005). Quantitative analysis of multi-species oral biofilms by TaqMan Real-Time PCR. *Clinical Medical Research*, Vol.3(No.3):176-185.

Yoshida, A., Suzuki, N., Nakano, Y., Oho, T., Kawada, M. & Koga, T. (2003a). Development of a 5' fluorogenic nuclease-based real-time PCR assay for quantitative detection of *Actinobacillus actinomycetemcomitans* and *Porphyromonas gingivalis*. *Journal of Clinical Microbiology*, Vol.41(No.2):863-866.

Yoshida, A., Suzuki, N., Nakano, Y., Kawada, M., Oho, T. & Koga, T. (2003b). Development of a 5' nuclease-based real-time PCR assay for quantitative detection of cariogenic dental pathogens *Streptococcus mutans* and *Streptococcus sobrinus*. *Journal of Clinical Microbiology*, Vol.41(No.9):4438-4441.

Yoshida, A., Kawada, M., Suzuki, N., Nakano, Y., Oho, T., Saito, T. & Yamashita, Y. (2004). TaqMan real-time polymerase chain reaction assay for the correlation of *Treponema denticola* numbers with the severity of periodontal disease. *Oral Microbiology and Immunology*, Vol.19(No.3):196-200.

Yoshida, A., Nagashima, S., Ansai, T., Tachibana, M., Kato, H., Watari, H., Notomi, T. & Takehara, T. (2005a). Loop-mediated isothermal amplification method for rapid detection of the periodontopathic bacteria *Porphyromonas gingivalis, Tannerella forsythia*, and *Treponema denticola. Journal of Clinical Microbiology*, Vol.43(No.5):2418-2424.

Yoshida, A., Tachibana, M., Ansai, T. & Takehara, T. (2005b). Multiplex polymerase chain reaction assay for simultaneous detection of black-pigmented *Prevotella* species in oral specimens. *Oral Microbiology and Immunology*, Vol.20(No.1):43-46.

Yoshida, A., Yoshimura, M., Ohara, N., Yoshimura, S., Nagashima, S., Takehara, T. & Nakayama, K. (2009). Hydrogen sulfide production from cysteine and homocysteine by periodontal and oral bacteria. *Journal of Periodontology*, Vol.80(No.11):1845-1851.

Williams, R.C. Periodontal disease. (1990). *New England Journal of Medicine*, Vol.322(No.6): 373-382.

Part 2

Pathogenesis of Periodontal Diseases

3

The Impact of Bacteria-Induced Adaptive Immune Responses in Periodontal Disease

Vincent K. Tsiagbe[1,2,3] and Daniel H. Fine[1,2]
[1]*Department of Oral Biology, New Jersey Dental School,*
[2]*Graduate School of Biomedical Science,*
[3]*Department of Pathology and Laboratory Medicine, New Jersey Medical School,*
University of Medicine and Dentistry of New Jersey,
Newark, NJ,
USA

1. Introduction

More than one microorganism causes periodontal disease, like many infectious diseases in humans. Because of the complexity of "polymicrobial infections", their study requires a multidisciplinary approach, employing specific in vitro techniques, and various animal models (Bakaletz 2004). Inherently, no one approach or animal model can completely elucidate the mechanisms of periodontal disease. Notwithstanding these difficulties, animal models do provide critically important information regarding periodontal disease pathogenesis (Graves 2008). Another layer of complexity resides in the fact that different strains of bacteria, as in the case of *P. gingivalis* (*Pg*)-induced disease, cause different levels of disease in the same mouse strain (Baker and Roopenian 2002). Similarly, differences in disease susceptibility can result from the same bacterium strain, as in the case of Aggregatibacter actinomycetemcomitans (*Aa*) infected rodents (Fine et al. 2009). Furthermore, different strains of rodents exhibit different susceptibilities to challenge from the same strain of bacterium, such as *Pg* (Baker et al. 2000). This finding also holds true for *Aa* (Schreiner et al. 2011). These observations resemble findings in human disease, especially in the case of *Aa*-related disease where the JP2 strain of *Aa* appears to be more virulent than other Aa strains, and where individuals of African heritage appear to be more susceptible to *Aa*–induced periodontal disease than Caucasian individuals (Haubek et al. 2008). The similarities between rodent and human bacterial-induced periodontal diseases lend credence to the validity of the animal model designed to assess this disease (Fine 2009).

The virulence factors elaborated by pathogenic microorganisms and the host immunologic responses to such factors play a major role in disease induction and progression. It has been established that *Aa*, a gram-negative facultative capnophilic rod, is the causative agent in localized juvenile periodontitis (LJP) (Zambon 1985). This agent is also a key pathogen for localized progressing and severe forms of adult periodontitis (Dzink et al. 1985; Zambon et al. 1988). *Aa* possesses several virulence factors, including endotoxin and leukotoxin (Fives-Taylor et al. 1999). *Aa* secretes a protein toxin, Leukotoxin (LtxA), which helps the bacterium evade the host immune response during infection, by specifically targeting white blood cells

(WBCs) (Kachlany 2010). The ability of LtxA to bind WBCs from humans and Old World primates, by interacting with lymphocyte function antigen-1 (LFA-1) on susceptible cells, has opened a window of opportunity for the use of LtxA as a novel therapeutic agent in leukemia (Kachlany et al. 2010). *Aa* also produces cytolethal distending toxin (Cdt), which is a potent immunotoxin that induces G2 arrest in human lymphocytes (Shenker et al. 2007). The immunologic and systemic impact of these bacterial toxins in periodontal disease is yet to be clarified.

The binding of *Aa* to buccal epithelial cells (BEC) was shown to be mediated by two Aa autotransporter adhesions (ApiA and Aae), which work, in concert to modulate *Aa* binding to BEC, specifically in humans and Old World Monkeys (Yue et al. 2007). The type and extent of the immunologic response mounted in response to oral pathogen will undoubtedly depend on the particular microbial pathogen(s), the virulence factors invoked and the genetic background of the host. The immunologic reactions mounted in response to oral pathogens have a potential to precipitate other unforeseen systemic diseases of grave importance. The connection between immunologic responses to oral pathogens and systemic diseases is mostly unexplored, at present.

2. Immune responses to microbial pathogens

Our understanding of periodontal pathogenesis has evolved over the years, and has transformed from periodontitis being considered an almost ubiquitous condition in which the role of plaque was thought to be the sole aetiologic factor to today where concepts of inflammation and individual susceptibility are considered (Preshaw and Taylor 2011). Neutrophils are a critical arm of the host defense in periodontitis, but bacterial evasion of neutrophil microbicidal machinery, together with delayed neutrophil apoptosis can transform neutrophil from defender to perpetrator (Nussbaum and Shapira 2011). In the recent Seventh European Workshop on Periodontology, aimed at understanding cellular and molecular mechanisms of host microbial interactions, a consensus was reached that "PMNs are important in the pathophysiology of periodontal disease but there is limited evidence on their much quoted destructive potential". Cytokine networks are enormously complex and we are really at the beginning of understanding their role in the disease process (Kinane, Preshaw and Loos 2011). Thus, there is an emerging appreciation for the complex role played by the adaptive immune system in responses to periodontal pathogens.

2.1 Humoral Immune responses to microbial pathogens

In early studies, significantly elevated serum immunoglobulin G (IgG) antibody levels to *B. gingivalis* were seen in adult and advanced destructive periodontitis patients, suggestive of distinctive host-parasite interactions in this disease (Ebersole and Cappelli 1994; Ebersole et al. 1986). Analysis of the proportion of various cell types present in gingival biopsies retrieved from subjects with severe chronic periodontitis showed that the proportion of B cells was larger than that of T cells, plasma cells and neutrophils. Furthermore, about 60% of the B cells were of the autoreactive B-1a sub-population ($CD19^{+}CD5^{+}$) (Donati et al. 2009). The plasma cells that developed were shown to derive from both B-2 cells (conventional B cells) and B-1a cells. There is strong evidence that B cells serve as antigen presenting cells in periodontitis (Gemmell et al. 2002; Mahanonda et al. 2002). Indeed, upregulation of the co-stimulatory molecule, CD86 (B7.2), and the dendritic cell marker, CD83, on B cells in periodontal lesions, have been reported (Gemmell et al. 2002). Thus, it is likely that the B cells found in periodontal tissue might present bacterial antigens to host T cells, leading to the elaboration of a whole range of cytokines, the nature of which would depend on the type of bacteria, and the host.

Altered CD4/CD8 T-cell ratios and autologous mixed-lymphocyte reaction in LJP, suggested a potential regulatory role of T cells in periodontitis. Using immunohistochemical and *in situ* hybridization techniques, a higher frequency of $CD4^{+}CD45RO^{+}$ cells expressing IL-4 has been seen in lesions from individuals with chronic periodontitis compared to normal tissue (Yamazaki et al. 1994). Comparing two different compartments (peripheral blood vs. periodontal tissue), it was noted that even though mRNA for IL-12 and IL-13 were similar between the two compartments, the level of IFN-γ was higher in circulating cells than in gingival cells. Inversely, IL-10 expression was higher in the gingival cells (Yamazaki et al. 1997). Moreover, the frequency of IL-10 expressing $CD14^{+}$ cells was higher in peripheral blood of chronic periodontitis, but not acute periodontitis patients, compared to healthy controls (Yamazaki et al. 1997).

In periodontal disease, the development of gingivitis involves Th1 cells, while in periodontitis, there is a shift toward Th2 cells (reviewed in (Berglundh and Donati 2005)). Autoimmune reactions do occur in periodontitis lesions; however, the role of autoantibodies in the regulation of host response in periodontitis needs to be clarified (Berglundh and Donati 2005). In studies conducted with *Aa*-induced periodontal disease rat model, we observed an early increase in serum IgG2a antibody 2-4 weeks post inoculation. This was accompanied by a concomitant increase in LtxA-specific IgG production, suggesting that the immune response was mediated by *Aa* (Li et al. 2010). An increase in B and CD4 T cell numbers in draining cervical and submandibular lymph nodes accompanied this *Aa*-specific antibody production. CD8 T cell numbers were not examined in this study (Li et al. 2010). In agreement with this observation, there was an increase in the expression of CD70 (TNFSF7) in B cells harvested from draining lymph nodes in rats infected by *Aa* (Li et al. 2010). CD70 has been shown to be expressed on a subpopulation of germinal center B cells (Hintzen et al. 1994).

2.2 Cytokines in periodontal disease

Innate immunity is mediated by macrophages, dendritic cells (DCs), neutrophils, monocytes, epithelial cells and endothelial cells that recognize and temporarily respond to pathogen associated molecular patterns (PAMPS), like LPS on gram-negative bacteria. The adaptive immune system, on the other hand, uses specific antigen recognition structures on T and B cell. Such responses are specific and maintained by the generation of memory. Various cytokines generated by macrophages and DCs create a milieu, which determines the differentiation of particular effector T-cell subsets as well as the class and subclass of immunoglobulin (Ig) antibodies synthesized. Cytokines act in concert with other signalling pathways and, especially, cell-to-cell interactions via antigen presentation and co-stimulatory molecules (Preshaw and Taylor 2011).

The role of inflammatory cytokines, such as interleukin (IL)-1β, tumor necrosis factor-α, and IL-6, has been the most understood (reviewed in (Preshaw and Taylor 2011). Inhibition of IL-1 and tumor necrosis factor (TNF) resulted in amelioration of bone loss in experimental periodontitis (Assuma et al. 1998; Graves et al. 1998). In our studies on *Aa*-induced periodontal disease, the early induction of *Aa*-specific IgG and IgG2a antibodies in *Aa*-fed rats is of interest since mRNA for Th1 cytokines TNF and lymphotoxin beta (LTβ) (Abbas,

Murphy and Sher 1996) were upregulated early (2-4 weeks) in the inflammatory response, which could explain the significant switch in *Aa*-specific antibody production to IgG2a. This is consistent with the observation that Th1 cytokines drive isotype switching to IgG2a in inflammatory responses of atherosclerosis (Schulte, Sukhova and Libby 2008).

2.2.1 Th1/Th2 paradigm

Cytokines mediate and sustain the development and function of $CD4^+$ Th cell subsets. In the original description of Th cell dichotomy, Th1 cells secrete interferon-γ (IFN-γ), and promote cell-mediated immunity by activating macrophages, natural killer (NK) cells and cytotoxic $CD8^+$ T-cells, whereas Th2 cells secrete IL-4, IL-5 and IL-13 and regulate humoral (antibody-mediated) immunity and mast cell activity (Mosmann and Coffman 1989). It was conjectured that the dynamic interaction between T-cell subsets might result in fluctuations in disease activity and that a Th1 response (providing protective cell-mediated immunity) underlies a "stable" periodontal lesion, and a Th2 response (leading to activation of B-cells) mediates a destructive lesion possibly through enhanced B-cell-derived IL-1β (Gemmell, Yamazaki and Seymour 2007; Seymour and Gemmell 2001). It is now becoming clearer that the Th1/Th2 model alone is inadequate to explain the role of T-cells in periodontal disease process (Gaffen and Hajishengallis 2008).

2.2.2 Role of Th17 cells

Th17 cells secrete the IL-17 cytokines (which have a number of pro-inflammatory activities in common with IL-1β and TNFα) and IL-22, and are crucial for immunity against extracellular bacteria (Miossec, Korn and Kuchroo 2009). Th17 cells have been implicated in the pathogenesis of several autoimmune and inflammatory disorders, and *in vitro* polarization of human and mouse Th17 cells is under the influence of Notch1 (Keerthivasan et al. 2011). Studies have shown that IL-17A produced by Th17 cells stimulate the development of osteoclasts (osteoclastogenesis) in the presence of osteoblasts (Zhang et al. 2011), and expression of IL-17 has been observed in gingiva from patients with periodontitis (Cardoso et al. 2009).

In our studies on *Aa*-induced rat model for periodontal disease, we observed upregulation in IL-17 in $CD4^+$ T cells (2.8 fold) and B cells (2 fold), in lymph nodes from *Aa*-infected rats, compared to control rats. This level of expression was below our stringent criterion of four-fold differential gene expression in this study. However, this finding is in conformity with the observation that IL-17 might be involved in inflammatory response and bone resorption in periodontal disease animal models (Oseko et al. 2009) (Xiong, Wei and Peng 2009). It should, however, be noted that T cells exhibit "functional plasticity" that is influenced by the cytokine milieu (Bluestone et al. 2009). For instance, Th17 cells can differentiate into Th1 cells, under the influence of IL-12 (Korn et al. 2009), and follicular T helper cells (Thf), present in the B cell follicles of lymph nodes, are dependent on IL-6 and IL-21 for their development, and are capable of secreting a cytokine profile corresponding to Th1, Th2 or Th17 cells (Korn et al. 2009).

2.2.3 Role of regulatory (Treg) cells

It has been established that naturally arising $Foxp3^+CD4^+CD25^+$ (Treg) cells play a central role in the maintenance of immunological tolerance (Sakaguchi 2005). Treg cells secrete transforming growth factor-β (TGF-β) and IL-10 which are critical in regulating other T-cell subsets and maintaining tolerance against self-antigens, thereby preventing autoimmunity (Josefowicz and Rudensky 2009). Gingival mononuclear cells from mice infected with *Pg* were found to exhibit increased levels of Treg cells 30 days post infection, suggesting that there are potential roles for Treg cells during the chronic stage of periodontitis in the regulation of gingival inflammation and alveolar bone loss (Kobayashi et al. 2011). $FoxP3^{+}CD8^{+}$ T cells, with suppressive function have recently been identified in simian immunodeficiency virus infected rhesus macaques, and in HIV-1 infected humans. Expansion of $CD8^{+}$ Tregs correlated directly with acute phase viremia and inversely with the magnitude of antiviral T cell response (Nigam et al. 2010). Using transgenic OT-I mice, the administration of ovalbumin (OVA) enabled osteoclasts to cross-present OVA to Ag-specific $CD8^{+}$ T cells to induce their proliferation, and secretion of of IL-2, IL-6, and IFN-γ. $CD8^{+}$ T cells activated by osteoclasts expressed FoxP3, CTLA4 and RANKL. Those $CD8^{+}$ T cells were found to be anergic and suppressed dendritic cell priming of naive responder $CD8^{+}$ T cells (Kiesel, Buchwald and Aurora 2009). The role of this novel group of $CD8^{+}$ Treg cells in periodontal disease requires further examination.

2.2.4 Novel cytokine roles in periodontal disease

In our studies on *Aa*-induced periodontal disease rat model, we observed upregulation in mRNA for a number of cytokines, not normally ascribed to periodontal disease. IL-16 was upregulated in CD4 T cells in the early phase of the response (Li et al. 2010). IL-16 has been shown to be involved in the selective migration of CD4 T cells, and participates in inflammatory diseases (Akiyama et al. 2009). It was detected in gingival crevicular fluid (Sakai et al. 2006). IL-19, a novel cytokine of the IL-10 family, was also upregulated in CD4 T cells in response to *Aa*. IL-19 produced by synovial cell in Rheumatoid arthritis (RA) patients promotes joint inflammation (Sakurai et al. 2008). IL-21, which has recently been shown to induce receptor activator of nuclear factor kappaB ligand (RANKL) and was implicated in arthritis (Jang et al. 2009), was upregulated in B cells responding to Aa. There was also an induction of IL-24 by 12 weeks in CD4 T cells responding to Aa. Studies conducted on RA showed an increase in IL-24 in the synovium of RA patients, and this cytokine was implicated in recruitment of neutrophil granulocytes (Kragstrup et al. 2008). B-cell-activating-factor (BAFF, or TNFSF13B) and a proliferation-inducing ligand (APRIL), members of the TNF family, were upregulated in B cells and CD4 T cells, respectively, in response to Aa infection. Both of these factors were found to be upregulated in children with atopic dermatitis (Jee et al. 2009), and thus would represent factors that characterize *Aa*-induced periodontal disease.

IL-23, a proinflammatory cytokine composed of IL-23p19 and IL-12/23p40 subunits, is known to promote the differentiation of Th17 cells. Studies showed that IL-23 and IL-12 were expressed at significantly higher levels in periodontal lesions than in control sites, suggesting that IL-23-induced Th17 pathway is stimulated in inflammatory periodontal lesions (Ohyama et al. 2009). IL-33 is a new member of the IL-1 family, which plays a role in inflammatory response. Injection of TNF transgenic mice, overexpressing human TNF, with IL-33 or IL-33R agonistic antibody inhibited the development of spontaneous joint inflammation and cartilage destruction. Furthermore, *in vitro*, IL-33 directly inhibits mouse and human M-CSF/receptor activator for NF-kβ ligand-driven osteoclast differentiation, suggesting an important role for IL-33 as a bone-protecting cytokine with potential for treating bone resorption (Zaiss et al. 2011).

2.2.5 Role of RANKL and related molecules

RANKL plays a role in T cell-mediated bone resorption. Interference with RANKL by systemic administration of osteoprotegerin (OPG), the decoy receptor for (and inhibitor of) RANKL, was found to result in abrogation of periodontal bone resorption in a rat model (Taubman et al. 2005). Studies in humans have demonstrated that RANKL levels in gingival crevicular fluid (GCF) were low in health or gingivitis, but increased in periodontitis. On the other hand, OPG levels were higher in health than periodontitis, or gingivitis groups (Bostanci et al. 2007). Thus, GCF RANKL and OPG levels were oppositely regulated in periodontitis, but not gingivitis, resulting in an enhanced RANKL/OPG ratio. In our studies with *Aa*-induced periodontal disease rat model, while the bone resorption protein RANKL (TNFSF11) was induced in CD4 T cells from *Aa*-fed rats, its soluble decoy receptor OPG (TNFSF11b) was also induced in the CD4 T cells (Li et al. 2010). Developments in the field of osteoimmunology, which examine the crosstalk of immune cells and bone, have uncovered a novel role for the RANKL-RANK-OPG system in other processes such as in controlling autoimmunity or immune responses in the skin (Leibbrandt and Penninger 2010). Despite the sustained upregulation of OPG, bone resorption still occurred. The critical balance between osteoblast-mediated bone formation and osteoclast-mediated bone resorption has been described as "coupling" of bone formation to bone resorption (Parfitt 1982).

2.2.6 Role of BMPs and GDFs in periodontal disease

Bone morphogenic proteins (BMPs) and growth differentiation factors (GDFs) are members of the transforming growth factor-β (TGF- β) superfamily. They play important roles during development and organogenesis in delivering positional information in both vertebrates and invertebrates, and are involved in the development of hard as well as soft tissue (Herpin, Lelong and Favrel 2004).

BMPs can also act locally on target tissues to affect proliferation and survival (Rosen 2006). BMP2, even though dispensable for bone formation, is a necessary component of the signaling cascade that governs fracture repair (Tsuji et al. 2006). In our studies, BMP2 was induced in B cells early (week 4) of an inflammatory process, at the same time that RANKL was induced in CD4 T cells (Li et al. 2010). This suggests that bone repair mechanisms were induced early, well ahead of impending bone resorption. However, by 12 weeks of infection by *Aa*, BMP2 was shut down, as bone resorption proceeded. BMP3 was also upregulated at week 4 in B cells responding to Aa. BMP3 has been shown to be a negative regulator in the skeleton, as mice lacking BMP3 have increased bone mass. Transgenic mice over-expressing BMP3 had altered endochondral bone formation resulting in spontaneous rib fractures (Gamer et al. 2009). On the other hand, it has been suggested that BMP2 and BMP3 might be co-regulated. BMP-2 was found to enhance BMP-3 and -4 mRNA expressions in primary cultures of fetal rat calvarial osteoblasts. The enhancement of BMP-3 and -4 mRNA expressions by BMP-2 was associated with an increased expression of bone cell differentiation marker genes (Chen et al. 1997). It is of interest that BMP2 and BMP3 were upregulated in B cells at the same time (4 weeks post infection), and were shut down at 12 weeks, at which time bone resorption was evident.

In our studies with *Aa*- rat model for periodontal disease, we found that B cells responding to *Aa* upregulated BMP10 at all time points (Li et al. 2010). BMP10 has been shown to regulate myocardial hypertrophic growth (Chen et al. 2006), and may function as a tumor suppressor and apoptosis regulator for prostate cancer (Ye, Kynaston and Jiang 2009). To our knowledge, our work is the first report on the production of BMP10 by B cells responding to infection. The expression pattern of BMP10 in our studies, suggests that it might be involved in inflammation, as well as in bone resorption. Furthermore, the involvement of BMP10 in cardiac hypertrophy and cancer, suggests that it might represent one of the possible "missing links" between periodontal disease and other systemic diseases like heart disease and cancer. Evidence for this is provided in the modeled biological interaction pathway depicted in Fig 1.

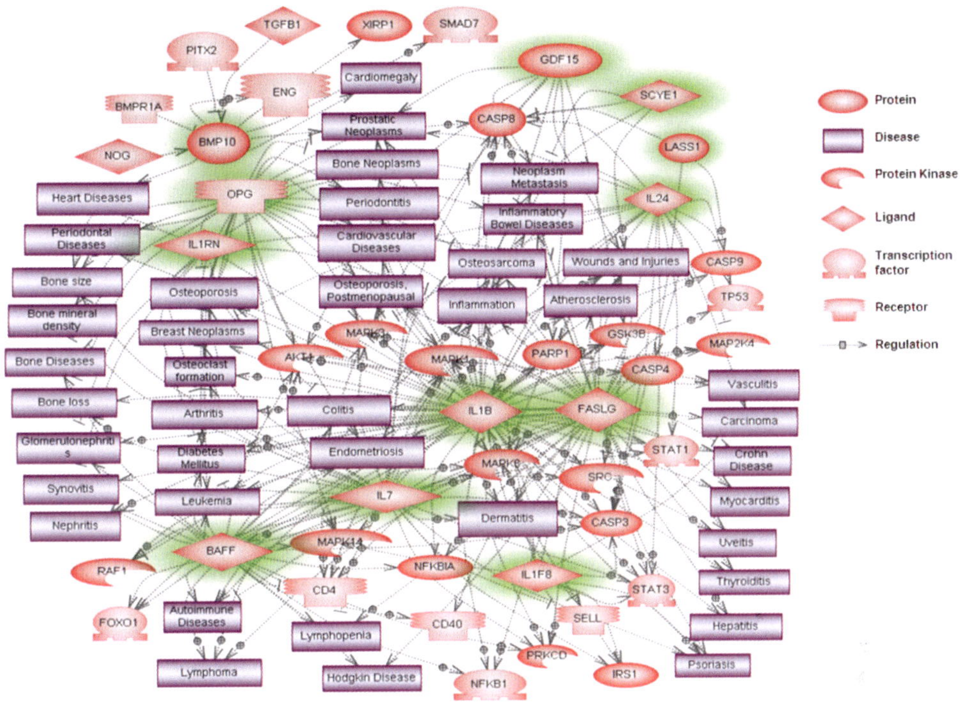

Fig. 1. Proposed biological interaction network of differentially expressed genes from B and CD4 T cells of *Aa*-fed rats at 12 weeks post infection by *Aa*, and their relationship to disease. Genes upregulated by at least four-fold (i.e. Log_2 fold greater than 2) in B and CD4 T cells derived from cervical and submandibular lymph nodes of *Aa*-fed rats, in comparison to B and CD4 T cells from control rats, were imported into Pathway Studio (Ariadne Genomics, Inc., Rockville, MD, USA) (Yuryev et al. 2006) for analyses. The picture shows interactions between upregulated genes in the expression data (shown as green highlights) and their interactions with related genes and diseases. The biological relationships revealed by the network are depicted in the pallets at the right of the figure. The relevance of the expression data to various diseases, as determined by the mining of the published Resnet 7 database in Pathway Studio, is indicated in the network. Reprinted with permission from Li Y *et al.* Molecular Oral Microbiology 2010; 25:275-292.

Growth differentiation factor 11 (GDF11) or BMP11, plays an important role in establishing embryonic axial skeletal patterns (McPherron, Lawler and Lee 1999). Transfection of GFF11 gene was found to stimulate a large amount of reparative dentin formation in amputated dental pulp of canine teeth in vivo (Nakashima et al. 2003). In our studies with *Aa*-induced periodontal disease rat model, GDF11 was upregulated at 12 weeks post infection, in both B and CD4 T cells, at the time of bone resorption. This suggests that GDF11 may have a novel role in bone resorption. The fact that GDF11 activation has been observed in cancer (Yokoe et al. 2007), may also provide another possible link between periodontal disease and cancer.
Growth differentiation factor 15 (GDF15), was upregulated in both B and CD4 T cells of Aa-infected rats at 12 week, coinciding with the time of bone resorption. However, there are conflicting reports on the role of GDF15 in bone resorption and other systemic diseases. Studies have shown that pure GDF15 and the GDF15-containing growth medium of 1,25(OH)2-vitamin D3-treated prostate adenocarcinoma LNCaP cells suppress osteoclast differentiation (Vanhara et al. 2009). In addition, elevation in GDF15 has been associated with cardiovascular disease (Kempf and Wollert 2009), and colorectal cancer metastasis (Xue et al.). Thus, GDF15 may also contribute another possible link between periodontal disease and systemic diseases.

3. Conclusions

The nature of the adaptive response to oral microbial insult is vastly dependent on the nature of the microbe, the host (including genetic background), as well as the milieu of prevailing cytokines and chemokines. The *Aa*-induced rat model and *Pg*-induced mouse model for periodontal disease have provided extensive knowledge about role of several previously uncharacterized genes in periodontal disease, however, much more work needs to be done. Therefore, examination of B and CD4 T cells from lymph nodes draining the oral cavity of *Aa*-fed rats showed that inflammatory processes are initially activated early (2-4 weeks) post infection. This, ultimately, leads to activation of bone resorption pathways that end in overt bone resorption by 12 weeks post infection. Apart from induction of known inflammatory cytokines (such as TNFα, IL-1β, and LTβ), other cytokines and TGF-β superfamily member genes, not previously associated with bone resorption, were found to be upregulated in B and/or CD4 T cells. Some of these genes have known effects on systemic diseases such as heart disease, cancer, autoimmune disease, and diabetes. The role of CD8 T cells in adaptive immune responses to periodontal pathogens is not yet clarified. This evidence suggests a subtle link between periodontal disease and other systemic diseases. In conclusion, animal studies have played an important role in unraveling key elements of our understanding of microbial pathogenesis in many human diseases (Shea et al. 2010). The availability of new and more complete data from mouse and rat genome studies coupled with the access to powerful tools that can uncover microbial and host expression can provide novel ways to examine periodontal disease pathogenesis. Application of these tools can allow for comparisons to common pathways with respect to other infectious diseases. This chapter has presented some data derived from the application of one of these new immune response pathway tools to microbial-induced periodontal disease in a rat model.

4. Acknowledgements

This work was supported by grants from the Foundation of University of Medicine and Dentistry of New Jersey (grant #36-08 and PC31-10), and by grant DE-016306 from the National Institute for Dental and Craniofacial Research.

5. References

Abbas, A. K., K. M. Murphy, and A. Sher. 1996. "Functional diversity of helper T lymphocytes." *Nature* 383(6603):787-93.

Akiyama, K., M. Karaki, R. Kobayshi, H. Dobashi, T. Ishida, and N. Mori. 2009. "IL-16 variability and modulation by antiallergic drugs in a murine experimental allergic rhinitis model." *Int Arch Allergy Immunol* 149(4):315-22.

Assuma, R., T. Oates, D. Cochran, S. Amar, and D. T. Graves. 1998. "IL-1 and TNF antagonists inhibit the inflammatory response and bone loss in experimental periodontitis." *J Immunol* 160(1):403-9.

Bakaletz, L. O. 2004. "Developing animal models for polymicrobial diseases." *Nat Rev Microbiol* 2(7):552-68.

Baker, P. J., M. Dixon, R. T. Evans, and D. C. Roopenian. 2000. "Heterogeneity of Porphyromonas gingivalis strains in the induction of alveolar bone loss in mice." *Oral Microbiol Immunol* 15(1):27-32.

Baker, P. J., and D. C. Roopenian. 2002. "Genetic susceptibility to chronic periodontal disease." *Microbes Infect* 4(11):1157-67.

Berglundh, T., and M. Donati. 2005. "Aspects of adaptive host response in periodontitis." *J Clin Periodontol* 32 Suppl 6:87-107.

Bluestone, J. A., C. R. Mackay, J. J. O'Shea, and B. Stockinger. 2009. "The functional plasticity of T cell subsets." *Nat Rev Immunol* 9(11):811-6.

Bostanci, N., T. Ilgenli, G. Emingil, B. Afacan, B. Han, H. Toz, G. Atilla, F. J. Hughes, and G. N. Belibasakis. 2007. "Gingival crevicular fluid levels of RANKL and OPG in periodontal diseases: implications of their relative ratio." *J Clin Periodontol* 34(5):370-6.

Cardoso, C. R., G. P. Garlet, G. E. Crippa, A. L. Rosa, W. M. Junior, M. A. Rossi, and J. S. Silva. 2009. "Evidence of the presence of T helper type 17 cells in chronic lesions of human periodontal disease." *Oral Microbiol Immunol* 24(1):1-6.

Chen, D., M. A. Harris, G. Rossini, C. R. Dunstan, S. L. Dallas, J. Q. Feng, G. R. Mundy, and S. E. Harris. 1997. "Bone morphogenetic protein 2 (BMP-2) enhances BMP-3, BMP-4, and bone cell differentiation marker gene expression during the induction of mineralized bone matrix formation in cultures of fetal rat calvarial osteoblasts." *Calcif Tissue Int* 60(3):283-90.

Chen, H., W. Yong, S. Ren, W. Shen, Y. He, K. A. Cox, W. Zhu, W. Li, M. Soonpaa, R. M. Payne, D. Franco, L. J. Field, V. Rosen, Y. Wang, and W. Shou. 2006. "Overexpression of bone morphogenetic protein 10 in myocardium disrupts cardiac postnatal hypertrophic growth." *J Biol Chem* 281(37):27481-91.

Donati, M., B. Liljenberg, N. U. Zitzmann, and T. Berglundh. 2009. "B-1a cells and plasma cells in periodontitis lesions." *J Periodontal Res* 44(5):683-8.

Dzink, J. L., A. C. Tanner, A. D. Haffajee, and S. S. Socransky. 1985. "Gram negative species associated with active destructive periodontal lesions." *J Clin Periodontol* 12(8):648-59.

Ebersole, J. L., and D. Cappelli. 1994. "Gingival crevicular fluid antibody to Actinobacillus actinomycetemcomitans in periodontal disease." *Oral Microbiol Immunol* 9(6):335-44.

Ebersole, J. L., M. A. Taubman, D. J. Smith, and D. E. Frey. 1986. "Human immune responses to oral microorganisms: patterns of systemic antibody levels to Bacteroides species." *Infect Immun* 51(2):507-13.

Fine, D. H. 2009. "Of mice and men: animal models of human periodontal disease." *J Clin Periodontol* 36(11):913-4.

Fine, D. H., H. Schreiner, C. Nasri-Heir, B. Greenberg, S. Jiang, K. Markowitz, and D. Furgang. 2009. "An improved cost-effective, reproducible method for evaluation of bone loss in a rodent model." *J Clin Periodontol* 36(2):106-13.

Fives-Taylor, P. M., D. H. Meyer, K. P. Mintz, and C. Brissette. 1999. "Virulence factors of Actinobacillus actinomycetemcomitans." *Periodontol 2000* 20:136-67.

Gaffen, S. L., and G. Hajishengallis. 2008. "A new inflammatory cytokine on the block: re-thinking periodontal disease and the Th1/Th2 paradigm in the context of Th17 cells and IL-17." *J Dent Res* 87(9):817-28.

Gamer, L. W., K. Cox, J. M. Carlo, and V. Rosen. 2009. "Overexpression of BMP3 in the developing skeleton alters endochondral bone formation resulting in spontaneous rib fractures." *Dev Dyn* 238(9):2374-81.

Gemmell, E., C. L. Carter, D. N. Hart, K. E. Drysdale, and G. J. Seymour. 2002. "Antigen-presenting cells in human periodontal disease tissues." *Oral Microbiol Immunol* 17(6):388-93.

Gemmell, E., K. Yamazaki, and G. J. Seymour. 2007. "The role of T cells in periodontal disease: homeostasis and autoimmunity." *Periodontol 2000* 43:14-40.

Graves, D. 2008. "Cytokines that promote periodontal tissue destruction." *J Periodontol* 79(8 Suppl):1585-91.

Graves, D. T., A. J. Delima, R. Assuma, S. Amar, T. Oates, and D. Cochran. 1998. "Interleukin-1 and tumor necrosis factor antagonists inhibit the progression of inflammatory cell infiltration toward alveolar bone in experimental periodontitis." *J Periodontol* 69(12):1419-25.

Haubek, D., O. K. Ennibi, K. Poulsen, M. Vaeth, S. Poulsen, and M. Kilian. 2008. "Risk of aggressive periodontitis in adolescent carriers of the JP2 clone of Aggregatibacter (Actinobacillus) actinomycetemcomitans in Morocco: a prospective longitudinal cohort study." *Lancet* 371(9608):237-42.

Herpin, A., C. Lelong, and P. Favrel. 2004. "Transforming growth factor-beta-related proteins: an ancestral and widespread superfamily of cytokines in metazoans." *Dev Comp Immunol* 28(5):461-85.

Hintzen, R. Q., S. M. Lens, G. Koopman, S. T. Pals, H. Spits, and R. A. van Lier. 1994. "CD70 represents the human ligand for CD27." *Int Immunol* 6(3):477-80.

Jang, E., S. H. Cho, H. Park, D. J. Paik, J. M. Kim, and J. Youn. 2009. "A positive feedback loop of IL-21 signaling provoked by homeostatic CD4+CD25- T cell expansion is essential for the development of arthritis in autoimmune K/BxN mice." *J Immunol* 182(8):4649-56.

Jee, H. M., K. W. Kim, J. Y. Hong, M. H. Sohn, and K. E. Kim. 2009. "Increased serum B cell-activating factor level in children with atopic dermatitis." *Clin Exp Dermatol.*

Josefowicz, S. Z., and A. Rudensky. 2009. "Control of regulatory T cell lineage commitment and maintenance." *Immunity* 30(5):616-25.

Kachlany, S. C. 2010. "Aggregatibacter actinomycetemcomitans leukotoxin: from threat to therapy." *J Dent Res* 89(6):561-70.

Kachlany, S. C., A. B. Schwartz, N. V. Balashova, C. E. Hioe, M. Tuen, A. Le, M. Kaur, Y. Mei, and J. Rao. 2010. "Anti-leukemia activity of a bacterial toxin with natural specificity for LFA-1 on white blood cells." *Leuk Res* 34(6):777-85.

Keerthivasan, S., R. Suleiman, R. Lawlor, J. Roderick, T. Bates, L. Minter, J. Anguita, I. Juncadella, B. J. Nickoloff, I. C. Le Poole, L. Miele, and B. A. Osborne. 2011. "Notch signaling regulates mouse and human th17 differentiation." *J Immunol* 187(2):692-701.

Kempf, T., and K. C. Wollert. 2009. "Growth-differentiation factor-15 in heart failure." *Heart Fail Clin* 5(4):537-47.

Kiesel, J. R., Z. S. Buchwald, and R. Aurora. 2009. "Cross-presentation by osteoclasts induces FoxP3 in CD8+ T cells." *J Immunol* 182(9):5477-87.

Kinane, D. F., P. M. Preshaw, and B. G. Loos. 2011. "Host-response: understanding the cellular and molecular mechanisms of host-microbial interactions--consensus of the Seventh European Workshop on Periodontology." *J Clin Periodontol* 38 Suppl 11:44-8.

Kobayashi, R., T. Kono, B. A. Bolerjack, Y. Fukuyama, R. S. Gilbert, K. Fujihashi, J. Ruby, K. Kataoka, M. Wada, and M. Yamamoto. 2011. "Induction of IL-10-producing CD4+ T-cells in chronic periodontitis." *J Dent Res* 90(5):653-8.

Korn, T., E. Bettelli, M. Oukka, and V. K. Kuchroo. 2009. "IL-17 and Th17 Cells." *Annu Rev Immunol* 27:485-517.

Kragstrup, T. W., K. Otkjaer, C. Holm, A. Jorgensen, M. Hokland, L. Iversen, and B. Deleuran. 2008. "The expression of IL-20 and IL-24 and their shared receptors are increased in rheumatoid arthritis and spondyloarthropathy." *Cytokine* 41(1):16-23.

Leibbrandt, A., and J. M. Penninger. 2010. "Novel Functions of RANK(L) Signaling in the Immune System." *Adv Exp Med Biol* 658:77-94.

Li, Y., C. Messina, M. Bendaoud, D. H. Fine, H. Schreiner, and V. K. Tsiagbe. 2010. "Adaptive immune response in osteoclastic bone resorption induced by orally administered Aggregatibacter actinomycetemcomitans in a rat model of periodontal disease." *Mol Oral Microbiol* 25(4):275-92.

Mahanonda, R., N. Sa-Ard-Iam, K. Yongvanitchit, M. Wisetchang, I. Ishikawa, T. Nagasawa, D. S. Walsh, and S. Pichyangkul. 2002. "Upregulation of co-stimulatory molecule expression and dendritic cell marker (CD83) on B cells in periodontal disease." *J Periodontal Res* 37(3):177-83.

McPherron, A. C., A. M. Lawler, and S. J. Lee. 1999. "Regulation of anterior/posterior patterning of the axial skeleton by growth/differentiation factor 11." *Nat Genet* 22(3):260-4.

Miossec, P., T. Korn, and V. K. Kuchroo. 2009. "Interleukin-17 and type 17 helper T cells." *N Engl J Med* 361(9):888-98.

Mosmann, T. R., and R. L. Coffman. 1989. "TH1 and TH2 cells: different patterns of lymphokine secretion lead to different functional properties." *Annu Rev Immunol* 7:145-73.

Nakashima, M., K. Tachibana, K. Iohara, M. Ito, M. Ishikawa, and A. Akamine. 2003. "Induction of reparative dentin formation by ultrasound-mediated gene delivery of growth/differentiation factor 11." *Hum Gene Ther* 14(6):591-7.

Nigam, P., V. Velu, S. Kannanganat, L. Chennareddi, S. Kwa, M. Siddiqui, and R. R. Amara. 2010. "Expansion of FOXP3+ CD8 T cells with suppressive potential in colorectal mucosa following a pathogenic simian immunodeficiency virus infection correlates with diminished antiviral T cell response and viral control." *J Immunol* 184(4):1690-701.

Nussbaum, G., and L. Shapira. 2011. "How has neutrophil research improved our understanding of periodontal pathogenesis?" *J Clin Periodontol* 38 Suppl 11:49-59.

Ohyama, H., N. Kato-Kogoe, A. Kuhara, F. Nishimura, K. Nakasho, K. Yamanegi, N. Yamada, M. Hata, J. Yamane, and N. Terada. 2009. "The involvement of IL-23 and the Th17 pathway in periodontitis." *J Dent Res* 88(7):633-8.

Oseko, F., T. Yamamoto, Y. Akamatsu, N. Kanamura, Y. Iwakura, J. Imanishi, and M. Kita. 2009. "IL-17 is involved in bone resorption in mouse periapical lesions." *Microbiol Immunol* 53(5):287-94.

Parfitt, A. M. 1982. "The coupling of bone formation to bone resorption: a critical analysis of the concept and of its relevance to the pathogenesis of osteoporosis." *Metab Bone Dis Relat Res* 4(1):1-6.

Preshaw, P. M., and J. J. Taylor. 2011. "How has research into cytokine interactions and their role in driving immune responses impacted our understanding of periodontitis?" *J Clin Periodontol* 38 Suppl 11:60-84.

Rosen, V. 2006. "BMP and BMP inhibitors in bone." *Ann N Y Acad Sci* 1068:19-25.

Sakaguchi, S. 2005. "Naturally arising Foxp3-expressing CD25+CD4+ regulatory T cells in immunological tolerance to self and non-self." *Nat Immunol* 6(4):345-52.

Sakai, A., M. Ohshima, N. Sugano, K. Otsuka, and K. Ito. 2006. "Profiling the cytokines in gingival crevicular fluid using a cytokine antibody array." *J Periodontol* 77(5):856-64.

Sakurai, N., T. Kuroiwa, H. Ikeuchi, N. Hiramatsu, A. Maeshima, Y. Kaneko, K. Hiromura, and Y. Nojima. 2008. "Expression of IL-19 and its receptors in RA: potential role for synovial hyperplasia formation." *Rheumatology (Oxford)* 47(6):815-20.

Schreiner, H., K. Markowitz, M. Miryalkar, D. Moore, S. Diehl, and D. H. Fine. 2011. "Aggregatibacter actinomycetemcomitans-induced bone loss and antibody response in three rat strains." *J Periodontol* 82(1):142-50.

Schulte, S., G. K. Sukhova, and P. Libby. 2008. "Genetically programmed biases in Th1 and Th2 immune responses modulate atherogenesis." *Am J Pathol* 172(6):1500-8.

Seymour, G. J., and E. Gemmell. 2001. "Cytokines in periodontal disease: where to from here?" *Acta Odontol Scand* 59(3):167-73.

Shea, P. R., K. Virtaneva, J. J. Kupko, 3rd, S. F. Porcella, W. T. Barry, F. A. Wright, S. D. Kobayashi, A. Carmody, R. M. Ireland, D. E. Sturdevant, S. M. Ricklefs, I. Babar, C. A. Johnson, M. R. Graham, D. J. Gardner, J. R. Bailey, M. J. Parnell, F. R. Deleo, and J. M. Musser. 2010. "Interactome analysis of longitudinal pharyngeal infection of cynomolgus macaques by group A Streptococcus." *Proc Natl Acad Sci U S A* 107(10):4693-8.

Shenker, B. J., M. Dlakic, L. P. Walker, D. Besack, E. Jaffe, E. LaBelle, and K. Boesze-Battaglia. 2007. "A novel mode of action for a microbial-derived immunotoxin: the cytolethal distending toxin subunit B exhibits phosphatidylinositol 3,4,5-triphosphate phosphatase activity." *J Immunol* 178(8):5099-108.

Taubman, M. A., P. Valverde, X. Han, and T. Kawai. 2005. "Immune response: the key to bone resorption in periodontal disease." *J Periodontol* 76(11 Suppl):2033-41.

Tsuji, K., A. Bandyopadhyay, B. D. Harfe, K. Cox, S. Kakar, L. Gerstenfeld, T. Einhorn, C. J. Tabin, and V. Rosen. 2006. "BMP2 activity, although dispensable for bone formation, is required for the initiation of fracture healing." *Nat Genet* 38(12):1424-9.

Vanhara, P., E. Lincova, A. Kozubik, P. Jurdic, K. Soucek, and J. Smarda. 2009. "Growth/differentiation factor-15 inhibits differentiation into osteoclasts--a novel factor involved in control of osteoclast differentiation." *Differentiation* 78(4):213-22.

Xiong, H., L. Wei, and B. Peng. 2009. "Immunohistochemical localization of IL-17 in induced rat periapical lesions." *J Endod* 35(2):216-20.

Xue, H., B. Lu, J. Zhang, M. Wu, Q. Huang, Q. Wu, H. Sheng, D. Wu, J. Hu, and M. Lai. "Identification of serum biomarkers for colorectal cancer metastasis using a differential secretome approach." *J Proteome Res* 9(1):545-55.

Yamazaki, K., T. Nakajima, E. Gemmell, B. Polak, G. J. Seymour, and K. Hara. 1994. "IL-4- and IL-6-producing cells in human periodontal disease tissue." *J Oral Pathol Med* 23(8):347-53.

Yamazaki, K., T. Nakajima, Y. Kubota, E. Gemmell, G. J. Seymour, and K. Hara. 1997. "Cytokine messenger RNA expression in chronic inflammatory periodontal disease." *Oral Microbiol Immunol* 12(5):281-7.

Ye, L., H. Kynaston, and W. G. Jiang. 2009. "Bone morphogenetic protein-10 suppresses the growth and aggressiveness of prostate cancer cells through a Smad independent pathway." *J Urol* 181(6):2749-59.

Yokoe, T., T. Ohmachi, H. Inoue, K. Mimori, F. Tanaka, M. Kusunoki, and M. Mori. 2007. "Clinical significance of growth differentiation factor 11 in colorectal cancer." *Int J Oncol* 31(5):1097-101.

Yue, G., J. B. Kaplan, D. Furgang, K. G. Mansfield, and D. H. Fine. 2007. "A second Aggregatibacter actinomycetemcomitans autotransporter adhesin exhibits specificity for buccal epithelial cells in humans and Old World primates." *Infect Immun* 75(9):4440-8.

Yuryev, A., Z. Mulyukov, E. Kotelnikova, S. Maslov, S. Egorov, A. Nikitin, N. Daraselia, and I. Mazo. 2006. "Automatic pathway building in biological association networks." *BMC Bioinformatics* 7:171.

Zaiss, M. M., M. Kurowska-Stolarska, C. Bohm, R. Gary, C. Scholtysek, B. Stolarski, J. Reilly, S. Kerr, N. L. Millar, T. Kamradt, I. B. McInnes, P. G. Fallon, J. P. David, F. Y. Liew, and G. Schett. 2011. "IL-33 shifts the balance from osteoclast to alternatively activated macrophage differentiation and protects from TNF-alpha-mediated bone loss." *J Immunol* 186(11):6097-105.

Zambon, J. J. 1985. "Actinobacillus actinomycetemcomitans in human periodontal disease." *J Clin Periodontol* 12(1):1-20.

Zambon, J. J., T. Umemoto, E. De Nardin, F. Nakazawa, L. A. Christersson, and R. J. Genco. 1988. "Actinobacillus actinomycetemcomitans in the pathogenesis of human periodontal disease." *Adv Dent Res* 2(2):269-74.

Zhang, F., H. Tanaka, T. Kawato, S. Kitami, K. Nakai, M. Motohashi, N. Suzuki, C. L. Wang, K. Ochiai, K. Isokawa, and M. Maeno. 2011. "Interleukin-17A induces cathepsin K and MMP-9 expression in osteoclasts via celecoxib-blocked prostaglandin E2 in osteoblasts." *Biochimie* 93(2):296-305.

4

Periodontal Disease and Gingival Innate Immunity – Who Has the Upper Hand?

Whasun Oh Chung and Jonathan Y. An
University of Washington, Seattle, WA
USA

1. Introduction

Dental plaque is a complex microbial biofilm that forms at high cell density in the oral cavity by the successive accumulation of hundreds of different species of bacteria. Both host immune and bacterial factors are involved in the progression from healthy to diseased state in plaque biofilm, and in the oral cavity, gingival epithelial cells (GECs) are one of the first host cell types that encounter colonizing bacteria. As a consequence, GECs respond to the presence of bacteria through an elaborate signaling network, producing antimicrobial peptides (AMPs) and cytokines, leading to host innate immune responses. Periodontal disease is a consequence of the imbalance between the pathogenic potential of the biofilm and host immune defense properties, resulting in an inflammatory reaction of the periodontium. As a part of host defense mechanism, GECs secrete specific endogenous serine protease inhibitors to prevent tissue damage from excessive proteolytic enzyme activity due to inflammation. Recent studies showed GECs induced different serine protease inhibitors in the presence of non-pathogenic bacteria, but these protease inhibitors were attenuated by periopathogens, whose main virulence factors are proteases. Furthermore, periodontal patients with periopathogens present in their plaque exhibited significantly lower protease inhibitors in gingival crevicular fluid in comparison to healthy controls. The degradation of protease inhibitors by periopathogens may result in decreased host protective capacity, and the balance between cellular protease inhibitors and their degradation by periodontal pathogens may be an important factor in susceptibility to breakdown from chronic infection. In addition to bacterial infection, genetic and environmental factors contribute to occurrence and progression of periodontal disease. Recent studies suggest that the manifestation and severity of periodontal disease may be influenced by epigenetic factors. Many patients with the same clinical symptoms respond differently to the same therapy, suggesting the inter-individual variability observed as a clinical outcome of the disease is influenced by genetic as well as epigenetic factors.

In this chapter, we will closely examine the mechanisms gingival epithelia utilize in inducing AMPs in response to bacterial presence and assess future therapeutic potential of AMPs. We will also focus on the impact the balance between the proteases and protease inhibitors has on oral health and how epigenetic modifications brought on by exposure to periodontal pathogens affect the progression of periodontal disease.

2. Microbial biofilm and innate immune responses of gingiva

Dental plaque is a complex microbial biofilm that forms at high cell density on tooth surfaces in the oral cavity by the successive accumulation of over 500 different species of bacteria (Kolenbrander, Andersen et al. 2002; Rickard, Gilbert et al. 2003). The early colonizers of the tooth surface are mainly non-pathogens comprised of Gram-positive facultative organisms, including *Streptococcus gordonii, Streptococcus sanguis* and *Streptococcus oralis*. These initial colonizers adhere to salivary pellicle on teeth, leading to successive colonization of Gram-negative anaerobes such as *Fusobacterium nucleatum* and finally to pathogens such as *Porphyromonas gingivalis*. The formation of plaque has been linked to the human oral diseases, caries and periodontitis (Socransky, Smith et al. 2002; Socransky and Haffajee 2005), and both host immune and bacterial factors are involved in the progression from healthy to diseased state in plaque biofilm.

Periodontitis is one of most common inflammatory diseases and can be of inflammatory, traumatic, metabolic, developmental and/or genetic origin. In most cases, periodontal disease results in an inflammatory reaction of the periodontium to pathogenic microorganisms. Among various species of microorganisms making up oral biofilm that accumulates on the tooth surface adjacent to the gingiva, Gram-negative anaerobic bacteria *P. gingivalis, Tannerella forsythia* and *Treponema denticola* in particular have been strongly associated with periodontal disease (Socransky, Haffajee et al. 1998; Armitage 1999; Socransky and Haffajee 2003). Bacteria first form a supra-gingival biofilm attached to the tooth surface, and once they have passed the junctional epithelium, bacteria may enter the gingival crevice to form sub-gingival biofilm, which provides an optimal environment for anaerobic bacteria to colonize and reproduce (Socransky and Haffajee 2003). The number of Gram-negative anaerobic bacteria increases during development and maturation of the dental biofilm. Both host immune and bacterial factors are involved in the progression from healthy to diseased state in plaque biofilm, thus periodontal disease is the result of the imbalance between the pathogenic potential of the biofilm and host immune defense properties. In addition, genetic and/or environmental factors, such as smoking, contribute to occurrence and progression of periodontal disease (Michalowicz, Aeppli et al. 1991; Michalowicz, Diehl et al. 2000; Kinane and Hart 2003; Loos, John et al. 2005).

P. gingivalis is an aggressive pathogen and considered an etiologic agent of severe adult periodontitis. Colonization of the oral cavity by *P. gingivalis* is facilitated by adherence to various oral surfaces, including epithelial cells, the salivary pellicle that coats tooth surfaces, and other oral bacteria that comprise the plaque biofilm (Socransky and Haffajee 1992). However, *P. gingivalis* is considered a secondary colonizer of plaque and rarely colonizes the tooth surface until initial plaque bacteria, such as *S. gordonii*, establish an appropriate environment. Adhesion between *S. gordonii* and *P. gingivalis* is mediated by *S. gordonii* cell-surface protein SspB and *P. gingivalis* minor fimbriae (Chung, Demuth et al. 2000). In the oral cavity, gingival epithelial cells are one of the first host cell types that encounter colonizing bacteria. As a consequence, epithelial cells respond to the presence of bacteria through an elaborate signaling network, producing antimicrobial peptides and cytokines, and at times stimulating apoptotic cell death. This bacterial-host communication takes place via a number of signal transduction pathways, but different bacteria may induce different signals from the host. Conversely, various host immune responses may interfere with the way commensals and pathogens communicate to form biofilm, although this means of defense is poorly understood.

Periodontal disease is of importance not only in oral health, but also in general health because of its association with an increased risk of preterm births and low birth weight babies (Offenbacher, Katz et al. 1996; Buduneli, Baylas et al. 2005). Thus, it is of importance to understand how oral bacteria alter host innate immune responses and how periodontal disease is affected by protective factors induced by the host.

3. The role of Antimicrobial Peptides in periodontal health

3.1 Antimicrobial Peptides (AMPs)

In the presence of diverse environment of microbial consortiums, epithelia express several natural antimicrobial peptides (AMPs) which work synergistically with a broad spectrum of activity against both Gram-negative and Gram-positive bacteria, as well as against yeast and some virus to maintain balance between health and disease (Hancock and Chapple 1999; Lehrer and Ganz 2002; Premratanachai, Joly et al. 2004). AMPs are small cationic peptides with molecular weights typically ranging between 3,500 and 6,500 Da (Dale 2002). They adopt amphiphilic topologies, which allows them to interact and selectively disrupt microbial cell membranes (Som, Vemparala et al. 2008). In humans these antimicrobial peptides include defensins and a cathelicidin family member LL-37 in skin and oral mucosa and other epithelia (Hancock and Scott 2000; Lehrer and Ganz 2002; Selsted and Ouellette 2005). The human defensins include the alpha-defensins of intestinal and neutrophil origin, and the beta-defensins of skin and oral mucosa and other epithelia. Alpha-defensins are expressed in neutrophils as part of their non-oxidative antimicrobial mechanisms (Lehrer, Lichtenstein et al. 1993; van Wetering, Sterk et al. 1999). Alpha-defensins are also found in Paneth cells in the intestine (Selsted 1992; Ouellette 1999). They are synthesized as precursors that are proteolytically activated and released during inflammation (Rock 1998; Wilson, Ouellette et al. 1999). The human beta-defensins (hBDs) are small, cationic antimicrobial peptides made primarily by epithelial cells and expressed in all human epithelia tested to date (Dale 2002). The beta-defensins are secreted in biological fluids, including urine, bronchial fluids, nasal secretions, saliva and gingival crevicular fluid (Valore, Park et al. 1998; Cole 1999; Sahasrabudhe 2000; Diamond, Kimball et al. 2001). hBDs were first identified in tracheal epithelial cells and subsequently found in many epithelia including kidney and urinary tract, oral mucosa and skin (Diamond, Russell et al. 1996; Zhao, Wang et al. 1996; Krisanaprakornkit, Weinberg et al. 1998; Valore, Park et al. 1998).

The expression of the cathelicidin, LL-37, is found in human tongue, buccal mucosa and saliva following inflammatory stimulation (Frohm Nilsson, Sandstedt et al. 1999; Murakami, Ohtake et al. 2002). It is kept inactive until proteases cleave the conserved proregion (Zanetti, Gennaro et al. 2000). Immunohistochemistry studies found that LL-37, derived from neutrophils, was detected in the junctional epithelium (Dale, Kimball et al. 2001). The defensins and LL-37 are localized in different sites in gingiva, which suggests that they may play different roles in specific sites in which they are expressed (Dale, Kimball et al. 2001). Because these AMPs have synergistic effects, their presence in saliva may provide natural antimicrobial barrier (Tao, Jurevic et al. 2005). Different sites within the oral cavity where various AMPs are predominantly expressed are depicted in Figure 1.

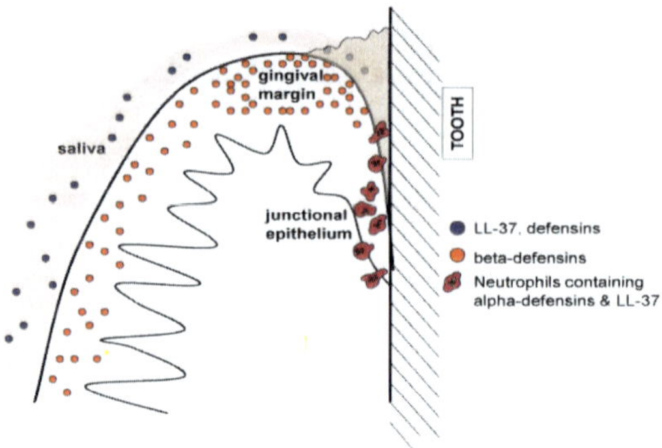

Fig. 1. Various sites in the oral cavity where different AMPs are predominantly expressed. Dale and Fredericks 2005; permission from Horizon Scientific Press

3.1.1 Alpha-defensins

Alpha- and beta-defensins are peptides with six disulfide-linked cysteines. Structurally, the difference between the two defensins lies within the length of peptide segments between the six cysteines and pairing of the cysteines (Bals and Wilson 2003). Six different human alpha-defensins have been identified so far, including four human neutrophil peptides, HNP1-4, and two others known as human defensins 5 and 6 (HD-5, HD-6) (Ganz, Selsted et al. 1985; Ganz and Lehrer 1994; Cunliffe 2003). Alpha-defensins are arginine-rich and localized in either neutrophil azurophilic granules or Paneth cells, which are the epithelia of the intestinal mucosa. During gingivitis, neutrophils dominate the lesion area, but the relative proportion compared to plasma cells and lymphocytes in neutrophils decreases during the transition to periodontitis (Kinane and Bouchard 2008; Nussbaum and Shapira 2011). Disorders in neutrophil production have been associated with destruction of periodontal tissue and eventual periodontal disease (Crawford, Wilton et al. 2000). Within neutrophils, human alpha-defensins are abundant and work together with the oral epithelium to provide a barrier to microbial colonization, particularly in the junctional epithelium of the tooth surface (Dale and Fredericks 2005). Studies have shown that two periodontal pathogens, *P. gingivalis* and *Aggregatibacter actinomycetemcomitans*, as well as non-pathogenic commensal bacteria *S. gordonii* are insensitive to alpha-defensin activity (Miyasaki, Bodeau et al. 1990; Zhong, Yang et al. 1998; Raj, Antonyraj et al. 2000). However, when extra amino acids were added to the N-terminus and C-terminus end of HNP2, an enhanced antibacterial activity against the same bacteria was shown, indicating the structural anatomy is a crucial determinant in this AMP's antibacterial activity (Raj, Antonyraj et al. 2000).

HNP 1-3 are detected in the junctional epithelium and the gingival crevicular fluid (GCF), and GCF from patients with aggressive and chronic periodontitis showed significantly elevated levels of HNP 1-3 compared to healthy patients (McKay, Olson et al. 1999; Dale, Kimball et al. 2001). Interestingly, the increased concentration of both alpha- and beta-defensins was correlated in patients with chronic periodontitis with the amount of periodontal pathogens *P. gingivalis*, *T. denticola*, and *T. forsythia* (Puklo, Guentsch et al. 2008). Recently, HNP1 and HNP2 were shown to decrease the response of pro-inflammatory cytokine IL-6, while enhancing antibody response to specific *P. gingivalis* adhesin in mice (Kohlgraf, Ackermann et al. 2010). Thus, alpha-defensins may play a key role as a mediator of innate immunity in gingiva against periopathogenic microbes.

3.1.2 Beta-defensins

Beta-defensins 1 and 2 (hBD-1 and hBD-2) are found in normal, uninflamed gingival tissues as part of the innate host defense mechanism (Krisanaprakornkit, Weinberg et al. 1998; Dale, Kimball et al. 2001). Furthermore, hBD-1 and hBD-2 are localized at the gingival margin where there is the most exposure to oral bacteria of the plaque on the tooth surface, but not in the junctional epithelium. Thus, the junctional epithelium is protected by alpha-defensins and LL-37 released from neutrophils, while the differentiated, stratified epithelia are protected by beta-defensins. Structurally a reduced hBD-1 differs from an oxidized hBD-1, and a reduction in the disulfide bridges of hBD-1 causes the peptide to become a potent AMP against opportunistic pathogen *Candida albicans* and *Lactobacillus* species (Schroeder, Wu et al. 2011). A structural modulation of hBD-1, dependent on the environment it exists in the oral cavity, could shield the healthy epithelium against colonization by commensal and periopathogenic bacteria. However, compared to other beta-defensins, hBD-1 only shows a minor effect against oral bacteria, such as *P. gingivalis, A. actinomycetemcomitans, Prevotella intermedia,* and *F. nucleatum* (Ouhara, Komatsuzawa et al. 2005).

In oral epithelia, the expression of hBD-2 is found in normal, uninflamed gingival tissues and is induced by various bacteria (Krisanaprakornkit, Kimball et al. 2000; Dale, Kimball et al. 2001; Chung and Dale 2004). The expression of hBD-2 after challenge from a commensal bacterium indicates that the normal oral epithelium is already at a heightened state to combat potentially harmful pathogens (Krisanaprakornkit, Kimball et al. 2000; Chung and Dale 2004).

hBD-3 has shown bactericidal activity against a wide range of oral bacteria, including periodontal pathogens *A. actinomycetemcomitans* and *P. gingivalis,* and cariogenic bacteria *Streptococcus mutans* (Maisetta, Batoni et al. 2003). Furthermore, both normal GECs and immortalized human oral epithelial cells showed an increase in hBD-3 levels upon exposure to *A. actinomycetemcomitans* (Feucht, DeSanti et al. 2003). Similar to HNPs, the peptide has also been detected in the GCF of healthy individuals, and a significant decrease in hBD-3 levels in GCF correlated with the stage of periodontitis, with a negative correlation between hBD-3 levels with the number of periopathogenic bacteria within the same site (Bissell, Joly et al. 2004; Brancatisano, Maisetta et al. 2011).

Studies on the regulation of the induction of beta-defensins reveal different ways gingival epithelia respond to the presence of pathogenic and non-pathogenic bacteria. Our group has reported the induction of hBD-2 by GECs in response to commensal bacteria like *F. nucleatum* and *S. gordonii* utilized p38 and JNK MAPK pathways, while in response to periopathogenic bacteria like *P. gingivalis* and *A. actinomycetemcomitans*, GECs utilized the NF-κB pathway in addition to the aforementioned MAPK (Krisanaprakornkit, Kimball et al. 2002; Chung and Dale 2008). Our group has further reported gingival innate immune response to *P. gingivalis* involves Protease-activated receptor-2 (PAR-2), a G-protein coupled receptor (Chung, Hansen et al. 2004; Dommisch, Chung et al. 2007). A study from another group reported mice given oral doses of *P. gingivalis* showed alveolar bone loss, but in PAR-2 deficient mice the amount of bone loss was significantly less, indicating PAR-2 may have a role in the inflammatory response against *P. gingivalis* (Holzhausen, Spolidorio et al. 2006). In addition, a recent study revealed that the expression of hBD-3 in response to another periodontal pathogen *T. denticola* is regulated via TLR2 (Shin, Kim et al. 2010). All these studies strongly suggest gingival epithelia are able to sense microbes, distinguish between commensal and periopathogenic bacteria, and regulate the appropriate responses for inflammation via regulation of AMPs.

3.1.3 Cathelicidin family – LL-37

Cathelicidin AMPs are heterogeneous and share similar characteristics with other AMPs, such as a basic residue, overall amphipathic nature, and a net positive charge at neutral pH (Dale and Fredericks 2005). LL-37, the only member in human cathelicidin family, is transcribed by *CAMP* (cathelicidin antimicrobial peptide) gene, which translates to an 18 kDa proprotein (Zanetti, Gennaro et al. 2000; Zaiou, Nizet et al. 2003). This AMP is detected and expressed in higher amounts within neutrophils that migrate through the junctional epithelium to the gingival sulcus (Dale, Kimball et al. 2001). This peptide is present in a different site than beta-defensins, suggesting they could serve different role in periodontium. The expression of LL-37 is detected in wide range of epithelia and other body sites, including junctional epithelium, inflamed epidermal keratinocytes, tongue, buccal mucosa and saliva following inflammatory stimulation (Frohm, Agerberth et al. 1997; Frohm Nilsson, Sandstedt et al. 1999; Dale, Kimball et al. 2001; Murakami, Ohtake et al. 2002; Howell 2007). Junctional epithelium also expresses IL-8, following a gradient that leads to directional migration of neutrophils into the gingival sulcus when exposed to bacteria (Tonetti, Imboden et al. 1994). Thus, it is plausible that neutrophil migration through the tissue may be the reason for the expression of LL-37 in gingival epithelium (Dale, Kimball et al. 2001; Dale and Fredericks 2005). LL-37 has shown antimicrobial activities against periodontal pathogen *A. actinomycetemcomitans* (Gomez-Garces, Alos et al. 1994), while is ineffective against some cariogenic bacteria, including *S. mutans, Streptococcus sobrinus* and *Actinomyces viscosus,* as well as periodontal pathogen *P. gingivalis* (Altman, Steinberg et al. 2006).

3.2 Differential expression of AMPs in periodontal health and disease

How the expression of various AMPs varies during gingival and periodontal inflammation has been reported by various groups, and these studies show high inter-individual variability in both gene and protein expression of AMPs in patient samples (Dunsche, Acil et al. 2002; Lu, Jin et al. 2004; Dommisch, Acil et al. 2005; Lu, Samaranayake et al. 2005). Analyses of gene expression by RT-PCR showed hBD-1 and hBD-2 mRNA expression was less frequently detected in tissues with gingivitis than in healthy gingiva. In biopsies from patients with gingivitis, mRNA of hBD-1 and hBD-2 was detectable in 66 % and 86 % of samples, respectively, while 100 % of all gingivitis samples showed the expression of hBD-3 mRNA (Dunsche, Acil et al. 2002). In addition, compared to the samples from healthy subjects, the level of beta-defensin mRNA expression was lower and less frequently found in samples from periodontitis patients (Dunsche, Acil et al. 2002; Bissell, Joly et al. 2004). Similar results have also been reported testing mRNA level by *in situ* hybridization and protein level using immunohistochemistry (Lu, Jin et al. 2004; Lu, Samaranayake et al. 2005; Hosokawa, Hosokawa et al. 2006). These studies suggest a decrease in the expression of hBD-2 and hBD-3 in both patient groups of gingivitis and periodontitis. However, other studies suggest differential expression of beta-defensins in patients with specific periodontal diseases, highlighting inter-individual variability in the expression of these AMPs. In samples collected from gingivitis and periodontitis patients, the amount of hBD-2 mRNA was up-regulated compared to the ones from healthy subjects, while the quantity of hBD-3 mRNA was equivalent in healthy and gingivitis groups, but increased in periodontitis samples (Dommisch, Acil et al. 2005). Quantitative RT-PCR analyses of hBD-1 and hBD-2 expression levels in gingiva of patients with gingivitis, aggressive periodontitis and chronic periodontitis found a significantly higher level of hBD-1 in chronic periodontitis group compared to gingivitis and aggressive periodontitis groups (Vardar-Sengul, Demirci et al. 2007). On the other hand, the expression level of hBD-2 was significantly higher in aggressive periodontitis group than in gingivitis and chronic periodontitis groups (Vardar-Sengul, Demirci et al. 2007). The localization of beta-defensin protein expression also varied among different patient groups. The protein expression of hBD-1 and hBD-2 was mostly found in the granular and spinous cell layer in healthy and diseased gingival tissue samples (Lu, Jin et al. 2004). On the contrary, the expression of hBD-3 was found in basal cell layer in healthy samples, while in the basal and spinous cell layers in samples from periodontal disease (Lu, Samaranayake et al. 2005).

The levels of AMPs in GCF are thought to be associated with periodontal disease, as demonstrated by Puklo et al. that the GCF HNP1-3 levels were higher in patients with aggressive or chronic periodontitis when compared to healthy controls (Puklo, Guentsch et al. 2008). Gingival tissue samples from chronic periodontitis patients showed elevated mRNA expression and higher immunostaining of LL-37 on neutrophils, while the LL-37 levels were also elevated in the GCF of periodontitis patients (Hosokawa, Hosokawa et al. 2006; Turkoglu, Emingil et al. 2009; Turkoglu, Kandiloglu et al. 2011). In addition, patients with morbus Kostmann syndrome, an inherited disorder that causes lower than normal levels of neutrophils, have been found to be more susceptible to periodontal disease, while those with a bone marrow transplant are not (Putsep, Carlsson et al. 2002). The patients with Kostmann syndrome lack LL-37 in saliva and have lower concentrations of HNP1-3, the latter of which is commonly found in patients with other neutrophil disorders (Ganz, Metcalf et al. 1988). However, when these patients receive a bone marrow transplant, normal concentration of LL-37 is found in their saliva (Putsep, Carlsson et al. 2002). Of interesting to note is when patients with Kostmann syndrome have their levels of neutrophils restored via treatment with recombinant granulocyte-colony stimulating factor, they still experience recurring periodontal infections (Putsep, Carlsson et al. 2002; Carlsson, Wahlin et al. 2006). All these studies suggest that the deficiency in salivary LL-37 is a likely reason for chronic periodontitis in patients with morbus Kostmann prior to bone marrow transplant and further suggests a potential protective role in host defense by LL-37.

All the studies presented in this section demonstrate that AMPs are differentially expressed in various stages of periodontal health and disease. These studies also suggest that there may be complex regulatory mechanisms involved in gingival innate immunity (Chung, Dommisch et al. 2007), and further suggest AMPs play a crucial role in the maintenance of gingival health and prevention of periodontal disease.

3.3 Potential therapeutic value of AMPs

How AMPs maintain the delicate balance between oral health and dental plaque containing microbial consortium is still a matter of conjecture. Some hypotheses include AMPs creating physical holes that cause cellular contents to leak out, fatal depolarization of normally energized bacterial membrane, or the activation of deadly processes such as the induction of hydrolases that degrade the cell wall (Som, Vemparala et al. 2008). Overall, the mode of antimicrobial activity of AMPs has been most commonly attributed to disruption of cell membranes (Ganz and Lehrer 1999; Hancock and Diamond 2000), but a recent study also reported that defensins can inhibit cell wall biosynthesis via binding and sequestering of lipid II, a building block of bacterial cell wall (Wilmes, Cammue et al. 2011).

Currently, a combination of antimicrobial and mechanical applications is used in treatment plans for periodontal disease, such as applying tetracycline or doxycline families in conjunction to scaling and root planning. Recently, a sub-antimicrobial dose doxycyline has been introduced where low doses are given to block matrix metalloproteinases (MMP), which are capable of degrading extracellular matrix proteins (Tuter, Kurtis et al. 2007; Payne, Golub et al. 2011). Yet, antibiotic treatment for periodontal disease still poses a risk of developing antibiotic-resistant periodontal bacteria in the subgingival plaque (van Winkelhoff, Herrera Gonzales et al. 2000; Handal, Caugant et al. 2003; Maestre, Bascones et al. 2007; Ardila, Granada et al. 2010). AMPs have several advantages as therapeutics, including the broad spectrum of antimicrobial activity and do not appear to induce antibiotic resistance. AMPs as therapeutics against microbes would be promising because the target of AMPs are the bacterial membrane, thus to combat AMPs the bacteria would need to redesign its membrane, which would be a "costly" solution for most species (Zasloff 2002). The possibility of alleviating bacterial infections related to cystic fibrosis through increasing physiological levels of LL-37, or re-engineering human macrophages to express beta-defensins to enhance efficacy against *Mycobacterium tuberculosis* have been proposed (Bals, Weiner et al. 1999; Kisich, Heifets et al. 2001). However, limitations as an effective therapeutic are stalled by high production costs and the susceptibility to proteolytic degradation, a mechanism which microbial pathogens secrete proteases to counter-measure the target of AMPs (Peters, Shirtliff et al. 2010). Due to these limitations, a new pursuit has been made to construct synthetic mimics of AMPs, which would capture the important properties of AMPs but also eliminate problems related to drug therapy. Structurally these AMP mimics would maintain its amphiphillic topology to eventually depolarize the membrane potential and ultimately kill bacteria, but also possess a non-natural backbone without amide or ester function so the peptide will not undergo proteolytic degradation from bacterial enzymes (Tew, Liu et al. 2002; Tew, Clements et al. 2006; Hua, Scott et al. 2010). A recent study showed one mimetic called mPE was able to exhibit potency against biofilm cultures of *A. actinomycetemcomitans* and *P. gingivalis*, while also inhibiting IL-1B-induced secretion of IL-8 in gingival epithelial cells (Hua, Scott et al. 2010). The anti-inflammatory activity was followed with a reduced activation of NF-κB, suggesting that these AMP mimics could act as an anti-biofilm and anti-inflammatory agent. Furthermore, it has been shown in bacterial resistance studies that *Staphylococcus aureus* showed increased minimum inhibitory concentration (MIC) for conventional antibiotics, but no change was observed with MIC for mPE (Beckloff, Laube et al. 2007; Hua, Scott et al. 2010). However, a current limitation of mimetic is that it has been tested on single bacterium but not on complex biofilm structures.

4. Proteases vs. protease inhibitors in periodontal health and disease

4.1 Various classes of protease inhibitors in gingival epithelia

Serine protease inhibitors play a critical role in host tissue homeostasis, as gingival epithelia secrete these protease inhibitors as a way to protect the tissue from excessive damage by proteases, which can be of pathogenic bacteria or of neutrophil origin. Thus, the balance between proteases and their inhibitors contributes to maintenance of tissue integrity (Magert, Drogemuller et al. 2005). These protease inhibitors include secretory leukocyte protease inhibitor (SLPI), elastase-specific inhibitor (ELAFIN) and squamous cell carcinoma antigen (SCCA). SLPI is found in a variety of mucous secretions, including in GCF from sites of periodontal disease (Minami 1999). This protease inhibitor protects tissues from destruction during an inflammatory response via regulating the activity of neutrophil elastase (Giannopoulou, Di Felice et al. 1990). ELAFIN, also known as skin-derived anti-leukoproteinase (SKALP), is expressed in human epithelia of the tongue, palate, lingual tonsils, pharynx as well as gingiva (Molhuizen and Schalkwijk 1995). ELAFIN has been shown to inhibit neutrophil elastase and proteinase 3, thus has a role in protecting tissue from degradation by the neutrophil enzymes (Ying and Simon 1993; Zani, Nobar et al. 2004). ELAFIN and SLPI are chelonianin family of serine protease inhibitors and share 40% sequence identity (Ying and Simon 1993; Zani, Nobar et al. 2004; Guyot, Butler et al. 2008). Both SLPI and ELAFIN have antimicrobial activity against Gram-positive as well as Gram-negative pathogens (Sallenave, Cunningham et al. 2003; McMichael, Maxwell et al. 2005; King, Wheelhouse et al. 2009).

SCCA1 and SCCA2 are members of the ovalbumin-serpin and serve as a marker for certain inflammatory conditions. Within the mucous membranes lined with squamous epithelia, co-expression of SCCA1 and 2 plays an important role in the coordinated regulation of certain serine and cysteine proteases associated with both normal and transformed cells (Cataltepe, Gornstein et al. 2000). SCCA1 and SCCA2 share 91% homology at the amino acid level, and both are induced by IL-4 and IL-13 (Yuyama, Davies et al. 2002; Mitsuishi, Nakamura et al. 2005). However, their functions differ: SCCA1 inhibits cysteine proteases such as cathepsin K, while SCCA2 inhibits serine proteases such as cathepsin G and human mast cell chymase (Silverman, Bird et al. 2001).

These protease inhibitors are expressed by various epithelial cells and act as an anti-protease to protect against tissue damages caused during inflammation (Alkemade, Molhuizen et al. 1994; Pfundt, van Ruissen et al. 1996; van Wetering, van der Linden et al. 2000). In addition, other studies demonstrated anti-bacterial and anti-inflammatory activities of ELAFIN that are independent of anti-protease activity (Simpson, Maxwell et al. 1999; Meyer-Hoffert, Wichmann et al. 2003). In the context of the periodontium, these protease inhibitors produced by GECs might protect against bacterial proteases and limit tissue damage due to neutrophil proteases associated with inflammation. Thus, the balance between protease inhibitors and proteases may be a factor in the progression of disease.

4.2 Regulation of protease inhibitors by periodontal pathogens

The development of periodontal disease is characterized by the transition of the subgingival flora from Gram-positive complex, such as Streptococci, to a Gram-negative complex including the presumptive pathogen, *P. gingivalis* (Kolenbrander, Andersen et al. 2002). *P. gingivalis* gingipains are cysteine proteases with specificity for cleavage at either arginine (Rgp) or lysine (Kgp) (Potempa, Pike et al. 1995; Potempa and Travis 1996). Rgp activates cellular responses of both epithelial cells and fibroblasts via PAR2 and up-regulates inflammatory and innate immune responses (Lourbakos, Potempa et al. 2001; Holzhausen, Spolidorio et al. 2006). In addition to *P. gingivalis*, periodontal pathogens *T. denticola* and *T. forsythia* also have serine or cysteine proteases as their main virulence factors, and these proteases play a role in periodontitis (Fenno, Lee et al. 2001; van der Reijden, Bosch-Tijhof et al. 2006). *F. nucleatum* is a common microorganism within the periodontium in both healthy and diseased tissue and serves as a bridging organism between commensals and pathogens. Previous studies reported *F. nucleatum* as well as commensal bacterium *S. gordonii* have serine-type proteases which are involved in the degradation of collagen and/or fibronectin (Juarez and Stinson 1999; Bachrach, Rosen et al. 2004). In addition to bacterial proteases, neutrophils also release proteases. In the normal epithelium, neutrophils flow into the space between the tooth and soft tissue due to the cytokine gradient. Although neutrophils serve as part of the continuous surveillance of the gingival sulcus, proteases released by neutrophils contribute to inflammation and tissue damage (Tonetti, Imboden et al. 1998; Nathan 2006).

Our laboratory previously showed that GECs exposed to *F. nucleatum* up-regulated expression of multiple protease inhibitors as well as antimicrobial peptides and other potentially protective factors (Table 1) (Yin and Dale 2007). Our data suggest that *F. nucleatum*, a bridging organism between non-pathogenic commensal and pathogenic bacteria, enhances expression of protease inhibitors that protect GECs in anticipation of virulent proteases secreted by pathogenic bacteria. Both host cell-derived proteases, such as neutrophil elastase, and pathogen-derived proteases, such as the gingipains, are targeted by these protease inhibitors, and therefore, the protease inhibitors may play an important role in maintaining the extent of inflammatory tissue damage (Into, Inomata et al. 2006; Williams, Brown et al. 2006; Yin, Swanson et al. 2010).

Protease Inhibitor	Target Protease	Potential Function	Fold Change*
ELAFIN	Elastase, PMN	Innate immunity, antimicrobial	14.31
SERPINB1	Elastase, Cathepsin G	Innate immunity, inhibits PMN proteases	3.2
SERPINB2	Thrombin	Regulates extravascular plasminogen activation	2.2
SCCA1	Cathepsin S, K, L	Inhibits Cathepsin S, K, L and modulates host immune response	19.4
SCCA2	Cathepsin G	Inhibits mast cell proteases	8.6
SLPI	Elastase, Trypsin, Cathepsin B	Stimulates wound healing, inhibits PMN proteases	4.3
Cystatin B	Stefin B	Protection against intracellular proteases	2.0

*Fold increase after stimulation with *F. nucleatum* cell wall extract for 24h compared to unstimulated.

Table 1. Changes in the induction level of various protease inhibitors in gingival epithelial cells following stimulation with *F. nucleatum* (Yin and Dale 2007).

These protease inhibitors are also affected by perio-pathogenic organism *P. gingivalis*, whose main virulence factors are cysteine proteases. A protective effect of these protease inhibitors in gingival health is shown by our study that demonstrated pre-treatment of GECs with SLPI, SCCA1 or SCCA2 partially attenuated antimicrobial proteins hBD-2 and CCL20 mRNA expression in response to *P. gingivalis* (Yin, Swanson et al. 2010). However, the same study showed the presence of *P. gingivalis* disrupted the function of these serine protease inhibitors, suggesting that the presence of an organism colonizing oral plaque prior to the establishment by pathogens enhances expression of protease inhibitors that protect GECs, while *P. gingivalis* secretes proteases that degrade cellular protease inhibitors (Yin, Swanson et al. 2010). It is of interest to note that various periodontal pathogens which secrete proteases (*P. gingivalis, T. forsythia, A. actinomycetemcomitans*) were tested, but *P. gingivalis* was most effective at degrading protease inhibitors (Figure 2) (Yin, Swanson et al. 2010). The degradation of protease inhibitors by *P. gingivalis* may result in decreased host protective capacity, and the balance between cellular protease inhibitors and their degradation by *P. gingivalis* and/or other periodontal pathogens may be an important factor in susceptibility to *P. gingivalis* infection. The dominance of *P. gingivalis* in the degradation of protease inhibitors is important to note, since during the formation of dental plaque, protease inhibitors may be induced as a host protective mechanism by the presence of non-pathogenic bacteria, but may become ineffective once protease-secreting pathogens are established.

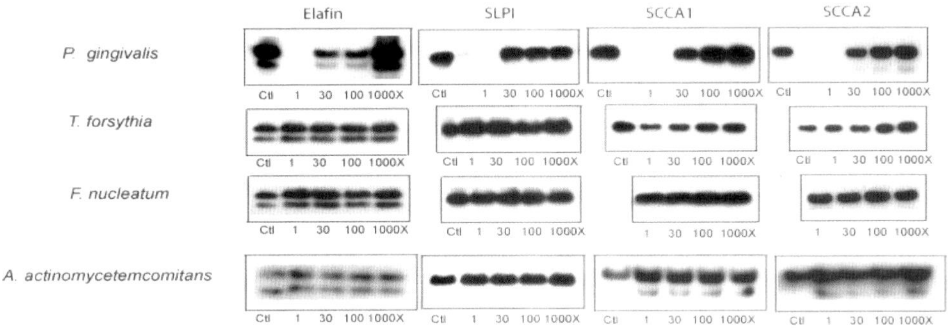

Fig. 2. Recombinant SLPI, ELAFIN, SCCA1, and SCCA2 are degraded by *P. gingivalis* supernatants *in vitro* in a dose-dependent manner. Western Blot analysis for each protease inhibitor using a constant concentration of recombinant protease inhibitor incubated with cell-free supernatants of oral bacteria for 15 min at RT. The undiluted supernatant (1) corresponds to MOI 100; increasing dilution factor is indicated below each protease inhibitor. Control: recombinant protein only. The controls shown with *P. gingivalis* also apply to the recombinant proteins treated with *T. forsythia* and *F. nucleatum* (Yin, Swanson et al. 2010). Permission from Co-Action Publishing.

In addition to exposure to proteases secreted by oral pathogenic bacteria, oral cavity may also be exposed to different neutrophil-derived serine proteases, such as human leukocyte elastase, cathepsin G and proteinase 3 (Sugawara, Uehara et al. 2001; Uehara, Muramoto et al. 2003). These neutrophil proteases may be secreted in response to the presence of oral bacteria, and thus oral cavity may be exposed to these neutrophil proteases prior to being exposed to proteases from periodontal pathogens. In addition, protease inhibitors are likely to have different effects on neutrophil proteases secreted by host vs. proteases secreted by periodontal pathogens: proteases secreted by pathogens may degrade host protease inhibitors; while proteases secreted by host neutrophils may maintain more natural balance in maintaining epithelial health. Proteases have to be at the right place at the right time to have an effect on the host, thus have to be tightly regulated by the host. Therefore, the balance between the proteases and protease inhibitors is crucial in the health of oral epithelia.

4.3 Changes in protease inhibitor levels in periodontitis

Periodontitis is a chronic inflammatory disease whose main etiologic agents include Gram-negative anaerobic bacteria and spirochetes (Haffajee and Socransky 1994). Among them, *P. gingivalis* in particular plays a significant role in the progression of chronic periodontitis (O'Brien-Simpson, Veith et al. 2004). Many virulence factors of this pathogen include proteases (gingipains), fimbriae and hemagglutinins (Amano 2003; Veith, Chen et al. 2004;

Into, Inomata et al. 2006). *P. gingivalis* gingipains have shown to degrade extracellular matrix components such as laminin, fibronectin, and collagen type III, IV, and V *in vitro* (Potempa, Banbula et al. 2000), and are thought to account for at least 85% of the general proteolytic activity displayed by *P. gingivalis* (Imamura 2003). Our previous *in vitro* study found that the secretion of SLPI and ELAFIN was significantly reduced in response to *P. gingivalis* and that *P. gingivalis* supernatants digested recombinant SLPI, ELAFIN, SCCA1 and 2 (Figure 2) (Yin, Swanson et al. 2010). These data suggest degradation of protease inhibitors by *P. gingivalis* may result in decreased host protective capacity and higher susceptibility to *P. gingivalis* infection (Yin, Swanson et al. 2010).

As a follow-up to this *in vitro* study, an *in vivo* study from our group correlated the amount of *P. gingivalis* in subgingival plaque of patients with chronic periodontitis with the level of protease inhibitors in GCF of healthy and periodontitis patients. Significantly lower levels of SLPI and ELAFIN were detected in subjects with periodontitis and *P. gingivalis* present in their plaque compare to healthy controls (Kretschmar, Yin et al. 2011). The level of SLPI was also decreased in GCF of periodontal patients without detectable level of *P. gingivalis* in their subgingival plaque. And an inverse correlation was observed between the ELAFIN and SLPI concentrations and the number of *P. gingivalis* present in subgingival plaque. Our findings showed that host-derived protease inhibitors SLPI and ELAFIN, which are secreted as a response to environmental and microbial stimuli, are decreased in concentration in periodontal pockets with *P. gingivalis.* The reduced concentrations of these protective protease inhibitors may contribute to the loss of host defense capacity and increase susceptibility to breakdown from chronic infection.

Similarly, a separate study reported when SLPI concentrations in GCF from active periodontitis patients and periodontitis patients in maintenance were compared, SLPI was significantly reduced in the group with high amount of *P. gingivalis* (Into, Inomata et al. 2006). The proteolytic activity of *P. gingivalis* gingipain isoform RgpA is thought to be responsible for this observation (Into, Inomata et al. 2006). Although the overall bacterial load in these samples was not specified, the data from this study is in agreement with our previous study utilizing *P. gingivalis* mutant strains lacking various gingipains (Yin, Swanson et al. 2010). In addition to the role RgpA may play in the degradation of SLPI, the bacterial biofilm may also play a role in the degradation of protease inhibitors, such as increased neutrophil elastase level as a result of high bacterial load in dental plaque.

5. Epigenetic regulation and its implication on periodontal disease

Epigenetics is heritable and reversible changes in gene expression without altering DNA sequence. Chromatin structure is made up of eight histone molecules (two each of H2A, H2B, H3 and H4) and DNA which winds around these proteins. Histones are subject to a number of post-translational modifications, such as acetylation, methylation, phosphorylation and ubiquitination (Hansen, Tse et al. 1998; Strahl and Allis 2000). The mechanisms of epigenetic modifications include histone acetylation, histone methylation and DNA methylation, and these modifications provide a way to control the expression of genes involved in various cellular functions as well as in cancer (Egger, Liang et al. 2004; Rodenhiser and Mann 2006). Enzymes involved in these epigenetic mechanisms are: histone acetyltransferases (HATs); histone deacetylases (HDACs); histone methyltransferases (HMTs); and DNA methyltransferases (DNMTs) (Figure 3). Modifications on chromatin structure can occur in response to diet, inherited polymorphisms in certain genes and to environmental toxins

(Sutherland and Costa 2003; Luch 2005; Rodenhiser and Mann 2006). When histones are acetylated, transcription factors can access DNA, leading to gene transcription, while deacetylated histones lead to condensed (or closed) chromatin structure, making DNA inaccessible to transcription factors and preventing gene expression (Figure 3). In addition, methylation of cytosine residues at CpG sites in DNA inhibits binding of transcription factors, leading to gene silencing. Methylation of gene promoter region is one of the most common epigenetic mechanisms in silencing tumor suppressor genes, and over-expression of DNMTs in humans is associated with a variety of cancers (Rodenhiser and Mann 2006). Furthermore, decreased methyltransferase activity and hypo-methylated DNA have been associated with autoimmune diseases (Richardson 2003; Oelke and Richardson 2004), and changes in the histone acetylation in central nervous system has been linked to cognitive decline in a mouse model (Peleg, Sananbenesi et al. 2010). Although various epigenetic mechanisms work in concert to produce long-term and stable regulation of gene expression, not much is known on how these processes are linked and how specific patterns of epigenetic modification are inherited.
A recent study reported that oral squamous cell carcinoma showed epigenetic changes associated with SERPINE1 expression (Gao, Nielsen et al. 2010), while other studies suggest that epigenetics play a critical role in regulating inflammatory responses and that the manifestation and severity of periodontal disease may be influenced by epigenetic factors (Bobetsis, Barros et al. 2007; Offenbacher, Barros et al. 2008). Many patients with the same clinical symptoms respond differently to the same therapy, suggesting the inter-individual variability observed as a clinical outcome of the disease is influenced by genetic (Schenkein 2002; Feinberg 2007) as well as epigenetic factors (Offenbacher, Barros et al. 2008). Epigenetic modifications alter patterns of gene expression, which in turn leads to various clinical outcomes. Furthermore, variations in epigenetic status will likely elicit diverse inflammatory responses. A new study from our group focused on finding answers to how epigenetic modifications brought on by exposure to oral bacteria, including periodontal pathogens, affect host innate immune responses and susceptibility to subsequent infections (Yin and Chung 2011).

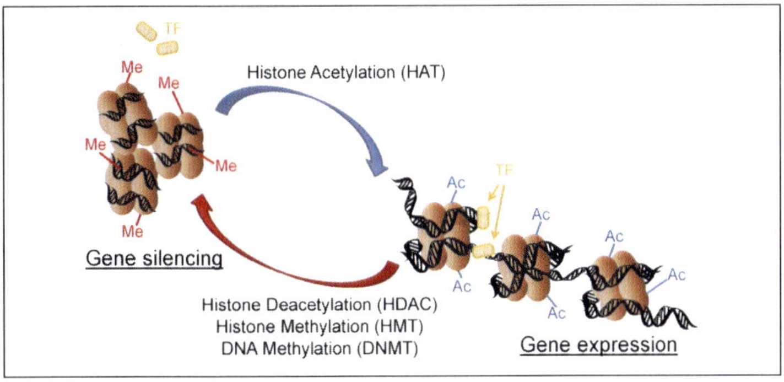

Fig. 3. Histone acetylation allows open chromatic structure, and transcription factors can access DNA. Deacetylation of histones as well as histone methylation and DNA methylation result in closed chromatin, thus transcription factors cannot access DNA, which results in gene silencing. Epigenetic modifications of histones and/or DNA via methylation lead to altered gene expression. TF: transcription factors; Ac: acetylation; Me: methylation; HAT: histone acetyltransferase; HDAC: histone deacetylase; HMT: histone methyltransferase; DNMT: DNA methyltransferase.

When any changes in the expression levels of enzymes involved in the epigenetic modification after GECs were exposed to oral bacteria were investigated, we found the expression of histone deacetylases and DNA methyltransferase changed in response to the presence of oral bacteria. Histone deacetylases (HDACs) remove acetyl groups from histone, leading to suppression of genes, while DNA methyltransferases (DNMTs) catalyze transfer of methyl groups onto DNA, which also leads to gene suppression (Figure 3). Quantitative real-time PCR analyses showed changes in the expression levels of these genes when GECs were treated with *P. gingivalis* or *F. nucleatum* at various multiplicities of infection for 1, 4, 24 and 48 h. The gene expression levels of DNMT1, HDAC1 and HDAC2 decreased in GECs treated with *P. gingivalis* or *F. nucleatum*, although the levels of decrease differed between bacterial species and/or exposure time (Yin and Chung 2011). As changes in the expression of enzymes catalyzing epigenetic modifications were observed, it was also of interest to note the changes in methylation levels of various genes in GECs after the cells were exposed to these oral bacteria. Studies utilizing methylation PCR Array showed a dose-dependent and statistically significant increase in methylation levels of the following genes after GECs were exposed to *P. gingivalis*: CD276, an immune regulator; elastase 2, a serine protease that plays a role in inflammatory diseases; INHBA, a tumor-suppressing protein; GATA 3, a putative tumor suppressor; TLR2; and IL-12A. Stimulation of GECs with *P. gingivalis* also resulted in hypo-methylation of ZNF287, a member of Zinc finger protein family. The up-regulation of Zinc finger proteins has been associated with cardiovascular disease (Dai and Liew 1999), thus this observation is in line with recent studies linking periodontal disease with increased risk of systemic disease (Persson and Persson 2008). GECs exposed to *P. gingivalis* also showed a decrease in the methylation of STAT5A, which mediates cellular responses to cytokines IL-2, IL-3, IL-7, GM-CSF and plays a role in progression of tumors. On the other hand, the methylation levels of elastase 2 and GATA3 decreased significantly after cells were stimulated with *F. nucleatum* (Yin and Chung 2011). Interestingly, only *F. nucleatum* induced hyper-methylation of MALT1 (Mucosa-associated lymphoid tissue lymphoma translocation gene) in GECs. MALT1 induces IKK catalytic activity, resulting in NFκB activation in immune cells (Schulze-Luehrmann and Ghosh 2006). The methylation of MALT1 is associated with silencing of MALT1 gene, which is consistent with our previous reports that *F. nucleatum* does not utilize the NFκB signaling pathway in the induction of innate immune responses (Chung and Dale 2004; Chung and Dale 2008). Taken together, these data suggest that epigenetic modification of genes, whose function is associated with growth control and inflammation, is differentially regulated by different oral bacteria (Yin and Chung 2011).

Modulations of chromatin structure play an important role in the regulation of transcription, and these modifications directly affect the accessibility of chromatin to transcription factors, thus on gene expression. When the changes in histone H3 level in GECs after exposure to periopathogen vs. non-pathogen were examined, the endogenous level of histone H3 that is tri-methylated at Lys4 was significantly decreased following stimulated with *P. gingivalis* compared to unstimulated control, while the level increased after exposure to *F. nucleatum* (Yin and Chung 2011). Our data suggest these two bacterial species, pathogen vs. non-pathogen, differentially regulate H3K4 methylation and further suggest bacterial infection in oral epithelia is associated with changes in H3K4 methylation (Yin and Chung 2011).

Gene promoter methylation is the most common epigenetic mechanism silencing tumor suppressor genes during oncogenesis. Almost all cancer-related signaling pathways are affected by methylation, and the number of genes affected in each major type of cancer is still rapidly growing. However, even the most relevant genes have not yet been correlated to individual cancer types for development of DNA methylation biomarkers. Recent studies reported that particular histone modifications are correlated with certain types of cancers and that histone modifications will be useful biomarkers for cancer (Su, Lucas et al. 2009; Manuyakorn, Paulus et al. 2010; Svotelis, Gevry et al. 2010). Since our recent data strongly suggest presence of oral bacteria affects chromatin modification in GECs, it is plausible periodontal patients with high number of periodontal pathogens recovered from the oral cavity will show altered chromatin modifications. Further studies are needed to identify epigenetic factors involved in development and pathogenesis of periodontitis, contributing to better defining of epigenetic modifications as an indicator of periodontal disease. It would be of importance in a periodontal treatment plan to identify a certain species of bacteria which induce epigenetic changes and subsequently modify host responses. Furthermore, better understanding of specific bacteria that show capacity to induce epigenetic changes would be of importance in developing specific therapeutic strategies for each patient.

6. Conclusion

Periodontitis is a disease that is not only caused by one single bacterium, but by a number of different bacterial species, organized in a complex biofilm and thereby exhibiting various properties. Understanding how gingival epithelia response to the presence of different commensals and pathogens, leading to induction of appropriate innate immune responses, will provide significant new insights into this complex biological system in the oral epithelia. Furthermore, better understanding the role of other factors influencing periodontal health, such as the balance between proteases and protease inhibitors, and the role epigenetic status plays in health and disease, will have direct implications for new understanding of oral innate immune responses and the development of potential new and innovative therapeutic interventions for periodontal disease.

7. Acknowledgments

Supported by NIH/NIDCR grants R01 DE013573 and DE19632

8. References

Alkemade, J. A., H. O. Molhuizen, et al. (1994). "SKALP/elafin is an inducible proteinase inhibitor in human epidermal keratinocytes." J Cell Sci 107 (Pt 8): 2335-42.

Altman, H., D. Steinberg, et al. (2006). "In vitro assessment of antimicrobial peptides as potential agents against several oral bacteria." J Antimicrob Chemother 58(1): 198-201.

Amano, A. (2003). "Molecular interaction of Porphyromonas gingivalis with host cells: implication for the microbial pathogenesis of periodontal disease." J Periodontol 74(1): 90-6.

Ardila, C. M., M. I. Granada, et al. (2010). "Antibiotic resistance of subgingival species in chronic periodontitis patients." J Periodontal Res 45(4): 557-63.

Armitage, G. C. (1999). "Development of a classification system for periodontal diseases and conditions." Ann Periodontol 4(1): 1-6.

Bachrach, G., G. Rosen, et al. (2004). "Identification of a Fusobacterium nucleatum 65 kDa serine protease." Oral Microbiol Immunol 19(3): 155-9.

Bals, R., D. J. Weiner, et al. (1999). "Transfer of a cathelicidin peptide antibiotic gene restores bacterial killing in a cystic fibrosis xenograft model." J Clin Invest 103(8): 1113-7.

Bals, R. and J. M. Wilson (2003). "Cathelicidins--a family of multifunctional antimicrobial peptides." Cell Mol Life Sci 60(4): 711-20.

Beckloff, N., D. Laube, et al. (2007). "Activity of an antimicrobial peptide mimetic against planktonic and biofilm cultures of oral pathogens." Antimicrob Agents Chemother 51(11): 4125-32.

Bissell, J., S. Joly, et al. (2004). "Expression of beta-defensins in gingival health and in periodontal disease." J Oral Pathol Med 33(5): 278-85.

Bobetsis, Y. A., S. P. Barros, et al. (2007). "Bacterial infection promotes DNA hypermethylation." J Dent Res 86(2): 169-74.

Brancatisano, F. L., G. Maisetta, et al. (2011). "Reduced human beta defensin 3 in individuals with periodontal disease." J Dent Res 90(2): 241-5.

Buduneli, N., H. Baylas, et al. (2005). "Periodontal infections and pre-term low birth weight: a case-control study." J Clin Periodontol 32(2): 174-81.

Carlsson, G., Y. B. Wahlin, et al. (2006). "Periodontal disease in patients from the original Kostmann family with severe congenital neutropenia." J Periodontol 77(4): 744-51.

Cataltepe, S., E. R. Gornstein, et al. (2000). "Co-expression of the squamous cell carcinoma antigens 1 and 2 in normal adult human tissues and squamous cell carcinomas." J Histochem Cytochem 48(1): 113-22.

Chung, W. O. and B. A. Dale (2004). "Innate immune response of oral and foreskin keratinocytes: utilization of different signaling pathways by various bacterial species." Infect Immun 72(1): 352-8.

Chung, W. O. and B. A. Dale (2008). "Differential utilization of nuclear factor-kappaB signaling pathways for gingival epithelial cell responses to oral commensal and pathogenic bacteria." Oral Microbiol Immunol 23(2): 119-26.

Chung, W. O., D. R. Demuth, et al. (2000). "Identification of a Porphyromonas gingivalis receptor for the Streptococcus gordonii SspB protein." Infect Immun 68(12): 6758-62.

Chung, W. O., H. Dommisch, et al. (2007). "Expression of defensins in gingiva and their role in periodontal health and disease." Curr Pharm Des 13(30): 3073-83.

Chung, W. O., S. R. Hansen, et al. (2004). "Protease-activated receptor signaling increases epithelial antimicrobial peptide expression." J Immunol 173(8): 5165-70.

Cole, A. M., P. Dewan, T. Ganz (1999). "Innate antimicrobial activity of nasal secretions." Infect Immun 67: 3267-3275.

Crawford, J. M., J. M. Wilton, et al. (2000). "Neutrophils die in the gingival crevice, periodontal pocket, and oral cavity by necrosis and not apoptosis." J Periodontol 71(7): 1121-9.

Cunliffe, R. N. (2003). "Alpha-defensins in the gastrointestinal tract." Mol Immunol 40(7): 463-7.

Dai, K. S. and C. C. Liew (1999). "Chromosomal, in silico and in vitro expression analysis of cardiovascular-based genes encoding zinc finger proteins." J Mol Cell Cardiol 31(9): 1749-69.

Dale, B. A. (2002). "Periodontal epithelium: a newly recognized role in health and disease." Periodontol 2000 30: 70-8.
Dale, B. A. and L. P. Fredericks (2005). Antimicrobial Peptides in the Oral Environment. Antimicrobial Peptides in Human Health and Disease. R. M. Gallo. San Diego, Horizon Bioscience: 223-252.
Dale, B. A. and L. P. Fredericks (2005). "Antimicrobial peptides in the oral environment: expression and function in health and disease." Curr Issues Mol Biol 7(2): 119-33.
Dale, B. A., J. R. Kimball, et al. (2001). "Localized antimicrobial peptide expression in human gingiva." J Periodontal Res 36(5): 285-94.
Diamond, D. L., J. R. Kimball, et al. (2001). "Detection of beta-defensins secreted by human oral epithelial cells." J Immunol Methods 256(1-2): 65-76.
Diamond, G., J. P. Russell, et al. (1996). "Inducible expression of an antibiotic peptide gene in lipopolysaccharide-challenged tracheal epithelial cells." Proc Natl Acad Sci U S A 93(10): 5156-60.
Dommisch, H., Y. Acil, et al. (2005). "Differential gene expression of human beta-defensins (hBD-1, -2, -3) in inflammatory gingival diseases." Oral Microbiol Immunol 20(3): 186-90.
Dommisch, H., W. O. Chung, et al. (2007). "Protease-activated receptor 2 mediates human beta-defensin 2 and CC chemokine ligand 20 mRNA expression in response to proteases secreted by Porphyromonas gingivalis." Infect Immun 75(9): 4326-33.
Dunsche, A., Y. Acil, et al. (2002). "The novel human beta-defensin-3 is widely expressed in oral tissues." Eur J Oral Sci 110(2): 121-4.
Egger, G., G. Liang, et al. (2004). "Epigenetics in human disease and prospects for epigenetic therapy." Nature 429(6990): 457-63.
Feinberg, A. P. (2007). "Phenotypic plasticity and the epigenetics of human disease." Nature 447(7143): 433-40.
Fenno, J. C., S. Y. Lee, et al. (2001). "The opdB locus encodes the trypsin-like peptidase activity of Treponema denticola." Infect Immun 69(10): 6193-200.
Feucht, E. C., C. L. DeSanti, et al. (2003). "Selective induction of human beta-defensin mRNAs by Actinobacillus actinomycetemcomitans in primary and immortalized oral epithelial cells." Oral Microbiol Immunol 18(6): 359-63.
Frohm, M., B. Agerberth, et al. (1997). "The expression of the gene coding for the antibacterial peptide LL-37 is induced in human keratinocytes during inflammatory disorders." J Biol Chem 272(24): 15258-63.
Frohm Nilsson, M., B. Sandstedt, et al. (1999). "The human cationic antimicrobial protein (hCAP18), a peptide antibiotic, is widely expressed in human squamous epithelia and colocalizes with interleukin-6." Infect Immun 67(5): 2561-6.
Ganz, T. and R. I. Lehrer (1994). "Defensins." Curr Opin Immunol 6(4): 584-9.
Ganz, T. and R. I. Lehrer (1999). "Antibiotic peptides from higher eukaryotes: biology and applications." Mol Med Today 5(7): 292-7.
Ganz, T., J. A. Metcalf, et al. (1988). "Microbicidal/cytotoxic proteins of neutrophils are deficient in two disorders: Chediak-Higashi syndrome and "specific" granule deficiency." J Clin Invest 82(2): 552-6.
Ganz, T., M. E. Selsted, et al. (1985). "Defensins. Natural peptide antibiotics of human neutrophils." J Clin Invest 76(4): 1427-35.

Gao, S., B. S. Nielsen, et al. (2010). "Epigenetic alterations of the SERPINE1 gene in oral squamous cell carcinomas and normal oral mucosa." Genes Chromosomes Cancer 49(6): 526-38.

Giannopoulou, C., R. Di Felice, et al. (1990). "Synthesis of alpha 2-macroglobulin in human gingiva: a study of the concentration of macroglobulin and albumin in gingival fluid and serum." Arch Oral Biol 35(1): 13-6.

Gomez-Garces, J. L., J. I. Alos, et al. (1994). "Bacteremia by multidrug-resistant Capnocytophaga sputigena." J Clin Microbiol 32(4): 1067-9.

Guyot, N., M. W. Butler, et al. (2008). "Elafin, an elastase specific inhibitor, is cleaved by its cognate enzyme neutrophil elastase in sputum from individuals with cystic fibrosis." J Biol Chem.

Haffajee, A. D. and S. S. Socransky (1994). "Microbial etiological agents of destructive periodontal diseases." Periodontol 2000 5: 78-111.

Hancock, R. E. and D. S. Chapple (1999). "Peptide antibiotics." Antimicrob Agents Chemother 43(6): 1317-23.

Hancock, R. E. and G. Diamond (2000). "The role of cationic antimicrobial peptides in innate host defences." Trends Microbiol 8(9): 402-10.

Hancock, R. E. and M. G. Scott (2000). "The role of antimicrobial peptides in animal defenses." Proc Natl Acad Sci U S A 97(16): 8856-61.

Handal, T., D. A. Caugant, et al. (2003). "Antibiotic resistance in bacteria isolated from subgingival plaque in a norwegian population with refractory marginal periodontitis." Antimicrob Agents Chemother 47(4): 1443-6.

Hansen, J. C., C. Tse, et al. (1998). "Structure and function of the core histone N-termini: more than meets the eye." Biochemistry 37(51): 17637-41.

Holzhausen, M., L. C. Spolidorio, et al. (2006). "Protease-activated receptor-2 activation: a major role in the pathogenesis of Porphyromonas gingivalis infection." Am J Pathol 168(4): 1189-99.

Hosokawa, I., Y. Hosokawa, et al. (2006). "Innate immune peptide LL-37 displays distinct expression pattern from beta-defensins in inflamed gingival tissue." Clin Exp Immunol 146(2): 218-25.

Howell, M. D. (2007). "The role of human beta defensins and cathelicidins in atopic dermatitis." Curr Opin Allergy Clin Immunol 7(5): 413-7.

Hua, J., R. W. Scott, et al. (2010). "Activity of antimicrobial peptide mimetics in the oral cavity: II. Activity against periopathogenic biofilms and anti-inflammatory activity." Mol Oral Microbiol 25(6): 426-32.

Imamura, T. (2003). "The role of gingipains in the pathogenesis of periodontal disease." J Periodontol 74(1): 111-8.

Into, T., M. Inomata, et al. (2006). "Arginine-specific gingipains from Porphyromonas gingivalis deprive protective functions of secretory leucocyte protease inhibitor in periodontal tissue." Clin Exp Immunol 145(3): 545-54.

Juarez, Z. E. and M. W. Stinson (1999). "An extracellular protease of Streptococcus gordonii hydrolyzes type IV collagen and collagen analogues." Infect Immun 67(1): 271-8.

Kinane, D. and P. Bouchard (2008). "Periodontal diseases and health: Consensus Report of the Sixth European Workshop on Periodontology." J Clin Periodontol 35(8 Suppl): 333-7.

Kinane, D. F. and T. C. Hart (2003). "Genes and gene polymorphisms associated with periodontal disease." Crit Rev Oral Biol Med 14(6): 430-49.

King, A. E., N. Wheelhouse, et al. (2009). "Expression of secretory leukocyte protease inhibitor and elafin in human fallopian tube and in an in-vitro model of Chlamydia trachomatis infection." Hum Reprod 24(3): 679-86.

Kisich, K. O., L. Heifets, et al. (2001). "Antimycobacterial agent based on mRNA encoding human beta-defensin 2 enables primary macrophages to restrict growth of Mycobacterium tuberculosis." Infect Immun 69(4): 2692-9.

Kohlgraf, K. G., A. Ackermann, et al. (2010). "Defensins attenuate cytokine responses yet enhance antibody responses to Porphyromonas gingivalis adhesins in mice." Future Microbiol 5(1): 115-25.

Kolenbrander, P. E., R. N. Andersen, et al. (2002). "Communication among oral bacteria." Microbiol Mol Biol Rev 66(3): 486-505, table of contents.

Kretschmar, S., L. Yin, et al. (2011). "Protease inhibitor levels in periodontal health and disease." J Perio Res, In press.

Krisanaprakornkit, S., J. R. Kimball, et al. (2002). "Regulation of human beta-defensin-2 in gingival epithelial cells: the involvement of mitogen-activated protein kinase pathways, but not the NF-kappaB transcription factor family." J Immunol 168(1): 316-24.

Krisanaprakornkit, S., J. R. Kimball, et al. (2000). "Inducible expression of human beta-defensin 2 by Fusobacterium nucleatum in oral epithelial cells: multiple signaling pathways and role of commensal bacteria in innate immunity and the epithelial barrier." Infect Immun 68(5): 2907-15.

Krisanaprakornkit, S., A. Weinberg, et al. (1998). "Expression of the peptide antibiotic human beta-defensin 1 in cultured gingival epithelial cells and gingival tissue." Infect Immun 66(9): 4222-8.

Lehrer, R. I. and T. Ganz (2002). "Defensins of vertebrate animals." Curr Opin Immunol 14(1): 96-102.

Lehrer, R. I., A. K. Lichtenstein, et al. (1993). "Defensins: antimicrobial and cytotoxic peptides of mammalian cells." Annu Rev Immunol 11: 105-28.

Loos, B. G., R. P. John, et al. (2005). "Identification of genetic risk factors for periodontitis and possible mechanisms of action." J Clin Periodontol 32 Suppl 6: 159-79.

Lourbakos, A., J. Potempa, et al. (2001). "Arginine-specific protease from Porphyromonas gingivalis activates protease-activated receptors on human oral epithelial cells and induces interleukin-6 secretion." Infect Immun 69(8): 5121-30.

Lu, Q., L. Jin, et al. (2004). "Expression of human beta-defensins-1 and -2 peptides in unresolved chronic periodontitis." J Periodontal Res 39(4): 221-7.

Lu, Q., L. P. Samaranayake, et al. (2005). "Expression of human beta-defensin-3 in gingival epithelia." J Periodontal Res 40(6): 474-81.

Luch, A. (2005). "Nature and nurture - lessons from chemical carcinogenesis." Nat Rev Cancer 5(2): 113-25.

Maestre, J. R., A. Bascones, et al. (2007). "Odontogenic bacteria in periodontal disease and resistance patterns to common antibiotics used as treatment and prophylaxis in odontology in Spain." Rev Esp Quimioter 20(1): 61-7.

Magert, H. J., K. Drogemuller, et al. (2005). "Serine proteinase inhibitors in the skin: role in homeostasis and disease." Curr Protein Pept Sci 6(3): 241-54.

Maisetta, G., G. Batoni, et al. (2003). "Activity of human beta-defensin 3 alone or combined with other antimicrobial agents against oral bacteria." Antimicrob Agents Chemother 47(10): 3349-51.

Manuyakorn, A., R. Paulus, et al. (2010). "Cellular histone modification patterns predict prognosis and treatment response in resectable pancreatic adenocarcinoma: results from RTOG 9704." J Clin Oncol 28(8): 1358-65.

McKay, M. S., E. Olson, et al. (1999). "Immunomagnetic recovery of human neutrophil defensins from the human gingival crevice." Oral Microbiol Immunol 14(3): 190-3.

McMichael, J. W., A. I. Maxwell, et al. (2005). "Antimicrobial activity of murine lung cells against Staphylococcus aureus is increased in vitro and in vivo after elafin gene transfer." Infect Immun 73(6): 3609-17.

Meyer-Hoffert, U., N. Wichmann, et al. (2003). "Supernatants of Pseudomonas aeruginosa induce the Pseudomonas-specific antibiotic elafin in human keratinocytes." Exp Dermatol 12(4): 418-25.

Michalowicz, B. S., D. Aeppli, et al. (1991). "Periodontal findings in adult twins." J Periodontol 62(5): 293-9.

Michalowicz, B. S., S. R. Diehl, et al. (2000). "Evidence of a substantial genetic basis for risk of adult periodontitis." J Periodontol 71(11): 1699-707.

Minami, M. (1999). "The levels of secretory leukocyte protease inhibitor and alpha 1-protease inhibitor in gingival crevicular fluid from adult periodontal patients." J Jpn Soc Periodontol 41: 28-35.

Mitsuishi, K., T. Nakamura, et al. (2005). "The squamous cell carcinoma antigens as relevant biomarkers of atopic dermatitis." Clin Exp Allergy 35(10): 1327-33.

Miyasaki, K. T., A. L. Bodeau, et al. (1990). "In vitro sensitivity of oral, gram-negative, facultative bacteria to the bactericidal activity of human neutrophil defensins." Infect Immun 58(12): 3934-40.

Molhuizen, H. O. and J. Schalkwijk (1995). "Structural, biochemical, and cell biological aspects of the serine proteinase inhibitor SKALP/elafin/ESI." Biol Chem Hoppe Seyler 376(1): 1-7.

Murakami, M., T. Ohtake, et al. (2002). "Cathelicidin antimicrobial peptides are expressed in salivary glands and saliva." J Dent Res 81(12): 845-50.

Nathan, C. (2006). "Neutrophils and immunity: challenges and opportunities." Nat Rev Immunol 6(3): 173-82.

Nussbaum, G. and L. Shapira (2011). "How has neutrophil research improved our understanding of periodontal pathogenesis?" J Clin Periodontol 38 Suppl 11: 49-59.

O'Brien-Simpson, N. M., P. D. Veith, et al. (2004). "Antigens of bacteria associated with periodontitis." Periodontol 2000 35: 101-34.

Oelke, K. and B. Richardson (2004). "Decreased T cell ERK pathway signaling may contribute to the development of lupus through effects on DNA methylation and gene expression." Int Rev Immunol 23(3-4): 315-31.

Offenbacher, S., S. P. Barros, et al. (2008). "Rethinking periodontal inflammation." J Periodontol 79(8 Suppl): 1577-84.

Offenbacher, S., V. Katz, et al. (1996). "Periodontal infection as a possible risk factor for preterm low birth weight." J Periodontol 67(10 Suppl): 1103-13.

Ouellette, A. J. (1999). "Paneth cell antimicrobial peptides and the biology of the mucosal barrier." American Journal of Physiology 277: G257-261.

Ouhara, K., H. Komatsuzawa, et al. (2005). "Susceptibilities of periodontopathogenic and cariogenic bacteria to antibacterial peptides, {beta}-defensins and LL37, produced by human epithelial cells." J Antimicrob Chemother 55(6): 888-96.

Payne, J. B., L. M. Golub, et al. (2011). "The effect of subantimicrobial-dose-doxycycline periodontal therapy on serum biomarkers of systemic inflammation: a randomized, double-masked, placebo-controlled clinical trial." J Am Dent Assoc 142(3): 262-73.

Peleg, S., F. Sananbenesi, et al. (2010). "Altered histone acetylation is associated with age-dependent memory impairment in mice." Science 328(5979): 753-756.

Persson, G. R. and R. E. Persson (2008). "Cardiovascular disease and periodontitis: an update on the associations and risk." J Clin Periodontol 35(8 Suppl): 362-79.

Peters, B. M., M. E. Shirtliff, et al. (2010). "Antimicrobial peptides: primeval molecules or future drugs?" PLoS Pathog 6(10): e1001067.

Pfundt, R., F. van Ruissen, et al. (1996). "Constitutive and inducible expression of SKALP/elafin provides anti-elastase defense in human epithelia." J Clin Invest 98(6): 1389-99.

Potempa, J., A. Banbula, et al. (2000). "Role of bacterial proteinases in matrix destruction and modulation of host responses." Periodontol 2000 24: 153-92.

Potempa, J., R. Pike, et al. (1995). "The multiple forms of trypsin-like activity present in various strains of Porphyromonas gingivalis are due to the presence of either Arg-gingipain or Lys-gingipain." Infect Immun 63(4): 1176-82.

Potempa, J. and J. Travis (1996). "Porphyromonas gingivalis proteinases in periodontitis, a review." Acta Biochim Pol 43(3): 455-65.

Premratanachai, P., S. Joly, et al. (2004). "Expression and regulation of novel human beta-defensins in gingival keratinocytes." Oral Microbiol Immunol 19(2): 111-7.

Puklo, M., A. Guentsch, et al. (2008). "Analysis of neutrophil-derived antimicrobial peptides in gingival crevicular fluid suggests importance of cathelicidin LL-37 in the innate immune response against periodontogenic bacteria." Oral Microbiol Immunol 23(4): 328-35.

Putsep, K., G. Carlsson, et al. (2002). "Deficiency of antibacterial peptides in patients with morbus Kostmann: an observation study." Lancet 360(9340): 1144-9.

Raj, P. A., K. J. Antonyraj, et al. (2000). "Large-scale synthesis and functional elements for the antimicrobial activity of defensins." Biochem J 347 Pt 3: 633-41.

Richardson, B. (2003). "DNA methylation and autoimmune disease." Clin Immunol 109(1): 72-9.

Rickard, A. H., P. Gilbert, et al. (2003). "Bacterial coaggregation: an integral process in the development of multi-species biofilms." Trends Microbiol 11(2): 94-100.

Rock, F. L., G. Hardiman, J.C. Timans, R.A. Kastelein, J.F. Bazan (1998). "A family of human receptors structurally related to Drosophila Toll." Proc Natl Acad Sci U S A 95: 588-593.

Rodenhiser, D. and M. Mann (2006). "Epigenetics and human disease: translating basic biology into clinical applications." CMAJ 174(3): 341-8.

Sahasrabudhe, K. S., J.R. Kimball, T. Morton, W. Weinberg, B.A. Dale (2000). "Expression of the antimicrobial peptide, human b-defensin 1, in duct cells of minor salivary glands and detection in saliva." Journal of Dental Research 79: 1669-1674.

Sallenave, J. M., G. A. Cunningham, et al. (2003). "Regulation of pulmonary and systemic bacterial lipopolysaccharide responses in transgenic mice expressing human elafin." Infect Immun 71(7): 3766-74.

Schenkein, H. A. (2002). "Finding genetic risk factors for periodontal diseases: is the climb worth the view?" Periodontol 2000 30: 79-90.

Schroeder, B. O., Z. Wu, et al. (2011). "Reduction of disulphide bonds unmasks potent antimicrobial activity of human beta-defensin 1." Nature 469(7330): 419-23.

Schulze-Luehrmann, J. and S. Ghosh (2006). "Antigen-receptor signaling to nuclear factor kappa B." Immunity 25(5): 701-15.

Selsted, M. E. and A. J. Ouellette (2005). "Mammalian defensins in the antimicrobial immune response." Nat Immunol 6(6): 551-7.

Selsted, M. E., S.I. Miller, A.H. Henschen, A.J. Ouellette (1992). "Enteric defensins: antibiotic peptide components of intestinal host defense." Journal of Cell Biology 118: 929-936.

Shin, J. E., Y. S. Kim, et al. (2010). "Treponema denticola suppresses expression of human {beta}-defensin-3 in gingival epithelial cells through inhibition of the toll-like receptor 2 axis." Infect Immun 78(2): 672-9.

Silverman, G. A., P. I. Bird, et al. (2001). "The serpins are an expanding superfamily of structurally similar but functionally diverse proteins. Evolution, mechanism of inhibition, novel functions, and a revised nomenclature." J Biol Chem 276(36): 33293-6.

Simpson, A. J., A. I. Maxwell, et al. (1999). "Elafin (elastase-specific inhibitor) has anti-microbial activity against gram-positive and gram-negative respiratory pathogens." FEBS Lett 452(3): 309-13.

Socransky, S. S. and A. Haffajee (2003). Microbiology of periodontal disease. Clin Periodontol Implant Dent. J. Lindhe. Oxford, Blackwell.

Socransky, S. S. and A. D. Haffajee (1992). "The bacterial etiology of destructive periodontal disease: current concepts." J Periodontol 63(4 Suppl): 322-31.

Socransky, S. S. and A. D. Haffajee (2003). Microbiology of periodontal disease. Clin Periodontol Implant Dent. J. Lindhe. Oxford, Blackwell. 4.

Socransky, S. S. and A. D. Haffajee (2005). "Periodontal microbial ecology." Periodontol 2000 38: 135-87.

Socransky, S. S., A. D. Haffajee, et al. (1998). "Microbial complexes in subgingival plaque." J Clin Periodontol 25(2): 134-44.

Socransky, S. S., C. Smith, et al. (2002). "Subgingival microbial profiles in refractory periodontal disease." J Clin Periodontol 29(3): 260-8.

Som, A., S. Vemparala, et al. (2008). "Synthetic mimics of antimicrobial peptides." Biopolymers 90(2): 83-93.

Strahl, B. D. and C. D. Allis (2000). "The language of covalent histone modifications." Nature 403(6765): 41-5.

Su, X., D. M. Lucas, et al. (2009). "Validation of an LC-MS based approach for profiling histones in chronic lymphocytic leukemia." Proteomics 9(5): 1197-206.

Sugawara, S., A. Uehara, et al. (2001). "Neutrophil proteinase 3-mediated induction of bioactive IL-18 secretion by human oral epithelial cells." J Immunol 167(11): 6568-75.

Sutherland, J. E. and M. Costa (2003). "Epigenetics and the environment." Ann N Y Acad Sci 983: 151-60.

Svotelis, A., N. Gevry, et al. (2010). "H2A.Z overexpression promotes cellular proliferation of breast cancer cells." Cell Cycle 9(2): 364-70.

Tao, R., R. J. Jurevic, et al. (2005). "Salivary antimicrobial peptide expression and dental caries experience in children." Antimicrob Agents Chemother 49(9): 3883-8.

Tew, G. N., D. Clements, et al. (2006). "Antimicrobial activity of an abiotic host defense peptide mimic." Biochim Biophys Acta 1758(9): 1387-92.

Tew, G. N., D. Liu, et al. (2002). "De novo design of biomimetic antimicrobial polymers." Proc Natl Acad Sci U S A 99(8): 5110-4.

Tonetti, M. S., M. A. Imboden, et al. (1994). "Localized expression of mRNA for phagocyte-specific chemotactic cytokines in human periodontal infections." Infect Immun 62(9): 4005-14.

Tonetti, M. S., M. A. Imboden, et al. (1998). "Neutrophil migration into the gingival sulcus is associated with transepithelial gradients of interleukin-8 and ICAM-1." J Periodontol 69(10): 1139-47.

Turkoglu, O., G. Emingil, et al. (2009). "Gingival crevicular fluid levels of cathelicidin LL-37 and interleukin-18 in patients with chronic periodontitis." J Periodontol 80(6): 969-76.

Turkoglu, O., G. Kandiloglu, et al. (2011). "Antimicrobial peptide hCAP-18/LL-37 protein and mRNA expressions in different periodontal diseases." Oral Dis 17(1): 60-7.

Tuter, G., B. Kurtis, et al. (2007). "Effects of scaling and root planing and sub-antimicrobial dose doxycycline on oral and systemic biomarkers of disease in patients with both chronic periodontitis and coronary artery disease." J Clin Periodontol 34(8): 673-81.

Uehara, A., K. Muramoto, et al. (2003). "Neutrophil serine proteinases activate human nonepithelial cells to produce inflammatory cytokines through protease-activated receptor 2." J Immunol 170(11): 5690-6.

Valore, E. V., C. H. Park, et al. (1998). "Human beta-defensin-1: an antimicrobial peptide of urogenital tissues." J Clin Invest 101(8): 1633-42.

van der Reijden, W. A., C. J. Bosch-Tijhof, et al. (2006). "prtH in Tannerella forsythensis is not associated with periodontitis." J Periodontol 77(4): 586-90.

van Wetering, S., P. J. Sterk, et al. (1999). "Defensins: key players or bystanders in infection, injury, and repair in the lung?" J Allergy Clin Immunol 104(6): 1131-8.

van Wetering, S., A. C. van der Linden, et al. (2000). "Regulation of SLPI and elafin release from bronchial epithelial cells by neutrophil defensins." Am J Physiol Lung Cell Mol Physiol 278(1): L51-8.

van Winkelhoff, A. J., D. Herrera Gonzales, et al. (2000). "Antimicrobial resistance in the subgingival microflora in patients with adult periodontitis. A comparison between The Netherlands and Spain." J Clin Periodontol 27(2): 79-86.

Vardar-Sengul, S., T. Demirci, et al. (2007). "Human beta defensin-1 and -2 expression in the gingiva of patients with specific periodontal diseases." J Periodontal Res 42(5): 429-37.

Veith, P. D., Y. Y. Chen, et al. (2004). "Porphyromonas gingivalis RgpA and Kgp proteinases and adhesins are C terminally processed by the carboxypeptidase CPG70." Infect Immun 72(6): 3655-7.

Williams, S. E., T. I. Brown, et al. (2006). "SLPI and elafin: one glove, many fingers." Clin Sci (Lond) 110(1): 21-35.

Wilmes, M., B. P. Cammue, et al. (2011). "Antibiotic activities of host defense peptides: more to it than lipid bilayer perturbation." Natural Product Reports May 27 E-published ahead of print.

Wilson, C. L., A. J. Ouellette, et al. (1999). "Regulation of intestinal alpha-defensin activation by the metalloproteinase matrilysin in innate host defense." Science 286(5437): 113-7.

Yin, L. and W. O. Chung (2011). "Epigenetic regulation of human beta-defensin 2 and CC chemokine ligand 20 expression in gingival epithelial cells in response to oral bacteria." Mucosal Immunol 4(4): 409-19.

Yin, L. and B. A. Dale (2007). "Activation of protective responses in oral epithelial cells by Fusobacterium nucleatum and human beta-defensin-2." J Med Microbiol 56(Pt 7): 976-87.

Yin, L., B. Swanson, et al. (2010). "Differential effects of periopathogens on host protease inhibitors SLPI, elafin, SCCA1, and SCCA2." Journal of Oral Microbiology Epub May 4.

Ying, Q. L. and S. R. Simon (1993). "Kinetics of the inhibition of human leukocyte elastase by elafin, a 6-kilodalton elastase-specific inhibitor from human skin." Biochemistry 32(7): 1866-74.

Yuyama, N., D. E. Davies, et al. (2002). "Analysis of novel disease-related genes in bronchial asthma." Cytokine 19(6): 287-96.

Zaiou, M., V. Nizet, et al. (2003). "Antimicrobial and protease inhibitory functions of the human cathelicidin (hCAP18/LL-37) prosequence." J Invest Dermatol 120(5): 810-6.

Zanetti, M., R. Gennaro, et al. (2000). "Structure and biology of cathelicidins." Adv Exp Med Biol 479: 203-18.

Zani, M. L., S. M. Nobar, et al. (2004). "Kinetics of the inhibition of neutrophil proteinases by recombinant elafin and pre-elafin (trappin-2) expressed in Pichia pastoris." Eur J Biochem 271(12): 2370-8.

Zasloff, M. (2002). "Antimicrobial peptides of multicellular organisms." Nature 415(6870): 389-95.

Zhao, C., I. Wang, et al. (1996). "Widespread expression of beta-defensin hBD-1 in human secretory glands and epithelial cells." FEBS Lett 396(2-3): 319-22.

Zhong, D., M. Yang, et al. (1998). "[In vitro sensitivity of oral gram-negative bacteria to the bactericidal activity of defensins]." Hua Xi Kou Qiang Yi Xue Za Zhi 16(1): 26-8.

5

Effects of Smoking and Smoking Cessation and Smoking Cessation Intervention

T. Hanioka[1], M. Ojima[2] and M. Nakamura[3]
[1]*Fukuoka Dental College,*
[2]*Graduate School of Dentistry, Osaka University,*
[3]*Osaka Medical Centre for Health Science and Promotion,*
Japan

1. Introduction

The three- to four-decade lag between peak in smoking prevalence and subsequent peak in smoking-related mortality was a major factor affecting public awareness of the substantial health hazards of tobacco use in developed countries (Lopez et al., 1994). This factor may be applicable to periodontal disease if this disease is chronically affected by smoking epidemic. We searched the literature electronically and plotted the number of journal articles on association between smoking and periodontal disease with the trend in cigarette consumption (for example, in the USA) and expected trend in periodontal disease epidemic due to smoking by the year group (Fig. 1). Both peaks of expected trend of the disease and the number of journals stand closely in the 1990'.

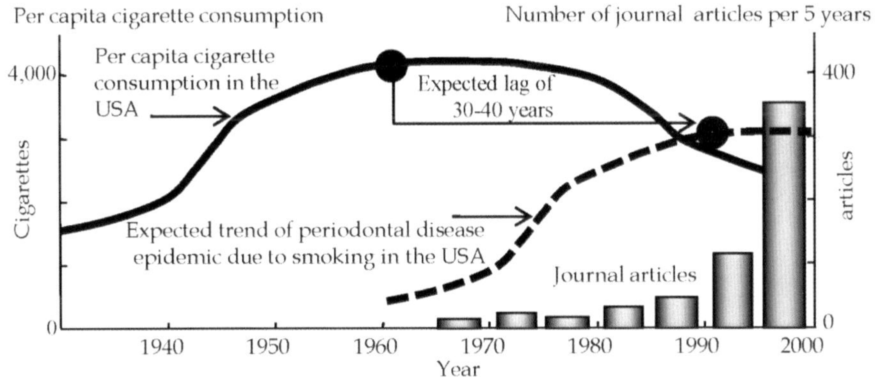

Fig. 1. Application of a descriptive model to the association of increase in smoking prevalence and smoking-related mortality with expected trends in smoking-attributable periodontal epidemic disease. The number of journal articles regarding smoking and periodontal disease followed the increase.

If this factor had been applied at an earlier stage in the series of periodontal research, practice of smoking cessation intervention in dental settings might have been more active.

The lag between the cigarette-smoking epidemic and epidemiological findings on the association of smoking with periodontal disease may have delayed public awareness of this association. Nevertheless, it is now well known that smoking is an independent risk factor of periodontal disease and influences the prognosis associated with periodontal treatments.
The validated association in the epidemiologic literature should be biologically plausible, since evidence supporting a causal association between smoking and periodontal disease has accumulated from clinical and basic studies over the past two decades. The underlying mechanism whereby smoking modulates components of the existing etiology of periodontal disease (Page & Kornman, 1997) has been largely clarified (Fig. 2). Though smokers are more susceptible to periodontal disease than non-smokers, bleeding on periodontal probing is less apparent in smokers than in non-smokers. The mechanisms underlying suppression of signs of clinical inflammation in smokers are under consideration for future studies.

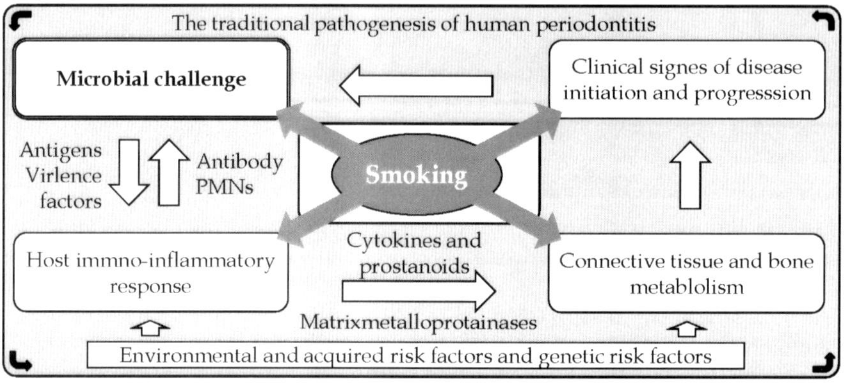

Fig. 2. Mechanisms by which smoking affects periodontal disease based on four components of the traditional pathogenesis of human periodontitis.

Smokers exhibit more periodontal tissue breakdown than non-smokers. These findings are based on the adjustment for confounding factors that are associated with periodontal disease and smoking. The underlying mechanisms include dysfunction of gingival fibroblasts, a decrease in microcirculatory function, and immune system deficiency. The more severe periodontal destruction in smokers than in non-smokers is attributable to impaired ability to repair damaged tissue rather than direct tissue damage.
Deeper understanding was provided by recent progress in molecular and genetic approaches (Ojima & Hanioka, 2010). Smokers exhibited overproduction of inflammatory molecules and suppression of anti-inflammatory molecules, thereby leading to inflammatory destruction of connective tissue and alveolar bone. Very recent studies using a novel method of bacterial identification revealed bacterial involvement in this process and provided an explanation of the connection between smoking and periodontal tissue breakdown in terms of pathogenic periodontal microorganisms.
The results of epidemiological and basic studies have led to periodontal disease now being considered a disease group in which there is sufficient evidence to infer its causal association with smoking. Special attention should be given to the treatment outcomes of periodontal disease in smokers. A negative response to periodontal treatment is consistently reported (Heasman et al., 2006). A more frequent recurrence of periodontal disease in

smokers than in non-smokers during periodontal maintenance was demonstrated (Carnevale et al., 2007). Evidence regarding the effects of smoking on periodontal disease and treatment indicates that smokers lose more tooth-supporting tissue than non-smokers. These effects lead to more rapid loss of tooth-supporting tissue in smokers than in non-smokers. An association between smoking and tooth loss during the periodontal maintenance period has recently been demonstrated (Chambrone et al., 2010). The number of journal articles on the association between smoking and tooth loss, as well as periodontal disease, has increased globally (Fig. 3), and evidence regarding the effect of smoking on tooth loss has accumulated. However, these reports are apparently limited to developed countries, possibly as a result of the lag between the smoking epidemic and occurrence of periodontal disease.

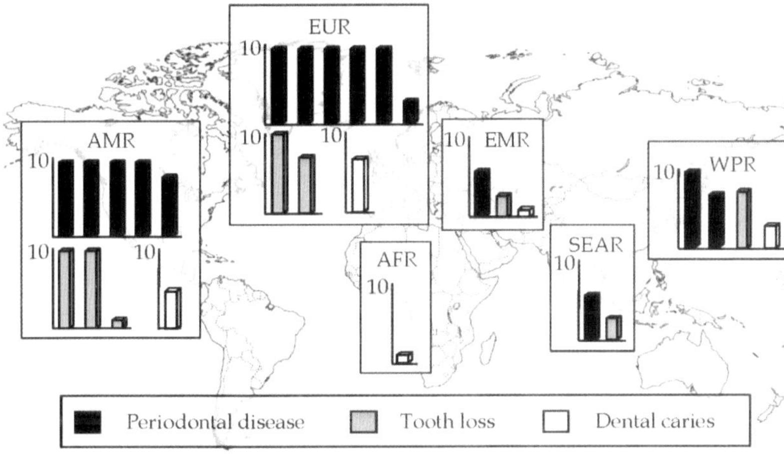

Fig. 3. Number of epidemiological articles addressing the association of smoking with periodontal disease, tooth loss, and dental caries in six WHO regions. The articles were extracted from MEDLINE in 2009 by searching for journal articles on periodontal disease, tooth loss, and dental caries by combining the key words "smoking" or "tobacco," and "periodontal disease" or "periodontitis," "tooth loss," and "dental caries," respectively.

A literature review of observational studies suggests that the evidence supporting a causal association between smoking and tooth loss is strong (Hanioka et al., 2011). Intervention for smoking cessation is an important practice not only for the prevention and treatment of periodontal disease but also for various important oral functions that may depend on the number of existing teeth. Several treatment modalities for tobacco dependence have been considered in the dental setting.

2. Epidemiological evidence

2.1 Periodontal disease and treatment

Effects of smoking and smoking cessation on periodontal disease and treatment responses were examined in observational studies. Data on the effects of adjunctive medications on treatment response in smokers were inconclusive. Benefits of smoking cessation in periodontal treatment were addressed recently.

2.1.1 Increased risk of periodontal disease due to smoking exposure

A comprehensive review in the Surgeon General's Report 2004 concluded that there is sufficient evidence to infer a causal relationship between smoking and periodontal disease (U.S. Department of Health and Human Services, 2004). In addition to studies in the review article, resent studies show a moderate to strong association (odds ratios ranging from 1.4 to 3.5, Warnakulasuriya et al., 2010). The effects on incidence and progression were also elucidated. Dose–response effects also demonstrated that heavy smokers had greater disease severity than light smokers in cross-sectional and cohort studies.

Representative populations were assessed in the USA, Japan, and Australia. The smoking-attributable fraction of periodontal disease ranged from 55.2% to 84% for current smokers and was 21.8% for former smokers. The population-attributable fraction ranged from 12.2% to 60% for current smokers and from 10.9% to 47% for former smokers (Tomar & Asma, 2000; Do et al., 2008). These variations may depend on different characteristics of the population, diversity of surrogate markers of periodontal disease, and confounding variables. An association has also been suggested in developing countries e.g., China, Thailand, and Brazil in terms of the cigarette-smoking epidemic. The consequences of the cigarette-smoking epidemic for oral health extend worldwide.

The effects of smoking on the young population are inconsistent. Smoking was significantly and independently associated with periodontal disease in the young population. A greater apparent association, with an odds ratio of 3.1, was shown in heavy smokers aged 14–29 years (Susin & Albandar, 2005) and in long-term smokers in a birth cohort study, which maintained a high follow-up rate (96%) and had high statistical power with a high incident odds ratio (5.2, Thomson et al., 2007). In contrast, association of smoking with periodontal diseases was not detected possibly due to lack of a sensitive marker such as attachment loss (Ojima et al., 2006).

Second-hand smoke inhalation potentiated bone loss during experimental periodontitis in rats. Data from the National Health and Nutrition Examination Survey (NHANES) III in the USA indicated that individuals exposed to second-hand smoke had greater odds (1.6 times) of having periodontal disease compared to individuals not exposed in the home and workplace (Arbes et al., 2001). Passive smokers, who were identified by salivary cotinine levels, showed a greater number of teeth with clinical attachment loss and higher levels of interleukin-1β, albumin, and aspartate aminotransferase in saliva than counterparts not exposed to passive smoke (Yamamoto et al., 2005). These findings were further confirmed by the research for dose-response relationship (Sanders et al., 2011). Smokeless tobacco users exhibited gingival recession and periodontal disease in the USA, Thailand, Bangladesh, and Sweden.

2.1.2 Decreased risk of periodontal disease due to smoking cessation

Decreased risk of periodontal disease due to smoking cessation is less clearly established than increased risk due to smoking exposure. Some studies suggest periodontal disease severity in former smokers falls between that of current and non-smokers. Very few studies demonstrate a dose–response relationship between risk reduction of periodontal disease and smoking cessation. Findings of the NHANES III revealed that the odds of periodontitis for former smokers who quit ≥11 years previously were indistinguishable from the odds for non-smokers (Tomar & Asma, 2000). In a study of senior employees and retired personnel of the electricity generating authority in Thailand, for light smokers, the odds for severe periodontitis reverted to the level of non-smokers when they had quit smoking for ≥10 years, and for moderate heavy smokers, the odds of having severe periodontitis did not differ from those of non-smokers when they had quit smoking for ≥20 years (Torrungruang et al., 2005).

2.1.3 Effects of smoking on treatment response

The effects of smoking on the response to periodontal treatment have been extensively reviewed (Heasman et al., 2006). A negative effect of smoking on the outcome of several periodontal treatment modalities has been demonstrated in recent studies, and the width of keratinized gingiva for gingival recession therapy, radiographic bone defect, subgingival microbial changes, inflammatory markers, and gingival blood flow in addition to the pocket probing depth, clinical attachment level, and bleeding on probing are used to examine treatment outcome. No significant difference was detected in the 10-year periodontal stability in recession defects of patients receiving guided tissue regeneration therapy and an immediate effect of instrumentation on the subgingival microflora between smokers and non-smokers. Smokers more frequently experienced a recurrence of periodontal disease than non-smokers during supportive periodontal therapy. Tooth loss is a tangible outcome of periodontal treatment and also reflects the recurrence of periodontal disease.

2.1.4 Effects of adjunctive medications on treatment response in smokers

Clinicians are required to use adjunct antimicrobial or host-modulation therapy for smokers. Adjunctive local medications were effective in reducing *Porphyromonas gingivalis,* the attachment level gain reduced with doxycycline, and red or orange-complex bacteria in current smokers and C-reactive protein concentration improved with minocycline. The effects of adjunctive systemic medications, however, are inconclusive. Low-dose doxycycline administration was shown to be effective on analysis of a smoking subgroup (Preshaw et al., 2005a), while no additional benefit was shown in smokers when a stricter analytical method with a multilevel model was used (Needleman et al., 2007). Adjunctive administration did not show an additional benefit compared to non-surgical treatment for azithromycin and surgical treatment for flurbiprofen, while adjunctive azithromycin administration adjunct to scaling and root planing contributed to treatment outcomes in smokers. These findings suggest inconclusive effects of adjunctive medications for smokers, indicating the importance of emphasizing the benefit of smoking cessation.

2.1.5 Benefits of smoking cessation in periodontal treatment

Observational studies comparing periodontal health between current, former, and non-smokers after periodontal treatment suggested that quitting smoking is beneficial to patients with periodontal diseases. Some studies showed that responses to treatment in ex-smokers were similar to those in people who had never smoked. However, there are limited data from long-term longitudinal clinical trials to demonstrate unequivocally the periodontal benefit of smoking cessation. An intervention study investigated longitudinally (12 months) the effect of quitting smoking on periodontal status when combined with non-surgical periodontal therapy in smokers with chronic periodontitis (Preshaw et al., 2005b). A new culture-independent assay for bacterial profiling quantifies the effect on subgingival pathogens. This method revealed an effect on subgingival microbial recolonization after smoking cessation.

Theoretical modeling of the cost-effectiveness of smoking cessation was described. The model revealed that a 10% increase in the number of cigarettes smoked per day increased the treatment costs of periodontal diseases by 0.7% and 0.2% for men and women, respectively (Sintonen & Tuominen, 1989). Adding smoking cessation to the concept of periodontitis prevention will enable significant cost savings to be made.

2.2 Tooth loss

Ten cross-sectional and five prospective cohort studies regarding smoking and tooth loss were selected for the evaluation of methodological quality among 496 citations obtained by a literature search and screening the database. Methodological quality of studies was assessed using a standardized scale; eight studies (six for cross-sectional and two for prospective cohort studies) were classified as high quality.

Three elements—the strength of association, experiment, and the dose-response relationship—were assessed in terms of consistency to allow the synthesis of evidence for each element. The evidence of association was evaluated for each element with respect to consistency through studies that examined 58,755 subjects in four countries; Germany, Italy, Japan, and the USA (Fig. 4). The association between current smoking and tooth loss was significant in all studies. The effect size in cross-sectional studies (odds ratio) varied from 1.69 to 4.04 and that in cohort studies (hazard ratio) was 2.1 and 2.3.

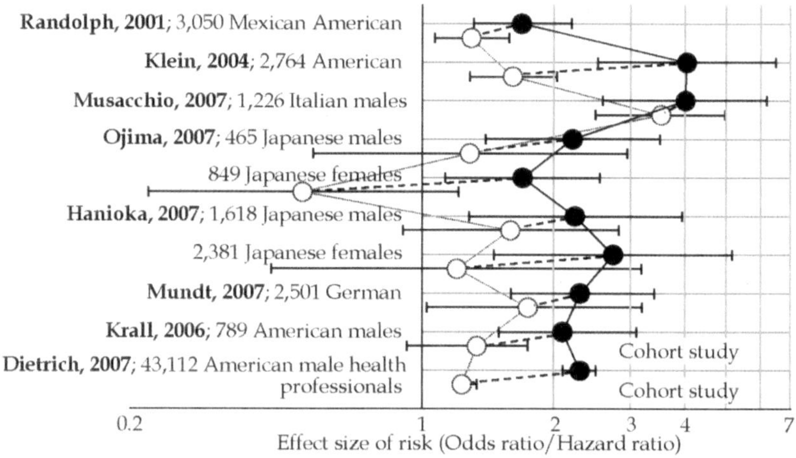

Fig. 4. Effect size (95% confidence interval) of risk of tooth loss in current (closed circles) and former smokers (open circles) relative to non-smokers.

The element of 'experiment' was evaluated by comparing the strength of association between former and current smokers relative to non-smokers, because interventional studies are difficult to conduct in humans. This surrogate element was named "natural experiment." The association between former smoking and tooth loss was not significant in four studies. Although another four studies reported a significant association, the effect size was consistently smaller for former smokers than for current smokers in all studies. The evidence from natural experiments for evaluating the association between smoking cessation and tooth loss was strong with respect to consistency. Two cohort studies with observational periods of 16 and 36 years on populations in the USA reported decreases in hazard ratios on the basis of years of abstinence (data not shown).

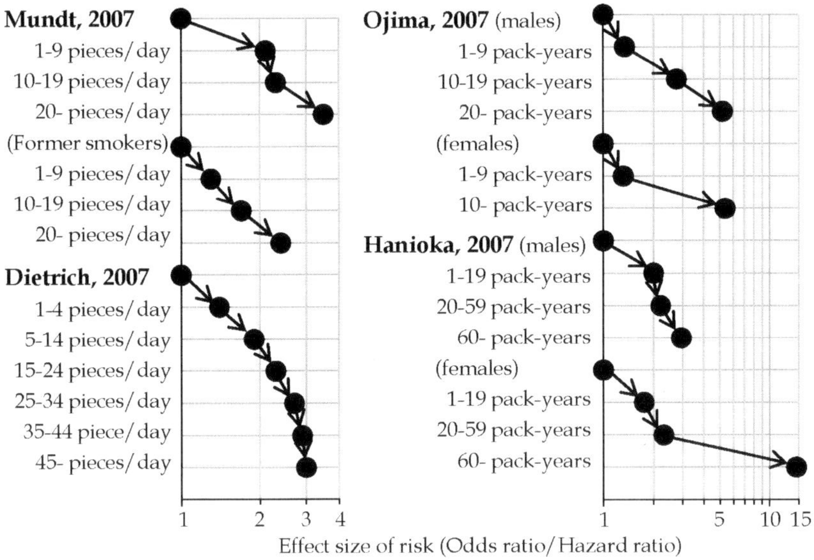

Fig. 5. Relationship between dose of exposure to smoking and effect size.

The dose–response relationship was reported in four high-quality studies, including one cohort study (Fig. 5). These studies examined 50,926 subjects in three countries; Germany, Japan, and the USA. One study in Germany examined the relationship in former smokers. The trend of the relationship between the level of exposure and effect size, i.e., odds ratio or hazard ratio, was obvious in all studies. Therefore, the evidence for a dose–response relationship between smoking and tooth loss was also strong with respect to consistency.

The results from the assessment of each element suggested that the evidence was strong in terms of consistency. This interpretation was based on consistent results with little or no evidence to the contrary in six cross-sectional and two prospective cohort studies. The inclusion of cohort studies indicates more convincing evidence for a causal association. Based on the consistent evidence from each element in the evaluation of this causal association with existing biological plausibility, the evidence supporting a causal association between smoking and tooth loss appears to be strong.

3. Biological plausibility

3.1 Molecular and genetic aspects

3.1.1 Microflora

The effect of smoking on the severity of periodontal disease with respect to the prevalence of specific periodontal pathogens is a controversial issue: some studies have shown differences in the microbial flora between smokers and non-smokers, but several other studies have not been able to demonstrate relevant differences. Differences in periodontal pathogen detection techniques, specimen sampling, and disease definition may explain these conflicting findings. DNA-based techniques have been employed for the detection of specific periodontal pathogens. The polymerase chain reaction (PCR) is a more sensitive and specific method for the detection of bacteria than conventional culture-based methods.

A series of recent studies (Preshaw et al., 2005b; Delima et al., 2010; Shchipkova et al., 2010) revealed a bacteriological mechanism by using a novel method for bacterial identification. The microbial profile of disease-associated and health-compatible organisms in smoking-associated periodontitis patients was significantly different from that in non-smokers. After non-surgical periodontal therapy and smoking cessation counseling, those who continued smoking had a microbial profile similar to that at baseline, while the subgingival microbiome in those who stopped smoking exhibited a healthy profile. These findings explain the connection between smoking and periodontal tissue breakdown by pathogenic periodontal microorganisms.

Another series of studies (Bagaitkar et al., 2009, 2010; Budneli et al., 2011) addressed the involvement of anaerobic bacterial periodontopathogens in the mechanism of suppression of the clinical inflammatory response in periodontal disease in smokers. As an environmental factor, the stress of cigarette smoke upregulates *P. gingivalis* fimbrial antigens and creates conditions that promote biofilm formation, though the proinflammatory response to the pathogen is inhibited. An reduced inflammatory response potential of oral microflora was indicated by alteration of fatty acid profiles in the saliva of smokers with chronic periodontitis.

3.1.2 Smoking-associated pathophysiological changes

Destructive effects of smoking on periodontal tissue are categorized with respect to vascular, immune, and inflammatory responses (Fig. 6). Smoking modulates the destruction of periodontal tissue through various responses; adverse vascular changes and suppression of host immune systems, and disorder of inflammation (Ojima & Hanioka, 2010).

Repeated vasoconstrictive attacks and impairment of revascularization due to cigarette smoking can influence immune function and the subsequent inflammatory reaction in the gingiva. In the inflamed gingival tissues of smokers, significantly fewer vessels were observed compared to non-smokers. Microcirculatory changes may be related to impairment of oxygen delivery to gingival tissue. Gingival blood flow increased after quitting smoking. Expression of intercellular adhesion molecule-1 (ICAM-1), a marker of endothelial dysfunction leading to damaging vascular disorders, was higher in smokers than in age-matched non-smoking controls. These vascular alterations due to cigarette smoking may contribute to disruption of the immune response and delay in the healing response.

Smoking may depress host immune responses, although there are some conflicting results. The number of neutrophils in gingival crevicular fluid (GCF) was lower or remained constant in smokers compared to non-smokers, while that in blood was higher in a dose-dependent manner. Adverse effects of smoking on the function of polymorphonuclear neutrophils, e.g., reduced viability and phagocytosis, were observed in periodontally healthy smokers. Smoking may influence lymphocyte numbers and antibody production. The serum level of Immunoglobulin G_2 (IgG_2), which was an important antibody against gram-negative periodontal pathogens, decreased in patients with periodontitis. Smoking may decrease the proliferative capacity of T cells or T-cell-dependent antibody responses that affect B-cell function and antibody generation.

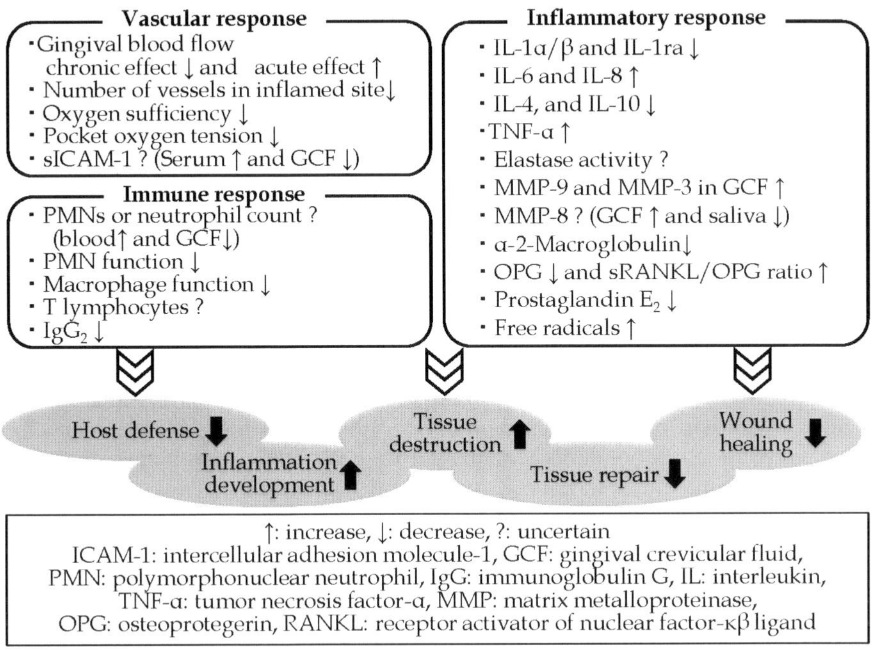

Fig. 6. Destructive effects of smoking on periodontal tissue.

Among several cytokines associated with periodontal disease, levels of interleukin (IL)-1 in GCF have been extensively compared between smokers and non-smokers. Smokers exhibited significantly lower concentrations of IL-1a and IL-1ra in GCF than nonsmokers. Smokers tend to exhibit excess production of inflammatory molecules, such as IL-6, IL-8, and tumor necrosis factor-α, and suppression of anti-inflammatory molecules, such as IL-4, IL-10, and IL-1ra; however, these findings are to some extent inconsistent. Findings regarding the effects of smoking on the level of neutrophil-derived proteolytic enzymes in oral specimens are inconsistent; however, smoking may increase their level in the systemic circulation.

Matrix metalloproteinase-9 (MMP-9) in plasma was higher in smokers than in non-smokers. Smokers had the higher level of elastase and MMP-3 in GCF, and MMP-8 expression in periodontal tissue than non-smokers, while the salivary MMP-8 level was significantly lower in current smokers than in former smokers. Smokers showed a significantly lower concentration of α-2-macroglobulin in GCF as well as total amounts of α-2- macroglobulin and α-1-antitrypsin than non-smokers. Smoking seems to disturb the balance between proteolytic and anti-proteolytic activities in periodontal tissue.

IL-1, IL-6, and TNF-α stimulated the expression of the receptor activator of nuclear factor-κβ ligand (RANKL) and the inhibitor protein osteoprotegerin (OPG), which are dominant regulators of bone resorption and remodeling. The OPG concentration was significantly lower and the sRANKL/OPG ratio was higher in smokers compared with non-smokers, in saliva as well as serum, explaining the greater potential for alveolar bone loss in smokers.

IL-1 and IL-6 induce production of prostaglandin E_2 (PGE_2) by neutrophils and macrophages, which could also accelerate alveolar bone resorption, although the level of PGE_2 in GCF and saliva in smokers was similar to that in non-smokers or even lower than that in non-smokers. The level of free oxygen radicals in periodontal tissues, which induces tissue damage by injuring cells such as fibroblasts, was higher in smokers than in non-smokers. Impairment of fibroblasts by smoking possibly leads to delay in tissue repair and wound healing in periodontal disease.

Most findings support the idea that smokers exhibit a greater burden of inflammatory responses to microbial challenges compared to non-smokers. However, limited evidence is available regarding the effects of quitting smoking on pathophysiological changes in periodontal tissue.

3.1.3 Gene-smoking relationship

Relationships between smoking and genetic susceptibility to periodontal diseases have been investigated with respect to genotypes associated with cytokines (IL-1, IL-6, and IL-10), the immune system (Fcγ receptor), bone metabolism (vitamin D receptor), and xenobiotics metabolism (N-acetyltransferase and myeloperoxidase).

IL-1 polymorphisms have been intensively studied using a cross-sectional design, except for one longitudinal study. Its relationship with respect to smoking is controversial. Several studies reported relationships between IL-1-positive genotypes and smoking; however, other studies demonstrated that the association of IL-1-positive genotypes with the severity of periodontal disease was independent of smoking, suggesting no relationship between smoking and IL-1 genotypes. Logistic regression analysis revealed that odds ratios of periodontal disease, in comparison with IL-1 genotype-negative non-smokers as a reference group, was 0.98 for genotype-positive non-smokers, 2.37 for genotype-negative smokers, and 4.50 for genotype-positive smokers, suggesting synergism between IL-1 polymorphism and smoking (Meisel et al., 2004).

An association between IL-6 and IL-10 genotype and periodontal status was more conspicuous in non-smokers. Fcγ receptors are important components in the binding and phagocytosis of IgG-sensitized cells. Genotypes for Fcγ receptor, FcγRIIa, and FcγRIIIb may be associated with periodontal disease in smokers (Yamamoto et al., 2004). Gene polymorphisms for enzymes that can metabolize smoking-derived substances may contribute to individual susceptibility to the risk of periodontitis among smokers. Subjects with the gene polymorphism for enzymes that can metabolize smoking-derived substances, e.g., cytochrome P450 1A1 M2 allele and the glutathione S-transferase M1 allele, exhibited an increased risk of periodontitis.

To date, gene-smoking relationships in periodontal disease are uncertain because of methodological limitations such as employment of subjects in a specific race, small sample size, and lack of detailed history of smoking and possible confounders. The gene-smoking relationships in periodontal disease may be bilateral; genetic susceptibility to periodontal disease is influenced by exposure to smoking, or the effect of smoking on periodontal disease is influenced by genetic susceptibility. Better understanding of gene–smoking relationship could contribute to the prevention of periodontal disease through personalized recommendation and targeted intervention in public and clinical dental programs.

4. Intervention of smoking cessation

4.1 Dental setting

Smoking cessation intervention is an important category in the dental practice. Smoking cessation intervention is performed in dental setting for a variety of purposes according to the oral condition of patients. Smoking cessation is effective in preventing not only oral diseases but also the progression of periodontal tissue breakdown. Smoking cessation intervention may be integrated in existing procedures of dental treatment because improvement of outcome of the treatment is expected by smoking cessation.

Periodontal practitioners should know the "5 A's" model for treating smoking and nicotine dependence (Fiore et al., 2008a). This model consists of five components for effective smoking cessation intervention: **Ask** about tobacco use; **Advise** about quitting; **Assess** willingness to make a quit attempt; **Assist** in the quit attempt; and **Arrange** follow-up. Although full implementation of the "5 A's" in clinical settings is superior to partial implementation, periodontal practitioners may be responsible for some parts of these components.

Several modalities of smoking cessation intervention have been proposed in the dental setting. The effectiveness of intervention modalities was examined with respect to the success rate of quitting. Since there are several pathways in both the clinical and social setting for smoking cessation, dental practitioners need to know about these pathways to assist patients routinely to choose an appropriate way to succeed in quitting in addition to improving the outcome of dental treatment specific to the patient.

Motivational interview strategies (Fiore et al., 2008a) such as "express empathy," "develop discrepancy," "roll with resistance," and "support self-efficacy" are specialized techniques. Dental hygienists may be able to accept these techniques because they routinely motivate dental patients about oral health behavior on the basis of these techniques. Another strategy that enhances future attempts to quit smoking is the "5 R's" (Table 1).

Relevance	Encourage the patient to indicate why quitting is **personally relevant**, being as **specific** as possible. Motivational information has the greatest impact if it is relevant to a patient's disease status or risk, family or social situation, health concerns, age, gender, and other important patient characteristics.
Risks	The clinician should ask the patient to identify potential negative consequences of tobacco use. The clinician may suggest and highlight those that seem **most relevant to the patient**.
Rewards	The clinician should ask the patient to **identify potential benefits** of stopping tobacco use. The clinician may suggest and highlight those that seem most relevant to the patient.
Roadblocks	The clinician should ask the patient to identify barriers or impediments to quitting and provide treatment that could address barriers.
Repetition	The motivational intervention should be **repeated every time** an unmotivated patient visits the clinic setting. Tobacco users who have failed in previous quit attempts should be told that most people make repeated quit attempts before they are successful.

Table 1. Motivational strategies to enhance attempts to quit smoking; the "5 R's."

The "5R's" strategy is available to dental practitioners. Particularly, four components of "relevance," "risks," "rewards," and "repetition" in the motivational strategies include some issues specific to dental practice. Various oral symptoms and dental treatments relevant to smoking may be used to motivate dental patients. For example, periodontal patients need to know the risk posed by continuing smoking for the development of periodontal tissue breakdown, because these patients are susceptible to smoking-associated periodontal disease. In other words, the issue of smoking and periodontal disease is personally relevant. Therefore, smoking cessation is recommended for the substantial benefit on the outcome of periodontal treatment. Periodontal practitioners can repeat motivational interventions when unmotivated patients visit for periodontal treatments. Periodontal practitioners need to acquire new knowledge about only one technique among the motivational strategies– roadblocks.

The level of willingness to quit smoking varies among dental patients. Dental practitioners need to know the stages of behavior change (Prochaska et al., 1992) and approaches that can be used to promote progress through the stages of behavior change. The theoretical model with behavioral approaches involves stage-based interventions. This model categorizes smokers into five different stages; precontemplation, contemplation, preparation, action, and maintenance.

The effectiveness of brief interventions by dental professionals using the feedback of oral symptoms and dental treatments personally relevant to smoking was examined with respect to quitting smoking and motivation for smoking cessation (Hanioka et al., 2007). Levels of changes in smoking behavior and cessation attempts were assessed using a standardized questionnaire. The questionnaires used at the first and final visits were analyzed for movement through the stages of behavior change. Experience with respect to quit attempts during the dental visits was surveyed in the questionnaire at the final visit. The intervention consisted of a brief explanation regarding dental events relevant to smoking, employing color charts. Patients in the non-intervention group received no intervention other than dental treatments.

The percentages of patients who attempted to quit among those who were not ready to quit were 9.1% and 3.3% in the intervention and non-intervention groups, respectively (Fig. 7). The percentages of patients who progressed through the stages were 22.6% and 17.7%, and the percentages of those who regressed through the stages were 7.7% and 15.8%, respectively. The differences between groups were all significant. The effects were not significant in patients who were ready to quit within 1 month (data not shown). However, the percentage of patients willing to quit was less than 10% (Fig. 8). Dental visits provide an important opportunity for health professionals to influence smokers with respect to motivation for smoking cessation.

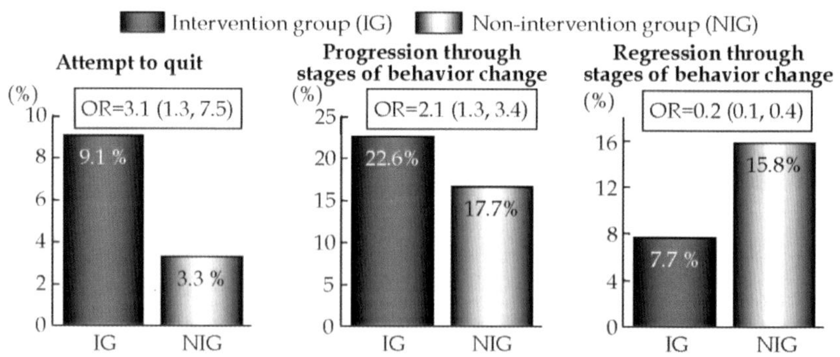

Fig. 7. Effects of a brief intervention using the dental strategy "5 R's" in patients who were not ready to quit.

Brief intervention for patients who are unwilling to quit

1. Motivating patients who are unwilling to quit by the dental "5R's" strategies
2. Presentation of smoking-associated symptoms specifically relevant to the patients
3. Presentation of a potential benefit of stopping smoking to periodontal treatment

Dental "5R's" strategies for 35% - 60% smokers who annually visit dental clinics in Japan

Precontemplation lacking interest to quit
29% of males, 19% of females ⇨ Precontemplation with interest to quit + Contemplation
64% of males, 71% of females ⇨ Preparation
7% of males
10% of females

Fig. 8. Intervention for patients unwilling to quit, and distribution of patients by stage of behavior change

Dental practitioners have the opportunity, by routine assessment, to find out whether the patient plans to attempt to quit during the motivational intervention or for another reason. Several strategies are available for patients willing to quit (Fig. 9). The dentist can assist the patient by offering medication and providing or referring for counseling or additional treatment, and arrange for follow-up contacts to prevent relapse (Fiore et al., 2008a). The success rate of smoking cessation differs among the different strategies. The cost and availability of each strategy and approved medication may be suited to the personality of the patient. Therefore, the provision of information about effective smoking cessation aids is an essential component of intervention for patients who are willing to quit.

Brief and intensive interventions and assistance of referral program for patients who are willing to quit

1. Provision of self-help materials
2. Behavioral approaches with/without NRTs (availabe as the OTC drug)
3. Assistance of another smoking cessation program including treatment of nicotine dependence in medical setting
4. Follow-up intervention for patients in short-term maintenace period

Action stage ⇨ Short-term maintenance period ⇨ Maintenace stage

NRT: Nicotine replacement therapy, OTC: Over-the- countor

Fig. 9. Intervention and assistance strategies for patients willing to quit.

A feasibility study was conducted to evaluate the potential effectiveness of an intensive smoking cessation intervention delivered by dental professionals with the outcome measure of abstinence rate (Hanioka et al., 2010). Patients who were willing to quit smoking were randomly assigned to either an intervention or a non-intervention group. Intensive intervention was provided, consisting of five counseling sessions, including an additional nicotine replacement regimen. Reported abstinence was verified by measuring the salivary cotinine level. On an intent-to-treat basis, 3-, 6-, and 12-month continuous abstinence rates in the intervention group were 51.5%, 39.4%, and 36.4%, respectively, while the rates in the non-intervention group were consistent at 13.0% (Fig. 10). Adjusted odds ratios (95% confidence interval) by logistic stepwise regression analyses were 7.1 (1.8, 28.5), 8.9 (1.7, 47.2), and 6.4 (1.3, 30.7), respectively.

Intensive smoking cessation intervention is effective in the dental setting. An intensive smoking cessation intervention conducted by dental hygienists was also successful (Binnie et al., 2007). Nicotine replacement therapy is, however, not allowed because of the limitation of the dental medication list (Action on Smoking and Health, 2008). The pharmaceutical approach may reduce withdrawal symptoms, which may include oral symptoms such as mouth ulcers, the prevalence of which is 40% (McEwen et al., 2006). Dentists are ideally placed to promote cessation because they are able explain the impact of tobacco on oral health to their patients, many of whom consider themselves to be perfectly healthy. The WHO oral health program has strengthened its support of countries that incorporate oral health into tobacco control (Petersen, 2003), and the FDI World Dental Federation has urged dental professionals to advise patients to quit smoking (FDI World Dental Federation, 2004). Referral programs for intensive intervention for smoking cessation are also available.

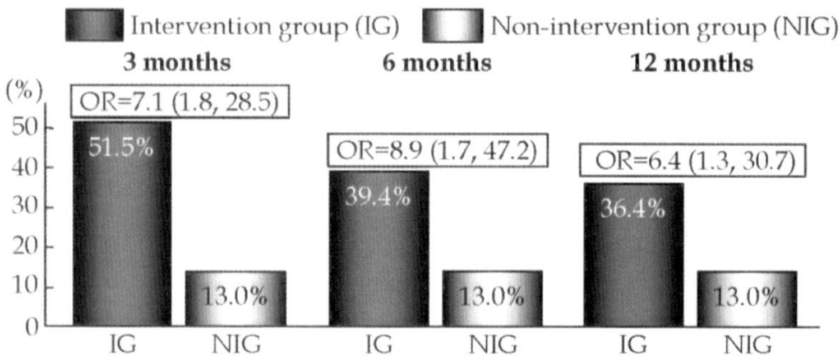

Fig. 10. Effects of intensive smoking cessation intervention in terms of abstinence rate in a feasibility study in a dental setting.

4.2 Referral services for intensive intervention

Intensive smoking cessation treatment is more effective than brief intervention. There is a strong dose–response relationship between counseling intensity and quitting success (Fiore et al, 2008b). Treatments may be made more intense by increasing the duration and number of individual treatment sessions. Many different types of providers (e.g., physicians, nurses, dentists, psychologists, and pharmacists) play substantial roles in increasing quit rates, and involving multiple providers can increase abstinence rates. Individual, group, and telephone counseling are effective formats for treatment of chronic tobacco use. Particular types of counseling strategies, like practical counseling (problem solving/skills training approaches) and the provision of intratreatment social support (emotional support during treatment) by providers, are especially effective and associated with significant increases in abstinence rates (Fiore et al, 2008b). In addition, pharmacological treatment with nicotine replacement therapy (NRT), bupropion, and varenicline consistently increase abstinence rates (Fiore et al, 2008a). A combination of counseling and pharmacotherapy also increases abstinence rates to a great extent.

Two major programs have proven to be effective referral services for smokers willing to quit, and are thus highly recommended(WHO report on the global tobacco epidemic, 2011):

1. free telephone help lines (known as quitlines)
2. treatment services with pharmacotherapy

4.2.1 Quitlines

Quitlines are telephone-based cessation support services and have been established in many countries since the late 1980s. In proactive quitlines, the call is initiated by the counselor, while reactive quitlines only respond to incoming calls. Services range from a single brief reactive counseling session, provided at the time a caller reaches the quitline, to intensive counseling via multiple proactive follow-up calls initiated by the counselor in addition to with self-help materials, web-based services, or pharmacotherapy for smoking cessation provided to the caller (McAfee, 2007; Centers for Disease Control and Prevention, 2004). The advent of quitlines indicates that intensive, specialist-delivered interventions are now available to smokers on an unprecedented basis (Fiore et al., 2008b).

Evidence regarding the effectiveness of proactive quitlines is well established, with a recent meta-analysis of randomized control trials (RCTs) demonstrating a higher likelihood of abstinence after 6 months or more of follow-up (risk ratio = 1.37; 95% confidence interval [CI], 1.26–1.50), but the evidence for reactive quitlines is not convincing (Stead, 2009). Adding telephone support to brief intervention or pharmacotherapy increases long-term abstinence rates when compared with brief intervention alone or pharmacotherapy alone (Stead, 2009). There is some evidence of a dose response; 1 or 2 brief calls are less likely to provide a measurable benefit when compared with a longer intervention. Three or more calls increase the chances of quitting when compared with a minimal intervention such as providing standard self-help materials or brief advice, or when compared with pharmacotherapy alone (Stead, 2009).

In addition to their effectiveness, quitlines have other advantages (Centers for Disease Control and Prevention, 2004): 1) easy access (quitlines reduce barriers in accessing traditional cessation services, including time, transportation difficulties, childcare responsibilities, financial costs, and the psychological barrier); 2) the benefits of centralization (quitlines can serve a large geographic area from a single, centralized base of operations, which leads to economy of scale, ease of promotion, better quality control, and ease of evaluation); and 3) acting as the hub of a network of cessation resources (quitlines serve not only as direct service providers but also as the hub of a comprehensive network of cessation resources in a community, and the coordinating function of the hub can include referral to appropriate resources for pharmacotherapy and intensive cessation programs in medical settings). These advantages increase the population impact of quitlines not only by providing effective counseling services, but also by enhancing the use of other available cessation resources. The U.S. Public Health Service-sponsored Clinical Practice Guideline and the Guide to Community Preventive Services recommend proactive quitlines as a way to help smokers quit (Fiore et al., 2008b; Task Force on Community Preventive Services, 2005).

Many clinicians find it hard to deliver all of the recommended 5As (ask, advise, assess, assist, and arrange) in a busy practice setting. One way of improving the efficiency of smoking cessation treatment delivered in primary care settings may be to give the physician a defined, but limited, role in delivery of the 5As (Bentz, 2006). This could be accomplished by incorporating quitlines.

QuitWorks is a free smoking cessation service developed by the Massachusetts Department of Public Health in collaboration with all major health plans in Massachusetts (Centers for Disease Control and Prevention, 2004; Massachusetts Department of Public Health). Nearly 22,000 patients have been referred to the QuitWorks program since its launch in April 2002. QuitWorks links healthcare providers and their patients who smoke to proactive telephone counseling and other smoking cessation services. Any physician, nurse, dentist, or other clinician can easily and quickly refer any smoking patient irrespective of health insurance status. The referral forms are faxed or electronically transmitted to the state-funded quitline service provider. Upon referral, the quitline counselor provides free multisession proactive counseling, internet counseling, and referral to community-based treatment programs. Every referring provider will receive reports about their patients. Within 1 month, a patient contact report is sent to confirm contact with the patient and the services accepted. About 6 months after the initial assessment, QuitWorks calls the patient to assess his or her smoking status and sends the provider a patient outcome report.

New Zealand's health system uses an ABC approach instead of the 5As model. ABC is a simple and easy tool for the guidance of all healthcare workers: Ask about smoking status, give Brief advice, and offer Cessation support, which implies face-to-face support with pharmacotherapy or referral to smoking cessation services, including quitlines (McRobbie, 2008). The national quitline assists more than 50,000 New Zealanders attempting to quit smoking each year. To promote smoking advice and assistance in healthcare settings, the Government introduced a health target of "better help for smokers to quit" as 1 of only 6 governmental priority health targets, with the ultimate goal being that 95% smokers who are admitted to a hospital should receive advice and assistance for quitting by July 2012 (WHO Framework Convention on Tobacco Control, 2011). Because of the success of this approach, it will be extended to primary healthcare services as well.

4.2.2 Treatment services with pharmacotherapy

In November 2010, WHO issued detailed guidelines for implementation of Article 14 of the Framework Convention on Tobacco Control (demand reduction measures with regard to tobacco dependence and cessation). These guidelines intend to encourage each government to strengthen or create a sustainable infrastructure to motivate quit attempts and to ensure wide access to smoking cessation treatment (WHO Framework Convention on Tobacco Control, 2011). The costs of smoking cessation treatment can be covered or reimbursed by public health services to reduce out-of-pocket expenses for people trying to quit. Eighty per cent high-income and 40% middle-income countries provide at least some cost coverage for smoking cessation treatment, including pharmacotherapy, while only 1 in 8 currently covers any costs of cessation services in low-income countries (WHO report on the global tobacco epidemic, 2011). Pharmacotherapy is generally more expensive and less cost-effective when compared with cessation advice in healthcare settings and quitlines; however, it has been shown to double or triple quit rates (Fiore et al., 2008a). NRT is usually available over the counter, whereas bupropion and varenicline require a doctor's prescription (WHO report on the global tobacco epidemic, 2009). NRT reduces withdrawal symptoms by replacing some of the nicotine absorbed from tobacco. Bupropion, an antidepressant, can reduce craving and other negative sensations when tobacco users stop their nicotine intake. Varenicline, a selective $\alpha 4\beta 2$ nicotinic acetylcholine-receptor partial agonist developed specifically for smoking cessation, relieves nicotine cravings and withdrawal effects while reducing the reinforcing effects of nicotine through its partial agonistic mechanism of action.

The UK offers the world's most comprehensive support for smokers wishing to quit (WHO report on the global tobacco epidemic, 2009). A national smoking cessation treatment service is universally available to all smokers, mainly free of charge, through the National Health Service (NHS). This service offers weekly support for at least the first 4 weeks of a quit attempt, with face-to-face intensive counseling and pharmacotherapy (McNeil, 2005). Typically, smokers are seen by smoking cessation counselors 1 week (maximum 2 weeks) before quitting and at weekly intervals for 4 weeks after quitting. Pharmacotherapy typically continues at weekly intervals for 8 weeks (Judge, 2005). Over 700,000 smokers per year (approximately 6%–7% of all smokers) set a quit date through the service and 49% smokers who set a quit date had successfully quit by self-report at the 4-week follow-up (NHS Health and Social Care Information Centre, 2010). Sixty-nine per cent smokers who successfully quit at the 4-week follow-up had their results validated with a carbon monoxide test. Most smokers who set a quit date received NRT (65%), whereas 23% received varenicline. The 1-year carbon monoxide-validated abstinence rate was 14.6%, rising to 17.7% when self-reported quitters were included (Ferguson, 2005).

In Japan, a smoking cessation treatment service for outpatients at registered medical institutions was started under public health insurance coverage in 2006. The reimbursed treatment program comprises 5 treatment sessions over a period of 12 weeks. Nicotine patches or varenicline can be prescribed under health insurance coverage during the treatment period. The number of registered medical institutions is increasing year by year. More than 12,800 institutions have now been registered. Access to treatment is improving but is still not satisfactory because the percentage of registered institutions is only 10 % among total medical institutions, limited to hospitals 20%.

According to the 2007 and 2009 surveys conducted by the Review Committee of the Central Social Insurance Medical Council of Japan (The Central Social Insurance Medical Council, 2008 and 2010), the self-reported continuous abstinence rate at randomly selected registered institutions was 32.6% (2007) and 29.7% (2009) after 9 months of completing smoking cessation treatment. If only those patients who received all 5 treatment sessions were considered, the rate was 45.7% (2007) and 49.1% (2009), respectively. These results indicate that smoking cessation treatment is functioning well.

The intervention factors related to the effectiveness of treatment services in the UK and Japan were examined using a large data sample of smokers using these services after adjusting for smoker characteristics (Brose, 2011; The Central Social Insurance Medical Council, 2010). In the UK, NRT alone was associated with higher success rates than no pharmacotherapy (Odds ratio [OR], 1.75; 95% CI, 1.39–2.22), whereas a combination of NRT and varenicline were more effective than NRT alone (OR, 1.42; 95% CI, 1.06–1.91 and OR, 1.78; 95% CI, 1.57–2.02). In addition, higher success rates were associated with group support than with one-to-one support (OR, 1.43; 95% CI, 1.16–1.76), and primary care settings were less successful than specialist clinics (OR, 0.80; 95% CI, 0.66–0.99). In Japan, a higher number of treatment sessions was associated with a higher success rate (OR, 1.78; $p < 0.05$). In addition, varenicline was more effective than NRT (OR, 1.24; $p < 0.05$), re-treatment was less successful than the initial treatment (OR, 0.68; $p < 0.05$), and physicians with greater experience in smoking cessation treatments were associated with higher success rates (OR, 1.03; $p < 0.05$). These findings using routine clinic data support those from RCTs.

To improve the quality of treatment services, England has established the NHS Centre for Smoking Cessation and Training for practitioners involved in smoking cessation activities. It offers certification to practitioners through its online training, which develops evidence-based competences (knowledge and skills) for treatment services. In Japan, the Japan Medical and Dental Association for Tobacco Control has developed e-learning programs to train healthcare providers, who can then administer reimbursed smoking cessation treatments as well as proactive brief intervention in routine healthcare settings.

5. References

Arbes, S.J., Agústsdóttir, H., & Slade, G.D. (2001). Environmental tobacco smoke and periodontal disease in the United States. *American Journal of Public Health,* Vol.91, No. 2, (February, 2001), pp.253-257, ISSN 0090-0036

Bagaitkar, J., Williams, L.R., Renaud, D.E., Bemakanakere, M.R., Martin, M., Scott, D.A., & Demuth, D.R. (2009). Tobacco-induced alterations to *Porphyromonas gingivalis*-host interactions. *Environmental Microbiology* Vol.11, No.5, (May, 2009), pp.1242-1253, ISSN 1462-2920

Bagaitkar, J., Demuth, D.R., Daep, C.A., Renaud, D.E., Pierce, D.L., & Scott, D.A. (2010) Tobacco upregulates *P. gingivalis* fimbrial proteins which induce TLR2 hyposensitivity. *PLoS ONE* Vol.5, No.5, (May, 2010), e9323, ISSN 1932-6203

Bentz, C.J., Bayley, K.B., Bonin, K.E., Fleming, L., Hollis, J.F., & McAfee, T. (2006). The feasibility of connecting physician offices to a state-level tobacco quit line. American Journal of Preventive Medicine, Vol. 30, No. 1, (January 2006), pp.31-37, ISSN 0749-3797

Binnie, V.I., McHugh, S., & Jenkins, W. (2007). A randomised controlled trial of a smoking cessation intervention delivered by dental hygienists: a feasibility study. *BMC Oral health* Vol.7, (May, 2007), 5, ISSN 1472-6831.

Brose, L.S., West, R., McDermott, M.S., Fidler, J.A., Croghan, E., & McEwen, A. (2011). What makes for an effective stop-smoking service?. Thorax, Published Online First, (June 2011), doi:10.1136/thoraxjnl-2011-200251, ISSN 0040-6376

Buduneli, N., Larsson, L., Bıyıkoğlu, B., Renaud, D.E., Bagaitkar, J. & Scott, D.A. (2011) Fatty acid profiles in smokers with chronic periodontitis. *Journal of Dental Research* Vol.90, No.1, (January, 2011), pp.47-52, ISSN 1544-0591

Carnevale, G., Cairo, F., & Tonetti, M.S. (2007). Long-term effects of supportive therapy in periodontal patients treated with fibre retention osseous respective surgery. I: recurrence of pockets, bleeding on probing and tooth loss. *Journal of Clinical Periodontology,* Vol.34, No.4, (April, 2007), pp.334-341, ISSN 0303-6979

Centers for Disease Control and Prevention. (September 2004). Telephone Quitlines: A Resource for Development, Implementation, and Evaluation. Department of Health and Human Services, Centers for Disease Control and Prevention, National Center for Chronic Disease Prevention and Health Promotion, Office on Smoking and Health, Atlanta, GA: U.S.

The Central Social Insurance Medical Council (July 9, 2008). Special survey (2007 fiscal year) on inspection by a Review Committee that assesses the outcome of medical fee revisions. A report of abstinence rates in registered medical institutions for reimbursement of nicotine dependence management fee. In: Ministry of Health, Labour and Welfare, August 19, 2011, Available from: <http://www.mhlw.go.jp/shingi/2008/07/dl/s0709-8k.pdf>, (in Japanese)

The Central Social Insurance Medical Council (June 2, 2010): Special survey (2009 fiscal year) on inspection by a Review Committee that assesses the outcome of medical fee revisions. A report of abstinence rates in registered medical institutions for reimbursement of nicotine dependence management fee · In: Ministry of Health, Labour and Welfare, August 19, 2011, Available from: http://www.mhlw.go.jp/shingi/2010/06/dl/s0602-3i.pdf>, (in Japanese)

Chambrone, L., Chambrone, D., Lima, L.A. & Chambrone, L.A. (2010). Predictors of tooth loss during long-term periodontal maintenance: a systematic review of observational studies. *Journal of Clinical Periodontology*, Vol.37, No.7, (July, 2010), pp. 675-684, ISSN 0303-6979

Delima, S.L., McBride, R.K., Preshaw, P.M., Heasman, P.A., & Kumar, P.S. (2010): Response of subgingival bacteria to smoking cessation. *Journal of Clinical Microbiology* Vol.48, No.7, (July, 2010), pp.2344-2349, ISSN 1098-660X

Do, L.G., Slade, G.D., Roberts-Thomson, K.F., & Sanders, A.E. (2008). Smoking-attributable periodontal disease in the Australian adult population. *Journal of Clinical Periodontology* Vol.35, No.5, (May, 2008), pp.398-404, ISSN 0303-6979

FDI World Dental Federation (2004). FDI policy statement: code of practice on tobacco control for oral health organizations. World Dental Press: Lowestoft, UK, pp. 1.

Fiore, M.C., Bailey, W.C., Cohen, S.J., Dorfman, S.F., Goldstein, M.G. et al. (2008a). Chapter 3 : Clinical interventions for tobacco use and dependence., In : *Treating tobacco use and dependence: clinical practice guideline. 2008 update*, USDHHS, PHS, 37-62, Rockville, MD, USA

Fiore, M.C., Bailey, W.C., Cohen, S.J., Dorfman, S.F., Goldstein, M.G. et al. (2008b). Chapter 4: Intensive interventions for tobacco use and dependence, In: *Treating tobacco use and dependence: clinical practice guideline. 2008 update*, pp.63-66, U.S. Department of Health and Human Services, Public Health Service, ISBN 1587633515, Rockville, MD, USA

Ferguson, J., Bauld, L., Chesterman, J., & Judge, K. (2005). The English smoking treatment services: one-year outcomes. Addiction.Vol. 100, Suppl. 2, (April 2005), pp.59-69. ISSN 0965-2140

Hanioka, T., Ojima, M., Hamajima, N., & Naito, M. (2007). Patient feedback as a motivating force to quit smoking. *Community Dentistry and Oral Epidemiology* Vol.35, No.4, (August, 2007), pp.310–317, ISSN 0301-5661

Hanioka, T., Ojima, M., Tanaka, H., Naito, M., Hamajima, N. & Matsuse, R. (2010). Intensive smoking-cessation intervention in the dental setting. *Journal of Dental Research* Vol.89, No.1, (January, 2010), pp.66-70, ISSN 1544-0591

Hanioka, T., Ojima, M., Tanaka, K., Matsuo, K., Sato, F., & Tanaka, H. (2011). Causal assessment of smoking and tooth loss: A systematic review of observational studies. *BMC Public Health*, Vol.11, (April, 2011), 221, ISSN 1471-2458

Heasman, L., Stacey, F., Preshaw, P.M., McCracken, G.I., Hepburn, S. & Heasman P.A. (2006). The effect of smoking on periodontal treatment response: a review of clinical evidence. *Journal of Clinical Periodontology*, Vol.33, No.4, (April, 2006), pp. 241-253, ISSN 0303-6979

Judge, K., Bauld, L., Chesterman, J., & Ferguson, J. (2005). The English smoking treatment services: short-term outcomes. Addiction. Vol. 100, Suppl. 2, (April 2005), pp.46-58, ISSN 0965-2140

Lopez, A.D., Collishaw, N.E., & Piha, T. (1994). A descriptive model of the cigarette epidemic in developed countries. *Tobacco Control* Vol.3, pp.242-247, ISSN 1468-3318

Massachusetts Department of Public Health. (August 11, 2011). QuitWorks: A solution for providers to help patients quit smoking. August 19, 2011, Available from: http://quitworks.makesmokinghistory.org>

McAfee, T.A. (2007). Quitlines a tool for research and dissemination of evidence-based cessation practices. American Journal of Preventive Medicine. Vol. 33, Suppl. 6, (December 2007), pp.357-367, ISSN 0749-3797

McEwen, A., Hajek, P., McRobbie, H. & West, R. (2006). Part Two: Practical Advice, 3 Brief interventions, 3.4 Reasons why stopping smoking can be difficult, 3.4.3 Tobacco withdrawal syndrome, In: Manual of smoking cessation: a guide for counselors and practitioners, pp. 47 ISBN 978-1-4051-3337-1, Blackwell Publishing Ltd, Oxford, UK, 2006

McNeill, A., Raw, M., Whybrow, J., & Bailey, P. (2005). A national strategy for smoking cessation treatment in England. Addiction. Vol. 100, Suppl. 2, (April 2005) pp.1-11, ISSN 0965-2140

McRobbie, H., Bullen, C., Glover, M., Whittaker, R., Wallace, B.M., & Fraser, T., New Zealand Guidelines Group. (2008). New Zealand smoking cessation guidelines. The New Zealand medical journal, Vol. 121, No. 1276, (June 2008), pp.57-70, ISSN 0028-8446

Meisel, P., Schwahn, C., Gesch, D., Bernhardt, O., John, U., & Kocher, T. (2004). Dose-effect relation of smoking and the interleukin-1 gene polymorphism in periodontal disease. *Journal of Periodontology*, Vol.75, No.2, (February, 2004), pp.236-242, ISSN 0022-3492

Needleman, I., Suvan, J., Gilthorpe, M.S., Tucker, R., St. George, G., Giannobile, W., Tonetti, M., & Jarvis, M. (2007). A randomized-controlled trial of low-dose doxycycline for periodontitis in smokers. *Journal of Clinical Periodontology*, Vol. 34, No. 4, (April, 2007), pp.325-333, ISSN 0303-6979

NHS Health and Social Care Information Centre. (August 19, 2010). Statistics on NHS Stop Smoking Services: England, April 2009 – March 2010. The Health and Social Care Information Centre, Retrieved from
<http://www.ic.nhs.uk/webfiles/publications/Health%20and%20Lifestyles/SSS_2009_10_revised.pdf>

Ojima, M., Hanioka, T., Tanaka, K., Inoshita, E., & Aoyama, H. (2006). Relationship between smoking status and periodontal conditions: findings from national databases in Japan. *Journal of Periodontal Research*, Vol.41, No.6, (December, 2006), pp.573-579, ISSN 0022-3484

Ojima, M. & Hanioka, T. (2010). Destructive effects of smoking on molecular and genetic factors of periodontal disease. *Tobacco Induced Diseases*, Vol.8, (February, 2010), 4, ISSN 1617-9625

Page, R.C. & Kornman, S. (1997). The pathogenesis of human periodontitis: an introduction, *Periodontology 2000*, Vol.14, (June, 1997), pp.9-11, ISSN 0906-6713

Petersen, P.E. (2003). Tobacco and oral health - the role of the World Health Organization. *Oral Health and Preventive Dentistry* Vol.1, No.4, (2003), pp.309-315, ISSN 1602-1622

Preshaw, P.M., Hefti, A.F., & Bradshaw, M.H. (2005a). Adjunctive subantimicrobial dose doxycycline in smokers and non-smokers with chronic periodontitis. *Journal of Clinical Periodontology*, Vol.32, No.6, (June, 2005), pp.610-616, ISSN 0303-6979

Preshaw, P.M., Heasman, L., Stacey, F., Steen, N., McCracken, G.I., & Heasman, P.A. (2005b). The effect of quitting smoking on chronic periodontitis. *Journal of Clinical Periodontology* Vol.32, No.4, (April, 2005), pp.869-879, ISSN 0303-6979

Prochaska, J.O., DiClemente, C.C., & Norcross, J.C. (1992). In search of how people change. Applications to addictive behaviors. *American Psychology* Vol.47, No.9, (September, 1992), pp.1102–1114, ISSN 0003-066X

Sanders, A.E., Slade, G.D., Beck, J.D., & Ágústsdóttir, H. (2011). Secondhand smoke and periodontal disease: atherosclerosis risk in communities study. *American Journal of Public Health* published online ahead of print May 5, 2011: e1–e8, ISSN 0090-0036

Shchipkova, A.Y., Nagaraja, H.N., & Kumar, P.S. (2010). Subgingival microbial profiles of smokers with periodontitis. *Journal of Dental Research* Vol.89, No.11, (November, 2010), pp.1247-1253, ISSN 1544-0591

Sintonen, H. & Tuominen, R. (1989). Exploring the determinants of periodontal treatment costs: a special focus on cigarette smoking. *Social Science & Medicine*, Vol.29, No.7, pp.835-844, ISSN 0277-9536

Stead, L.F., Perera, R., & Lancaster, T. (March 17, 2009). Telephone counselling for smoking cessation. The Cochrane Library 2009, Issue 3, John Wiley & Sons, Ltd., Retrieved from<http://www.thecochranelibrary.com/userfiles/ccoch/file/World%20No%20Tobacco%20Day/CD002850.pdf>

Susin, C., Albandar, J.M. (2005). Aggressive periodontitis in an urban population in southern Brazil. *Journal of Periodontology*, Vol.76, No.3, (March, 2005), pp.468-475, ISSN 0022-3492

Task Force on Community Preventive Services. (February 17, 2005). Chapter 1: Tobacco Reducing Initiation, Increasing Cessation, Reducing Exposure to Environmental Tobacco Smoke., In: The Guide to Community Preventive Services: What Works to Promote Health?. pp.3-79, Oxford University Press, ISBN 0195151097, New York, USA

Thomson, W.M., Broadbent, J.M., Welch, D., Beck, J.D., Poulton, R. (2007). Cigarette smoking and periodontal disease among 32-year-olds: a prospective study of a representative birth cohort. *Journal of Clinical Periodontology*, Vol.34, No.10, (Octobers, 2007), pp.828-834. 1, ISSN 0303-6979

Tomar, S.L. & Asma, S. (2000). Smoking-attributable periodontitis in the United States: findings from NHANES III. National Health and Nutrition Examination Survey. *Journal of Periodontology*, Vol.71, No.5, (May, 2000), pp. 743-751, ISSN 0022-3492

Torrungruang, K., Nisapakultorn, K., Sutdhibhisal, S., Tamsailom, S., Rojanasomsith, K., Vanichjakvong, O., Prapakamol, S., Premsirinirund, T., Pusiri, T., Jaratkulangkoon, O., Kusump, S., Rajatanavin, R. (2005). The effect of cigarette smoking on the severity of periodontal disease among older Thai adults. *Journal of Periodontology*, Vol.76, No.4, (April, 2005), pp.566-72, ISSN 0022-3492

U.S. Department of Health and Human Services (2004). *The Health Consequences of Smoking: A Report of the Surgeon General.* Atlanta, GA: U.S. Department of Health and Human Services, Centers for Disease Control and Prevention, National Center for Chronic Disease Prevention and Health Promotion, Office on Smoking and Health, (June, 2004), ISBN 0160515762

Warnakulasuriya, S., Dietrich, T., Bornstein, M.M., Casals Peidró, E., Preshaw, P.M., Walter, C., Wennström, J.L., Bergström, J.(2010). Oral health risks of tobacco use and effects of cessation. *International Dental Journal*, Vol.60, No.1, (February, 2010), pp.7-30, ISSN 0020-6539

WHO Framework Convention on Tobacco Control. (2011). Guidelines for implementation of Article 14 of the WHO Framework Convention on Tobacco Control. Demand reduction measures concerning tobacco dependence and cessation. World Health Organization, ISBN 9789241501316, Geneva, Switzerland

World Health Organization (2009). WHO report on the global tobacco epidemic, 2009. Implementing smoke-free environments, World Health Organization, ISBN 9789241563918 , Geneva, Switzerland

World Health Organization (2011). WHO report on the global tobacco epidemic, 2011. Warning about the dangers of tobacco, Geneva, World Health Organization, ISBN 9789241564267, Geneva, Switzerland

Yamamoto, K., Kobayashi, T., Grossi, S., Ho, A.W., Genco, R.J., Yoshie, H., & De Nardin, E. (2004). Association of Fcgamma receptor IIa genotype with chronic periodontitis in Caucasians. *Journal of Periodontology*, Vol.75, No.4, (April, 2004), pp.517-522, ISSN 0022-3492

Yamamoto, Y., Nishida, N., Tanaka, M., Hayashi, N., Matsuse, R., Nakayama, K., Morimoto, K., Shizukuishi, S. (2005). Association between passive and active smoking evaluated by salivary cotinine and periodontitis. *Journal of Clinical Periodontology*, Vol.32, No.10, (October, 2005), pp1041-1046, ISSN 0303-6979

Part 3

Relationship Between Periodontal Disease and Systemic Health

6

The Emerging Concepts on the Impact of Periodontitis on Systemic Health

S. Anil[1,5], S. V. Varma[2], R.S. Preethanath[1], P. S. Anand[3] and A. Al Farraj Aldosari[4]
[1]*Department of Periodontics and Community Dentistry, College of Dentistry, King Saud University, Riyadh,*
[2]*Sri Sankara Dental College, Trivandrum, Kerala,*
[3]*People's College of Dental Sciences & Research Centre, Bhanpur, Bhopal, Madhya Pradesh,*
[4]*Department of Prosthetic Science, College of Dentistry, King Saud University, Riyadh,*
[5]*Dental Implant and Osseointegration Research Chair, King Saud University, Riyadh,*
[1,4,5]*Saudi Arabia*
[2,3]*India*

1. Introduction

Look to thy mouth; diseases enter here - George Herbert (1593-1632)

Oral health is an integral component of general health and well-being of an individual. Knowledge about the link between periodontal disease and systemic health is growing rapidly. Increasing evidence is available indicating periodontitis as a risk factor for various systemic diseases such as cardiovascular diseases, diabetes mellitus, low birth weight infants and pulmonary diseases (Cullinan et al., 2009; Scannapieco et al., 2010). To date, the bulk of evidence points to the higher levels of circulating periodontal bacterial components, such as endotoxins, that could travel via blood to other organs in the body and cause harm (Dave and Van Dyke, 2008). The relationship between periodontal bacteria and systemic diseases was investigated extensively during the past two decades. More recently, a wealth of epidemiological, clinical and laboratory studies have provided irrefutable evidence that periodontal disease negatively impacts systemic health and proposed mechanisms by which such an association may occur (Fisher et al., 2008; Marakoglu et al., 2008). It is now widely accepted that periodontitis can induce pro-inflammatory cytokines, chemokines and mediators which may play a major role in the development of a variety of systemic conditions (Kuo et al., 2008). However, with the knowledge of possible links between periodontal disease and systemic conditions, patients with advanced periodontitis could be considered systemically compromised even in the absence of overt clinical symptoms or illness.

As science discovers new ways to identify the specific disease process and pathogens, the dental profession discovers new ways to manage the disease from a medical approach. This chapter is focused on evaluating and updating the current status of oral infections, especially periodontitis, as a causal factor for systemic diseases, such as cardiovascular diseases, diabetes mellitus, respiratory disorders, preterm low birth weight and osteoporosis.

2. Periodontal etiopathogenesis

The pathogenesis of human periodontitis was placed on a rational footing for the first time by Page and Schroeder (1976). The destructive process is initiated by the bacterial lipopolysaccharides (LPS) but propagated by the host. Microorganisms such as *Porphyromonas gingivalis, Tannerella forsythia* (formerly *Bacteroides forsythus),* and *Aggregatibacter actinomycetemcomitans* (formerly *Actinobacillus actinomycetemcomitans)* produce enzymes that breakdown the extra cellular matrix such as collagen and host cell membrane to produce nutrients for their growth and further tissue invasion, thereby, initiating an immune and inflammatory process which stimulates the host to release various pro-inflammatory cytokines, MMPs, prostaglandins and host enzymes. They break up the collagen and tissues, creating inroads for further leukocytic infiltration. As periodontal disease progresses, collagen fibres and connective tissue attachment to the tooth are destroyed and epithelial cells proliferate apically deepening the periodontal pockets. This leads to migration of junctional epithelium apically, thereby, exposing the alveolar bone resulting in the activation of osteoclasts initiating bone destruction.

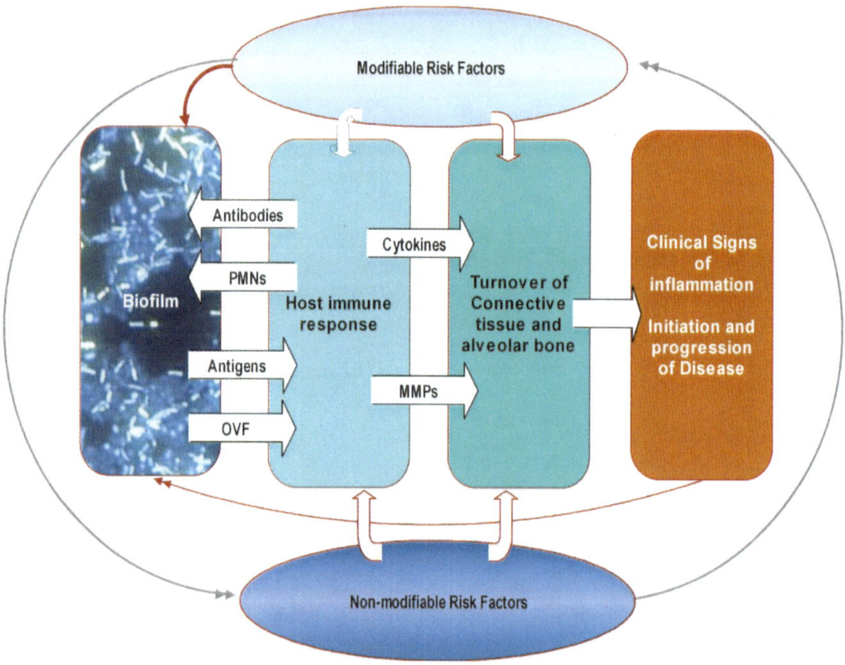

Fig 1. Pathogenesis of Periodontitis – the interplay of modifiable and non-modifiable risk factors (LPS - Lipopolysaccharide, OVF-Other virulence factors, MMP-Matrix metalloproteinases, PMN-Polymorphonuclear leukocytes).

3. Focal infection: The changing concepts

The theory of focal infection, which was promulgated during the 19th and early 20th centuries, stated that "foci" of sepsis were responsible for the initiation and progression of a variety of inflammatory diseases such as arthritis, peptic ulcers and appendicitis (Scannapieco, 1998). Therapeutic edentulation or the "clean-sweep" was common as a result of the popularity of the focal infection theory. Since many teeth were extracted without evidence of infection, thereby providing no relief of symptoms, the theory was discredited and largely ignored for many years (Dussault and Sheiham, 1982). However, it has become increasingly clear that the oral cavity can act as the site of origin for dissemination of pathogenic organisms to distant body sites, especially in immune-compromised hosts such as patients suffering from malignancies, diabetes, rheumatoid arthritis or having corticosteroid and other immunosuppressive treatment. A number of epidemiological studies have suggested that oral infection, especially marginal and apical periodontitis may be a risk factor for systemic diseases (Li et al., 2000). The anatomic closeness of this oral microflora to the bloodstream can facilitate bacteremia and systemic spread of bacterial products, components and immune complexes.

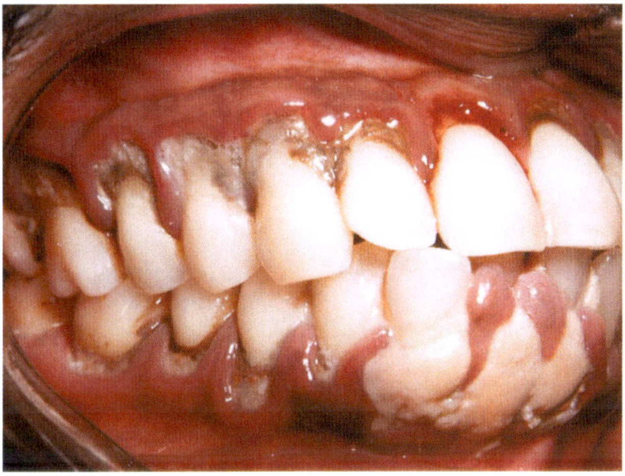

Fig. 2. A case of periodontitis showing the inflammatory process and destruction of the supporting tooth structures.

3.1 Possible pathways of oral infections and non-oral diseases

Pathway for oral infection	Possible non oral diseases
Metastatic infection from oral cavity via transient bacteremia	Subacute infective endocarditis, acute bacterial myocarditis, brain abscess, cavernous sinus thrombosis, sinusitis, lung abscess/infection, Ludwig's angina, orbital cellulitis, skin ulcer, osteomyelitis, prosthetic joint infection
Metastatic injury from circulation of oral microbial toxins	Cerebral infarction, acute myocardial infarction, abnormal pregnancy outcome, persistent pyrexia, idiopathic trigeminal neuralgia, toxic shock syndrome, systemic granulocytic cell defects, chronic meningitis
Metastatic inflammation caused by immunological injury from oral organisms	Behcet's syndrome, chronic urticaria, uveitis, inflammatory bowel disease, Crohn's disease

Table 1.

3.2 Emergence of periodontal medicine

Most studies concerning the relationship between oral infection and systemic diseases are related to periodontal disease, by far the most common oral infection. The term periodontal disease is used to describe a group of conditions that cause inflammation and destruction of the supporting structures of the teeth. Periodontal disease is caused by bacteria found in the dental plaque and about 10 species have been identified as putative pathogens. *A. actinomycetemcomitans*, *P. gingivalis* and *T. forsythia* are the gram-negative bacteria most commonly associated with periodontitis (Haffajee and Socransky, 1994).

The term Periodontal medicine as suggested by Offenbacher, is defined as a rapidly emerging branch of periodontology focusing on the wealth of new data establishing a strong relationship between periodontal health or disease and systemic health or disease. Logically included in this definition would be new diagnostic and treatment strategies that recognize the relationship between periodontal disease and systemic disease (Williams and Offenbacher, 2000).

Page (1998) proposed that periodontitis may affect the host's susceptibility to systemic disease in three ways: by **shared risk factors**, by **subgingival biofilms acting as reservoirs of gram-negative bacteria** and **through the periodontium acting as a reservoir of inflammatory mediators.**

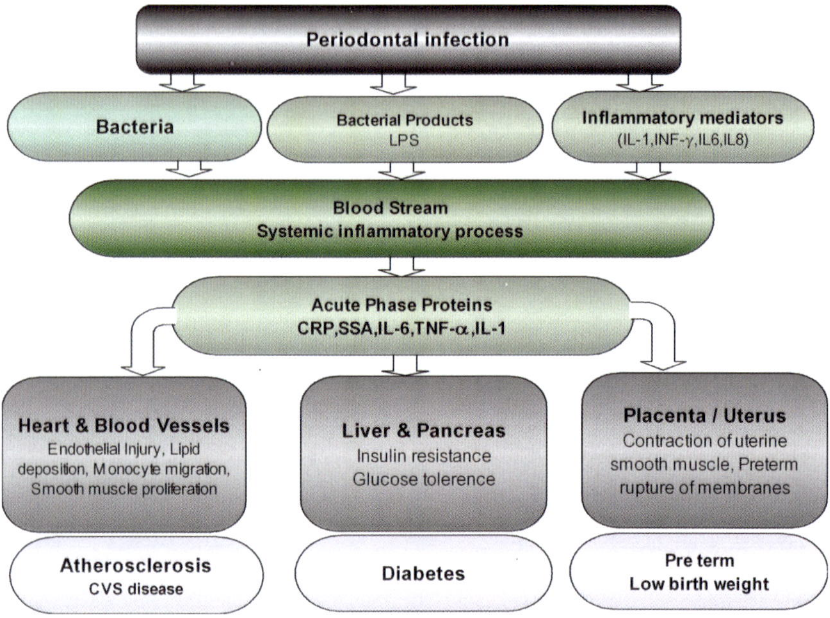

Fig. 3. Periodontal infection and systemic conditions - Potential linkage and possible pathogenic mechanisms (CRP-C-reactive protein, LPS- lipopolysaccharide, IL-1- interleukin-1,IL-6 - interleukin-6, IL-8 - interleukin-8, SSA – Sjogrens's antibodies , INF-γ-Interferon-gamma, TNF-α Tumor necrosis factor-alpha).

3.2.1 Shared risk factors
Factors that place individuals at high risk for periodontitis may also place them at high risk for systemic diseases such as cardiovascular disease. Among the environmental risk factors and indicators shared by periodontitis and systemic disease (cardiovascular disease) are tobacco smoking, stress, aging, race or ethnicity and male gender (Page, 1998).

3.2.2 Subgingival biofilms
Presence of subgingival biofilms constitutes an enormous and constant bacterial load. They present continually renewing reservoir of LPS and other gram-negative bacteria with ready access to the periodontal tissues and the circulation. Systemic challenge with gram-negative bacteria or LPS induces major vascular responses, including an inflammatory cell infiltrate in the vessel walls, intravascular coagulation, vascular smooth muscle proliferation and fatty degeneration. (Mattila, 1989; Marcus and Hajjar, 1993). LPS upregulates expression of endothelial cell adhesion molecules and secretion of interleukin-1 (IL-1), tumor necrosis factor alpha (TNF-α) and thromboxane, which results in platelet aggregation and adhesion, formation of lipid-laden foam cells and deposition of cholesterol and cholesterol esters.

3.2.3 Periodontium as a cytokine reservoir
The pro-inflammatory cytokines TNF-α, IL-1β, and gamma interferon as well as prostaglandin E_2 (PGE_2) reach high tissue concentrations in periodontitis (Page, 1998). The periodontium can therefore serve as a renewing reservoir for spill-over of these mediators, which can enter the circulation and induce as well as perpetuate systemic effects. IL-1β favors coagulation and thrombosis and retards fibrinolysis (Clinton et al., 1991). These mediators emanating from the diseased periodontium may also account for preterm labor and low-birth-weight infants.

4. Periodontitis and cardiovascular system

Cardiovascular diseases such as atherosclerosis and myocardial infarction occur as a result of a complex set of genetic and environmental factors (Herzberg and Weyer, 1998). The genetic factors include age, lipid metabolism, obesity, hypertension, diabetes, increased fibrinogen levels and platelet-specific antigen Zwb ($P1^{A2}$) polymorphism. Environmental risk factors include socioeconomic status, exercise, stress, diet, non- steroidal anti-inflammatory drugs, smoking and chronic infection.

4.1 Epidemiology of periodontal disease and cardiovascular disease
According to the National Health and Nutrition Examination Survey (NHANES III) carried out between 1988 and 1994, 34.5% of dentate U.S. citizens 30 years or older had periodontitis. The prevalence of periodontitis increased with increasing age (Albandar et al., 1999) in developed countries. Cardiovascular disease accounts for 50% of deaths (WHO, 1995) and is considered the leading cause of death in the United States (Rosenberg et al., 1996).

4.2 Dental plaque to atherosclerotic plaque
Several mechanisms have been proposed to explain how periodontal disease initiated by the microorganisms in the dental plaque can contribute to the development of cardiovascular

diseases. The mechanisms associating plaque microorganisms to periodontal disease are discussed in the following section.

4.2.1 First mechanism

Oral bacteria such as *Streptococcus sanguis, P. gingivalis* have collagen like molecule (platelet aggregation associated protein) on their surface (Herzberg et al., 1994) which induces platelet aggregation leading to thrombus formation (Herzberg and Meyer, 1996). When *S. sanguis* is injected intravenously into rabbits, a heart attack-like series of events occur. Antibodies which are reactive to periodontal organisms localize in the heart and trigger complement activation, leading to a series of events causing sensitized T cells and heart disease (Herzberg and Meyer, 1996). Deshpande et al (1998) showed that *P. gingivalis* can actively adhere to and invade fetal bovine heart endothelial cells, bovine aortic endothelial cells and human umbilical vein endothelial cells. Potempa et al(2003) studied proteolytic enzymes referred to as "gingipains R", which when released in large quantities from *P. gingivalis* enter the circulation and activate factorX, prothrombin and protein C, promoting platelet aggregation, finally resulting in intravascular clot formation. *P. gingivalis* and *S. sanguis*, may be isolated from atherosclerotic plaques taken from human carotid endarterectomy specimen (Chiu, 1999; Haraszthy et al., 2000). Putative periodontal pathogens that have been investigated for the development of cardiovascular disease include *Chlamydia pneumoniae, Helicobacter pylori,* Herpes Simplex Virus (HSV), Hepatitis A virus (HAV) and Cytomegalovirus (CMV)

4.2.2 Second mechanism

Patients with certain forms of periodontal disease, such as early-onset periodontitis and refractory periodontitis, possess a hyper inflammatory monocyte phenotype which is an exaggerated host response to a given microbial or LPS challenge. Peripheral blood monocytes from these individuals with the hyper inflammatory monocyte phenotype secrete 3 to 10 fold greater amounts of PGE_2, TNF- α, and IL-1β in response to LPS than those from normal monocyte phenotype individuals (Hernichel-Gorbach et al., 1994; Offenbacher et al., 1994).

4.2.3 Third mechanism

LPS from periodontal pathogens transferred to the serum as a result of bacteremia or bacterial invasion may have a direct effect on endothelia thereby promoting atherosclerosis (Pesonen et al., 1981). LPS may also elicit recruitment of inflammatory cells into major blood vessels and stimulate proliferation of vascular smooth muscle, vascular fatty degeneration, intravascular coagulation and blood platelet function. These changes are the result of the action of various biologic mediators, such as PGs, ILs, and TNF-α on vascular endothelium and smooth muscle (Thom et al., 1992; Beck et al., 1996). The increase in fibrinogen and WBC count noted in periodontitis patients may be a secondary effect of the above mechanisms or a constitutive feature of those at risk for both cardiovascular disease and periodontitis (Kweider et al., 1993).

4.2.4 Fourth mechanism

An elevated level of C-reactive protein, a non-specific marker of inflammation, has been associated with an increased risk of cardiovascular disease. Periodontitis as an infection may stimulate the liver to produce C-reactive protein (CRP), which in turn will form deposits on injured blood vessels. CRP binds to cells that are damaged and fixes complement, which activates phagocytes, including neutrophils. These cells release nitric oxide, thereby contributing to atheroma formation (Genco et al., 2002). In a study of 1,043 apparently healthy men, baseline plasma concentrations of CRP predicted the risk of future myocardial infarction and stroke (Ridker et al., 1997). Ebersole et al (1997) found that patients with adult periodontitis had higher levels of CRP and haptoglobin which declined significantly after periodontal therapy when compared to subjects without periodontitis. In a study by Loos et al (2000) among 153 systemically healthy subjects consisting of 108 untreated periodontitis patients and 45 control subjects, it was found that mean plasma CRP levels were higher among periodontitis patients. They also reported that patients with severe periodontitis had significantly higher CRP levels than mild-periodontitis patients, and both had significantly higher levels than the controls. Another study by Genco et al (2001) evaluated the relationship of cardiovascular disease and CRP. Groups of adults who had neither periodontal nor cardiovascular disease, one of these diseases, or both of them were assembled. In those with both heart disease and periodontal disease, the mean level of CRP (8.7 g/ml) was significantly different from that (1.14 g/ml) in controls with neither disease. The study revealed that treatment of the periodontal disease caused a 65% reduction in the level of CRP at 3 months.

4.2.5 Fifth mechanism

A specific heat shock protein, Hsp65, has been reported to link cardiovascular risks and host responses. Heat shock proteins are important for the maintenance of normal cellular function and may have additional roles as virulence factors for many bacterial species (Young and Elliott, 1989). In animal studies, Xu et al (1993) demonstrated that immunization of rabbits with bacterial Hsp65 induces atherosclerotic lesions. Bacterial infection stimulates the host response to Hsp65, which is a major immunodominant antigen of many bacterial species. The interaction between expressed Hsp65 and the immune response induced by bacterial infection is hypothesized to be responsible for the initiation of the early atherosclerotic lesion (Xu et al., 1993). It has been suggested that chronic oral infection stimulates high levels of Hsp65 in subjects with high cardiovascular risk (Loesche and Lopatin, 1998). Thus, if antibodies directed towards bacterial heat shock proteins cross-react with heat shock proteins expressed by the host tissue, especially those found in the lining of blood vessels, then some oral species might well be the link between oral infection and cardiovascular disease (Loesche and Lopatin, 1998).

4.2.6 Sixth mechanism

MMPs: MMPs, including the collagenases, likely play an important role in periodontal tissue breakdown (Lee et al., 2004) as well as destabilization of atheromas leading to heart failure and the deleterious changes in extracellular matrix in the myocardium. In fact, there is increasing evidence that inhibition of MMPs, already shown to be effective for inhibition of periodontal attachment loss, can also inhibit the development of cardiac failure (Matsumura et al., 2005).

4.3 Common risk factors for periodontal disease and cardiovascular disease

The difficulty in drawing a cause and effect relationship between periodontitis and cardiovascular disease stems from the fact that the two groups of diseases share many risk factors. Risk factors, such as smoking, genetics, stress and increasing age, could independently lead to periodontal disease and cardiovascular disease.

4.3.1 Smoking

Smoking is a significant risk factor for both diseases. Current evidence suggests that an important component of cigarette smoke, aryl hydrocarbons (Singh et al., 2000), have the ability to inhibit bone formation, particularly in the presence of periodontal disease-causing bacterial co-factors (Singh et al., 2000). As such, these data could help to explain, in part, how cigarette smoking might lead to periodontal bone loss. Interestingly, we now also have data to suggest that these same aryl hydrocarbons may promote vascular disease, as measured by vascular calcification (Usman, 2004). Thus, a common risk factor, smoking/aryl hydrocarbons, mitigates negative effects in two disparate systems: the periodontium and vascular tissues.

4.3.2 Association between periodontal disease and atherosclerosis

Atherosclerosis has been defined as a progressive disease process that involves the large- to medium-sized muscular and large elastic arteries. The advanced lesion is the atheroma, which consists of elevated focal intimal plaques with a necrotic central core containing lysed cells, cholesterol ester crystals, lipid-laden foam cells and surface plasma proteins, including fibrin and fibrinogen (Boon et al., 1995). The presence of atheroma tends to make the patient thrombosis-prone because the associated surface enhances platelet aggregation and thrombus formation that can occlude the artery or be released to cause thrombosis, coronary heart disease and stroke. A study report indicated that atherosclerotic plaques are commonly infected with gram-negative periodontal pathogens, including *A. actinomycetemcomitans* and *P. gingivalis* (Haraszthy et al., 2000).

5. Periodontal disease and diabetes mellitus

Diabetes mellitus represents a group of complex metabolic disorders characterized by hyperglycemia resulting from defects in insulin secretion, insulin action or both resulting in inability of glucose to be transported from blood stream into tissues and a consequent excretion of sugar in the urine (Harmel et al., 2004).

Diabetes occurs in two major forms: **Type 1 diabetes** previously called as **'insulin-dependent diabetes mellitus'** is the result of a reduction in or the elimination of insulin production by beta cells in the pancreas. Reduced insulin production is most often the result of destruction of the beta cells, probably due to autoimmune or viral disease. Individuals with type 1 diabetes require daily insulin supplementation to properly regulate glucose use. Insulin delivery is usually by injection, although progress has been made with the use of insulin pumps and pancreatic transplantation that provides an endogenous source of insulin. **Type 2 diabetes** previously called **'non-insulin-dependent diabetes mellitus'** is characterized by a deficient response to insulin by target cells, although insulin production is typically normal or even enhanced in these individuals. This impairment may be due to changes in the structure or number of the cell receptors for insulin. It is suggested that type 2 diabetes may be a disorder of the innate immune system and results from a chronic, low-level inflammatory process (Pickup and Crook, 1998). This form of diabetes is by far the most common (estimated to be 85%-90% of all diabetes). Although the precise etiology is still uncertain in both types of primary diabetes, environmental factors interact with genetic susceptibility to determine which of those with the genetic predisposition actually develop the clinical syndrome and the timing of its onset. Environmental factors in insulin-dependent diabetes include virus, diet, immunological factors and pancreatic disease. In non-insulin-dependent diabetes, environmental factors such as lifestyle, age, pregnancy, pancreatic pathology, insulin secretion and resistance are included.

5.1 Inter-relationships between periodontal diseases and diabetes mellitus

The interrelationship between diabetes and periodontal disease is established through a number of pathways and is bidirectional. Diabetes is a risk factor for gingivitis and periodontitis. Blood sugar control is an important variable in the relationship between diabetes and periodontal disease. Individuals who have poor glycemic control have a greater prevalence and severity of gingival and periodontal inflammation. It has been suggested that hyperglycemia promotes periodontitis and its progression.

One plausible biologic mechanism for why diabetics have more severe periodontal disease is that glucose-mediated advanced glycation end-products (AGE) accumulation affects the migration and phagocytic activity of mononuclear and polymorphonuclear phagocytic cells, resulting in the establishment of a more pathogenic subgingival flora. The maturation and gradual transformation of the subgingival microflora into an essentially gram-negative flora will in turn constitute, via the ulcerated pocket epithelium, a chronic source of systemic challenge. This in turn triggers both an "infection-mediated" pathway of cytokine upregulation, especially with secretion of TNF-α and IL-1, and a state of insulin resistance, affecting glucose-utilizing pathways. The interaction of mononuclear phagocytes with AGE-modified proteins induces upregulation of cytokine expression and induction of oxidative stress. Thus, monocytes in diabetic individuals may be "primed" by AGE-protein binding. Periodontal infection challenge to these primed phagocytic cells may, in turn, amplify the magnitude of the macrophage response to AGE-protein, enhancing cytokine production and oxidative stress. Simultaneously, periodontal infection may induce a chronic state of insulin resistance, contributing to the cycle of hyperglycemia, nonenzymatic irreversible glycation, AGE-protein binding and accumulation, amplifying the classical pathway of diabetic connective tissue degradation, destruction and proliferation. Hence, the relationship between diabetes mellitus and periodontal disease or infection becomes bi-directional. A self-feeding two-way system of catabolic response and tissue destruction ensues, resulting in more severe periodontal disease and increased difficulty in controlling blood sugar.

Studies on Pima Indians, who have a very high rate of diabetes, show a higher prevalence and incidence of periodontal attachment loss and alveolar bone loss than control populations (Nelson et al., 1990). Both diseases have a relatively high incidence in the general population and are polygenic disorders featuring some degree of immune system dysfunction (Anil et al., 1990a; Anil et al., 1990b). Most of the early studies tended to consider the relationship between the two diseases as unidirectional, with a higher incidence and severity of periodontitis in patients with diabetes. Studies have suggested evidence for a bidirectional adverse interrelationship between diabetes and periodontal diseases (Taylor et al., 2004). In particular, individuals susceptible to diabetes and those with poor metabolic control may experience one or more complications in multiple organs and tissues. The evidence for a bidirectional relationship between the two conditions comes from studies conducted in distinctly different settings worldwide (Taylor, 2001).

A model was presented by Grossi and Genco (1998), in which severe periodontal disease increases the severity of diabetes mellitus and complicates metabolic control. They proposed that an infection-mediated upregulation cycle of cytokine synthesis and secretion by chronic stimulus from LPS and products of periodontopathic organisms may amplify the magnitude of the AGE-mediated cytokine response that is operative in diabetes mellitus. The combination of these two pathways, infection and AGE-mediated cytokine upregulation, helps explain the increase in tissue destruction seen in diabetic periodontitis and how periodontal infection may complicate the severity of diabetes and the degree of metabolic control, resulting in a two-way relationship between diabetes mellitus and periodontal disease or infection. Overall, the evidence supports the view that the relationship between diabetes and periodontal diseases is bidirectional. Further, rigorous systematic studies are warranted to firmly establish that treating periodontal infections can contribute to glycemic management and possibly to a reduction in the complications of DM.

5.2 Periodontal treatment and the glycemic control in diabetic patients

It has been made clear that severe periodontitis is associated with poor blood sugar control and that effective periodontal treatment can improve some complications of diabetes, especially hyperglycemia. Periodontal treatment has been shown to improve the metabolic control of diabetic patients, thereby influencing a reduction in glycated and glycemic hemoglobin levels (Faria-Almeida et al., 2006).

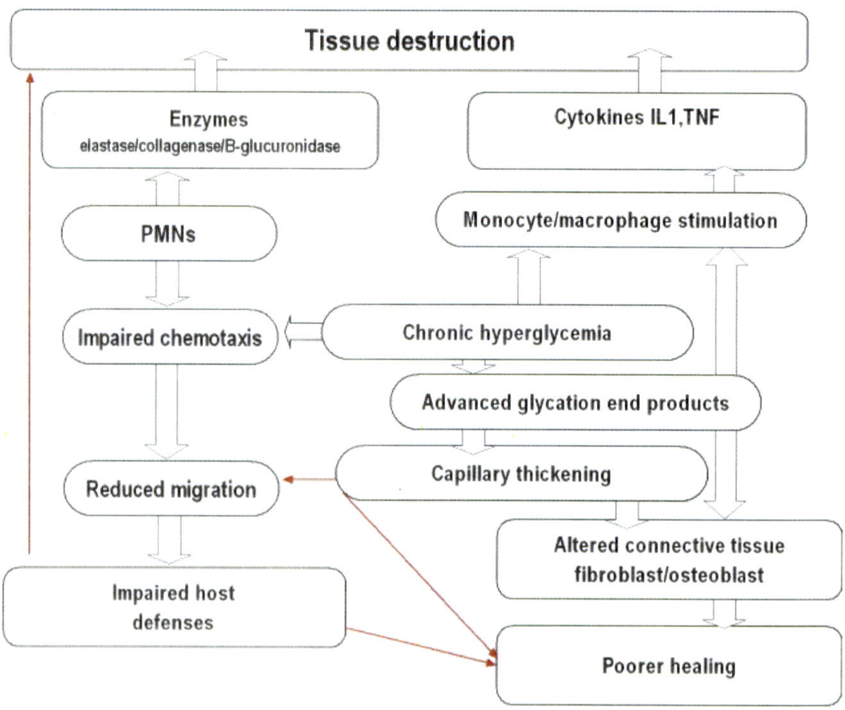

Fig. 4. Effect of diabetes mellitus on host response.

The majority of periodontal treatment studies have shown some improvement in diabetic control as measured by a reduction in HbA_{1c} levels, but some of these studies only had small numbers of patients. A recent meta-analysis of 456 patients has shown that the reductions in HbA_{1c} were small and not statistically significant. Hence, further studies with larger sample sizes and including only type 2 diabetics are needed before definite conclusions can be drawn. Even so, HbA_{1c} levels tend to increase over time in diabetics, and so even a small reduction may be of clinical significance for individual patients, especially as the studies do seem to show a lot of inter-individual variation.

A systematic review of the literature by Grossi et al (1994) concluded that the effect on diabetic status was dependent upon the treatment modality. Studies that investigated the effect of only mechanical debridement were unable to demonstrate any effect on blood glucose level or glycated hemoglobin level regardless of periodontal disease severity or degree of diabetes control. However, all three studies that added systemic antibiotics to mechanical debridement demonstrated improved metabolic control of diabetes. Results from a randomized clinical trial conducted on the Pima population indicated that all subjects that were treated with doxycycline experienced a reduction in glycated hemoglobin. These results suggest that periodontal antimicrobial treatment may reduce the level of glycated hemoglobin in diabetic subjects and may ultimately hold the potential to reduce diabetic sequelae.

There is a strong bidirectional relationship between periodontal diseases and diabetes. Not only are populations and patients with uncontrolled diabetes more susceptible to periodontal diseases, but the presence of active periodontal disease can worsen glycemic control. Effective periodontal therapy combined with systemic antibiotics appears to have a dual effect for diabetic patients, by reducing periodontal infection and improving glycemic status. Dental professionals should also monitor the patient's glycemic control in order to provide optimal dental care.

6. Periodontal disease and adverse pregnancy outcomes

There is emerging evidence of a relationship between periodontal health and adverse pregnancy outcomes, particularly preterm birth (PTB)/preterm low-birth-weight infants (PLBW). PTB and low birth weight (LBW) are considered to be the most relevant biological determinants of newborn infants survival, both in developed and in developing countries. The term "adverse pregnancy outcomes" include conditions such as preterm low-birth weight (PLBW) infants, infants born small for gestational age, miscarriage, and pre-eclampsia (Bobetsis et al., 2006). According to the World Health Organization, low birth weight (LBW) is defined as a birth weight <2500g. This low birth weight may be either due to pre-term birth or full term infants who had intra-uterine growth restriction (IUGR) which results in the infant being born small for gestational age (Kramer, 2003). Pre-term births occur mainly because of premature rupture of membranes of preterm labor.

Infection of the chorioamnionic, or extraplacental membrane, may lead to chorioamnionitis, a condition strongly associated with a premature membrane rupture and preterm delivery (Mueller-Heubach et al., 1990). This suggests that distant sites of infection or sepsis may be targeting the placental membranes. PLBW is a major cause of infant mortality and morbidity that poses considerable medical and economic burden on the society (Alves and Ribeiro, 2006). PTB remains a significant public health issue and it is the leading cause of neonatal death and other health problems including neurodevelopmental disturbances (Williams et al., 2000).

Many risk factors have been proposed to cause preterm rupture of membranes and preterm labor. Identified risk factors for PLBW include maternal age; African-American ancestry, low socio-economic status, inadequate prenatal care, drug, alcohol and tobacco abuse; hypertension, genitourinary tract infection, diabetes mellitus (DM), previous PLBW and multiple pregnancies. Smoking during pregnancy has been linked to 20-30% of LBW births and 10% of fetal and infant deaths (Boutigny et al., 2005). Infection is also considered as a major cause of PLBW deliveries, accounting for 30% and 50% of all cases (Offenbacher et al., 1998; Marakoglu et al., 2008).

It has been proposed that one important factor contributing to the continuing prevalence of infants with PLBW is the effect of maternal burden of infection. In this context, periodontal infection may be of importance. Studies have shown that conditions such as bacterial infection of the genitourinary tract, bacterial vaginosis and a high prevalence of maternal lower genitourinary tract infections are associated with adverse pregnancy outcomes. It is also possible that infectious processes occurring elsewhere in the body may contribute to neonatal morbidity and mortality which suggests that periodontal disease may be one such infection.

6.1 Pathogenic mechanisms linking periodontal disease to adverse pregnancy outcomes

Evidence suggests a role for inflammation and endothelial activation in the pathophysiology of preeclampsia (Roberts et al., 1989); periodontal infection is one of many potential stimuli for these host responses. The risk for PLBW may be increased by distant infections which result in translocation of bacteria or their components. Distant sites of infection or sepsis such as periodontal disease may target the placental membranes through biological mechanisms involving bacterially induced activation of cell-mediated immunity leading to cytokine production and ensuing synthesis and release of prostaglandin, which can trigger preterm labor (Hillier et al., 1988). Cytokines such as IL-1, IL-6, and TNF-α are all potent inducers of both prostaglandin synthesis and labor and the levels of these cytokines have been found to be elevated in the amniotic fluid of patients in preterm labor with amniotic fluid infection (Romero et al., 2006). Intra-amnionic levels of PGE_2 and TNF-α rise steadily throughout pregnancy until a critical threshold is reached to induce labor, cervical dilation, and delivery (Offenbacher et al., 1996). Since these cytokines function as physiological mediators of labor and delivery, any condition that results in an increase in their levels may have the potential of resulting in PTB and LBW. As a remote gram-negative infection, periodontal disease may have the potential to affect pregnancy outcome through these mechanisms. The gram-negative bacteria associated with progressive disease can produce a variety of bioactive molecules that can directly affect the host. One microbial component, LPS, can activate macrophages and other cells to synthesize and secrete a wide array of molecules, including the cytokines IL-Iβ, TNF-α, IL-6, PGE_2 and matrix metalloproteinases (Darveau et al., 1997). During pregnancy, the ratio of anaerobic gram-negative bacterial species to aerobic species increases in dental plaque in the second trimester (Kornman and Loesche, 1980), and this may lead to an increased production of these cytokines. If they escape into the general circulation and cross the placental barrier, they could augment the physiologic levels of PGE_2 and TNF-α in the amniotic fluid and induce premature labor. Moreover, it has been demonstrated in a rabbit model that chronic maternal exposure to the periodontal pathogen *P. gingivalis* results in systemic dissemination, transplacental passage, and fetal exposure (Boggess et al., 2005). Studies on murine models have shown that *P. gingivalis* infection during pregnancy results in systemic dissemination of the organism which was associated with IUGR, placenta-specific

translocation of *P. gingivalis*, increased maternal TNF-α and *P. gingivalis*-specific serum IgG levels and a shift in the placental Th1/Th2 cytokine balance (Lin et al., 2003).
Significantly elevated levels of *T. forsythia* and *Campylobacter rectus* among PLBW mothers was reported in a study conducted among African-American and Hispanic subjects (Mitchell-Lewis et al., 2001). These findings suggest that periodontal infection caused by gram negative species which produce LPS may be associated with an increased risk of PLBW. Buduneli et al (2005) compared the periodontal microflora of PLBW mothers and controls in a Turkish population and reported that the bacterial loads of certain species including important periodontal pathogens such as *P. gingivalis, A. actinomycetemcomitams, P. intermedia, and Streptococcus intermedius* were significantly higher among controls than among cases (Buduneli et al., 2005). Although the occurrence rates of *P. intermedia, Fusobacterium nucleatum, Peptostreptococcus micros, C. rectus, Eikenella corrodens, Selenomonas noxia, and S. intermedius* were higher among cases, the differences were not statistically significant. Logistic regression analysis revealed that *P. micros* and *C. rectus* significantly increased the risk of PLBW while *Prevotella nigrescens* and *A. actinomycetemcomitans* decreased the risk.

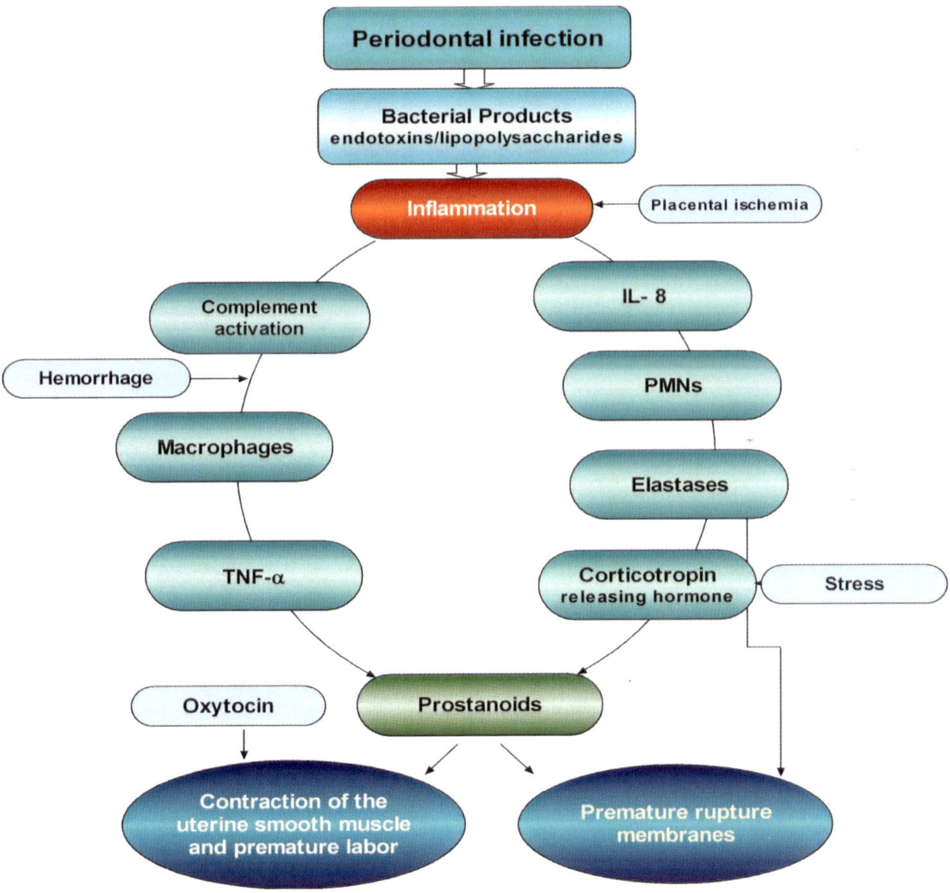

Fig. 5. Proposed biological mechanisms for induction of premature birth.

In a study evaluating the relationship between fetal inflammatory and immune responses to oral pathogens and risk for PTB, umbilical cord blood specimens were examined for presence of fetal immunoglobulin M (IgM) antibody against oral pathogens and levels of C-reactive protein, IL-β, IL-6, TNF-α, PGE_2, and 8-isoprostane. The results showed that the presence of IgM antibodies to oral pathogens and increased levels of TNF-α and 8-isoprostane were associated with increased rates of PTB, and that the combined effects of fetal IgM, C-reactive protein, TNF-α, PGE_2, and 8-isoprostane resulted in a significantly increased risk for PTB (Boggess et al., 2005). An elevated level of CRP among pregnant patients with periodontitis compared to periodontally healthy subjects has been reported by other investigators (Pitiphat et al., 2006; Horton et al., 2008).

Studies have shown that elevated levels of serum and placental soluble VEGF receptor-1 are associated with an increased risk of pre-eclampsia (Koga et al., 2003; Romero et al., 2008). Elevated levels of soluble VEGF receptors have also been reported in mothers with periodontitis who gave birth to PLBW infants (Sert et al., 2011). Subjects with periodontitis have been shown to have elevated levels of β2-glycoprotein I-dependent anti-cardiolipin autoantibodies; a class of antibodies associated with adverse pregnancy outcomes and fetal loss as well as elevated levels of markers of vascular inflammation (Schenkein et al., 2007).

7. Periodontal infection and gastrointestinal diseases

The oral cavity provides a gateway between the external environment and the gastrointestinal tract and facilitates both food ingestion and digestion. Oral hygiene and tooth loss can potentially affect gastrointestinal flora and nutritional status, and thus, they have implications for the development of chronic gastro-intestinal diseases. Poor dental health, tooth loss, or both have been associated with increased risk for chronic gastritis, peptic ulcer and gastrointestinal malignancies, including oral, esophageal and gastric cancers (Abnet et al., 2005; Kossioni and Dontas, 2007).

7.1 *Helicobacter pylori* infection

Helicobacter pylori (*H. pylori*) is one of the most common bacterial infections of humans (Blaser, 1997). The presence of the organism *H. pylori* (initially termed *Campylobacter pyloridis*) in the antral mucosa of humans was first reported in 1983 (Warren and Marshall, 1983). *H. pylori have* been closely linked to chronic gastritis, peptic ulcer, gastric cancer and mucosa-associated lymphoid tissue (MALT) lymphoma (Dunn et al., 1997; Wang et al., 2002). Although the mode of transmission of *H. pylori* is not yet clear, it has been suggested that oral-oral and fecal-oral routes are the most likely routes (Moreira et al., 2004). The microorganism may be transmitted orally and has been detected in dental plaque and saliva (Krajden et al., 1989; Dowsett et al., 1999). But the role of oral cavity and dental plaque as extra-gastric reservoirs of *H. pylori* is not yet clear. If the oral cavity is an extra-gastric reservoir of the *H. pylori*, it may have a bearing on the treatment of *H. pylori* associated gastric disease on account of the fact that the dental plaque provides protection to the resident microflora (Al Asqah et al., 2009).

Dental plaque has been suggested as a reservoir for *H. pylori(Avcu et al., 2001)*.The presence of *H. pylori* has been universally associated with chronic gastritis, and strongly with duodenal ulcer. Previous studies have also identified the microorganism in dental plaque and saliva, which would implicate the oral cavity as a potential reservoir for *H. pylori* or as a possible route of transmission to other sites. Presently, it is not clear whether the oral cavity permanently harbors viable *H. pylori* or merely serves as the route of transmission to other sites (Kim et al., 2000). In a survey of Dye et al (2002) periodontal disease, specifically periodontal pocket depth, was associated with seroprevalence of *H. pylori*. Furthermore, gastric carriage of *H. pylori* is a known risk factor for gastric cancer, with the cytotoxin-associated gene-A-positive (CagA+) strain having a greater propensity for inflammation, ulceration and malignancy (Stolzenberg-Solomon et al., 2003). The question as to whether the oral cavities, in general, and dental plaque, specifically, are reservoir of *H. pylori,* has been controversial. Desai et al (1991) suggested dental plaque as a permanent reservoir of *H. pylori*. Other investigators, however, would argue against the notion that the oral cavity and dental plaque are permanent reservoirs for *H.* pylori (Kamat et al., 1998). The detection of *H. pylori* by polymerase chain reaction in dental plaque, however, would indicate that the oral cavity may act as a reservoir or sanctuary for the organism (Oshowo et al., 1998).

7.2 *H. pylori* and periodontal disease

Among the various studies that have evaluated the relationship between periodontal disease and *H. pylori* infection, some have reported a positive association between the two conditions, while findings from other studies did not support this association. A large scale epidemiological study to evaluate the relationship between *H. pylori* infection and abnormal periodontal conditions was conducted by Dye et al (2002) utilizing the data from the first phase of the third National Health and Nutrition Examination Survey. The authors reported that this association is comparable to the studies on independent effects of poverty on *H. pylori* and concluded that poor periodontal health, characterized by advanced periodontal pockets, may be associated with *H. pylori* infection in adults, independent of poverty status.

7.3 *H. pylori* eradication therapy and oral *H. pylori*

Studies have shown that chemotherapy usually employed for the management of *H. pylori*-associated gastric disease, although is successful in eradication of the organism from the gastric mucosa, seldom has any effect on the organism in the dental plaque. In a study in which *H. pylori* was detected in dental plaque and in gastric antral and body mucosa in 98%, 67% and 70%, respectively, of 43 consecutive patients with dyspepsia, triple drug therapy was administered for 15 days to 24 patients. *H. pylori* was eliminated from the gastric mucosa in all 24 patients but persisted in dental plaque in all of them indicating that dental plaque is unaffected by triple drug therapy. Miyabayashi et al (2000) analyzed the correlation between the success of gastric eradication and the prevalence of *H. pylori* in the oral cavity in 47 patients with *H. pylori*-gastritis. Presence of *H. pylori* was determined by nested polymerase chain reaction (PCR) before and after eradication therapy. Of the 24 patients who tested negative for oral *H. pylori* before eradication therapy, *H. pylori* were completely eradicated from the stomach in 22 (92%). None of these patients experienced recurrence during the mean follow-up period of 19.7 months (range 1-48 months). In contrast, 4 weeks after initial therapy, complete eradication of gastric *H. pylori* was achieved for only 12 (52%) of the 23 patients who tested positive for oral *H. pylori*. Of these 12 cases, 7 remained oral positive and 5 became oral negative and 2 of the oral positive cases relapsed within 2 years of initial therapy. Among the 23 patients, oral *H. pylori* were eradicated by therapy only in 8 cases (35%) and one of these relapsed within 2 years of initial therapy. The prevalence of *H. pylori* colonization in dental plaque and tongue scrapings of patients with chronic gastritis and the effect of systemic treatment upon this colonization and eradication of *H. pylori* from gastric mucosa were studied by Ozdemir et al (2001). Among the 81 patients examined for the study, chronic gastritis was diagnosed in 63 (77.7%) of 81 patients while dental plaque samples of 64 (79%) patients and tongue scraping samples of 48 (59.2%) patients were urease positive. Of the 63 patients with chronic gastritis, dental plaque and tongue scrapings were urease positive in 52 (83%) and 37 (59%) patients, respectively. After 14 days of triple drug therapy (omeprazole, clarithromycin, and amoxicillin), *H. pylori* was eradicated from the gastric mucosa of almost all of the patients, whereas no changes were detected in dental plaque and tongue scrapings by CLO test examination.

7.4 Effects of periodontal therapy on the management of *H. pylori*-associated gastric disease

If the hypothesis that oral cavity, dental plaque in particular, is a reservoir for *H. pylori*, then plaque control or periodontal therapy may hold potential benefits in the management of *H. pylori*-associated gastric disease. Very few studies have evaluated the benefits of periodontal therapy in the management of *H. pylori*-associated gastric disease. However, studies conducted in this regard have shown encouraging results. Recently it was reported that plaque control results in lesser prevalence of *H. pylori* in the gastric mucosa (Jia et al., 2009). Another study reported that 77.3% of the patients treated using a combination of periodontal treatment and triple therapy exhibited successful eradication of gastric *H. pylori*, compared with 47.6% who underwent only triple therapy (Zaric et al., 2009).

8. Periodontal disease and respiratory disease

The anatomical continuity between the lungs and the oràl cavity makes the latter a potential reservoir of respiratory pathogens. The micro-organisms may enter the lung by inhalation, but the most common route of infection is aspiration of what pneumologists have long referred to as oropharyngeal secretions. Therefore, it is plausible that oral micro-organisms might infect the respiratory tract. However, only recently has the role of the oral flora in the pathogenesis of respiratory infection been examined closely (Mojon, 2002).

Current evidence suggests that periodontal disease may be associated with systemic diseases. Respiratory diseases is the term for diseases of the respiratory system, including lung, pleural cavity, bronchial tubes, trachea and upper respiratory tract. They range from a common cold to life threatening conditions such as bacterial pneumonia or chronic obstructive pulmonary disease (COPD), which are important causes of death worldwide (Weidlich et al., 2008). COPD is currently the fourth leading cause of death in the world and further increase in the prevalence and mortality of the disease can be predicted in the coming decades (Pauwels et al., 2001). Chronic bronchitis and emphysema are the most common forms of COPD.

COPD is a pathological and chronic obstruction of airflow through the airways or out of the lungs, and includes chronic bronchitis and emphysema. Its main risk factor is smoking, but air pollution and genetic factors are also strongly implicated. *Chronic bronchitis is an inflammatory condition associated with excessive mucus production sufficient to cause cough with expectoration for at least 3 months of the year for 2 or 3 years. Emphysema is the destruction of the air spaces distal to terminal bronchioles.*

Pneumonia (both community-acquired and hospital acquired) is an acute infection of the lung and is characterized by cough, breath shortness, sputum production and chest pain. It is caused by the micro-aspiration of oropharyngeal secretions containing bacteria into the lung, and failure of the host to clear the bacteria (Weidlich et al., 2008).

8.1 Relationship between periodontal infection and respiratory disease

There is increasing evidence that a poor oral health can predispose to respiratory diseases, especially in high-risk patients. The oral cavity is contiguous with the trachea and may be a portal for respiratory pathogen colonization. Dental plaque can be colonized by respiratory pathogens (Didilescu et al., 2005) which may be aspirated from the oropharynx into the upper airway and then reach the lower airway and adhere to bronchial or alveolar epithelium (Scannapieco, 1999). A systematic review done by Azarpazhooh and Leake (2006) concluded that there is fair evidence of an association of pneumonia with oral health, but there is poor evidence of a weak association between COPD and oral health. A prospective study conducted with 697 elderly individuals observed that the adjusted mortality due to pneumonia was 3.9 times higher in subjects with periodontal disease (Awano et al., 2008). Scannapieco *et al* (2003) conducted a systematic review about the effectiveness of oral decontamination to prevent pneumonia. An association between poor oral health and chronic obstructive pulmonary disease (COPD) was observed on analysis of existing large databases such as the Veterans Administration Normative Aging Study and the National Health and Nutrition Examination Survey III (NHANES III), after controlling for confounding variables such as smoking, sex, age and socioeconomic status(Scannapieco and Ho, 2001). Awano et al (2008) conducted a study which concluded that an increase in teeth with periodontal pockets in the elderly may be associated with increased mortality from pneumonia. A systematic review of 21 studies reports on the impact of periodontal disease and other indicators of poor oral health on the initiation or progression of pneumonia (Scannapieco et al., 2003).

8.2 Mechanism of infection

Several biological mechanisms are hypothesized to explain the link between poor oral health and pneumonia. Two routes exist for oral micro-organisms to reach the lower respiratory tract: hematogenous spread and aspiration.

Hematogenous spread of bacteria is an inevitable adverse effect of some dental treatments and may occur even after simple prophylactic procedures. Nonetheless, this route of infection seems rare.

Aspiration: Three mechanisms of infection related to aspiration of material from the upper airway can be envisioned. First, periodontal disease or poor oral hygiene might result in a higher concentration of oral pathogens in the saliva. These pathogens would then be aspirated into the lung, overwhelming the immune defences. Second, under specific conditions, the dental plaque could harbour colonies of pulmonary pathogens and promote their growth. Finally, periodontal pathogens could facilitate the colonization of the upper airways by pulmonary pathogens. Cytokines and enzymes induced from the periodontally inflamed tissues by the oral biofilm may also be transferred into the lungs where they may stimulate local inflammatory process preceding colonization of pathogens and the actual lung infection (Scannapieco et al., 2001). Other possible mechanisms of pulmonary infection are inhalation of airborne pathogens or translocation of bacteria from local infections via bacteremia. The possibility that bacteria in oral biofilms influence respiratory infection suggests that good oral hygiene may prevent the aspiration of large numbers of oral bacteria into the lower airway and thus prevent initiation or progression of respiratory infection in susceptible individuals. Further studies are required to verify the importance of oral conditions in the pathogenesis of lung diseases such as COPD (Teng et al., 2002).

8.3 Microbiological similarities between organisms infecting the lungs and oral flora

The vast majority of pulmonary diseases are due to aerobic bacteria that are found in the oral flora but are not related to any oral diseases. In contrast, the list of anaerobes that are implicated in the destruction of periodontal tissues and that have also been isolated from infected lungs is quite long. For example, *Actinobacillus actinomycetemcomitans* and *Fusobacterium nucleatum* have both been isolated from infected lungs, whereas *Pseudomonas aeruginosa*, a known pulmonary pathogen, has been isolated from patients with "refractory" periodontitis (Slots et al., 1990). The pulmonary pathogenicity of *P. gingivalis* has been confirmed in an animal model simulating aspiration (Nelson et al., 1986). Common potential respiratory pathogens (PRPs) such as *Streptococcus pneumoniae*, *Mycoplasma pneumoniae*, and *Haemophilus influenza* can colonize the oropharynx and will be aspirated into the lower airways.

9. Periodontitis and osteoporosis

Osteoporosis is a skeletal disorder characterized by low bone mass and micro-architectural deterioration with a resulting increase in bone fragility and susceptibility to fracture (Cummings and Melton, 2002). It is the most common type of metabolic bone disease, characterized by compromised bone strength. Osteoporosis and periodontal diseases have several risk factors in common, such as increased disease prevalence with increased age, negative impacts of smoking on disease development and severity and impaired tissue healing as a result of the disease. Therefore, it would be interesting for dental professionals to examine the relationship between osteoporosis and periodontal diseases.

9.1 Inter-relationships and interactions between periodontal diseases and osteoporosis

Several potential mechanisms have been proposed to explain the association between osteoporosis and periodontal diseases. First, osteoporosis results in loss of BMD throughout the body, including the maxilla and the mandible. The resulting low density in the jawbones leads to increased alveolar porosity, altered trabecular pattern and more rapid alveolar bone resorption following invasion by periodontal pathogens. Second, systemic factors affecting bone remodeling may also modify the local tissue response to periodontal infection, such as increased systemic release of IL-1 and IL-6.

The majority of the literature has investigated the role of osteoporosis in the onset and progression of periodontitis and tooth loss (Weyant et al., 1999; Tezal et al., 2000; Lundstrom et al., 2001). However, chronic infection around multiple teeth could contribute significantly to elevations in circulating IL-6 levels, a predictor of bone loss (Scheidt-Nave et al., 2001). In an animal study, elevated levels of IL-6 were found in the serum and gingival tissues adjacent to deep periodontal pockets (Johnson et al., 1997). Therefore, it is at least theoretically possible that chronic periodontitis may contribute to the development or progression of osteoporosis. Whether individuals with oral osteopenia are at risk for systemic osteopenia and osteoporosis remains to be determined. Medications used for the treatment and prevention of osteoporosis have the potential to reduce alveolar bone loss (Persson et al., 2002; Yoshihara et al., 2004). It has been shown that estrogen used in hormone replacement therapy of postmenopausal women is associated with reduced gingival inflammation and a reduced frequency of gingival attachment loss in osteoporotic women in early menopause (Krall, 2001). The use of bisphosphonate alendronate, an antiresorptive drug has been shown to lower the risk of bone loss in adults with periodontal disease (El-Shinnawi and El-Tantawy, 2003). There is a possible relationship between osteoporosis and periodontitis which need further investigations.

9.2 Effects of periodontal infection on systemic bone loss

Although periodontal diseases have historically been deemed to be the result of an infectious process, others have suggested that periodontal diseases may be an early manifestation of osteoporosis (Whalen and Krook, 1996). The link between these two diseases may be the bone-resorptive process. Increased local production of cytokines associated with periodontal diseases could accelerate systemic bone resorption by modulating the host response. Pro-inflammatory cytokine IL-6, produced by osteoblasts, may play a pivotal role in this potential mechanism. In normal bone homeostasis, IL-6 production stimulates osteoclastic activity resulting in bone resorption. Many of the effects on BMD may also be modulated through IL-6 (Reddy, 2001).

Genetic factors that predispose an individual to systemic bone loss may also predispose them to periodontal destruction. Among several factors that down regulate IL-6 gene expression are estrogen and testosterone. After menopause, IL-6 levels are elevated, even in the absence of infection, trauma or stress. The increased gene expression of IL-6 with age may be the reason why both osteoporosis and chronic periodontal diseases are age related (Ershler and Keller, 2000). Certain lifestyle factors, such as smoking and low calcium intake, may influence the risk of developing osteoporosis and periodontal diseases (Payne et al., 2000).

A growing body of literature has accumulated to investigate the association between osteoporosis and periodontal diseases. Although significant advances have been made in determining the relationship between periodontal disease and osteoporosis, further studies are needed to clarify this correlation. Compared to other systemic diseases, the research done in elucidating the association is limited, and many researchers have highlighted and stressed in their publications this great need for a better understanding of the relationship. Another issue is that periodontal disease is diagnosed largely in males whereas osteoporosis is a disorder predominantly diagnosed in females.

Most published studies explaining the relationship between osteoporosis and periodontal diseases support a positive association between these two common diseases. However, the conclusions drawn from these studies need to be interpreted with caution due to the limitations of the study design, small sample sizes and inadequate control of other confounding factors. Additional well-controlled, large-scale, prospective studies are needed to clarify the situation and to provide a better understanding of the mechanisms by which osteoporosis and periodontal diseases are associated.

10. Rheumatoid arthritis and periodontitis

Rheumatoid arthritis (RA) is an autoimmune disease that affects several organs and systems and it is also associated with destruction of joint connective tissue and bone. It has been reported that the patterns of hard and soft tissue destruction in RA is similar to that seen in chronic periodontitis. Besides the similarity in tissue destruction, the two conditions also share certain pathogenic mechanisms such as release of inflammatory mediators which mediate the tissue destruction. This similarity of clinical and pathologic features led to the hypothesis of a bidirectional association between RA and periodontitis which involves RA affecting the pathogenesis of periodontitis and vice-versa (Mercado et al., 2000; Ribeiro et al., 2005). Both conditions are associated with destruction of bone, mediated by inflammatory cytokines such as interleukin-1, tumor necrosis factor and prostaglandin E2 (Bozkurt et al., 2000). During the inflammatory response, cytokines and matrix metalloproteinases, factors that are essential in the pathogenesis of both diseases, are released from the inflammatory cells (Birkedal-Hansen, 1993; Kjeldsen et al., 1993). An altered function of the inflammatory response and the metabolism of soft and hard tissues may turn out to be identical pathogenic factors (Kornman et al., 1997). A novel cytokine termed Secreted osteoclastogenic factor of activated T cells (SOFAT) has been suggested as factor which may exacerbate inflammation and/or bone turnover under inflammatory conditions such as RA and periodontitis (Rifas and Weitzmann, 2009). An experimental study in which adjuvant arthritis was induced in rats showed that the development of arthritis was associated with an elevation of joint tissue MMPs, TNF-α, and IL-1β compared to control rats. In the gingival tissues of arthritic rat's gelatinase, collagenase, TNF-α and IL-1β were elevated. There was also a significant increase in periodontal bone loss and tooth mobility in arthritic rats (Ramamurthy et al., 2005).

Rheumatoid arthritis also influences the pathogenesis of periodontitis through its motor and emotional impairment (Persson et al., 1999). Motor impairment may make it more difficult to perform adequate oral hygiene. The salivary flow reduction due to medication or secondary Sjogren syndrome may increase supragingival plaque formation in these individuals (Bozkurt et al., 2000). Psychological alterations found among RA patients were suggested as risk indicators for periodontitis (Genco et al., 1999).

Periodontitis might interfere with the pathogenesis of RA through bacteremia, presence of inflammatory mediators, bacterial antigens and immunoglobulins in the serum. It has been demonstrated that RA patients have higher levels of serum antibodies to periodontopathogenic bacteria such as *P. gingivalis, T. forsythia, P. intermedia,* and *Prevotella melaninogenica* (Mikuls et al., 2009). Elevated levels of antibodies to *P. intermedia* and *T. forsythia* have been reported in the synovial fluid samples of RA patients (Moen et al., 2003). Elevated levels of antibodies to *P. gingivalis* have been correlated with RA-related autoantibody and CRP concentrations (Mikuls et al., 2009). Moreover, periodontitis may have systemic repercussions with increased inflammatory mediator levels and frequent transitory bacteremia occurring over a prolonged period of time.

Periodontitis and RA present an imbalance between pro-inflammatory and anti-inflammatory cytokines, which is deemed responsible for the tissue damage. Hence it can be assumed that both these conditions possibly have a common genetic trait (Ribeiro et al., 2005). HLA-DR4 antigens and their subtypes are directly associated with both these diseases (Marotte et al., 2006). The findings of the existing studies on the association between rheumatoid arthritis and periodontitis are conflicting. Sjostrom et al (1989) even described a tendency for better periodontal conditions among rheumatoid arthritis patients. This finding may be explained by a significantly reduced amount of plaque and calculus compared with the control group. Other studies are based on the number of remaining or missing teeth (Malmstrom and Calonius, 1975; Laurell et al., 1989) but, the value of tooth loss as a measure of periodontal infection is questionable. Although a causal relationship between periodontitis and rheumatoid arthritis is not supported by these data, persons with rheumatoid arthritis may, in fact, be more likely to experience advanced periodontitis than non-arthritic persons. Kasser et al (1997) showed that patients with long-standing active rheumatoid arthritis had increased gingival bleeding (50%), greater probing depth (26%), greater attachment loss (173%), and a higher number of missing teeth (29%) compared with controls. The study controlled for relevant risk factors such as oral hygiene, smoking, male gender and age. Mercado et al (2001) showed that rheumatoid arthritis patients were more than twice as likely to have moderate-to-severe periodontal bone loss and probing depth. The study also showed that rheumatoid arthritis patients with moderate-to-severe periodontitis had more swollen joints. Ishi Ede et al (2008) reported that RA patients had fewer teeth, higher prevalence of sites presenting dental plaque and a higher frequency of sites with advanced attachment loss compared to healthy controls. A self-reported health questionnaire survey combined with an evaluation of oral radiographs in patients referred for periodontal treatment indicated that the prevalence of moderate-to-severe periodontitis was significantly elevated in individuals suffering from rheumatoid arthritis receiving medical treatment of the disease (Mercado et al., 2000). Conversely, individuals referred for periodontal treatment had a higher prevalence of rheumatoid arthritis compared with the general population.

Since periodontitis and rheumatoid arthritis share pathogenic factors at the inflammatory level, it has been suggested that dual purpose therapies which can treat both these conditions may be beneficial in modulating the tissue destructive aspects of the host response. If so, then the latest achievements in treating rheumatoid arthritis with biologic drugs inhibiting proinflammatory cytokines such as TNF and IL-1, also may be beneficial adjuvants in the treatment of periodontitis (Sjostrom et al., 1989). In a study among 40 patients with RA and periodontitis, it was observed that patients receiving non-surgical periodontal therapy demonstrated a significant reduction in RA disease activity score and erythrocyte sedimentation rate compared to patients not receiving periodontal therapy (Ortiz et al., 2009). In the same study, it was also observed that in the 20 patients receiving anti-TNF-α therapy, there was a significant improvement in clinical attachment level, probing depth, bleeding on probing and gingival index scores. Conversely, in another study, it was reported that, in patients with RA and periodontitis, although non-surgical periodontal therapy resulted in reduction of ESR, CRP, and α-1 acid glycoprotein, the reductions were not statistically significant. However, in another group in the same study comprising of periodontitis patients who did not have RA, non-surgical periodontal therapy resulted in improvement of periodontal parameters with associated significant improvements in ESR, CRP, and α-1 acid glycoprotein levels suggesting that RA is a multi-factorial disease (Pinho Mde et al., 2009).

11. Periodontitis and cancer

The American Cancer Society estimated 30,990 new oral cancers and 7320 deaths from these cancers in 2006. Dental profession can play a major role in controlling the oral neoplasms. It is estimated that between 65% and 75% of patients with oral cancer initially present to a dentist (Tezal et al., 2007). About 50% of those who are diagnosed will die within 5 years of diagnosis. Because of the well-recognized phenomenon of "field cancerization" in the head and neck region, persons with primary tumours of the oral cavity and pharynx are also more likely to develop cancers of the esophagus, larynx, lung, and stomach. In addition, those with oral cancer often have multiple primary lesions and have up to a 20-fold increased risk of having a second primary oral cancer (Schwartz et al., 1994).

Epidemiological studies have shown a link between periodontal disease and head and neck squamous cell carcinoma. In a case-control study conducted over a period of 6 years to determine the association between periodontal disease and risk of tongue cancers, it was found that each millimetre of alveolar bone loss was associated with a 5.23-fold increase in the risk of tongue cancer (Tezal et al., 2007). In this study, besides periodontitis, other oral health conditions such as dental caries, tooth loss, restorations, and endodontic treatment were also evaluated and the results showed that periodontitis was the only variable that was significantly associated with oral cancer. Another study by the same investigators revealed that each millimetre of alveolar bone loss was associated with a more than 4-fold increase in the risk of head and neck squamous cell carcinoma (Tezal et al., 2009). In both these studies, the use of alveolar bone loss as a measure of periodontitis was beneficial in establishing the temporal sequence by showing that periodontal disease preceded the diagnosis of cancer.

Data from two multi-centre case control studies conducted in Europe and Latin America also demonstrated that periodontal disease and mouthwash use may be independent risk factors for cancers of head, neck, and oesophagus (Guha et al., 2007). In centres in central Europe, it was found that in subjects with poor oral hygiene, the odds ratio of having oral cancer was 4.51, pharyngeal cancer was 7.66, and laryngeal cancer was 1.95 and cancers of all the 3 sites pooled together was 2.89. Regarding missing teeth, in subjects missing 6-15 teeth, the odds ratio was 0.85, 1.04, 1, and 1.09 for oral cancer, pharyngeal cancer, laryngeal cancer, and for all sites respectively and in subjects missing >15 teeth, there was no significant increase in the risk for cancer. In the centres in Latin America, a similar trend was observed regarding poor oral hygiene. However, the risk for cancer increased with increasing number of missing teeth for subjects missing 6 teeth or more. The authors suggested that the lack of increase in the risk of cancer after loss of more than 15 teeth may be due to the absence of a periodontal pathogen or due to presence of little or no remaining teeth.

Studies have also shown that periodontal disease is also associated with other cancers such as pancreatic, colorectal, prostate, uterine and breast cancers (Michaud et al., 2007; Arora et al., 2010; Soder et al., 2011).

11.1 Mechanisms underlying association between periodontal diseases and cancer

Chronic infections such as periodontitis, can play a direct or indirect role in carcinogenesis.

Role of microorganisms: Microbial infections have been known to be associated with increased risk for cancer. *H. pylori* infection is a well characterized example of increased cancer risk in the setting of bacterial infection. Periodontitis is a chronic oral infection thought to be caused by gram-negative anaerobic bacteria in the dental biofilm (Loesche and Grossman, 2001). However, recently, the presence of viruses such as human papilloma virus (HPV) (Hormia et al., 2005), cytomegalovirus and Epstein-Barr virus (Saygun et al., 2005), which have been implicated in the etiology of oral cancer, have been reported to be present in dental plaque and periodontal pockets. Inflammation caused by bacterial infection has been shown to increase cancer risk. This has been correlated with aberrant DNA methylation in gastric epithelial cells in the case of *H. pylori* infection. In the periodontal setting with a large variety of microorganisms, bacteria and their products such as endotoxins, enzymes and metabolic by-products which are toxic to surrounding cells may directly induce mutations in tumor suppressor genes and proto-oncogenes or alter signalling pathways that affect cell proliferation and/or survival of epithelial cells.

Indirect effect through inflammation: The connection between inflammation and cancer has been suggested as consisting of 2 mechanisms: extrinsic and intrinsic mechanisms. In the extrinsic mechanism, a chronic inflammatory state increases the risk of cancer while in the intrinsic mechanism, acquired genetic alterations trigger tumor development. Chronic infection may stimulate the formation of epithelial-derived tumors through an indirect mechanism involving activation of surrounding inflammatory cells. It may also expose epithelial cells to mutagens. Microorganisms associated with the inflammatory process as well as their products can activate host cells such as inflammatory cells, fibroblasts, and epithelial cells to generate a variety of substances which can induce DNA damage in epithelial cells. Chronic inflammatory processes are frequently associated with the release of large amounts of cytokines, chemokines, growth factors, and other signals that provide an environment for cell survival, proliferation, migration, angiogenesis, and inhibition of apoptosis. This environment may help epithelial cells to accumulate mutations and drive these mutant epithelial cells to proliferate, migrate, and give them a growth advantage (Tezal et al., 2007).

The association between periodontal disease and oral neoplasms is biologically plausible and may be explained by the following mechanisms (Tezal et al., 2007).

- Broken mucosal barrier in the presence of periodontal disease and consequent enhanced penetration of carcinogens such as tobacco and alcohol.
- Increased cellularity in blood vessels and connective tissue in chronic inflammation. Association between chronic inflammation and cancer is coupled with the development of chronic diffuse epithelial hyperplasia which is regarded as a common precursor to intraepithelial neoplasia.
- Immunosupression as a common mechanism leading both to periodontal disease and oral cancer. For example, major concentrations of defensins (which have antibacterial, antiviral, and antitumor activities and are likely to play an important role in killing periodontal pathogens) found in neutrophils and epithelia suggest potential implications for critical immune surveillance within periodontal attachment (Biragyn et al., 2002; Zhang et al., 2002)
- Viruses such as Human Papilloma Virus (HPV) and Herpes Simplex Virus 1 (HSV 1) or *Candida albicans* found both in oral cancer and periodontal disease.
- Bacterial overgrowth in patients with poor oral hygiene may lead to an increased rate of metabolites with possible carcinogenic potential. For example, higher microbial production of carcinogenic acetaldehyde from ethanol has been shown in patients with poor oral hygiene (Homann et al., 2001).
- Shared genetic risk factors: Studies have shown that in dizygotic twins, baseline periodontal disease results in a significant increase in cancer risk while in monozygotic twins, this association was markedly attenuated (Arora et al., 2010).

In summary, substantial evidence supports an association between chronic infections and increased risk of cancer. A specific association between chronic periodontitis and oral cancer is plausible and needs to be explored. Oral cancer is dismissed as benign ulcers, traumatic lesions, or other soft tissue aberrations. Despite the advances in treatment, survival rate from oral cancer has not improved during the last few decades mainly due to advanced stage of oral cancer at the time of diagnosis, remaining around 50%. Thus, identification of high risk populations and early diagnosis appears to be the single most important way to control oral cancer (Tezal et al., 2005).

12. Summary

Although periodontal diseases have been traditionally considered as inflammatory diseases of the supporting tissues of the teeth, scientific evidence gathered during the last couple of decades have shown that the detrimental effects of these diseases can affect distant organs and adversely impact the systemic health of periodontitis patients. Moreover, studies have shown that periodontal therapy in patients with systemic diseases may be potentially beneficial in improving the overall health of systemically diseased individuals. Although the relationship of periodontal disease with systemic diseases is still being actively investigated, in the light of currently available evidence, it may be considered prudent to include oral health care programmes in the management of patients with systemic diseases. Thus, the role of dental professionals in the public healthcare system becomes more crucial, and prevention as well as treatment of periodontal diseases should be an important initiative in this respect.

13. References

Abnet CC, Qiao YL, Dawsey SM, Dong ZW, Taylor PR, Mark SD. 2005. Tooth loss is associated with increased risk of total death and death from upper gastrointestinal cancer, heart disease, and stroke in a Chinese population-based cohort. Int J Epidemiol 34:467-474.

Al Asqah M, Al Hamoudi N, Anil S, Al Jebreen A, Al-Hamoudi WK. 2009. Is the presence of *Helicobacter pylori* in dental plaque of patients with chronic periodontitis a risk factor for gastric infection? Can J Gastroenterol 23:177-179.

Albandar JM, Brunelle JA, Kingman A. 1999. Destructive periodontal disease in adults 30 years of age and older in the United States, 1988-1994. J Periodontol 70:13-29.

Alves RT, Ribeiro RA. 2006. Relationship between maternal periodontal disease and birth of preterm low weight babies. Braz Oral Res 20:318-323.

Anil S, Remani P, Vijayakumar T, Hari S. 1990a. Cell-mediated and humoral immune response in diabetic patients with periodontitis. Oral Surg Oral Med Oral Pathol 70:44-48.

Anil S, Remani P, Vijayakumar T, Joseph PA. 1990b. Total hemolytic complement (CH50) and its fractions (C3 and C4) in the sera of diabetic patients with periodontitis. J Periodontol 61:27-29.

Arora M, Weuve J, Fall K, Pedersen NL, Mucci LA. 2010. An exploration of shared genetic risk factors between periodontal disease and cancers: a prospective co-twin study. American journal of epidemiology 171:253-259.

Avcu N, Avcu F, Beyan C, Ural AU, Kaptan K, Ozyurt M, Nevruz O, Yalcin A. 2001. The relationship between gastric-oral *Helicobacter pylori* and oral hygiene in patients with vitamin B12-deficiency anemia. Oral Surg Oral Med Oral Pathol Oral Radiol Endod 92:166-169.

Awano S, Ansai T, Takata Y, Soh I, Akifusa S, Hamasaki T, Yoshida A, Sonoki K, Fujisawa K, Takehara T. 2008. Oral health and mortality risk from pneumonia in the elderly. J Dent Res 87:334-339.

Azarpazhooh A, Leake JL. 2006. Systematic review of the association between respiratory diseases and oral health. J Periodontol 77:1465-1482.

Beck J, Garcia R, Heiss G, Vokonas PS, Offenbacher S. 1996. Periodontal disease and cardiovascular disease. J Periodontol 67:1123-1137.

Biragyn A, Ruffini PA, Leifer CA, Klyushnenkova E, Shakhov A, Chertov O, Shirakawa AK, Farber JM, Segal DM, Oppenheim JJ, Kwak LW. 2002. Toll-like receptor 4-dependent activation of dendritic cells by beta-defensin 2. Science 298:1025-1029.

Birkedal-Hansen H. 1993. Role of cytokines and inflammatory mediators in tissue destruction. J Periodontal Res 28:500-510.

Blaser M. 1997. Ecology of Helicobacter pylori in the human stomach. Journal of Clinical Investigation 100:759.

Bobetsis YA, Barros SP, Offenbacher S. 2006. Exploring the relationship between periodontal disease and pregnancy complications. J Am Dent Assoc 137 Suppl:7S-13S.

Boggess KA, Madianos PN, Preisser JS, Moise KJ, Jr., Offenbacher S. 2005. Chronic maternal and fetal Porphyromonas gingivalis exposure during pregnancy in rabbits. Am J Obstet Gynecol 192:554-557.

Boon N, Fox K, Bloomfield P. 1995. Disease of the cardiovascular system. Davidson's principles and practice of medicine, 17th ed Churchill Livingstone, New York, NY:191–312.

Boutigny H, Boschin F, Delcourt-Debruyne E. 2005. Maladies parodontales, tabac et grossesse. Journal de Gynecologie Obstetrique et Biologie de la Reproduction 34:74-83.

Bozkurt FY, Berker E, Akkus S, Bulut S. 2000. Relationship between interleukin-6 levels in gingival crevicular fluid and periodontal status in patients with rheumatoid arthritis and adult periodontitis. J Periodontol 71:1756-1760.

Buduneli N, Baylas H, Buduneli E, Turkoglu O, Kose T, Dahlen G. 2005. Periodontal infections and pre-term low birth weight: a case-control study. J Clin Periodontol 32:174-181.

Chiu B. 1999. Multiple infections in carotid atherosclerotic plaques. Am Heart J 138:S534-536.

Clinton SK, Fleet JC, Loppnow H, Salomon RN, Clark BD, Cannon JG, Shaw AR, Dinarello CA, Libby P. 1991. Interleukin-1 gene expression in rabbit vascular tissue in vivo. Am J Pathol 138:1005-1014.

Cullinan MP, Ford PJ, Seymour GJ. 2009. Periodontal disease and systemic health: current status. Aust Dent J 54 Suppl 1:S62-69.

Cummings SR, Melton LJ. 2002. Epidemiology and outcomes of osteoporotic fractures. Lancet 359:1761-1767.

Darveau RP, Tanner A, Page RC. 1997. The microbial challenge in periodontitis. Periodontol 2000 14:12-32.

Dave S, Van Dyke T. 2008. The link between periodontal disease and cardiovascular disease is probably inflammation. Oral Dis 14:95-101.

Desai HG, Gill HH, Shankaran K, Mehta PR, Prabhu SR. 1991. Dental plaque: a permanent reservoir of *Helicobacter pylori*? Scand J Gastroenterol 26:1205-1208.

Deshpande RG, Khan MB, Genco CA. 1998. Invasion of aortic and heart endothelial cells by Porphyromonas gingivalis. Infect Immun 66:5337-5343.

Didilescu AC, Skaug N, Marica C, Didilescu C. 2005. Respiratory pathogens in dental plaque of hospitalized patients with chronic lung diseases. Clinical Oral Investigations 9:141-147.

Dowsett S, Archila L, Segreto V, Gonzalez C, Silva A, Vastola K, Bartizek R, Kowolik M. 1999. Helicobacter pylori infection in indigenous families of Central America: serostatus and oral and fingernail carriage. Journal of clinical microbiology 37:2456.

Dunn BE, Cohen H, Blaser MJ. 1997. *Helicobacter pylori*. Clin Microbiol Rev 10:720-741.

Dussault G, Sheiham A. 1982. Medical theories and professional development. The theory of focal sepsis and dentistry in early twentieth century Britain. Soc Sci Med 16:1405-1412.

Dye BA, Kruszon-Moran D, McQuillan G. 2002. The relationship between periodontal disease attributes and *Helicobacter pylori* infection among adults in the United States. Am J Public Health 92:1809-1815.

Ebersole JL, Machen RL, Steffen MJ, Willmann DE. 1997. Systemic acute-phase reactants, C-reactive protein and haptoglobin, in adult periodontitis. Clin Exp Immunol 107:347-352.

El-Shinnawi UM, El-Tantawy SI. 2003. The effect of alendronate sodium on alveolar bone loss in periodontitis (clinical trial). J Int Acad Periodontol 5:5-10.

Ershler WB, Keller ET. 2000. Age-associated increased interleukin-6 gene expression, late-life diseases, and frailty. Annu Rev Med 51:245-270.

Faria-Almeida R, Navarro A, Bascones A. 2006. Clinical and metabolic changes after conventional treatment of type 2 diabetic patients with chronic periodontitis. J Periodontol 77:591-598.

Fisher MA, Taylor GW, Shelton BJ, Jamerson KA, Rahman M, Ojo AO, Sehgal AR. 2008. Periodontal disease and other nontraditional risk factors for CKD. Am J Kidney Dis 51:45-52.

Genco R, Offenbacher S, Beck J. 2002. Periodontal disease and cardiovascular disease: epidemiology and possible mechanisms. J Am Dent Assoc 133 Suppl:14S-22S.

Genco RJ, Glurich I, Haraszthy V, Zambon J, DeNardin E. 2001. Overview of risk factors for periodontal disease and implications for diabetes and cardiovascular disease. Compend Contin Educ Dent 22:21-23.

Genco RJ, Ho AW, Grossi SG, Dunford RG, Tedesco LA. 1999. Relationship of stress, distress and inadequate coping behaviors to periodontal disease. J Periodontol 70:711-723.

Grossi SG, Genco RJ. 1998. Periodontal disease and diabetes mellitus: a two-way relationship. Ann Periodontol 3:51-61.

Grossi SG, Zambon JJ, Ho AW, Koch G, Dunford RG, Machtei EE, Norderyd OM, Genco RJ. 1994. Assessment of risk for periodontal disease. I. Risk indicators for attachment loss. J Periodontol 65:260-267.

Guha N, Boffetta P, Wunsch Filho V, Eluf Neto J, Shangina O, Zaridze D, Curado MP, Koifman S, Matos E, Menezes A, Szeszenia-Dabrowska N, Fernandez L, Mates D, Daudt AW, Lissowska J, Dikshit R, Brennan P. 2007. Oral health and risk of squamous cell carcinoma of the head and neck and esophagus: results of two multicentric case-control studies. American journal of epidemiology 166:1159-1173.

Haffajee AD, Socransky SS. 1994. Microbial etiological agents of destructive periodontal diseases. Periodontol 2000 5:78-111.

Haraszthy VI, Zambon JJ, Trevisan M, Zeid M, Genco RJ. 2000. Identification of periodontal pathogens in atheromatous plaques. J Periodontol 71:1554-1560.

Harmel AP, Mathur R, Davidson MB. 2004. Davidson's diabetes mellitus : diagnosis and treatment, 5th ed. Philadelphia, Pa.: W.B. Saunders.

Hernichel-Gorbach E, Kornman KS, Holt SC, Nichols F, Meador H, Kung JT, Thomas CA. 1994. Host responses in patients with generalized refractory periodontitis. J Periodontol 65:8-16.

Herzberg M, MacFarlane G, Liu P, Erickson P. 1994. The platelet as an inflammatory cell in periodontal diseases: interactions with *Porphyromonas gingivalis*. Molecular pathogenesis of periodontal disease Washington, DC: American Society for Microbiology:247.

Herzberg MC, Meyer MW. 1996. Effects of oral flora on platelets: possible consequences in cardiovascular disease. J Periodontol 67:1138-1142.

Herzberg MC, Weyer MW. 1998. Dental plaque, platelets, and cardiovascular diseases. Ann Periodontol 3:151-160.

Hillier SL, Martius J, Krohn M, Kiviat N, Holmes KK, Eschenbach DA. 1988. A case-control study of chorioamnionic infection and histologic chorioamnionitis in prematurity. N Engl J Med 319:972-978.

Homann N, Tillonen J, Rintamaki H, Salaspuro M, Lindqvist C, Meurman JH. 2001. Poor dental status increases acetaldehyde production from ethanol in saliva: a possible link to increased oral cancer risk among heavy drinkers. Oral oncology 37:153-158.

Hormia M, Willberg J, Ruokonen H, Syrjanen S. 2005. Marginal periodontium as a potential reservoir of human papillomavirus in oral mucosa. J Periodontol 76:358-363.

Horton AL, Boggess KA, Moss KL, Jared HL, Beck J, Offenbacher S. 2008. Periodontal disease early in pregnancy is associated with maternal systemic inflammation among African American women. J Periodontol 79:1127-1132.

Ishi Ede P, Bertolo MB, Rossa C, Jr., Kirkwood KL, Onofre MA. 2008. Periodontal condition in patients with rheumatoid arthritis. Braz Oral Res 22:72-77.

Jia CL, Jiang GS, Li CH, Li CR. 2009. Effect of dental plaque control on infection of Helicobacter pylori in gastric mucosa. J Periodontol 80:1606-1609.

Johnson RB, Gilbert JA, Cooper RC, Dai X, Newton BI, Tracy RR, West WF, DeMoss TL, Myers PJ, Streckfus CF. 1997. Alveolar bone loss one year following ovariectomy in sheep. J Periodontol 68:864-871.

Kamat AH, Mehta PR, Natu AA, Phadke AY, Vora IM, Desai PD, Koppikar GV. 1998. Dental plaque: an unlikely reservoir of Helicobacter pylori. Indian J Gastroenterol 17:138-140.

Kasser UR, Gleissner C, Dehne F, Michel A, Willershausen-Zonnchen B, Bolten WW. 1997. Risk for periodontal disease in patients with longstanding rheumatoid arthritis. Arthritis Rheum 40:2248-2251.

Kim N, Lim SH, Lee KH, You JY, Kim JM, Lee NR, Jung HC, Song IS, Kim CY. 2000. *Helicobacter pylori* in dental plaque and saliva. Korean J Intern Med 15:187-194.

Kjeldsen M, Holmstrup P, Bendtzen K. 1993. Marginal periodontitis and cytokines: a review of the literature. J Periodontol 64:1013-1022.

Koga K, Osuga Y, Yoshino O, Hirota Y, Ruimeng X, Hirata T, Takeda S, Yano T, Tsutsumi O, Taketani Y. 2003. Elevated serum soluble vascular endothelial growth factor receptor 1 (sVEGFR-1) levels in women with preeclampsia. J Clin Endocrinol Metab 88:2348-2351.

Kornman KS, Crane A, Wang HY, di Giovine FS, Newman MG, Pirk FW, Wilson TG, Jr., Higginbottom FL, Duff GW. 1997. The interleukin-1 genotype as a severity factor in adult periodontal disease. J Clin Periodontol 24:72-77.

Kornman KS, Loesche WJ. 1980. The subgingival microbial flora during pregnancy. J Periodontal Res 15:111-122.

Kossioni AE, Dontas AS. 2007. The stomatognathic system in the elderly. Useful information for the medical practitioner. Clin Interv Aging 2:591-597.

Krajden S, Fuksa M, Anderson J, Kempston J, Boccia A, Petrea C, Babida C, Karmali M, Penner J. 1989. Examination of human stomach biopsies, saliva, and dental plaque for *Campylobacter pylori*. Journal of clinical microbiology 27:1397.

Krall EA. 2001. The periodontal-systemic connection: implications for treatment of patients with osteoporosis and periodontal disease. Ann Periodontol 6:209-213.

Kramer MS. 2003. The epidemiology of adverse pregnancy outcomes: an overview. J Nutr 133:1592S-1596S.

Kuo LC, Polson AM, Kang T. 2008. Associations between periodontal diseases and systemic diseases: a review of the inter-relationships and interactions with diabetes, respiratory diseases, cardiovascular diseases and osteoporosis. Public Health 122:417-433.

Kweider M, Lowe GD, Murray GD, Kinane DF, McGowan DA. 1993. Dental disease, fibrinogen and white cell count; links with myocardial infarction? Scott Med J 38:73-74.

Laurell L, Hugoson A, Hakansson J, Pettersson B, Sjostrom L, Berglof FE, Berglof K. 1989. General oral status in adults with rheumatoid arthritis. Community Dent Oral Epidemiol 17:230-233.

Lee HM, Ciancio SG, Tuter G, Ryan ME, Komaroff E, Golub LM. 2004. Subantimicrobial dose doxycycline efficacy as a matrix metalloproteinase inhibitor in chronic periodontitis patients is enhanced when combined with a non-steroidal anti-inflammatory drug. J Periodontol 75:453-463.

Li X, Kolltveit KM, Tronstad L, Olsen I. 2000. Systemic diseases caused by oral infection. Clin Microbiol Rev 13:547-558.

Lin D, Smith MA, Elter J, Champagne C, Downey CL, Beck J, Offenbacher S. 2003. Porphyromonas gingivalis infection in pregnant mice is associated with placental dissemination, an increase in the placental Th1/Th2 cytokine ratio, and fetal growth restriction. Infect Immun 71:5163-5168.

Loesche WJ, Grossman NS. 2001. Periodontal disease as a specific, albeit chronic, infection: diagnosis and treatment. Clin Microbiol Rev 14:727-752, table of contents.

Loesche WJ, Lopatin DE. 1998. Interactions between periodontal disease, medical diseases and immunity in the older individual. Periodontol 2000 16:80-105.

Loos BG, Craandijk J, Hoek FJ, Wertheim-van Dillen PM, van der Velden U. 2000. Elevation of systemic markers related to cardiovascular diseases in the peripheral blood of periodontitis patients. J Periodontol 71:1528-1534.

Lundstrom A, Jendle J, Stenstrom B, Toss G, Ravald N. 2001. Periodontal conditions in 70-year-old women with osteoporosis. Swed Dent J 25:89-96.

Malmstrom M, Calonius PE. 1975. Teeth loss and the inflammation of teeth-supporting tissues in rheumatoid disease. Scand J Rheumatol 4:49-55.

Marakoglu I, Gursoy UK, Marakoglu K, Cakmak H, Ataoglu T. 2008. Periodontitis as a risk factor for preterm low birth weight. Yonsei Med J 49:200-203.

Marcus AJ, Hajjar DP. 1993. Vascular transcellular signaling. J Lipid Res 34:2017-2031.

Marotte H, Farge P, Gaudin P, Alexandre C, Mougin B, Miossec P. 2006. The association between periodontal disease and joint destruction in rheumatoid arthritis extends the link between the HLA-DR shared epitope and severity of bone destruction. Ann Rheum Dis 65:905-909.

Matsumura S, Iwanaga S, Mochizuki S, Okamoto H, Ogawa S, Okada Y. 2005. Targeted deletion or pharmacological inhibition of MMP-2 prevents cardiac rupture after myocardial infarction in mice. J Clin Invest 115:599-609.

Mattila KJ. 1989. Viral and bacterial infections in patients with acute myocardial infarction. J Intern Med 225:293-296.

Mercado F, Marshall RI, Klestov AC, Bartold PM. 2000. Is there a relationship between rheumatoid arthritis and periodontal disease? J Clin Periodontol 27:267-272.

Mercado FB, Marshall RI, Klestov AC, Bartold PM. 2001. Relationship between rheumatoid arthritis and periodontitis. J Periodontol 72:779-787.

Michaud DS, Joshipura K, Giovannucci E, Fuchs CS. 2007. A prospective study of periodontal disease and pancreatic cancer in US male health professionals. Journal of the National Cancer Institute 99:171-175.

Mikuls TR, Payne JB, Reinhardt RA, Thiele GM, Maziarz E, Cannella AC, Holers VM, Kuhn KA, O'Dell JR. 2009. Antibody responses to *Porphyromonas gingivalis (P. gingivalis)* in subjects with rheumatoid arthritis and periodontitis. Int Immunopharmacol 9:38-42.

Mitchell-Lewis D, Engebretson SP, Chen J, Lamster IB, Papapanou PN. 2001. Periodontal infections and pre-term birth: early findings from a cohort of young minority women in New York. Eur J Oral Sci 109:34-39.

Miyabayashi H, Furihata K, Shimizu T, Ueno I, Akamatsu T. 2000. Influence of oral *Helicobacter pylori* on the success of eradication therapy against gastric *Helicobacter pylori*. Helicobacter 5:30-37.

Moen K, Brun JG, Madland TM, Tynning T, Jonsson R. 2003. Immunoglobulin G and A antibody responses to *Bacteroides forsythus* and *Prevotella intermedia* in sera and synovial fluids of arthritis patients. Clin Diagn Lab Immunol 10:1043-1050.

Mojon P. 2002. Oral health and respiratory infection. J Can Dent Assoc 68:340-345.

Moreira E, Santos R, Nassri V, Reis A, Guerra A, Alcântara A, Matos J, Carvalho W, Moura C, Silvani C. 2004. Risk factors for *Helicobacter pylori* infection in children: is education a main determinant? Epidemiology and infection 132:327-335.

Mueller-Heubach E, Rubinstein DN, Schwarz SS. 1990. Histologic chorioamnionitis and preterm delivery in different patient populations. Obstet Gynecol 75:622-626.

Nelson RG, Shlossman M, Budding LM, Pettitt DJ, Saad MF, Genco RJ, Knowler WC. 1990. Periodontal disease and NIDDM in Pima Indians. Diabetes care 13:836-840.

Nelson S, Laughon BE, Summer WR, Eckhaus MA, Bartlett JG, Jakab GJ. 1986. Characterization of the pulmonary inflammatory response to an anaerobic bacterial challenge. The American review of respiratory disease 133:212-217.

Offenbacher S, Beck JD, Lieff S, Slade G. 1998. Role of periodontitis in systemic health: spontaneous preterm birth. J Dent Educ 62:852-858.

Offenbacher S, Collins J, Yalta B, Haradon G. 1994. Role of prostaglandins in high-risk periodontitis patients. Molecular pathogenesis of periodontal disease American Society for Microbiology, Washington, DC:203–214.

Offenbacher S, Katz V, Fertik G, Collins J, Boyd D, Maynor G, McKaig R, Beck J. 1996. Periodontal infection as a possible risk factor for preterm low birth weight. J Periodontol 67:1103-1113.

Ortiz P, Bissada NF, Palomo L, Han YW, Al-Zahrani MS, Panneerselvam A, Askari A. 2009. Periodontal therapy reduces the severity of active rheumatoid arthritis in patients treated with or without tumor necrosis factor inhibitors. J Periodontol 80:535-540.

Oshowo A, Gillam D, Botha A, Tunio M, Holton J, Boulos P, Hobsley M. 1998. Helicobacter pylori: the mouth, stomach, and gut axis. Ann Periodontol 3:276-280.

Ozdemir A, Mas MR, Sahin S, Saglamkaya U, Ateskan U. 2001. Detection of *Helicobacter pylori* colonization in dental plaques and tongue scrapings of patients with chronic gastritis. Quintessence Int 32:131-134.

Page RC. 1998. The pathobiology of periodontal diseases may affect systemic diseases: inversion of a paradigm. Annals of periodontology 3:108-120.

Page RC, Schroeder HE. 1976. Pathogenesis of inflammatory periodontal disease. A summary of current work. Lab Invest 34:235-249.

Pauwels RA, Buist AS, Calverley PM, Jenkins CR, Hurd SS. 2001. Global strategy for the diagnosis, management, and prevention of chronic obstructive pulmonary disease. NHLBI/WHO Global Initiative for Chronic Obstructive Lung Disease (GOLD) Workshop summary. American journal of respiratory and critical care medicine 163:1256-1276.

Payne JB, Reinhardt RA, Nummikoski PV, Dunning DG, Patil KD. 2000. The association of cigarette smoking with alveolar bone loss in postmenopausal females. J Clin Periodontol 27:658-664.

Persson LO, Berglund K, Sahlberg D. 1999. Psychological factors in chronic rheumatic diseases--a review. The case of rheumatoid arthritis, current research and some problems. Scand J Rheumatol 28:137-144.

Persson RE, Hollender LG, Powell LV, MacEntee MI, Wyatt CC, Kiyak HA, Persson GR. 2002. Assessment of periodontal conditions and systemic disease in older subjects. I. Focus on osteoporosis. J Clin Periodontol 29:796-802.

Pesonen E, Kaprio E, Rapola J, Soveri T, Oksanen H. 1981. Endothelial cell damage in piglet coronary artery after intravenous administration of E. coli endotoxin. A scanning and transmission electron-microscopic study. Atherosclerosis 40:65-73.

Pickup JC, Crook MA. 1998. Is type II diabetes mellitus a disease of the innate immune system? Diabetologia 41:1241-1248.

Pinho Mde N, Oliveira RD, Novaes AB, Jr., Voltarelli JC. 2009. Relationship between periodontitis and rheumatoid arthritis and the effect of non-surgical periodontal treatment. Braz Dent J 20:355-364.

Pitiphat W, Joshipura KJ, Rich-Edwards JW, Williams PL, Douglass CW, Gillman MW. 2006. Periodontitis and plasma C-reactive protein during pregnancy. J Periodontol 77:821-825.

Potempa J, Sroka A, Imamura T, Travis J. 2003. Gingipains, the major cysteine proteinases and virulence factors of *Porphyromonas gingivalis*: structure, function and assembly of multidomain protein complexes. Current Protein and Peptide Science 4:397-407.

Ramamurthy NS, Greenwald RA, Celiker MY, Shi EY. 2005. Experimental arthritis in rats induces biomarkers of periodontitis which are ameliorated by gene therapy with tissue inhibitor of matrix metalloproteinases. J Periodontol 76:229-233.

Reddy MS. 2001. Osteoporosis and periodontitis: discussion, conclusions, and recommendations. Ann Periodontol 6:214-217.

Ribeiro J, Leao A, Novaes AB. 2005. Periodontal infection as a possible severity factor for rheumatoid arthritis. J Clin Periodontol 32:412-416.

Ridker PM, Cushman M, Stampfer MJ, Tracy RP, Hennekens CH. 1997. Inflammation, aspirin, and the risk of cardiovascular disease in apparently healthy men. N Engl J Med 336:973-979.

Rifas L, Weitzmann MN. 2009. A novel T cell cytokine, secreted osteoclastogenic factor of activated T cells, induces osteoclast formation in a RANKL-independent manner. Arthritis Rheum 60:3324-3335.

Roberts JM, Taylor RN, Musci TJ, Rodgers GM, Hubel CA, McLaughlin MK. 1989. Preeclampsia: an endothelial cell disorder. American journal of obstetrics and gynecology 161:1200-1204.

Romero R, Espinoza J, Goncalves LF, Kusanovic JP, Friel LA, Nien JK. 2006. Inflammation in preterm and term labour and delivery. Semin Fetal Neonatal Med 11:317-326.

Romero R, Nien JK, Espinoza J, Todem D, Fu W, Chung H, Kusanovic JP, Gotsch F, Erez O, Mazaki-Tovi S, Gomez R, Edwin S, Chaiworapongsa T, Levine RJ, Karumanchi SA. 2008. A longitudinal study of angiogenic (placental growth factor) and anti-angiogenic (soluble endoglin and soluble vascular endothelial growth factor receptor-1) factors in normal pregnancy and patients destined to develop preeclampsia and deliver a small for gestational age neonate. J Matern Fetal Neonatal Med 21:9-23.

Rosenberg HM, Ventura SJ, Maurer JD, Heuser RL, Freedman MA. 1996. Births and deaths: United States, 1995. Monthly vital statistics report 45:1-39.

Saygun I, Kubar A, Ozdemir A, Slots J. 2005. Periodontitis lesions are a source of salivary cytomegalovirus and Epstein-Barr virus. J Periodontal Res 40:187-191.

Scannapieco FA. 1998. Position paper of The American Academy of Periodontology: periodontal disease as a potential risk factor for systemic diseases. J Periodontol 69:841-850.

Scannapieco FA. 1999. Role of oral bacteria in respiratory infection. J Periodontol 70:793-802.

Scannapieco FA, Bush RB, Paju S. 2003. Associations between periodontal disease and risk for nosocomial bacterial pneumonia and chronic obstructive pulmonary disease. A systematic review. Annals of Periodontology 8:54-69.

Scannapieco FA, Dasanayake AP, Chhun N. 2010. "Does periodontal therapy reduce the risk for systemic diseases?". Dental clinics of North America 54:163-181.

Scannapieco FA, Ho AW. 2001. Potential associations between chronic respiratory disease and periodontal disease: analysis of National Health and Nutrition Examination Survey III. J Periodontol 72:50-56.

Scannapieco FA, Wang B, Shiau HJ. 2001. Oral bacteria and respiratory infection: effects on respiratory pathogen adhesion and epithelial cell proinflammatory cytokine production. Ann Periodontol 6:78-86.

Scheidt-Nave C, Bismar H, Leidig-Bruckner G, Woitge H, Seibel MJ, Ziegler R, Pfeilschifter J. 2001. Serum interleukin 6 is a major predictor of bone loss in women specific to the first decade past menopause. J Clin Endocrinol Metab 86:2032-2042.

Schenkein HA, Best AM, Brooks CN, Burmeister JA, Arrowood JA, Kontos MC, Tew JG. 2007. Anti-cardiolipin and increased serum adhesion molecule levels in patients with aggressive periodontitis. J Periodontol 78:459-466.

Schwartz LH, Ozsahin M, Zhang GN, Touboul E, De Vataire F, Andolenko P, Lacau-Saint-Guily J, Laugier A, Schlienger M. 1994. Synchronous and metachronous head and neck carcinomas. Cancer 74:1933-1938.

Sert T, Kirzioglu FY, Fentoglu O, Aylak F, Mungan T. 2011. Serum Placental Growth Factor (PIGF), Vascular Endothelial Growth Factor (VEGF), Soluble VEGF Receptor -1 and -2 Levels In Periodontal Disease and Adverse Pregnancy Outcomes. J Periodontol.

Singh SU, Casper RF, Fritz PC, Sukhu B, Ganss B, Girard B, Jr., Savouret JF, Tenenbaum HC. 2000. Inhibition of dioxin effects on bone formation in vitro by a newly described aryl hydrocarbon receptor antagonist, resveratrol. J Endocrinol 167:183-195.

Sjostrom L, Laurell L, Hugoson A, Hakansson JP. 1989. Periodontal conditions in adults with rheumatoid arthritis. Community Dent Oral Epidemiol 17:234-236.

Slots J, Feik D, Rams TE. 1990. Prevalence and antimicrobial susceptibility of Enterobacteriaceae, Pseudomonadaceae and Acinetobacter in human periodontitis. Oral microbiology and immunology 5:149-154.

Soder B, Yakob M, Meurman JH, Andersson LC, Klinge B, Soder PO. 2011. Periodontal disease may associate with breast cancer. Breast cancer research and treatment 127:497-502.

Stolzenberg-Solomon RZ, Dodd KW, Blaser MJ, Virtamo J, Taylor PR, Albanes D. 2003. Tooth loss, pancreatic cancer, and Helicobacter pylori. Am J Clin Nutr 78:176-181.

Taylor GW. 2001. Bidirectional interrelationships between diabetes and periodontal diseases: an epidemiologic perspective. Ann Periodontol 6:99-112.

Taylor GW, Manz MC, Borgnakke WS. 2004. Diabetes, periodontal diseases, dental caries, and tooth loss: a review of the literature. Compend Contin Educ Dent 25:179-184, 186-178, 190; quiz 192.

Teng YT, Taylor GW, Scannapieco F, Kinane DF, Curtis M, Beck JD, Kogon S. 2002. Periodontal health and systemic disorders. J Can Dent Assoc 68:188-192.

Tezal M, Grossi SG, Genco RJ. 2005. Is periodontitis associated with oral neoplasms? J Periodontol 76:406-410.

Tezal M, Sullivan MA, Hyland A, Marshall JR, Stoler D, Reid ME, Loree TR, Rigual NR, Merzianu M, Hauck L, Lillis C, Wactawski-Wende J, Scannapieco FA. 2009. Chronic periodontitis and the incidence of head and neck squamous cell carcinoma. Cancer epidemiology, biomarkers & prevention : a publication of the American Association for Cancer Research, cosponsored by the American Society of Preventive Oncology 18:2406-2412.

Tezal M, Sullivan MA, Reid ME, Marshall JR, Hyland A, Loree T, Lillis C, Hauck L, Wactawski-Wende J, Scannapieco FA. 2007. Chronic periodontitis and the risk of tongue cancer. Archives of otolaryngology--head & neck surgery 133:450-454.

Tezal M, Wactawski-Wende J, Grossi SG, Ho AW, Dunford R, Genco RJ. 2000. The relationship between bone mineral density and periodontitis in postmenopausal women. J Periodontol 71:1492-1498.

Thom DH, Grayston JT, Siscovick DS, Wang SP, Weiss NS, Daling JR. 1992. Association of prior infection with *Chlamydia pneumoniae* and angiographically demonstrated coronary artery disease. Jama 268:68-72.

Usman OA. 2004. The effects of aryl hydrocarbon on vascular calcification in the warfarin-vitamin K rat model. . In. Toronto: University of Toronto.

Wang R, Wang T, Chen K, Wang J, Zhang J, Lin S, Zhu Y, Zhang W, Cao Y, Zhu C. 2002. Helicobacter pylori infection and gastric cancer: evidence from a retrospective cohort study and nested case-control study in China. World Journal of Gastroenterology 8:1103-1107.

Warren J, Marshall B. 1983. Unidentified curved bacilli on gastric epithelium in active chronic gastritis. Lancet 1:1273-1275.

Weidlich P, Cimoes R, Pannuti CM, Oppermann RV. 2008. Association between periodontal diseases and systemic diseases. Braz Oral Res 22 Suppl 1:32-43.

Weyant RJ, Pearlstein ME, Churak AP, Forrest K, Famili P, Cauley JA. 1999. The association between osteopenia and periodontal attachment loss in older women. J Periodontol 70:982-991.

Whalen JP, Krook L. 1996. Periodontal disease as the early manifestation of osteoporosis. Nutrition 12:53-54.

WHO WHO. 1995. The World Health Report 1995: Bridging the Gap. Executive Summary: World Health Organization.

Williams CE, Davenport ES, Sterne JA, Sivapathasundaram V, Fearne JM, Curtis MA. 2000. Mechanisms of risk in preterm low-birthweight infants. Periodontol 2000 23:142-150.

Williams RC, Offenbacher S. 2000. Periodontal medicine: the emergence of a new branch of periodontology. Periodontol 2000 23:9-12.

Xu Q, Kleindienst R, Waitz W, Dietrich H, Wick G. 1993. Increased expression of heat shock protein 65 coincides with a population of infiltrating T lymphocytes in atherosclerotic lesions of rabbits specifically responding to heat shock protein 65. J Clin Invest 91:2693-2702.

Yoshihara A, Seida Y, Hanada N, Miyazaki H. 2004. A longitudinal study of the relationship between periodontal disease and bone mineral density in community-dwelling older adults. J Clin Periodontol 31:680-684.

Young RA, Elliott TJ. 1989. Stress proteins, infection, and immune surveillance. Cell 59:5-8.

Zaric S, Bojic B, Jankovic L, Dapcevic B, Popovic B, Cakic S, Milasin J. 2009. Periodontal therapy improves gastric *Helicobacter pylori* eradication. J Dent Res 88:946-950.

Zhang L, Yu W, He T, Yu J, Caffrey RE, Dalmasso EA, Fu S, Pham T, Mei J, Ho JJ, Zhang W, Lopez P, Ho DD. 2002. Contribution of human alpha-defensin 1, 2, and 3 to the anti-HIV-1 activity of CD8 antiviral factor. Science 298:995-1000.

7

Systemic Effects of Periodontal Diseases: Focus on Atherosclerosis

Emil Kozarov and John Grbic
Columbia University College of Dental Medicine, Section of Oral and Diagnostic Sciences, New York, NY, USA

1. Introduction

Periodontitis is a bacterially induced, localized, chronic inflammatory disease of periodontium that destroys connective tissues and bone supporting the teeth and may lead to tooth exfoliation and edentulism. Periodontitis is one of the most prevalent infectious diseases in humans. Mild forms affect 30% to 50% of adults and the severe generalized form affects 5% to 15% of the US adults (Periodontology, 2005). It is associated with specific bacterial groups, components of the dental biofilm, one of them (the "red complex") closely related to clinical measures of periodontal disease (Socransky et al., 1998).
Periodontal pathogens normally inhabit the oral cavity as constituents of the dental biofilm. Since they are in intimate contact with the gingival epithelial tissues, they, however, can breach the gingival mucosal barrier at the ulcerative lesion and enter the circulation. Indeed, these organisms have been implicated in infections at distant sites, such as the central nervous system (Ewald et al., 2006), and measures of periodontitis (tooth loss) has been linked to subclinical atherosclerotic vascular disease (carotid artery plaque prevalence) (Desvarieux et al., 2003).
Systemic dissemination can be a result of tissue invasion, or of dental procedures including personal oral hygiene, leading to bacteremia. Tissue invasion is very likely a key virulence factor for a bacterium since it provides a "privileged niche" (Falkow, 1997) with access to host nutritional and iron substrates and a shelter from the host humoral and cellular immune response. Intracellular localization also brings about bacterial persistence, critical property of a causative agent of a chronic disease.
Atherosclerosis is a chronic inflammatory focal proliferative lesion of the arteries associated with conventional risk factors such as hypercholesterolemia, hypertension, diabetes and smoking, in addition to genetic factors (Libby and Theroux, 2005). However, the incidence of AS is not fully explained by these risk factors. It is now accepted that inflammation as a key integrative process playing a major role in the initiation and progression of atherosclerotic lesions, with the active participation of smooth muscle cells, leukocytes, growth factors and inflammatory mediators. A dynamic and progressive process, atherogenesis begins with endothelial dysfunction ("response to injury" model) that also interacts with the standard risk factors (Van Dyke and Kornman, 2008), (Libby et al., 2009).
Novel diagnostic and treatment modalities targeting vascular inflammation are dependent on further investigations of the origins of the inflammation. The focus of this review is the

contribution of periodontal pathogens to atherosclerotic inflammations, based on the latest communications.

Inflammation is involved in all stages of the atherosclerosis, from initiation through progression and, ultimately, the thrombotic complications (Libby et al., 2002). The role of inflammation as a direct causative factor in atherosclerotic vascular disease is intensely investigated (Libby et al., 2011). Thus, increased concentrations of high sensitivity C-reactive protein (hsCRP) have been shown to predict future acute myocardial infarction (MI) (de Beer et al., 1982). hsCRP levels were significantly elevated in 90% in unstable angina pectoris patients compared to 13% of stable angina patients; the average CRP values were significantly different ($p = 0.001$) for the unstable angina group (2.2 +/- 2.9 mg/dl) compared to the stable angina (0.7 +/- 0.2 mg/dl) groups (normal is less than 0.6 mg/dl) (Berk et al., 1990). Further, after adjustment for lipid and non-lipid factors, elevated CRP levels were significantly related to an increased risk of coronary heart disease (CHD), with relative risk 1.79 [(at CRP levels ≥3.0 mg per liter, as compared with subjects with levels of <1.0 mg per liter (95% CI, 1.27 to 2.51; P for trend <0.001)] (Pai et al., 2004). Overall, the recognition of inflammatory character of atherosclerosis led to the successful application of hsCRP as acute-phase marker for cardiovascular risk assessment (Libby et al., 2010).

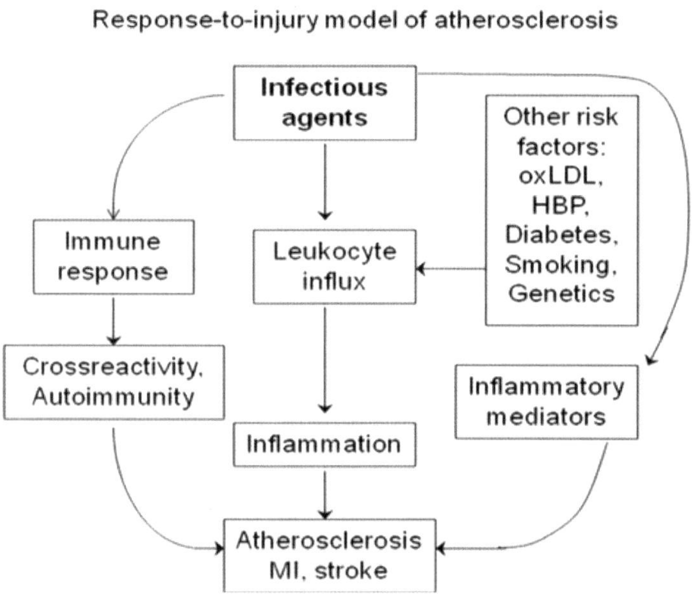

Fig. 1. Simplified chart representing the response to injury model of infectious agents-induced initiation and progression of the atherogenesis. Inflammation drives the initiation, progression, and eventually, the rupture of atherosclerotic plaques. The process involves inflammatory mediators and innate and adaptive immunity. A constant or repetitive injury may ultimately lead to necrosis, plaque rupture, myocardial infarction (MI) or stroke.

Pathogen burden. Since the incidence of atherosclerosis is only partially explained by the accepted risk factors, the attention was turned to infections as a potential cause of AS, focusing on the total infectious burden (Ridker, 2002), (Epstein et al., 2009). The accumulated evidence suggests that the aggregate burden of the chronic infections, rather than a single pathogen, may contribute to increased risk of AS and clinical vascular events (Elkind, 2010). Indeed, an abundance of epidemiological evidence is presented in support of this notion (Ross, 1999), (Libby et al., 2002), and particularly in respect to periodontal infections [Desvarieux, 2005 #2905], (Demmer and Desvarieux, 2006), (Kebschull et al., 2010). The pathogen-initiated inflammatory process leading to endothelial cell activation, leukocyte rolling, adhesion and diapedesis, growth factor release, smooth muscle cell (SMC) proliferation and foam cell formation (Libby et al., 2010) all form the basis of the "response to injury" model of atherogenesis (Fig. 1).

Periodontitis as a risk factor for adverse ischemic events. Epidemiological and seroepidemiological studies addressed the association between these conditions relatively recently. The first **epidemiological** association was found between dental health and acute myocardial infarction (MI), where the former was significantly worse in 100 patients with MI than in 102 controls after adjustment for age, social class, smoking, serum lipid concentrations, and the presence of diabetes (Mattila et al., 1989). The results from the Oral Infections and Vascular Disease Epidemiology Study (INVEST) of 657 subjects with no history of stroke or myocardial infarction indicated that chronic infections, including periodontitis, may predispose to cardiovascular disease (CVD) (Desvarieux et al., 2005). In that study, mean carotid artery intima-media thickness (IMT) was related to the total bacterial burden, the periodontal bacterial burden, and to the relative predominance of periodontal over other bacteria in the subgingival plaque. After adjustments for age, race/ethnicity, gender, education, body mass index, smoking, diabetes, systolic blood pressure, and LDL and HDL cholesterol, it was demonstrated that periodontal bacterial burden was related to the carotid IMT, a measure of subclinical atherosclerosis ($P=0.002$). In other investigations, using a multivariate logistic regression model, periodontal bone loss was associated with a ~ 4-fold increase in risk for carotid atherosclerosis (adjusted OR, 3.64; CI, 1.37 to 9.65) (Engebretson et al., 2005) and edentulousness was independently associated with the risk of aortic stenosis in a cohort of 2341 individuals (Volzke et al., 2005).

Using **seroepidemiology**, a study of 572 patients showed that the extent of atherosclerosis (using coronary angiography, carotid duplex sonography, and ankle-arm index) and CVD mortality were associated with elevated IgA and IgG titers to infectious agents. After adjustment for age, sex, classical risk factors and high hsCRP, infectious burden was significantly associated with advanced atherosclerosis, with an odds ratio (95% CI) of 1.8 (1.2 to 2.6) for 4 to 5 seropositivities ($P<0.01$) and 2.5 (1.2 to 5.1) for 6 to 8 seropositivities ($P<0.02$) (Espinola-Klein et al., 2002). Elevated levels of he periodontal patrhogens *Porphyromonas gingivalis* and *Aggregatibacter actinomycetemcomitans* – specific serum IgG were associated with atherosclerosis (Colhoun et al., 2008). Interestingly, IgM antibodies specific for phosphorylcholine (PC), hapten-like epitope found on oxLDL and also on bacteria are atheroprotective; low PC-antibody titers are associated with an increased risk for CVD (Frostegard, 2010). Recently, in a study of 313 cases and 747 controls, using immunofluorescence microscopy and species-specific antibodies, the presence of six periodontal pathogens, *P. gingivalis, Tannerella forsythensis, Prevotella intermedia, Campylobacter recta, Fusobacterium nucleatum,* and *Eubacterium saburreum,* and their co-occurrence (0-6) was compared with the odds of having MI. Suggesting a role for a total periodontal microbial burden, subjects with ≥ 3 periodontal pathogens species had about 2-fold increase in odds of having nonfatal MI than those who did not have any type of bacterial species [OR = 2.01 (1.31-3.08)], also suggesting that specifically the presence of *T. forsythensis* and *P. intermedia* was associated with increased odds of having MI (Andriankaja et al., 2011).

Interestingly, there is some noticeable discrepancy between the effects of periodontal infections on MI compared to ischemic stroke, even within the same populations and databases. While one such investigation found stronger association of periodontitis with stroke than with CHD (hazard rate 3.52; 95% confidence interval [CI], 1.59-7.81) (Jimenez et al., 2009), another study of 8032 subjects did not find "convincing evidence of a causal association between periodontal disease and CHD risk" (Hujoel et al., 2000). Still, using data from a total of 10,146 participants from the Third National Health and Nutrition Examination Survey (1988-1994), the link between periodontal health (gingival bleeding index, calculus index, and periodontal disease status, defined by pocket depth and attachment loss) and CVD risk factors (serum total and high density lipoprotein cholesterol, C-reactive protein, and plasma fibrinogen) was examined, showing a significant relation between indicators of poor periodontal status and increased CRP (Wu et al., 2000).

The results from these investigations vary significantly for variety of reasons, such as variations in study populations, differing measures - clinical (such as pocket depth and bleeding on probing) - and non-clinical (systemic antibody response or alveolar bone loss radiography) of periodontitis. These discrepancies suggest confounding factors common for periodontitis and CVD such as smoking that would interfere with the association between the conditions (Hujoel, 2002). Therefore, specific studies using multivariate and stratified analyses have been designed to address the confounding (Demmer and Desvarieux, 2006) and few meta-analyses have been published. One such analysis of PubMed, Cochrane Controlled Trials Register, EMBASE, and SCOPUS databases for references on periodontitis and CVD showed strong association between them, with a summary odds ratio of 1.75 (95% confidence interval (CI): 1.32 to 2.34; P <0.001), compared to periodontally healthy subjects (Mustapha et al., 2007). Another meta-analysis of seven cohort studies supported the association and shows that periodontitis is a risk factor or marker for CHD, independent of traditional risk factors (Humphrey et al., 2008). Taken together, the epidemiological and seroepidemiological data suggest further investigation of the periodontal component of CVD.

Bacteremia. Since there are 10^8 - 10^{12} bacteria found per diseased periodontal site, large numbers of oral bacterial species, including periodontal can enter the circulation through the microvasculature following tooth brushing and other dental procedures (Iwai, 2009). Using PCR, hematogenous spread of bacteria was demonstrated in blood samples taken from 30 patients after ultrasonic scaling, periodontal probing and tooth brushing at 23%, 16% and 13% of the patients, respectively (Kinane et al., 2005). Further supporting the notion that periodontal organisms gain access to the circulation during dental hygiene procedures, another investigation of 194 patients demonstrated that periodontal site bleeding after tooth brushing was associated with ~8-fold increase in bacteremia (Lockhart et al., 2009). Unlike the clinical measures of periodontitis, the bleeding on probing was more associated with systemic inflammation than attachment loss (Beck and Offenbacher, 2002) and most associated with bacteremia (Lockhart et al., 2009).

2. Periodontal pathogen-accelerated endothelial injury and atherogenesis

The **"response to injury"** hypothesis presents atherosclerosis as an inflammatory disease, bearing similarity to a bacterial infection where the innate and adaptive arms of the immune systems are involved. In addition to the initiation and progression of the atheromas, inflammation is also related to the end stage of the disease, characterized by plaque rupture, atherothrombosis and acute ischemic events (Libby, 2007).

Several plausible models have emerged focusing on the pro-atherogenic mechanisms of action of periodontal pathogens. The immune response to periodontitis that may contribute to atherogenesis via pro-atherogenic systemic inflammatory response (immunological sounding) and autorecognition (autoimmunity, molecular mimicry) has been thoroughly reviewed elsewhere (Gibson et al., 2008), (Hayashi et al., 2010), (Teles and Wang, 2011).

Microbial invasion and its sequelae. In addition to immunological mechanisms, there are two metastatic avenues that periodontal organisms can exploit to reach vascular endothelia, direct invasion as a consequence of bacteremia and dissemination via internalization in migrating phagocytic cells (the "Trojan horse" approach).

Direct invasion. Periodontal bacteria have evolved elaborate strategies to invade non-professional phagocytes. Invasion of host cells is very likely a key virulence mechanism for a bacterium since intracellular residence provides "privileged niche" with 1) a nutrient-rich reducing environment with access to host protein and iron substrates, 2) partial protection from dental hygiene procedures including scaling and root planing (Johnson et al., 2008), 3) sequestration from the humoral and cellular immune responses, crucial at early stages of infection, 4) a means for replication and persistence that provides a reservoir and is essential for a chronic disease, and 5) protection from drug treatment (Eick and Pfister, 2004). Most available information regarding the invasive ability of periodontopathic bacteria concerns *P. gingivalis* [Lamont, 1995 #1268], (Dorn et al., 2001) and *A. actinomycetemcomitans* (Fives-Taylor et al., 1999), (Tomich et al., 2007). *Eikenella corrodens* and *Prevotella intermedia* were also shown to invade human primary endothelial and SM cells (Dorn et al., 1999). Collectively, it appears that the intracellular localization is a viable option for variety of periodontal pathogens (Tribble and Lamont, 2010).

Dissemination via internalization in migrating phagocytic cells (the "Trojan horse" approach). Unlike direct bacteremic dissemination, where bacteria spread in the circulation subject to opsonization and clearing by the humoral and cellular immune response, bacteria can metastasize after internalization in monocytes/macrophages or in dendritic cells (DCs) at the diseased site. Using such a "Trojan horse" approach, pathogens are able to disseminate and gain reach of endothelia, where due to extravasation of the carrier phagocytes they can localize at the activated endothelium in the arterial wall. A recently proposed model describes how *P. gingivalis* may exploit DCs to spread from the oral sites and gain access to systemic circulation. Thus, *P. gingivalis* may contribute to atherogenesis via subverting normal DC function, promoting a semimature, highly migratory, and immunosuppressive DC phenotype that contributes to the inflammatory development of atherosclerosis and, eventually, to plaque rupture (Zeituni et al., 2010). Supporting this suggestion, the infection with invasive *P. gingivalis* strain was shown to induce monocyte migration and significantly enhance the production of the pro-inflammatory cytokines (Pollreisz et al., 2010).

Bacterial transmission between vascular endothelial and smooth muscle cells. In the only thorough investigation of *P. gingivalis* invasion of primary human endothelial and SM cells, it was shown that the organism can spread intercellularly in vascular cell types (Li et al., 2008). This property has been previously demonstrated with a monoculture of gingival epithelial cells (Yilmaz et al., 2006). Using vascular cell cultures and immunofluorescence, the study demonstrates that bacteria can transmit between the same as well as between different cell types, from infected to fresh cells, leading to spreading of the infection that in clinical setting could lead to chronicity of disease (Li et al., 2008).

2.1 Proatherogenic consequences of bacterial presence in vascular cells

Activation of endothelial and smooth muscle cells. Endothelial cell activation is a pivotal moment in initiation of atherogenesis. It was shown that infection with *P. gingivalis,* but not with non-invasive non-fimbriated mutant induced the expression of intercellular adhesion molecule 1 (ICAM-1), vascular cell adhesion molecule 1 (VCAM-1) and P- and E-selectins in human endothelial cells (Khlgatian et al., 2002). Further, it was shown that *P. gingivalis* fimbria elicit chemokine production in human aortic endothelial cells via actin cytoskeletal rearrangements and that the pro-inflammatory IL-1β, IL-8 and MCP-1 were induced in these cells (Takahashi et al., 2006). *P. gingivalis* infection activates host cells via TLR2 and TLR4 - mediated cell signaling (Hajishengallis et al., 2006), (Hayashi et al., 2010).
The smooth muscle cells (SMC) were found to respond to bacteria in a prothrombotic or in a proliferative manner (Roth et al., 2009), (Wada and Kamisaki, 2010). In the latter communication, it was shown that SMC proliferation in distal aorta aneurysms was associated with presence of *P. gingivalis* in the dental plaque of the patients.
Prothrombotic effects of bacteria and plaque rupture. An alternative mechanism through which bacteremias (or bacteria present in ruptured plaque) may contribute to vascular thrombosis is the triggering of the coagulation cascade (Herzberg et al., 2005), (Iwai, 2009). The potential adverse role of bacteria in atherothrombosis has been shown using human aortic SMC. Live invasive *P. gingivalis,* but not heat-killed or non-invasive mutant specifically suppressed tissue factor pathway inhibitor (TFPI) produced by vascular cells. The results suggested a procoagulant response of the host cells to bacteria (Roth et al., 2009).Plaque rupture, leading to exposure of the prothrombotic plaque core to the circulation and thrombus formation can be attributed to bacteria-dependent release of metalloproteinases (MMPs) with concomitant suppression of the MMP antagonist, tissue inhibitor of MMPs (TIMP) (Sato et al., 2009), (Guan et al., 2009).
Animal models furnish a useful research tool and are indispensable in testing hypotheses at a pre-clinical stage (Graves et al., 2008). In a study of wild-type *P. gingivalis* and a non-invasive $FimA^-$ mutant, both strains were detected in blood and aortic tissue of $ApoE^{-/-}$ mice by PCR after challenge, however only the invasive strain accelerated atherosclerosis in the animal model [Gibson, 2004 #2679]. Importantly, a prevention of *P. gingivalis*-accelerated atherosclerosis via immunization to control *P. gingivalis*-elicited periodontitis was demonstrated in the same study. Furthermore, using a mouse model of atherosclerosis and metronidazole administration followed by *P. gingivalis* i.v. inoculation, it was shown that 1) the lack of invasion ability of the mutant prevents the formation of aortic lesions in the animals inoculated with fimbriae-deficient strain (DPG3) compared to wild-type strain (381), and that 2) metronidazole, common antibacterial used in anaerobic periodontal infections, completely prevents the formation of *P. gingivalis* – associated arterial lesions (Amar et al., 2009). The results indicate that this oral pathogen can exert a critical damage on the vessels, and that drugs are viable treatment options. It further suggests that the bacterial

- endothelia interaction and activation causing phagocyte recruitment to the infection site may represent a key step in atherogenesis.

In addition, rabbit model with experimentally induced periodontitis developed fatty streaks in the aorta faster than in periodontally healthy animals, suggesting direct contribution of periodontitis to atherosclerosis (Jain et al., 2003) and recurrent *P. gingivalis* bacteremia induced aortic and coronary lesions in normocholesterolemic pigs and increases atherosclerosis in hypercholesterolemic pigs (Brodala et al., 2005). Altogether, variety of animal models have been used to demonstrate the adverse effect of periodontal bacteria on vascular health.

3. Association of periodontal bacteria with atheromata: Are we finally having "the smoking gun"?

Bacterial fingerprints in atheromas. As outlined above, there is strong evidence that oral bacteria can spread in the circulation during dental procedures such as tooth brushing (Lockhart et al., 2009). Since more than 700 bacterial species are identified in the mouth (Dewhirst et al., 2010), (Parahitiyawa et al., 2010), it is expected that many species, including *P. gingivalis* are disseminated to large vessels. Identification of the pathogens associated with atherosclerotic lesions can be performed using PCR and metagenomic approaches. Indeed, DNA from periodontal organisms, including *A. actinomycetemcomitans* and *P. gingivalis* were detected in atheromas by PCR [Haraszthy, 2000 #2237]. Using 16S rDNA PCR, it was also found that 1.5-2.2% of the total DNA in the atheromatous samples was bacterial, where large proportion of it was of oral origin, especially in the elderly group of individuals (mean age, 67 years). *P. gingivalis* was reported to be the most represented among the 10 species tested in this study (Kozarov et al., 2006), which is in line with its invasive properties described above (Dorn et al., 1999). It was also expected, since severe periodontal diseases ($\geq$ 4 mm attachment loss) increase in prevalence with age (approximately 50% of 55-64 years old individuals have severe disease), and this is the age with the highest incidence of acute ischemic events.

Using clone libraries, in a comprehensive 16S rDNA PCR signatures study of atherosclerotic tissue from 38 CHD patients and 26 controls, bacterial DNA was found only in (all) CHD patients but not in controls. Presence of bacteria was confirmed by fluorescence in situ hybridization. A bacterial diversity of >50 different species was demonstrated, with a high mean bacterial diversity in atheromas, 12.33 +/- 3.81 (range, 5 to 22) (Ott et al., 2006).The broad spectrum of bacterial signatures encompassed species from the human barrier organs, the skin and the oral cavity.

Focus on causality. Cardiovascular disease is the leading cause of death and disability in industrialized countries. Although bacterial DNA has been recovered from atheromatous lesions and a link between inflammatory burden and atherogenesis has been established, there has been limited evidence that bacterial agents can be cultivated from atheromatous lesions. However, to fulfill Koch's postulate for infectious disease and to provide mechanistic data linking infectious agents to CVD, the cultivation of microorganisms from atheromatous tissue must be demonstrated.

Such cultivation has been eluding the biomedical community for decades. As a result (with the exception of *Chlamydophila pneumoniae*), clinical strains could not be cultivated to provide key mechanistic link (Fiehn et al., 2005).

After viable *P. gingivalis* and *A. actinomycetemcomitans* in atheromatous vascular tissue were detected for the first time [Kozarov, 2005 #2700], bacterial transmission between primary vascular cell types was shown (Li et al., 2008) and finally, periodontal organisms including *Propionibacteruim acnes, Staphylococcus epidermidis, Streptococcus infantis* and *P. gingivalis* were recently cultivated from atheromatous tissue (Rafferty et al., 2011). In addition to *P. gingivalis*, a major periodontal pathogen, the identified species are no strangers to inflamed periodontium. *P. acnes* has been recovered from root canals and from blood samples taken during and after endodontic treatment (Debelian et al., 1998) and is the most prevalent species in apical periodontitis (Fujii et al., 2009). Importantly, using multivariable regression models, it has been shown that among patients with 25 or more teeth, those with two or more endodontic therapies had 1.62 times the odds (95% CI, 1.04-2.53) of prevalent coronary disease compared with those reporting never having had endodontic therapy (Caplan et al., 2009). *Staphylococcus* or *Streptococcus*, found in the oral cavity, are also detected in other systemic infections, in prosthetic valve endocarditis (Nataloni et al., 2010) and in heart valves and atheromas, respectively (Nakano et al., 2006), (Kozarov et al., 2006).

4. Atherosclerosis microbiome, the latest and most critical segment of the human microbiome may have a large periodontal component

Impact of genomics. Although multiple human microbiome projects have been launched, genomic studies of the atherosclerosis microbiome have not been initiated. Of note, out of 1,843 microbial genomes funded by the Human Microbiome Project by July 2011 (http://www.hmpdacc-resources.org/cgi-bin/hmp_catalog/main.cgi), none are associated with atherosclerosis. For comparison, 464 GI tract genomes have been selected for sequencing. A project targeting vascular inflammation-associated bacterial pathogens (the atherosclerosis microbiome) is conspicuously missing. This is simply due to the inability, until now, of the researchers to recover clinical isolates from diseased vascular tissue. Importantly, this segment of the human microbiome may represent a subset of the oral (and, possibly, gut) microbiome.
Focus on viable microbes. Identification of *viable* bacterial pathogens, members of the atherosclerosis microbiome, associated with human atheromatous tissue is critical for complete clarification of the potential for infectious etiologies of atherosclerosis and for reconsidering application of antibacterials in CVD treatment trials. Using a cellular immunology approach (Rafferty et al., 2011) allowing for cultivation of heretofore "uncultivable" bacteria from atheromatous tissue of vascular surgery patients, the community is now for the first time in a position to comprehensively address the bacterial component in vascular inflammations, the atherosclerosis microbiome.
With this approach, the identification of DNA from dead bacteria will be eliminated and only *bona fide* live organisms will be identified and investigated as the most likely targets for association with disease. The approach currently used, PCR of total atheroma DNA with species-specific primers or with universal primers followed by cloning of the amplification products and sequencing the resulting plasmid libraries (Ott et al., 2006) generates a large number of hits and is inconclusive. Bacterial DNA presence in the atheromata may be due to macrophages carrying their refuse, phagocytized bacteria from distant sites of the body, leading to many 16S rDNA bacterial signatures that may be false positives. The recovered by Rafferty et el isolates belong to four species only, both anaerobic and facultative. This approach will significantly decrease the complexity of the problem of false positives and obviate the need for investing in expensive or newly designed methods and equipment such as isolating a single bacterial cell from a specimen and sequencing its chromosome.

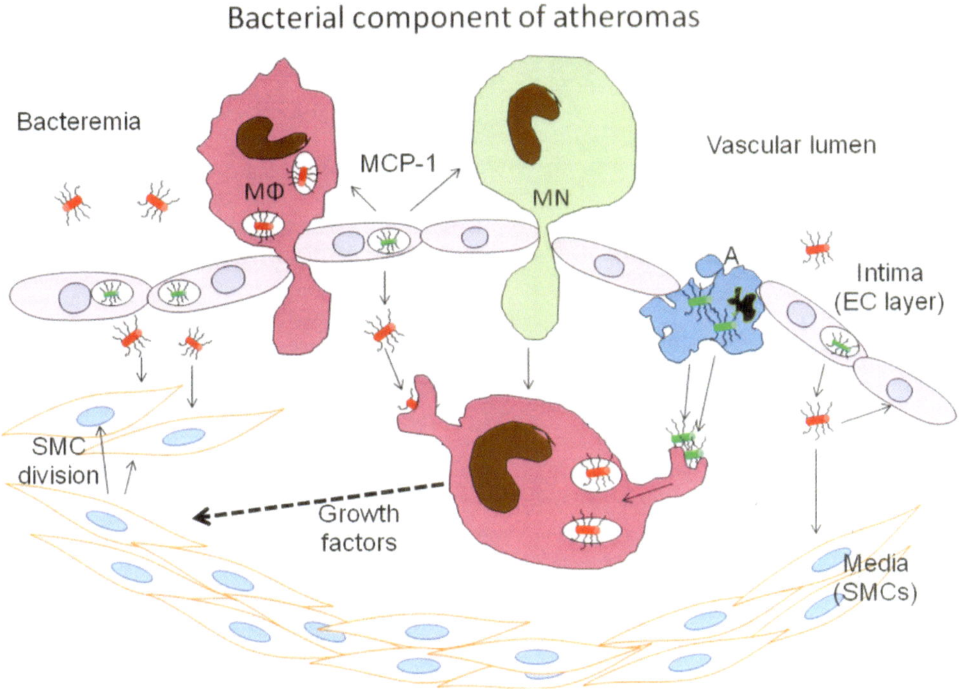

MN, monocyte. MΦ, macrophage with internalized bacteria. EC, endothelial cell. SMC, smooth muscle cell. A, apoptotic endothelial cell releasing intracellular bacteria.

Fig. 2. Bacterial infection-mediated model of atherogenesis presenting a bacteremic and macrophage-mediated tissue infection. Depicted are the tunica intima, a monolayer of endothelial cells (ECs) over a basal lamina that contains SMCs and the tunica media containing SMCs. Represented at left is the bacteremic microbial invasion of ECs. Within 24-72 hours the invading intracellular bacteria turn into non-cultivable state (in green). Endothelial activation is represented as release in the vascular lumen of proinflammatory mediators such as MCP-1. They activate circulating monocytes (MN) and macrophages (MΦ), promote their local adhesion and diapedesis into the lesion (in the center). MΦ can carry internalized persisting bacteria, thus contributing to the bacterial spreading. The activation of non-cultivable bacteria during vascular cell-cell transmission and the spreading of infection to adjacent ECs is and to SMCs is shown at right and left. Additional bacteria are released in the atherosclerotic core following apoptosis and necrosis of host cells (at right). The phagocytosis of bacteria by a monocyte maturating into macrophage and the activation of dormant non-cultivable bacteria into active invasive stage (resuscitation, from green to red), following their ingestion is shown in the center. Growth factors released from the phagocytes promote SMC proliferation and migration (neointimal formation). For clarity, vasa vasorum neovascularization, lipids, foam cell formation, plaque rupture and blood coagulation/thrombus formation are not presented.

5. The heart of the matter: Current model of bacterial infection-accelerated atherogenesis, plaque rupture and acute ischemic events

A model of atherogenesis now emerges where (periodontal) bacteria invade endothelia either directly, following bacteremia, or are carried by phagocytes migrating from the primary infection site (the "Trojan horse" approach) (Figure 2). Upon invasion of endothelial cells, bacterial pathogens such as *P. gingivalis* are able to reside intracellularly for extended period of time, activating the endothelia and initiating the atherogenic process. Within 24-72 hours however, in order to sustain and persist, the bacteria switch into a dormant uncultivable stage (Li et al., 2008). Still facing a hostile environment (phagolysosomal fusion), some bacteria escape from the dormant stage, exiting into intracellular space and invading adjacent host cells, becoming transiently invasive and cultivable, and perpetuating persistent low-grade inflammation. The return to cultivable state specifically can occur after internalization by phagocytes (Rafferty et al., 2011). This leads to additional metastatic dissemination, injurious response, apoptosis and necrosis that are hallmarks of a chronic disease. Importantly, dormant bacteria have low metabolic activity, therefore targets for antibiotics are lacking and the organisms can become drug-tolerant. Using such mechanism, intracellular pathogens residing in atheromas could control their population yet allow for the observed persistent infection.

In conclusion, the epidemiological and seroepidemiological analyses, the in vitro and in vivo investigations, the presence in atheromata of live bacteria, some of them unique for periodontal lesions, and the clinical trials conducted so far, largely defend the argument that periodontal infections can be an exacerbating component of vascular inflammations. The latest data presented here expand the existing model of infectious component of atherosclerosis, identifying for the first time possible members of atherosclerosis microbiome, suggesting a novel mechanism for bacterial persistence in diseased tissue and for recurrence of disease and possibly explaining the failure of antibiotics to ameliorate the outcome after treatment of cardiovascular disease patients.

6. References

Amar, S., Wu, S.C., and Madan, M. (2009). Is *Porphyromonas gingivalis* cell invasion required for atherogenesis? Pharmacotherapeutic implications. J Immunol *182*, 1584-1592.

Andriankaja, O., Trevisan, M., Falkner, K., Dorn, J., Hovey, K., Sarikonda, S., Mendoza, T., and Genco, R. (2011). Association between periodontal pathogens and risk of nonfatal myocardial infarction. Community Dent Oral Epidemiol *39*, 177-185.

Beck, J.D., and Offenbacher, S. (2002). Relationships among clinical measures of periodontal disease and their associations with systemic markers. Ann Periodontol *7*, 79-89.

Berk, B.C., Weintraub, W.S., and Alexander, R.W. (1990). Elevation of C-reactive protein in "active" coronary artery disease. Am J Cardiol *65*, 168-172.

Brodala, N., Merricks, E.P., Bellinger, D.A., Damrongsri, D., Offenbacher, S., Beck, J., Madianos, P., Sotres, D., Chang, Y.L., Koch, G., *et al.* (2005). *Porphyromonas gingivalis* bacteremia induces coronary and aortic atherosclerosis in normocholesterolemic and hypercholesterolemic pigs. Arterioscler Thromb Vasc Biol *25*, 1446-1451.

Caplan, D.J., Pankow, J.S., Cai, J., Offenbacher, S., and Beck, J.D. (2009). The relationship between self-reported history of endodontic therapy and coronary heart disease in the Atherosclerosis Risk in Communities Study. J Am Dent Assoc *140*, 1004-1012.

Colhoun, H.M., Slaney, J.M., Rubens, M.B., Fuller, J.H., Sheiham, A., and Curtis, M.A. (2008). Antibodies to periodontal pathogens and coronary artery calcification in type 1 diabetic and nondiabetic subjects. J Periodontal Res *43*, 103-110.

de Beer, F.C., Hind, C.R., Fox, K.M., Allan, R.M., Maseri, A., and Pepys, M.B. (1982). Measurement of serum C-reactive protein concentration in myocardial ischaemia and infarction. Br Heart J *47*, 239-243.

Debelian, G.J., Olsen, I., and Tronstad, L. (1998). Anaerobic bacteremia and fungemia in patients undergoing endodontic therapy: an overview. Ann Periodontol *3*, 281-287.

Demmer, R.T., and Desvarieux, M. (2006). Periodontal infections and cardiovascular disease: the heart of the matter. J Am Dent Assoc *137 Suppl*, 14S-20S; quiz 38S.

Desvarieux, M., Demmer, R.T., Rundek, T., Boden-Albala, B., Jacobs, D.R., Jr., Papapanou, P.N., and Sacco, R.L. (2003). Relationship between periodontal disease, tooth loss, and carotid artery plaque: the Oral Infections and Vascular Disease Epidemiology Study (INVEST). Stroke *34*, 2120-2125.

Desvarieux, M., Demmer, R.T., Rundek, T., Boden-Albala, B., Jacobs, D.R., Jr., Sacco, R.L., and Papapanou, P.N. (2005). Periodontal microbiota and carotid intima-media thickness: the Oral Infections and Vascular Disease Epidemiology Study (INVEST). Circulation *111*, 576-582.

Dewhirst, F.E., Chen, T., Izard, J., Paster, B.J., Tanner, A.C., Yu, W.H., Lakshmanan, A., and Wade, W.G. (2010). The human oral microbiome. J Bacteriol *192*, 5002-5017.

Dorn, B.R., Dunn, W.A., Jr., and Progulske-Fox, A. (1999). Invasion of human coronary artery cells by periodontal pathogens. Infect Immun *67*, 5792-5798.

Dorn, B.R., Dunn, W.A., Jr., and Progulske-Fox, A. (2001). *Porphyromonas gingivalis* traffics to autophagosomes in human coronary artery endothelial cells. Infect Immun *69*, 5698-5708.

Eick, S., and Pfister, W. (2004). Efficacy of antibiotics against periodontopathogenic bacteria within epithelial cells: an in vitro study. J Periodontol *75*, 1327-1334.

Elkind, M.S. (2010). Infectious burden: a new risk factor and treatment target for atherosclerosis. Infect Disord Drug Targets *10*, 84-90.

Engebretson, S.P., Lamster, I.B., Elkind, M.S., Rundek, T., Serman, N.J., Demmer, R.T., Sacco, R.L., Papapanou, P.N., and Desvarieux, M. (2005). Radiographic measures of chronic periodontitis and carotid artery plaque. Stroke *36*, 561-566.

Epstein, S.E., Zhu, J., Najafi, A.H., and Burnett, M.S. (2009). Insights into the role of infection in atherogenesis and in plaque rupture. Circulation *119*, 3133-3141.

Espinola-Klein, C., Rupprecht, H.J., Blankenberg, S., Bickel, C., Kopp, H., Rippin, G., Victor, A., Hafner, G., Schlumberger, W., and Meyer, J. (2002). Impact of infectious burden on extent and long-term prognosis of atherosclerosis. Circulation *105*, 15-21.

Ewald, C., Kuhn, S., and Kalff, R. (2006). Pyogenic infections of the central nervous system secondary to dental affections--a report of six cases. Neurosurg Rev *29*, 163-166; discussion 166-167.

Falkow, S. (1997). Perspectives series: host/pathogen interactions. Invasion and intracellular sorting of bacteria: searching for bacterial genes expressed during host/pathogen interactions. J Clin Invest *100*, 239-243.

Fiehn, N.E., Larsen, T., Christiansen, N., Holmstrup, P., and Schroeder, T.V. (2005). Identification of periodontal pathogens in atherosclerotic vessels. J Periodontol *76*, 731-736.

Fives-Taylor, P.M., Meyer, D.H., Mintz, K.P., and Brissette, C. (1999). Virulence factors of *Actinobacillus actinomycetemcomitans*. Periodontol 2000 *20*, 136-167.

Frostegard, J. (2010). Low level natural antibodies against phosphorylcholine: a novel risk marker and potential mechanism in atherosclerosis and cardiovascular disease. Clin Immunol *134*, 47-54.

Fujii, R., Saito, Y., Tokura, Y., Nakagawa, K.I., Okuda, K., and Ishihara, K. (2009). Characterization of bacterial flora in persistent apical periodontitis lesions. Oral Microbiol Immunol *24*, 502-505.

Gibson, F.C., 3rd, Ukai, T., and Genco, C.A. (2008). Engagement of specific innate immune signaling pathways during *Porphyromonas gingivalis* induced chronic inflammation and atherosclerosis. Front Biosci *13*, 2041-2059.

Graves, D.T., Fine, D., Teng, Y.T., Van Dyke, T.E., and Hajishengallis, G. (2008). The use of rodent models to investigate host-bacteria interactions related to periodontal diseases. J Clin Periodontol *35*, 89-105.

Guan, S.M., Shu, L., Fu, S.M., Liu, B., Xu, X.L., and Wu, J.Z. (2009). *Prevotella intermedia* upregulates MMP-1 and MMP-8 expression in human periodontal ligament cells. FEMS Microbiol Lett *299*, 214-222.

Hajishengallis, G., Tapping, R.I., Harokopakis, E., Nishiyama, S., Ratti, P., Schifferle, R.E., Lyle, E.A., Triantafilou, M., Triantafilou, K., and Yoshimura, F. (2006). Differential interactions of fimbriae and lipopolysaccharide from *Porphyromonas gingivalis* with the Toll-like receptor 2-centred pattern recognition apparatus. Cell Microbiol *8*, 1557-1570.

Hayashi, C., Gudino, C.V., Gibson, F.C., 3rd, and Genco, C.A. (2010). Review: Pathogen-induced inflammation at sites distant from oral infection: bacterial persistence and induction of cell-specific innate immune inflammatory pathways. Mol Oral Microbiol *25*, 305-316.

Herzberg, M.C., Nobbs, A., Tao, L., Kilic, A., Beckman, E., Khammanivong, A., and Zhang, Y. (2005). Oral streptococci and cardiovascular disease: searching for the platelet aggregation-associated protein gene and mechanisms of *Streptococcus sanguis*-induced thrombosis. J Periodontol *76*, 2101-2105.

Hujoel, P.P. (2002). Does chronic periodontitis cause coronary heart disease? A review of the literature. J Am Dent Assoc *133 Suppl*, 31S-36S.

Hujoel, P.P., Drangsholt, M., Spiekerman, C., and DeRouen, T.A. (2000). Periodontal disease and coronary heart disease risk. JAMA *284*, 1406-1410.

Humphrey, L.L., Fu, R., Buckley, D.I., Freeman, M., and Helfand, M. (2008). Periodontal disease and coronary heart disease incidence: a systematic review and meta-analysis. J Gen Intern Med *23*, 2079-2086.

Iwai, T. (2009). Periodontal bacteremia and various vascular diseases. J Periodontal Res *44*, 689-694.

Jain, A., Batista, E.L., Jr., Serhan, C., Stahl, G.L., and Van Dyke, T.E. (2003). Role for periodontitis in the progression of lipid deposition in an animal model. Infect Immun *71*, 6012-6018.

Jimenez, M., Krall, E.A., Garcia, R.I., Vokonas, P.S., and Dietrich, T. (2009). Periodontitis and incidence of cerebrovascular disease in men. Ann Neurol *66*, 505-512.

Johnson, J.D., Chen, R., Lenton, P.A., Zhang, G., Hinrichs, J.E., and Rudney, J.D. (2008). Persistence of extracrevicular bacterial reservoirs after treatment of aggressive periodontitis. J Periodontol *79*, 2305-2312.

Kebschull, M., Demmer, R.T., and Papapanou, P.N. (2010). "Gum bug, leave my heart alone!"--epidemiologic and mechanistic evidence linking periodontal infections and atherosclerosis. J Dent Res *89*, 879-902.

Khlgatian, M., Nassar, H., Chou, H.H., Gibson, F.C., 3rd, and Genco, C.A. (2002). Fimbria-dependent activation of cell adhesion molecule expression in *Porphyromonas gingivalis*-infected endothelial cells. Infect Immun *70*, 257-267.

Kinane, D.F., Riggio, M.P., Walker, K.F., MacKenzie, D., and Shearer, B. (2005). Bacteraemia following periodontal procedures. J Clin Periodontol *32*, 708-713.

Kozarov, E., Sweier, D., Shelburne, C., Progulske-Fox, A., and Lopatin, D. (2006). Detection of bacterial DNA in atheromatous plaques by quantitative PCR Microbes Infect *8*, 687-693.

Li, L., Michel, R., Cohen, J., DeCarlo, A., and Kozarov, E. (2008). Intracellular survival and vascular cell-to-cell transmission of *Porphyromonas gingivalis*. BMC Microbiol *8, Feb 6*, 26-36.

Libby, P. (2007). Inflammatory mechanisms: the molecular basis of inflammation and disease. Nutr Rev *65*, S140-146.

Libby, P., Okamoto, Y., Rocha, V.Z., and Folco, E. (2010). Inflammation in atherosclerosis: transition from theory to practice. Circ J *74*, 213-220.

Libby, P., Ridker, P.M., and Hansson, G.K. (2009). Inflammation in atherosclerosis: from pathophysiology to practice. J Am Coll Cardiol *54*, 2129-2138.

Libby, P., Ridker, P.M., and Hansson, G.K. (2011). Progress and challenges in translating the biology of atherosclerosis. Nature *473*, 317-325.

Libby, P., Ridker, P.M., and Maseri, A. (2002). Inflammation and atherosclerosis. Circulation *105*, 1135-1143.

Libby, P., and Theroux, P. (2005). Pathophysiology of coronary artery disease. Circulation *111*, 3481-3488.

Lockhart, P.B., Brennan, M.T., Thornhill, M., Michalowicz, B.S., Noll, J., Bahrani-Mougeot, F.K., and Sasser, H.C. (2009). Poor oral hygiene as a risk factor for infective endocarditis-related bacteremia. J Am Dent Assoc *140*, 1238-1244.

Mattila, K.J., Nieminen, M.S., Valtonen, V.V., Rasi, V.P., Kesaniemi, Y.A., Syrjala, S.L., Jungell, P.S., Isoluoma, M., Hietaniemi, K., and Jokinen, M.J. (1989). Association between dental health and acute myocardial infarction. Brit Med J *298*, 779-781.

Mustapha, I.Z., Debrey, S., Oladubu, M., and Ugarte, R. (2007). Markers of systemic bacterial exposure in periodontal disease and cardiovascular disease risk: a systematic review and meta-analysis. J Periodontol *78*, 2289-2302.

Nakano, K., Inaba, H., Nomura, R., Nemoto, H., Takeda, M., Yoshioka, H., Matsue, H., Takahashi, T., Taniguchi, K., Amano, A., *et al.* (2006). Detection of cariogenic *Streptococcus mutans* in extirpated heart valve and atheromatous plaque specimens. J Clin Microbiol *44*, 3313-3317.

Nataloni, M., Pergolini, M., Rescigno, G., and Mocchegiani, R. (2010). Prosthetic valve endocarditis. J Cardiovasc Med (Hagerstown) *2010 Feb 11*. .

Ott, S.J., El Mokhtari, N.E., Musfeldt, M., Hellmig, S., Freitag, S., Rehman, A., Kuhbacher, T., Nikolaus, S., Namsolleck, P., Blaut, M., *et al.* (2006). Detection of diverse bacterial signatures in atherosclerotic lesions of patients with coronary heart disease. Circulation *113*, 929-937.

Pai, J.K., Pischon, T., Ma, J., Manson, J.E., Hankinson, S.E., Joshipura, K., Curhan, G.C., Rifai, N., Cannuscio, C.C., Stampfer, M.J., *et al.* (2004). Inflammatory markers and the risk of coronary heart disease in men and women. N Engl J Med *351*, 2599-2610.

Parahitiyawa, N.B., Scully, C., Leung, W.K., Yam, W.C., Jin, L.J., and Samaranayake, L.P. (2010). Exploring the oral bacterial flora: current status and future directions. Oral Dis *16*, 136-145.

Periodontology, A.A.o. (2005). Epidemiology of periodontal diseases (position paper). J Periodontol *76*, 1406 -1419.

Pollreisz, A., Huang, Y., Roth, G.A., Cheng, B., Kebschull, M., Papapanou, P.N., Schmidt, A.M., and Lalla, E. (2010). Enhanced monocyte migration and pro-inflammatory cytokine production by *Porphyromonas gingivalis* infection. J Periodontal Res *45*, 239-245.

Rafferty, B., Jönsson, D., Kalachikov, S., Demmer, R.T., Nowygrod, R., Elkind, M.S., Bush, H., Jr., and Kozarov, E. (2011). Impact of monocytic cells on recovery of uncultivable bacteria from atherosclerotic lesions. Journal of Internal Medicine, 2011 Mar 3.

Ridker, P.M. (2002). On evolutionary biology, inflammation, infection, and the causes of atherosclerosis. Circulation *105*, 2-4.

Ross, R. (1999). Mechanisms of Disease: Atherosclerosis -- An Inflammatory Disease. N Engl J Med *340*, 115-126.

Roth, G.A., Aumayr, K., Giacona, M.B., Papapanou, P.N., Schmidt, A.M., and Lalla, E. (2009). *Porphyromonas gingivalis* infection and prothrombotic effects in human aortic smooth muscle cells. Thromb Res *123*, 780-784.

Sato, Y., Kishi, J., Suzuki, K., Nakamura, H., and Hayakawa, T. (2009). Sonic extracts from a bacterium related to periapical disease activate gelatinase A and inactivate tissue inhibitor of metalloproteinases TIMP-1 and TIMP-2. Int Endod J *42*, 1104-1111.

Socransky, S.S., Haffajee, A.D., Cugini, M.A., Smith, C., and Kent, R.L., Jr. (1998). Microbial complexes in subgingival plaque. J Clin Periodontol *25*, 134-144.

Takahashi, Y., Davey, M., Yumoto, H., Gibson, F.C., 3rd, and Genco, C.A. (2006). Fimbria-dependent activation of pro-inflammatory molecules in *Porphyromonas gingivalis* infected human aortic endothelial cells. Cell Microbiol *8*, 738-757.

Teles, R., and Wang, C.Y. (2011). Mechanisms involved in the association between peridontal diseases and cardiovascular disease. Oral Dis.

Tomich, M., Planet, P.J., and Figurski, D.H. (2007). The *tad* locus: postcards from the widespread colonization island. Nat Rev Microbiol *5*, 363-375.

Tribble, G.D., and Lamont, R.J. (2010). Bacterial invasion of epithelial cells and spreading in periodontal tissue. Periodontol 2000 *52*, 68-83.

Van Dyke, T.E., and Kornman, K.S. (2008). Inflammation and factors that may regulate inflammatory response. J Periodontol *79*, 1503-1507.

Volzke, H., Schwahn, C., Hummel, A., Wolff, B., Kleine, V., Robinson, D.M., Dahm, J.B., Felix, S.B., John, U., and Kocher, T. (2005). Tooth loss is independently associated with the risk of acquired aortic valve sclerosis. Am Heart J *150*, 1198-1203.

Wada, K., and Kamisaki, Y. (2010). Roles of oral bacteria in cardiovascular diseases--from molecular mechanisms to clinical cases: Involvement of *Porphyromonas gingivalis* in the development of human aortic aneurysm. J Pharmacol Sci *113*, 115-119.

Wu, T., Trevisan, M., Genco, R.J., Falkner, K.L., Dorn, J.P., and Sempos, C.T. (2000). Examination of the relation between periodontal health status and cardiovascular risk factors: serum total and high density lipoprotein cholesterol, C-reactive protein, and plasma fibrinogen. Am J Epidemiol *151*, 273-282.

Yilmaz, O., Verbeke, P., Lamont, R.J., and Ojcius, D.M. (2006). Intercellular spreading of *Porphyromonas gingivalis* infection in primary gingival epithelial cells. Infect Immun *74*, 703-710.

Zeituni, A.E., Carrion, J., and Cutler, C.W. (2010). *Porphyromonas gingivalis*-dendritic cell interactions: consequences for coronary artery disease. J Oral Microbiol 2.

8

One for All™: How to Tackle with Diabetes, Obesity and Periodontal Diseases

Ayse Basak Cinar
Faculty of Health Sciences, Dental Institute, University of Copenhagen
Denmark

1. Introduction

Diabetes, obesity, and oral diseases (dental caries and periodontal diseases), largely preventable chronic diseases, are described as global pandemic due their distribution and severe consequences.[1-4] WHO calls for a global action for prevention and promotion regarding these diseases as a vital investment in urgent need.[1-4]

Current scientific evidence provides a strong and plausible basis to assert that diabetes, obesity and oral diseases have common risk factors (poor dietary habits, a sugar-rich diet, smoking)[5-9] and biologic mechanisms.[10-17] Current research supports that there is a bidirectional relationship between type 2 diabetes (DM2) and oral health: Poor oral health negatively contributes to glycemic control whereas poor DM2 management negatively affects oral health.[17] Thus, they lead to poor systemic health conditions.[18] Obesity is a triggering risk factor both for DM2 and oral diseases, namely periodontal diseases.[10-12]

Diabetes and obesity, showing an increasing trend, lead to disabilities and negatively affect the quality of life through life-course along with oral diseases.[19, 20] WHO projects that there are almost 200 million people with diabetes at present, and 3,2 million deaths/year are attributable to diabetes complications, and both will double worldwide by 2030.[19,21-23] Globally, more than 1 billion adults are overweight; almost 300 million of them are clinically obese. Being obese or overweight raises steeply the likelihood of developing DM2; approximately 85% of people with diabetes are DM2, and of these 90% are obese or overweight.[22] Promoting a good oral health is significantly essential for preventing and reducing the negative consequences of DM2 and obesity.[24]

Key to successful maintenance of a high glycemic control, DM2 management and obesity, and good oral health is adherence to the regime of daily treatment and self-care practices.[25-28] However, many patients find or feel themselves unable to follow recommended lifestyles (a healthy diet, physical exercise, no smoking, medications, twice daily toothbrushing), which makes them more prone to diabetes-related complications, poor oral health and obesity; therefore leading a poor quality of life.

WHO,[2] International Diabetes Federation (IDF),[29] The World Dental Federation (FDI),[30] and Council of European Dentists,[31] American Dental Association[32] underline a need to adopt a common-risk factor approach[33] for oral and general health promotion; a need for interventions integrating oral health into chronic disease management. WHO highly recommends behavioral interventions to meet this need.[34]

Health Coaching (HC), a health promotion tool, is a new and innovative `behavioral intervention that facilitates individuals in establishing and attaining health promoting goals in order to change lifestyle-related behaviors, with the intend of reducing health risks, improving self-management of chronic-conditions, and increasing health-related quality of life.[35] HC is demonstrated as an effective behavioral technique associated with positive behavioral outcomes (smoking cessation,[36] obesity,[37-40] and diabetes management[40-42]) but it has not been used as a holistic intervention for oral health and DM2 and obesity.
The theory of self-efficacy was developed within the Social Cognitive Theory by Bandura,[43] in which health is determined by the interactions between behavioral, environmental and individual factors. [43] Self-efficacy is the belief in one's capabilities to learn, to organize and to perform healthy behaviors across different challenging situations. The perception of self-efficacy plays a crucial role at adoption, maintenance, and improvement of health behaviors as people engage in activities that they believe they can manage but avoid the ones that they perceive as more than they can cope with.[44] In terms of diabetes management, diabetes-related self-efficacy has been found to predict compliance with diabetes treatment and patients´ understanding of glycemic control.[45,46] Little is known about how self-efficacy can play an intermediate role between oral health and diabetes management; thus better perception of dental self-efficacy was found to associate with better glycemic control and higher tooth-brushing frequency among patients with diabetes type 1.[47] As oral diseases and DM2 are defined as behavioral diseases, dental self-efficacy a may play a crucial role in management of both diseases. However, this has not been studied yet.
The aim of the current chapter is to introduce and to discuss an oral health focused HC model based on improving self-efficacy among patients with DM2, under the framework of a research project. The project refers to an intervention study which aims to assess the impact of oral health focused HC on oral and general health (DM2, obesity, quality of life) in two countries, Turkey and Denmark, by using subjective (self-reports) and objective (clinical) measurements. The new oral health focused HC aims to provide "One for All™"; a new translational health coaching model applicable in real life settings for the patients and an effective transformational leadership tool to improve the patient-health professional communication.

2. Methods

The study is an international prospective intervention study including DM2 adult patients, Turkey (n=200) and Denmark (n=200). Patients will be selected by a random sampling from hospitals. In Turkey, it is planned to recruit patients through advertisement by a web site and from the hospitals` outpatient clinics (Turkish Diabetes Association, S.B. Kartal Research and Education Hospital). In Denmark, patients visiting the dental clinics of School of Dentistry, University of Copenhagen are to be included in the study. General practioners working at the participating medical settings are to be asked to refer their patients to the study. Key inclusion and exclusion criteria are shown in Figure 1.
Invitation for participation and a written informed consent along with an informative pamphlet will be distributed at the clinics and mailed (including postage paid envelopes) to eligible patients. All patients, including those who decline, will be asked to return the consents and response, allowing a comparison of participant and non-participant-groups. Participating patients will be randomly allocated to intervention (coaching) or control

(formal training) group, stratified by gender and age. Comparison of these two groups in terms of training format is shown in Table 1.

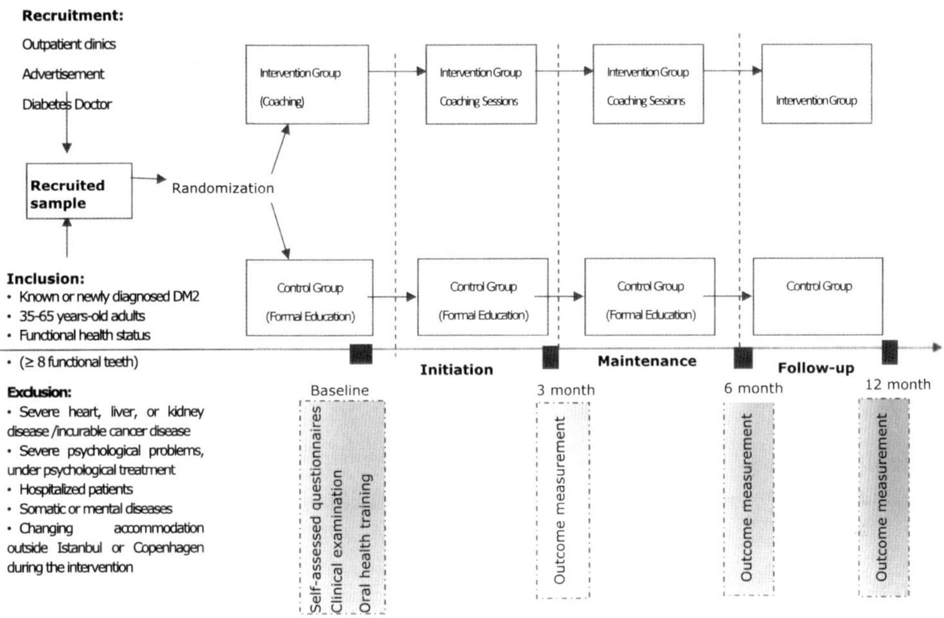

Fig. 1. Schematic representation of the study design.

All patients will be called for clinical examinations (oral and general health) and on the day of clinical examinations, questionnaires will be distributed and collected back. Then clinical oral health examinations (caries, CPI, Periodontal attachment loss) and measurements for BMI and body-fat will be performed. Then clinical measures (HbA1c, fasting blood glucose, postprandial glucose, cholesterol) from the last current patient records of the hospitals will be taken. Salivary samples to measure streptococcus mutans and lactobacillus counts will be taken by CRT® kit (IVOCLAR Vivadent, Plandent, Denmark). Within one week, all patients will be invited to a short seminar about oral diseases and their relation with diabetes and obesity. Then patients will be invited for periodontal cleaning; thus will be performed by two dentists in Turkey and two dental hygienists in Denmark.

3. The intervention

Two dentists in Turkey and two dental hygienists in Denmark, with professional ICC (International Coaching Council) training, will run the coaching sessions which will be modified from ICC manual. Sessions in format of individual,telephone and group coaching will start one week after the clinical examination. They will continue as two 3-months interventions and a 6-months follow-up. The sessions will be modified and adjusted by a multi-disciplinary team of professional health coaches, community dentistry professionals, and diabetes specialist nurse, physician and dietician.

Aspect	Control Group (Traditional Health Education)	Intervention group (Health Coaching Approach)
Orientation	Task-oriented (**The focus is on the tasks such** as tooth-brushing, regular physical exercise, adherence to dietary regimes)	Patient-oriented (**The focus is on the patient** such that if s/he can do regular tooth-brushing and physical exercise, and have the healthy diet. Focus is on the challenges and facilitators that patient faces up when s/he is to adopt positive health behaviors)
Most common techniques used	Advice-giving by the dental hygienist, information sharing between the dental hygienist and the patient: dentist /dental hygienist advises on regular tooth-brushing and healthy diet. She also asks and advises the patient about adherence to regular physical exercise and dietary regimes prescribed by the medical profession.	Expression of empathy, rolling with resistance of the patient to have healthy lifestyles, supporting self-efficacy: The patient sets up health goals, focusing on the oral health as the first, and then s/he works on how to achieve the goal together with the coach- professionally trained dental hygienist) There is an action plan within a set-up time frame, set up by patient and supported by the coach.
Technique used	None	Motivational Interviewing, self-efficacy, NLP
Decision-making process about to improve oral health and diabetes	Dentist /dental hygienist advises/tells what is best for the patient using evidence-based practice guidelines	Collaborative effort between dental hygienist and the patient Dental hygienist guides and supports the patient towards exploring how to improve oral health and diabetes. Dental hygienist facilitates movement of the patient through positive health behavior change.

Table 1. Comparison of the control and intervention.

The HC concept will be introduced at first session focusing on building the rapport between the coach and the patient. Knowledge and early experiences about health management, expectations and needs will be discussed to define health-targeted goals, specified by the patient. Coaching will focus on empowerment of patients for daily health-related practices, compliance to diabetes- and oral health care regimes and visits. The specific target will be improving skills for capacity building and self-monitoring, and taking responsibility for health and quality of life. A specific plan of action to be achieved until the next coaching session will be defined by the patient under the guidance and empowerment of a coach. Each HC session, the foundation for the next coaching session, is used for subsequent monitoring of patient's progress towards the achievement of the target goal. Pre-set time frame for HC sessions is 20-60 minutes, determined by needs, expectations, hindrances, and progress of each patient. Each session will be supported by telephone coaching sessions.

The HC intervention, focusing on improvement health behaviors for successful management of DM2 and oral health, targets to achieve 0.1% reduction on current HbA1c levels, reduced level of stress, increased self-efficacy and self-esteem, no gingival bleeding and no calculus as outcomes.

4. The coaching model: A continuous coaching cycle

Oral health focused HC follows a continuous empowerment cycle for adoption of positive health behaviors and a better lifestyle (Figure 2).

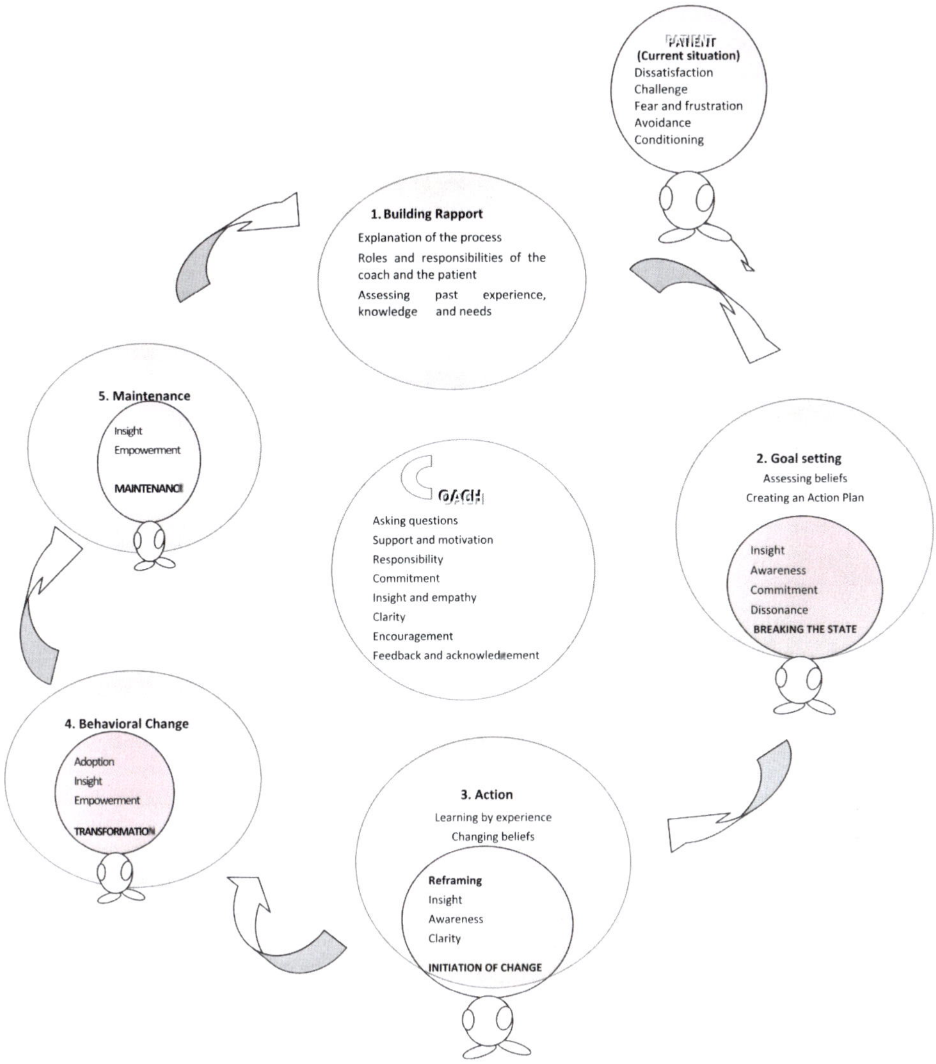

Fig. 2. Coaching cycle and its stages.

Stage 1. Building rapport and trust: The first session includes a letter of welcoming to the patient to the program and written information about coaching sessions. An informed consent between coach and patient is signed to set the framework for responsibilities and expectations of each. The first session is launched as an individual coaching, thus the patient shares his/her experiences about mainly oral health and diabetes. The coach asks questions about oral health, diabetes, weight management, and quality of life. Visual analog scales are used to enable better assessment of current health situation by each patient. The log-book with the name and contact details of his/her coach is given to each patient to monitor own progress.

Stage 2. Goal setting, assessing of beliefs and creating action plan: During the first session, the patient is asked for questions to set up his/her goal, mainly for oral health. In case the patient's priority is other specific health issue concerning diabetes, then the session will be scheduled based on this need and expectation. Hindering and empowering beliefs to achieve the goal are questioned by a coach and the patient is led through a self-brainstorming process. Beliefs, knowledge, and attitudes about earlier experiences concerning health and relevant learning practices are to be discussed. Needs and expectations of the patient are to be assessed. An action plan is set by the patient under the framework of the coaching programme. Specific action plan and empowerment tools are attached in the log-book at the end. In addition, a monitoring schedule for blood glucose measurement and oral health behavior (toothbrushing) is included.

Following the first session, each patient is coached by telephone call (8-10 minutes) after 10-15 days for motivation, encouragement and support for specific behavioral change which was determined by the patient as a personal health goal. A bilateral agreement for the schedule and content is provided for the next session. Depending on his/her needs and health situation, patient may be coached and supported to consult a health professional concerning diabetes, nutrition, and/or dentist.

Stage 3. Changing beliefs, experiencing and learning. During the following coaching session patient adherence to the negotiated action plan and relevant obstacles are evaluated. Beliefs, attitudes, challenges and enablers experienced following the first coaching session are assessed by the questions. Reinforcement is provided to empower the patient for achieving the health-related goal. If the patient mostly fails at achievements, then struggles and challenges of the patient are clarified. The goal and action plan are re-evaluated by the patient under the supervision of the coach. Empowerment by telephone coaching is provided after the session. Depending on the patient's progress, a further individual coaching session may be launched. Summary of the coaching sessions is noted on the patient's log-book by himself. This stage may be so called as `transition` as the patient moves from his health-related past experiences and beliefs to new beliefs and knowledge by self-practice.

Stage 4. Behavioral Change. Based on the self-regulation and self-learning practices, the patient performs a new positive health behavior including structuring and anchoring, so a transformation takes place. New experiences are shared by a group coaching session, and interactive learning from personal experiences is used for anchoring and empowering the new positive health behaviors and beliefs. Patients are encouraged to discuss about the patterns - action plan - to maintain and to improve the new behavioral patterns with each other. Visual analog scales for self-assessment are used for better evaluation of the current stage. Evaluation of the coaching sessions are summarized and shared. Bilateral agreement on further sessions is to be decided by the patient and the coach.

Stage 5. Behavioral Maintenance: The patient is on the stage of self-monitoring for newly adopted health behavior. As positive health behaviors, so called health enhancing behaviors, cluster together, patient will be on the process of practicing new positive health behaviors while he/she is practicing the newly adopted one. Insight and awareness of positive outcomes of the new behavior will be a gateway to experience the other health enhancing behaviors. Empowerment and support by the coach will enable to better assess changes in self-regulation. At this stage the coach follows up the patient and provides coaching sessions less frequently as the patient is on the process of learning to be a `coach` of himself/herself; thus he/she adopts and maintains positive health behaviors.

5. The control (education) group

The control group receives the formal education focused on oral health and its relation with diabetes, obesity and quality of life. Two dentists, participated in post-graduate oral public health training by Turkish Dentists Chamber, will give oral health education in the format of seminars to patients. In Denmark, two dental hygienists will be consulted about the curriculum of the formal education and then they will perform the oral health training with the patients. A diabetes specialist a nurse, a physician and a dietician will participate in the education programme in both countries, and their sessions will include diabetes, education self blood glucose monitoring, the importance of physical activity, healthy diet, weight loss, medication and smoking cessation, and late complications of DM2. Educative pamphlets about oral health and diabetes will be posted to the patients following the training sessions to support the learning environment. Training will be performed face to face twice in a month supported by phone sessions once in a month. Patients will be asked and advised on telephone by the trainers about any possible change regarding their beliefs, knowledge and behavior concerning mainly oral health, diabetes and weight management.

6. Outcome measures and data collection

The outcome measures are clinical, psycho-social and behavioral. The clinical measures are as follows: HbA1c, postprandial glucose, fasting glucose, body-fat composition, BMI, dental (DMFT) and periodontal health (CPI, periodontal attachment loss) status along with streptococcus mutans and lactobacillus counts. Measurement of these species for caries risk assessment may enable assessing the diabetes risk groups as poor oral health is a risk factor diabetes and glycemic control. All outcome measures are collected at baseline and at the end of the two 3-month interventions and at the end of follow-up after 6-months.

The self-administered questionnaires to measure psycho-social and behavioral and socioeconomic were modified from several scales (PAID,[48] Summary of Diabetes Self-Care Activities,[49] Appraisal of Diabetes Scale,[50] WHO Quality of Life,[51] and WHO HPQ[52]), and Health Behavior Questionnaire.[53]

A pilot study was conducted among 60 DM2 patients in Istanbul, Turkey, December 2009-January 2010 to test the reliability and validity of the questionnaires, in collaboration with the Oral Public Health Department (Yeditepe Dental Faculty) and The Diabetes Association. The response rate was 56%. The results are under analysis; preliminary results were submitted for presentation to IADR Congress.[53]

7. Sample size considerations and statistical measures

The size of the study is estimated by G*Power statistical power analysis software program[54, 55] (Power =0.95 α, significance level 0.05) based on the mean group difference (0.7, moderate level Cohen's d), thus may be detected as 150 for each group. Considering the possible drop-outs and non-attendance, the initial sample will target 200 patients in each group. Neither patients nor study personnel are blinded to treatment assignment. The study statisticians carrying out the data analysis on the outcomes will be blinded and will not have any contact with the patients.

Descriptive statistics (means ± SD, or median and percentile ranges, as appropriate) will be used to describe the study sample with regards to baseline characteristics. The analysis will be performed according to the intention-to-treat principles using the statistical software SPSS 17. Comparisons of outcomes between the two groups will be analyzed by values measured after the two 3-month interventions and the follow-up, using appropriate parametric tests for variables fulfilling the normal distribution criteria or appropriate non-parametric tests for variables not fulfilling the normal distribution criteria. When relevant, changes in outcomes from 3-month interventions to 6-months follow-up will be assessed. The patients will be allocated according to their oral health risk groups (streptococcus mutans and lactobacillus counts and CPI), and those groups will be analyzed and compared for the recommended goal for HbA1c and better health outcomes such as reduced body-fat ratio and stress, healthy BMI and increased quality of life. Statistical significance is set at $P < 0.05$.

8. Ethics

The study will be conducted according to the principles of the Helsinki declaration. The approval from the Danish National Committee on Biomedical Research Ethics and the Danish Data Protection Agency is in process. The permission from The Turkish Biomedical Research Ethics Committee was taken in May 2010.

9. Discussion

In Turkey, the prevalence and severity of oral diseases is high;[56-59, 26] thus 88-92% of adults experience dental caries and they have almost no healthy gums compared to the whole population (Oktay I. National Oral Health Survey 2009. Personal Communication, April 2010).[56,59] In Denmark, mean caries experience among Danish adult population is 46.6 DMF-S with an increasing prevalence among the elderly (104.1 DMF-S, 65-74-year-olds) and those with low education[60]. A study among Danish adults aged 35-44-year olds has found out that bleeding is about one fourth of the teeth and one third of the study population has at least one shallow pocket (4-5mm), most severe sign of periodontal disease, while deep pockets (at least 6mm) are about 6%.[61,62]

Inflammation in the periodontium in early old age tends to be associated with mortality in older age.[63] As people with diabetes are more likely to have periodontal disease than those without diabetes, most probably due to the increased susceptibility to contracting infections,[64-66] these people may have high risk for having a healthy life-course. However, the current periodontal health status of DM2 patients in Turkey and Denmark does not seem to be known –to our knowledge-.

DM2 is increasing in both Turkey [current prevalence: 14.7%; Oğuz A. PURE (Prospective Urban and Rural Epidemiological Study) 2010. Personal communication, April 2010] and Denmark (4.6%).[67,68] It is expected that the number of patients with diabetes almost to triple up to year of 2030.[68-70] Many individuals in Turkey and Denmark die each year because of diabetes and its complications, thus the number increases considering the interrelation of diabetes with CVD, and obesity.[69, 70] DM2 represents 90-95% of the total number of people with diabetes.[22] However, the deaths and the complications are preventable by at least 40% by improving the lifestyles.[70] Poor lifestyles (increased consumption of fat and carbohydrates, physical inactivity) contribute to DM2, accompanied mostly by obesity,[1, 3] and oral diseases.[2, 26] Thus, DM2 and oral diseases may be called lifestyle diseases so the assessment of patient's health behavior by its psychosocial and environmental determinants is crucial. Relevant studies in Turkey and Denmark are scarce.

Psychological support is needed for successful life-long management of diabetes and better quality of life.[71,72] Good psychological well-being is a prerequisite for a healthy diet, improved glycemic control, regular diabetic self-care[72, 73] and oral health care. Respective studies for oral health speak that dental caries is interrelated with self-esteem, school performance and obesity among adolescents. In addition, self-efficacy is a significant contributor for healthy eating patterns and twice daily toothbrushing.[2, 8, 9, 74] However, interventions considering patient's psychology (e.g. structuring the patient goals and motivation) on oral health and diabetes management are scarce. The present research, -to our knowledge for the first time-, is structured on capacity building skills of patients focusing on a common risk factor approach for management of both oral health and DM2 among adults.

This prospective, controlled and randomized study tests whether an oral health focused HC compared to the formal oral health training provides better health outcomes considering diabetes, oral health, obesity and quality of life among DM2 patients. Both groups receive formal oral health and diabetes training at the initial stage, further process speaks for HC for the intervention group and formal advice giving for the control group about mainly oral health, and partially diabetes, weight, and quality of life management. The major difference between two groups is that in oral HC, the patient first explores his/her `self` and then sets a health goal based on his/her expectations, needs, and beliefs. The task of the coach is to ask specific questions to guide the patient in finding out his/her own solutions and action plan. The coach empowers and supports the positive actions and change for adopting the new positive health behavior.

There are many researches in the field of health promotion and prevention of DM2 and oral health; however, there is not any research in that field speaking for both chronic diseases by HC based intervention, as well by assessing both oral health and diabetes-related subjective and clinical outcomes. The study, first in the field of oral health coaching, is unique -to our knowledge-.

10. Relevance of the project to clinical dentistry

Even 1% reduction at HbA1c has significant effects at decreasing the risk of developing complications (18%, myocardial infarction; 25%, deaths).[75] Clinical treatment of periodontal disease supported by HC intervention by dental chair-side may speak for at least 1% reduction at DM2 complications. That may enlighten the significant and frontier role of dentistry at provision of quality of life and general health among DM2 patients.

In addition, possible association/interrelation between

1. HbA1c and periodontal disease, and between caries and BMI, may provide evidence that clinical oral health examination should take a frontier role at holistic medical diagnosis: Diagnosis of DM2 at early stages and also monitoring the progress of DM2 by periodontal health status may prevent further DM2 complications. That will increase the long-term success and effectiveness of the dental and medical treatments which will reduce more complex treatments and their relevant costs.
2. HbA1c, BMI, body-fat ratio and cariogenic bacteria can provide evidence and enlighten the need of specific dental preventive regimes and oral health promotion among DM2 patients.

HC may increase the patient compliance which is a major challenge in dentistry. That will reduce the further complex treatments and therefore their costs. Evidence for the success of HC may bring a dental therapy concept that can be integrated to clinical dentistry; thus will provide new resources for clinical dentistry in terms of treatment success, finance and cost-effectiveness.

11. Relevance of the project for interdisciplinary research

HC speaks for integration of medical sciences, business administration, psychology and sociology. It is based on NLP, motivational interviewing and cognitive psychology which are currently accepted as the most effective resources for adoption, change and maintenance of positive health behaviors, leading to a healthy lifestyle. Positive health behaviors and healthy lifestyles are the main concerns of many international and national organizations; thus HC goes far beyond building a bridge between certain disciplines by connecting different stakeholders whose concern is health. Present study, based on both clinical and community dentistry, speaks for an interdisciplinary research and common concern of different organizations; that is one of the first, to our knowledge.

12. Conclusion

The study, to our knowledge, is the first that settles up a common health promotion and intervention for DM2 and oral health, in line with the declaration of IDF and FDI (2007).[29,30] Besides, it uses also for the first time an oral health focused HC as an intervention tool for chronic disease management under an umbrella. The findings of the research may provide a new approach for the holistic management of oral diseases and DM2. As there is a growing evidence that the dentistry can play a pioneer role in DM2 diagnosis and as well in prevention of further complications of DM2, the findings of the study may answer some of the questions regarding "why" and "how" dentistry can take a significant role in DM2 management. The study further underlines the need for a strong collaboration between various stake holders (universities, hospitals, government) and professionals (diabeticians, physicians, dentists, coaches) to improve the quality of life among DM2 patients and as well their families.

13. Acknowledgements

The present research study is being run at the outpatient clinics of the S.B. Kartal Research and Education Hospital and Turkish Diabetes Association under the auspicies of the Department of Oral Public Health, Yeditepe Dental Faculty, Turkey and School of Dentistry, University of Copenhagen, Denmark since September 2010. I am grateful to the coordinators of the project; Prof. Inci Oktay (Head, the Department of Oral Public Health, Yeditepe Dental Faculty) and Prof. Lone Schou (Head, School of Dentistry, University of Copenhagen, Denmark). I also express my deepest thanks to Prof. Nazif Bagriacik (Head, Turkish Diabetes Association), and Associate Prof. Mehmet Sargin and Head Diabetes Nurse Sengul Isik (Diabetes Unit, S.B. Kartal Research and Education Hospital) for all their support and help during the research process.

I am also thankful to all colleagues and friends at S.B. Kartal Research and Education Hospital and Turkish Diabetes Association for all their continuous and friendly support. I also thank to my colleagues Duygu Ilhan and Arzu Beklen for their valuable contributions to the study.

Numerous people in the Istanbul Provincial Health Directory help me during the process of official permission. Also Turkish Dentist Chamber supports the study. I thank them for their invaluable help. I also express my thanks to Prof.Aytekin Oguz for his help on the preparation of the documents for the ethical permission.

I am thankful to my coaching trainer Christian Dinesen for his perfect teaching and continuous professional support all the way through research.
I also would like to thank ZENDIUM for oral health care kits, SPLENDA (TR) for the promotional tools, ChiBall World Pty Ltd for exercising chi-balls, and to IVOCLAR Vivadent, Plandent, Denmark for the help at provision of CRT kits.
Many thanks are due to my patients for their participation and cooperation. I can never thank my mother for their love, support, and encouragement.
The research project is supported by FDI and the International Research Fund of University of Copenhagen.

14. References

[1] Preventing chronic diseases: a vital investment. Geneva: WHO; 2005. http://www.who.int/chp/chronic_disease_report/contents/en/index.html. Accessed July 2010.
[2] Petersen PE. The World Oral Health Report 2003: continuous improvement of oral health in the 21st century-the approach of the WHO Global Oral Health Programme. Community Dent Oral Epidemiol. 2003; 31 Suppl 1:3-23.
[3] Global Strategy on Diet, Physical Activity and Health: Facts related to chronic diseases. WHO; 2010. http://www.who.int/dietphysicalactivity/publications/facts/chronic/en/index.html. Accessed July 2010.
[4] Australian Government, Australian Institute of Health and Welfare. Chronic diseases; 2007. http://www.aihw.gov.au/cdarf/diseases_pages/index.cfm. Accessed July 2010.
[5] Marshall TA, Eichenberger-Gilmore JM, Broffitt BA, et al. Dental caries and childhood obesity: roles of diet and socio-economic status. Community Dent Oral Epidemiol. 2007; 35:449-458.
[6] Alm A, Fahreus C, Wendt LK, et al. Body adiposity status in teenagers and snacking habits in early childhood in relation to proximal caries at 15 years of age. Int J Paediatr Dent. 2008; 18:189-186.
[7] WHO. Diet nutrition and the prevention of chronic diseases. Report of the joint WHO/FAO expert consultation, WHO Technical Report Series, No.916 (TRS 916). WHO: Geneva; 2003.
[8] Cinar AB, Murtomaa H. Clustering of Obesity and Dental Health with Life-Style Factors among Turkish and Finnish Pre-adolescents. Obesity Facts. 2008; 1:196-202
[9] Cinar AB, Murtomaa H. Interrelation between obesity, oral health and life-style factors among Turkish school children. Clin Oral Investig. 2010 Jan. [Epub ahead of print]
[10] Pischon N, Heng N, Bernimoulin JP, et al. Obesity, inflammation, and periodontal disease. J Dent Res. 2007; 86:400-409.
[11] Al-Zahrani MS. Obesity and Periodontal Disease in Young, Middle-Aged, and Older Adults J Periodontol. 2003; 74: 610-615.
[12] Genco RJ, Grossi SG, Ho A, et al. A proposed model linking inflammation to obesity, diabetes, and periodontal infections. J Periodontol 2005; 76(11 Suppl): 2075-2084.
[13] Ashley J, Brigette R. Obesity and its role in oral health. The Internet Journal of Allied Health and Practice Sciences. 2007; 5 (1). http://ijahsp.nova.edu/articles/vol5num1/cooper.pdf.
[14] Lundin M, Yucel-Lindberg T, Dahllöf G,et al. Correlation between TNFalpha in gingival crevicular fluid and body mass index in obese subjects. Acta Odontol Scand 2004;62:273-277.

[15] Ritchie CS, Kinane DF. Nutrition, inflammation, and periodontal disease. Nutrition 2003; 19:475-476.
[16] Nishimura F, Soga Y, Iwamoto Y, et al. Periodontal disease as part of the insulin resistance syndrome in diabetic patients. J Int Acad Periodontol. 2005; 7:16-20.
[17] Nishimura F, Kono T, Fujimoto C, et al. Negative effects of chronic inflammatory periodontal disease on diabetes mellitus. J Int Acad Periodontol 2000; 2 :49-55.
[18] Santacroce L, Carlaio RG, Bottalico L. Does it Make Sense that Diabetes is Reciprocally Associated with Periodontal Disease? Endocr Metab Immune Disord Drug Targets; 2010. [Epub ahead of print]
[19] WHO. The global burden of chronic diseases. WHO, 2010. http://www.who.int/nutrition/topics/2_background/en/index.html
[20] Ostberg AL, Andersson P, Hakeberg M. Oral impacts on daily performances: associations with self-reported general health and medication. Acta Odontol Scand. 2009; 22:1-7.
[21] WHO. Diabetes. WHO, 2010. http://www.who.int/mediacentre/factsheets/fs312/en/. Accessed July 2010.
[22] Global Strategy on Diet, Physical Activity and Health: Facts related to diabetes. WHO, 2010. http://www.who.int/dietphysicalactivity/publications/facts/diabetes/en/. Accessed July 2010.
[23] Global Strategy on Diet, Physical Activity and Health: Facts related obesity. WHO, 2010. http://www.who.int/dietphysicalactivity/publications/facts/obesity/en/. Accessed July 2010.
[24] WHO European Region. Health21: the health for all policy framework for the WHO European Region. Denmark: WHO;1999.
[25] Funnell MM. Peer-based behavioural strategies to improve chronic disease self-management and clinical outcomes: evidence, logistics, evaluation considerations and needs for future research. Family Practice. 2009. doi:10.1093/fampra/cmp027.
[26] Cinar AB. Preadolescents and Their Mothers as Oral Health-Promoting Actors: Non-biologic Determinants of Oral Health among Turkish and Finnish Preadolescents. Doctorate Thesis. Helsinki: University of Helsinki; 2008.
[27] Bhuyan KK. Health promotion through self-care and community participation: Elements of a proposed programme in the developing countries. BMC Public Health. 2004. doi:10.1186/1471-2458-4-11
[28] Minet L, Møller S, Vach W, et al. Mediating the effect of self-care management intervention in type 2 diabetes: A meta-analysis of 47 randomised controlled trials. Patient Educ Couns. 2009. doi:10.1016/j.pec.2009.09.33
[29] IDF; 2009. Diabetes and oral health. Available at: http://www.idf.org/diabetes-and-oral-health. Accessed July 2010.
[30] FDI. People with diabetes need to pay special attention to oral health; 2007. http://www.fdiworldental.org/content/people-diabetes-need-pay-special-attention-oral-health. Accessed July 2010.
[31] Council of European Dentists; 2007. http://ec.europa.eu/health/ph_overview/strategy/docs/R-031.pdf. Accessed July 2010.
[32] American Dental Association; 2010. http://ebd.ada.org/. Accessed July 2010.
[33] Sheiham A, Watt RG. The common risk factor approach: a rational basis for promoting oral health. Community Dent Oral Epidemiol. 2000; 28:399-406.
[34] WHO; 2010. Facts related to chronic diseases. http://www.who.int/dietphysicalactivity/publications/facts/chronic/en/. Accessed July 2010.

[35] Butterworth SW, Linden A, McClay W. Health coaching as an intervention in health management programs. Dis Manage Health Outcomes. 2007; 15: 299-307.
[36] Lancaster T, Stead LF. Individual behavioural counselling for smoking cessation. Cochrane Database Syst Rev. 2005: 2.
[37] Stevens VJ, Glasgow RE, Toobert DJ, et al. One-year results from a brief, computer-assisted intervention to decrease consumption of fat and increase consumption of fruits and vegetables. Prev Med., 2003; 3: 594-600.
[38] Klesges RC, Kumanyika SK, Murray DM et al. Child- and parent-targeted interventions: the Memphis GEMS pilot study. Ethn Dis. 2003;13(1 Suppl 1):S40-53.
[39] Bacon L, Stern JS, Van Loan MD, Keim NL. Size acceptance and intuitive eating improve health for obese, female chronic dieters. J Am Diet Assoc. 2005; 105: 929-936.
[40] Sarvestani RS, Jamalfard MH, Kargar M, Kaveh MH, Tabatabaee HR. Effect of dietary behaviour modification on anthropometric indices and eating behaviour in obese adolescent girls. J Adv Nurs. 2009; 65: 1670-1675.
[41] Whittemore R, D'Eramo Melkus G, Grey M. Metabolic control, self-management and psychosocial adjustment in women with type 2 diabetes. J Clin Nurs. 2005; 14: 195-203.
[42] Whittemore R, Melkus GD, Sullivan A, Grey M. A nurse-coaching intervention for women with type 2 diabetes. Diabetes Educ. 2004; 30: 795-804.
[43] Bandura A. Social Learning Theory. USA: Prentice-Hall 1977; 1-55.
[44] Bandura A. Self-efficacy: The exercise of control. USA: WH Freeman and Company 1997; 79-160, 279-313.
[45] Skelly AH, Marshall JR, Haughey BP, Davis PJ, Dunford RG. Self-efficacy and confidence in outcomes as determinants of self-care practices in inner-city, African-American women with non-insulin-dependent diabetes. Diabetes Educ 1995;21:38-46.
[46] Krichbaum K, Aarestad V, Buethe M.Exploring the connection between self-efficacy and effective diabetes self-management. Diabetes Educ 2003; 29:653-62.
[47] Syrjälä AM, Kneckt MC, Knuuttila ML. Dental self-efficacy as a determinant to oral health behaviour, oral hygiene and HbA1c level among diabetic patients.J Clin Periodontol 1999; 26:616-21.
[48] Polonsky WH, Anderson BJ, Lohrer PA, et al. Assessment of diabetes-related distress. Diabetes Care. 1995; 18:754-776.
[49] Toobert DJ, Hampson SE, Glasgow RE .The Summary of Diabetes Self-Care Activities Measure. Diabetes Care. 2000: 23; 943-950.
[50] Carey MO, Jorgensen RS, Weinstock RS, et al. Reliability and validity of the appraisal of diabetes scale. J Behav Med. 1991; 14: 43-51.
[51] WHO.WHO Quality of Life-BREF (WHOQOL-BREF), 2005. http://www.who.int/substance_abuse/research_tools/whoqolbref/en/index.html. Accessed July 2010.
[52] WHO. World Health Organization Health and Performance Questionnaire (HPQ): Clinical Trials Baseline Version. http://www.HC p.med.harvard.edu/hpq/ftpdir/survey_clinical_7day.pdf
[53] Cinar AB, Oktay I, Schou L. The role of self-efficacy in oral health behavior and diabetes. IADR, General Session, Barcelona, Spain, 14-17 July 2010 (accepted).
[54] Baguley TS. Understanding statistical power in the context of applied research. Applied Ergonomics. 2004; 35: 73-80.
[55] Buchner A, Erdfelder E, Faul F. Teststärkeanalysen [Power analysis]. In Erdfelder ER, Mausfeld T, Meiser & G. Ruding (Eds.). Handbuch Quantitative Methoden. Weinheim: Psychologie Verlags Union;1996.

[56] Saydam G, Oktay İ, Möller İ. Türkiye'de ağız diş sağlığı durum analizi (National Oral Health Survey in cooperation with WHO). İstanbul; 1990.

[57] Bostanci V, Develioglu H, Çinar Z. The comparison of the periodontal treatment needs and filling needs of the students aged between 12-17 years from private and public schools from Sivas city center. Cumhuriyet Üniversitesi Diş Hekimliği Fakültesi Dergisi. 2008:11 (2). (Abstract in English)

[58] Sarıbay A. Ankara ili Çankaya ilçesinde MEB'na bağlı pilot olarak seçilmiş baz ortaöğretim kurumlarında öğrenim gören 13-19 yaş grubundaki bireylerde Juvenil Periodontitis görülme sıklığı (The prevalence of Juvenile Periodontiris among 13-19 year-old school children in a province of Ankara-Cankaya-). Doktora Tezi (Doctoral Thesis). Ankara: A. Ü. Sağlık Bilimleri Enstitüsü; 1999.

[59] Gökalp S, Doğan GB, Tekcicek M, Berbereoglu A, Ünlüer S. Oral Health Profile among the Adults and Elderly-Turkey-2004 (Abstract in English). Hacettepe Dis Hekimligi Dergisi 2007b; 31: 11-18.

[60] Krustrup U, Petersen PE. Dental caries prevalence among adults in Denmark-the impact of socio-demographic factors and use of oral health services. Community Dent Health. 2007; 24:225-32.

[61] Krustrup U, Petersen PE. Periodontal conditions in 35-44 and 65-74-year-old adults in Denmark. Acta Odontologica Scandinavica. 2006; 64: 65-73.

[62] Juel K, Sørensen J, Brønnum-Hansen H. Risk factors and public health in Denmark. National Institute of Public Health, University of Southern Denmark; 2007.

[63] Avlund K, Schultz-Larsen K, et al. Effect of inflammation in the periodontium in early old age on mortality at 21-year follow-up. J Am Geriatr Soc. 2009; 57: 1206-1212.

[64] Sandberg GE, Sundberg HE, Fjellstrom CA, et al. Type 2 diabetes and oral health: a comparison between diabetic and non-diabetic subjects. Diabetes Res Clin Pract. 2000; 50:27-34.

[65] Taylor GW, Burt BA, Becker MP, et al. Non-insulin dependent diabetes mellitus and alveolar bone loss progression over 2 years. J Periodontol. 1998; 69: 76-83.

[66] American Academy of Periodontology, 2010. Gum Disease and Diabetes. http://www.perio.org/consumer/mbc.diabetes.htm. Accessed July 2010

[67] Onat A, Hergenç G, Uyarel H, Can G, Ozhan H. Prevalence, incidence, predictors and outcome of type 2 diabetes in Turkey. Anadolu Kardiyol Derg. 2006; 6: 314-321.

[68] Danish Diabetes Association, 2009. http://www.accu-chek.dk/dk/fakta/diabetesidanmark.html. Accessed July 2010.

[69] WHO; 2010. http://www.who.int/diabetes/facts/en/index.html. Accessed July 2010.

[70] WHO; 2010. http://www.who.int/chp/chronic_disease_report/turkey.pdf. Accessed July 2010

[71] Savli H, Sevinc A.The evaluation of the Turkish version of the Well-being Questionnaire (WBQ-22) in patients with Type 2 diabetes: the effects of diabetic complications. J Endocrinol Invest. 2005;28:683-691.

[72] Akinci F, Yildirim A, Gözü H, Sargin H, Orbay E, Sargin M. Assessment of health-related quality of life (HRQoL) of patients with type 2 diabetes in Turkey. Diabetes Res Clin Pract.2008;79:117-123.

[73] Eren I, Erdi O, Sahin M. The effect of depression on quality of life of patients with type II diabetes mellitus. Depress Anxiety. 2008; 25:98-106.

[74] Cinar AB, Tseveenjav B, Murtomaa H. Oral health-related self-efficacy beliefs and toothbrushing: Finnish and Turkish pre-adolescents' and their mothers' responses. Oral Health Prev Dent. 2009; 7: 173-81.

[75] University of Koc and SANERC. Manual for Training of Diabetes Nurses.2009

9

Diabetes Mellitus Impact on Periodontal Status in Children and Adolescents

Liliana Foia[1], Vasilica Toma[1] and Petra Surlin[2]
[1]*University of Medicine and Pharmacy "Gr. T. Popa" Iasi,*
[2]*University of Medicine and Pharmacy Craiova,*
Romania

1. Introduction

Diabetes mellitus is a systemic disease with several major complications affecting both the quality and length of life. One of these complications is periodontal disease. Periodontal disease (periodontitis) is much more than a localized oral infection, recent data indicating that periodontitis may cause changes in systemic physiology. The interrelationships between periodontitis and diabetes provide an example of systemic disease predisposing to oral infection, and once that infection is established, the oral infection exacerbates systemic disease. The relationship between periodontitis and diabetes has been extensively investigated over the last years, but despite of the numerous scientific studies on the influence of periodontal treatments on glycemic control, there is limited knowledge on the impact of glycemic control upon periodontal status. Moreover, the impact of periodontal treatment on sugar metabolic control in diabetics has not been fully elucidated, the present chapter intending an outlining of the features that governs the interrelationship diabetes mellitus - periodontal disease, a discussion of the present scientific evidences, mainly focusing on clinic-biological research in juvenile groups of population.

2. Diabetes mellitus

Diabetes mellitus represents a metabolic disease usually characterized by the classic triad of polyuria, polydipsia and polyphagia, resulted from homeostasis disruption due to impaired glucose metabolism.

2.1 Classification

There are two basic types of diabetes mellitus described: insulin-dependent diabetes mellitus (IDDM- type 1) and noninsulin-dependent diabetes mellitus (NIDDM-type 2). The prevalence of type 1 diabetes mellitus exhibits a wide range, with an ever increasing rate within Europe (Neubert et al., 2011). This classification does not designate exclusively the need for exogenous insulin, sometimes the hormone being also required by type-2 diabetic patients. Type-1 diabetes is produced by the destruction of insulin-producing cells, whereas type-2 results from the combination of an increase in cell resistance to endogenous insulin with a defective secretion of this substance. Diabetes mellitus consist of an even more alarming public health problem, the prevalence of the metabolic disorder recording significant regional and ethnic variations, and a risk factor for several conditions.

2.2 Etiology and pathogenesis

The main pivotal mechanisms related to the etiology and pathogenesis of the diabetic complications include: 1) increased oxidative stress with excessive production of reactive oxygen and nitrogen species (Robertson & Harmon, 2006) and decreased antioxidants (Simmons, 2006); 2) the polyol pathway, resulting in toxic complications induced by sorbitol and 3) production of advanced glycosylation end products (AGEs) associated to impaired lipid metabolism. This last theory proposes that glucose binds, by non enzymatic reaction, to proteins such as hemoglobin, collagen, or albumin, determining certain complications triggered by the AGEs-released mediators. Diabetes complications, long time exclusively assigned to hyperglycemia can be equally determined by lipid metabolism impairment, characterized by serum LDL (low density lipoprotein), TG (triglycerides) and FA (fatty acids) level augmentation. Lipid imbalances may be related to monocytes function disorder, monocytes being able to elicit suppression of growth factors production, therefore expressing an inflammatory phenotype (rather than a proliferative one), consecutive stimulation by the pathogenic bacteria endotoxin (lipopolysaccharide). Moreover most of the evidences from the literature prove that higher levels of serum triglycerides induce stimulation of monocytes production of pro inflammatory interleukins on one hand, and of chemotactic and phagocytic abilities of neutrophils on the other hand (Iacopino, 2001).

3. Periodontal disease

Among the others cavities of the body, the oral cavity represents a distinctive ecosystem endowed with critical important biological functions, the fluids that bathes the mentioned ecosystem possessing an impressive number of components. Among the inflammatory disorders, periodontal disease-PD represents gram-negative anaerobic infections that involve tooth supporting tissues, the structures that form the periodontium (gingiva, alveolar ligament, root cementum, and alveolar bone). These alterations have mainly episodic evolution affecting first the gingiva and followed by possible secondary alteration of the surrounding connective tissue.

3.1 Classification

The most widely used classification was the American Association of Periodontology classification that distinguishes six categories: gingival disease, chronic periodontitis, aggressive periodontitis, periodontitis as manifestation of systemic disease, necrotizing periodontal disease, and periodontal abscess (Armitage, 1999). Actually, being no well-defined clinical criteria for the diagnosis, periodontal disease cannot be classified according only to the etiology, the designation periodontal disease including both reversible, soft form of inflammation, gingivitis, and irreversible, more extensive processes, periodontitis, tightly associated not only to the connective tissue of the tooth support destruction, but also accompanied by apical migration of the whole apparatus. It is one of the most widespread diseases in the world, the clinical importance of periodontal disease deriving partly from its very high prevalence, both in developed and developing countries. The main representative clinical manifestation of periodontal disease is the appearance of periodontal pockets, real favorable niche for microbiological colonization, relative facile to be revealed by clinical investigation with the periodontal probe and paraclinical X-ray imaging.

3.2 Etiology and pathogenesis

It is well known the fact that, although necessary in initiating the state of disease, bacteria represent insufficient criteria to determine its progression in the absence of an associated immune response. Also, despite the fact that the response of the host and environmental factors are important in manifesting the state of disease, nor gingivitis, neither periodontitis can onset in the absence of bacterial triggered mechanisms (Noda et al., 2007). The inflammatory reaction in the context of periodontal disease, initiated by the accumulation of bacterial plaque, starts in early childhood and reflects the special significance of the bacterial impact on the host, in a systemic context. At most children, the inflammatory process of the gum remains superficial - at the clinic stage of gingivitis, but there are cases where the balance between the bacterial aggression and the host response is impaired, leading to destructive processes which induce attachment loss, and even lost of the teeth. Moreover, Armitage (2000) includes in his classification the pre pubertal periodontitis, juvenile periodontitis and the fast progressive forms of manifestation of periodontal disease at children and teenagers, in the aggressive periodontitis class, because of the fast progression and severe impairment of periodontal tissues. This is why, tracking down the disorder as early as possible, is essential for an early establishment of a specific therapy, but especially for preventing the installing and evolution toward more severe forms of disease. On the other hand, the inconsistency between the aggression of periodontal destruction at child and teenager and the reduced quantity of biofilm (in some forms of tooth decay), determined some scientists to claim that the bacterial challenge represents an essential condition, although not sufficient in developing periodontitis, the decisive factor being actually, host susceptibility (Tabholz et al., 2010). Today, it is well known that both genetic and contracted factors are determinants of periodontitis presence, progression and severity in adults, Pihlstrom attributing to genetic causes almost half of the risk in developing a periodontal disease during life (and probable to be revealed even during childhood).

3.3 Gingival crevicular fluid as a diagnostic fluid

Present in the gingival sulcus, gingival crevicular fluid (GCF) has been studied since 1955 for its diagnostic potential. Since several decades, gingival fluid reentered into the specialists' attention, its components being analyzed as non-aggressive means of host reaction examination at the periodontal level and early diagnosis of the periodontal breakdown. The gingival crevicular fluid has numerous advantages versus blood and saliva, in particular because of the ability of designation and collection of convenient samples from specific sites containing components derived both from host (in the form of plasma, cellular components, tissue of connection) and bacterial plaque. GCF can thus be considered a true "battle field" (the center of interaction host-microorganism) between the external aggressors (especially of bacterial plaque) and internal aggressors (host derived). Besides, the trend of current understanding of the periodontal pathology suggests that destruction of the periodontal tissue is modulated by host response (Van Dyke, 2009), that release products representing real periodontal destructive markers, suitable for monitoring both, within plasma and gingival fluid. The correct determination of such sensitive markers of destructive periodontium imposes itself as a need for settling the management of the disease on more rational and less empirical bases. Gingival crevicular fluid (GCF) reflects the complexity of the host-bacteria interaction and offers information, referring not only the equilibrium between the infected germs and the host, but also specific dates concerning involved pathogenic mechanisms (Champagne et al., 2003). Therefore, GCF that reflects both, these influences at the systemic and host level on one side, and the local modulation of these responses following specific bacteria interactions on the other side, appears as a representative biologic sample for searching these indicators and predictors of the bidirectional interplay diabetes-periodontal disease.

4. Study approach

The anatomic and functional particularities of the marginal periodontium in child and adolescent, the variety of clinical expression of disease, and also the heterogeneity of etiology and the complexity of the pathogenic mechanisms, make the periodontal disease in child and adolescent to keep being a subject with many unknowns, interesting both the researchers and also practitioners. The lack of concordance between the aggression of periodontal destructions in child and adolescent and the amount of bacterial plaque in some forms of periodontal disease determined a series of researchers to state that bacteria, although absolutely necessary for developing the periodontal disease, are insufficient for developing periodontitis, thus susceptibility of the host being also involved (Kinane et al., 2007). Therefore, the prevalence, onset, progression and especially pathology of periodontal diseases can be modified by numerous endogenous factors. Soluble chemical mediators (prostaglandins, cytokines) or enzymes, sharing significant expression on the oral fluids level, are important in evaluation of the metabolic response within the active stage of the disease. The dental plaque-mediated inflammatory reaction onset within the periodontal breakdown takes place in early stages of childhood, and reflects the important signification of bacterial impact upon the host tissues within systemic context. In most of the children, the gingival inflammation remains superficial, but sometimes further destruction occurs, with loss of periodontal attachment. Over the last years, there has been an emerging interest in the bidirectional relationship diabetes mellitus and oral health. Postulated as a disruption in homeostasis of glucose metabolism, type 1-diabetes is often associated to periodontal disease, inflammation representing the common pathophysiologic feature.

4.1 Objectives

Starting from the alarming 2008 World Health Organization reports concerning the continuously increasing incidence of insulin dependent diabetes mellitus in the juvenile population, we focused much of our attention on the binomial relationship between IDDM and periodontal disease within this age group of individuals, considering both the potential of investigation and prevention of this malady and its complications within the juvenile population. The main preoccupations of the present research targeted the following aspects: a. study of the periodontal pathology in child and adolescent, through determination of the role and diagnostic value of certain cytokines determination, within the complex program of identification, evaluation and treatment of the patients with periodontal disease and unaffected general state (control group) and systemically affected individuals; b. analysis of impact on periodontal breakdown pathogenesis of the interleukins IL-1β, IL-2, IL-10 and interferon gamma (IFN-γ), and their expression as potential indicators or predictors of diagnostic and evolution of periodontal disease in systemic context.

4.2 Materials and methods

4.2.1 Subject population

The evaluation was carried out on 84 subjects, age 6 - 18 years, divided into two groups, both with several degree of periodontal alteration: 42 non-diabetic subjects who did not suffer from any systemic disease (control group), and 42 IDDM subjects. The subjects were evaluated and divided into subgroups, according to the prepubertal (6-10years old), pubertal (11-14 years) or juvenile age (15-18 years old), and metabolic control of the disease. The diabetic group enrolled in this study comprised half well-controlled (glycosylated hemoglobin levels ≤7%) and half poorly controlled (glycosylated hemoglobin levels >7%). All subjects were submitted blood collection, GCF sampling and clinical periodontal index evaluation. Data on blood glucose, lipid profile and glycosylated hemoglobin (HbA1c) were collected from the medical records. Considering the bivalent nature of the relationship between DM and PD, the evaluation of the gingival fluid comprised records of several immune-chemical inflammatory mediators: interleukin 1β - Il-1β, IL-2, IL-10 and IFN-γ, in parallel with serum mediator determinations. Total amounts and concentrations of serum and gingival crevicular cytokines were analyzed by enzyme-linked immunosorbent assay and flow cytometry. Diabetic patients were recruited from the Metabolic and nutrition diseases department of the University Children Hospital "Sf. Maria" Iasi, and selected based on the following criteria: aged between 6 and 18 years old, diagnosed with type 1 DM. Patients were excluded if they had non-type 1 diabetes, any inflammatory diseases, liver or renal impairment (depending of the blood creatinine levels), a periodontal treatment in the last 6 months prior to the assessment, any severe pathology of the teeth or were receiving medication that could influence the studied parameters (corticosteroids, antibiotics). The age matched control group was selected among the non-diabetic individuals that followed regular treatment in the dental unit of the Pediatric Dental Clinic. Informed consent was obtained in all cases, the local ethics committee approving the protocol deemed to conform to the guidelines issued in the Helsinki Declaration.

4.2.2 Clinical study design

Periodontal status was assessed by clinical evaluations of plaque index (PI), papillary bleeding index (PBI) and clinical attachment loss (CAL), and correlation with the degree of metabolic control (levels of glycemia and glycosylated hemoglobin). The mentioned periodontal parameters were evaluated in a randomized half mouth examination on six sites of each tooth (mesiobuccal, buccal, distobuccal, mesiolingual, lingual and distolingual) by a calibrated examiner. The level of oral hygiene was estimated with a plaque index - Quigley Heine index (based on the score from 0 to 5) (Silness & Löe, 1964). The scores of the plaque index were calculated according to the formula: per person = sum of individual scores/number of teeth present for each person, subsequently, the group scores being subtracted. Other clinical records consisted of papillary bleeding index evaluation, based on gentle probing and clinical attachment loss determinations of the total teeth in the mouth by periodontal probe exploration. PBI score (Saxter and Muhleman) was recorded based on four different grades of bleeding intensities subsequent to careful probing. Subsequent of completed probing, the bleeding intensity was scored in four grades: grade 0 = no bleeding; grade 1 = appearance of a single bleeding point; grade 2 = a fine line of blood or several bleeding points become visible at the gingival margin; grade 3 = blood filled interdental triangle; grade 4 = profuse bleeding consecutive probing. The bleeding value was given by the sum of the recorded scores and PBI by dividing the bleeding value to the total number of examined papilla. CAL, the distance from the cementoenamel junction to the base of the periodontal pocket, a measure of the amount of alveolar bone lost due to periodontal disease, was measured to the nearest millimeter using a North Carolina periodontal probe. Measurements of 1-2 mm were considered to be slight, 3-4 mm moderate, and ≥5 mm severe (Costa et al., 2007).

4.2.3 Gingival crevicular fluid and serum sampling

Collection and analysis of GCF represent noninvasive methods for the evaluation of host response in periodontal disease. Gingival crevicular fluid samples were obtained from the mesiobuccal site of every tooth (excluding third molars) from two randomly selected contralateral quadrants. Consecutive plaque evaluation and following isolation of the site with cotton rolls, supragingival plaque was removed, and the tooth air dried. GCF sample was collected on periopaper strips (Periopaper®, Amityville, NY) gently inserted 1-2 mm subgingivally, into the periodontal pocket. Gingival fluid volume was assessed using an electronic device, Periotron 8000® (Oraflow Inc., Plainview, NY). Collected samples were immediately placed into sterilized plastic tubes on ice, shipped to the laboratory and stored at −80°C till the day of determination. GCF samples were always collected prior to clinical measurements and samples contaminated with blood were discarded. Using the venipuncture technique, approximately 5 ml of venous blood was also drawn from the antecubital vein, using the vacutainer system (Becton Dickinson, NJ, USA), and analyzed for the lipid and carbohydrate metabolic profile. The degree of metabolic control was evaluated considering the glycosylated hemoglobin values (HbA1c), measured by high performance liquid chromatography (HPLC). Good metabolic control was taken to be represented by HbA1c ≤ 7%, while poor control was defined as HbA1c > 7%, (American Diabetes Association), normal values being considered for HbA1c < 6%.

4.2.4 Measurement and quantification of cytokines using multiplex cytometric bead array

Serum and local gingival fluid cytokine levels were determined using the high sensitivity human CBA cytokine multiplex (Cytometric Bead Array®, BD Pharmingen, San Diego) for flow cytometry. Prior to assay, GCF samples were eluted into 50 μl of the assay buffer by vortexing for 30 minutes and further 10 minutes centrifugation at 8,000 rpm. Flow cytometry is an investigation method that allows various cells sorting according to size, granularity, and specific markers expression. Cytometric investigation of cytokines has substantial advantages compared to ELISA immunoassay method, allowing simultaneous detection of multiple cytokines, fast and with very small sample volumes (50μl). CBA kit contains microspheres coated on the outside with anti-cytokine monoclonal antibodies. Each type of microsphere has a characteristic fluorescence level detectable on third channel (FL 3) of the cytometer. Detection of cytokine amount is performed through the second category of anti-analyte antibody, marked with a fluorescent protein, phycoerythrin, whose fluorescence is detectable on channel FL 2. The FACS Caliber (BD Biosciences, San Jose, CA, USA) monitors the spectral properties of the beads to distinguish the different antigens, simultaneously measuring the amount of fluorescence associated with phycoerythrin and reported as median fluorescence intensity. The concentrations of the assessed cytokines were estimated using a standard curve obtained following the manufacturer's instructions, by testing standard samples included in the kit and expression as pg/ml.

4.2.5 Data analysis and statistics

Periodontal parameters of subjects according to the age group were described by means of standard deviation and analyzed by analysis of variance (ANOVA).

Clinical data were collected from 6 sites per tooth for visible plaque, papillary bleeding index, and CAL. The levels of each inflammatory mediator were measured for up to 14 GCF samples per subject and expressed as pg/ml. Interactions between variables were studied using Pearson's correlation. The Mann–Whitney *U* test was used to compare values between groups. Paired non-parametric (Wilcoxon) *t* tests established significance for cytokine level within gingival fluid and serum from the same individual, while $p<0.05$ established significance.

4.3 Results

The association between DM and periodontal disease has been debated over decades, with conflicting conclusions. Most of the recent studies tend to support a higher prevalence and severity of periodontitis in diabetic adult patients, less literature data being available in what concerns insulin dependent diabetes upregulation of periodontal breakdown in children and adolescents. It has been shown that diabetes strongly influences the production of inflammatory mediators, cytokines and chemokines (Joo & Lee, 2007) resulting in abnormal immune inflammatory reaction and tissue injury in patients with periodontitis. Periodontal disease represents a group of alterations with episodic evolution that affects gingiva and could secondly alter the surrounding connective tissue.

The main goal of the present study was to examine the interplay between the local and systemic cytokine profile, and immune-inflammatory mediated clinical response, in systemically healthy and insulin dependent diabetes mellitus young subjects. In order to achieve this goal we employed flow cytometric techniques to characterize the levels of some pro and anti inflammatory cytokines both in serum and gingival fluid. In addition, the study tempted to reflect the clinical changes in the oral health within children and adolescents with type 1 diabetes mellitus, to assess the rate of gingival inflammation accompanying the systemic disorder and to contribute to the incidence data on periodontal disease for groups of patients where factors attributable to aging are not confounding variables.

The investigation was carried out on 84 subjects age 6-18 years, divided into two main groups: The first group (diabetic group) consisted of 42 subjects with type 1 diabetes mellitus diagnosed with marginal chronic periodontitis (n=6), aggressive periodontitis (n=6) and gingivitis (n=30). The diabetic group was subdivided according to the level of metabolic control, into well control diabetes, glycosylated hemoglobin levels ≤7% (n=22), and poor control diabetes with glycosylated hemoglobin levels > 7% (n=20). In the second group (non diabetes group=ND), there were 42 age-matched subjects who did not suffer from any systemic disease, most of them experiencing the mildest form of periodontal breakdown, gingivitis (n=36), followed by marginal chronic periodontitis (n=4) and aggressive periodontitis (n=2).

4.3.1 Statistics on periodontal breakdown in the two groups

After setting up lots of study, analysis of parameters related to distribution, diagnosis and age reveals the highest prevalence of gingivitis, the mildest form of plaque-induced inflammatory disease (85,7%), followed by breakdown of the superficial periodontal support (chronic superficial marginal periodontitis) (9,5%) and aggressive periodontitis

(4.8%) in the non diabetes group. Considering the diabetes group, there were different incidences of periodontal disease in the two subgroups: children and adolescents with good metabolic control (n=22) displayed generalized bacterial gingivitis in a proportion of 81% (n=18) and 19% aggressive periodontitis (n=4), while in the poorly controlled diabetes group, besides bacterial gingivitis (60%, n=12), 30% were diagnosed with chronic superficial marginal periodontitis (n=6) and 10% with aggressive periodontitis (n=2). Thus, despite of some previous results that founded no significant correlation between gingival condition and glycosylated hemoglobin levels (De Pomereau et al., 1992), our data suggest that at young ages, there is a higher incidence and severity of periodontal breakdown in poorly controlled diabetes, where the incidence rate increases after puberty and continuously increases by age, with an overall elevation in resorption of the bone and epithelial attachment, and predisposition to infection.

4.3.2 Oral hygiene levels

The level of oral hygiene was assessed for all the patients by plaque index evaluation (Quigley Heine index), based on the score from 0 to 5. Our results highlighted high incidence of values in the 2-3 range for the non diabetes group compared with the distribution of values in other groups. In the analysis presented in figure 1, statistical indicators display a high average of plaque index in poorly controlled diabetic patients (3.293 ± 1.06) compared to mean values calculated for the non diabetes group (2.995 ± 0.58) and individuals with well controlled diabetes (2.881 ± 0.857), respectively. Standard deviation registers the minimum value for the nondiabetics (SD = 0.58) while for the group with poorly controlled diabetes, standard deviation reaches a maximum value (SD=1.06).

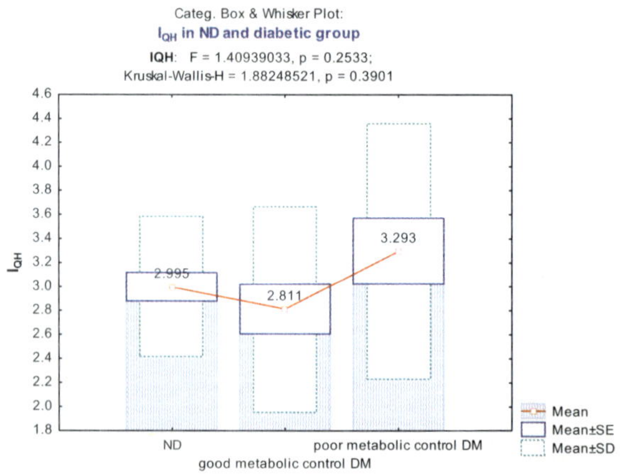

Fig. 1. Mean values of Quigley Heine Index in nondiabetics (ND), good control- and poor control DM groups.

ANOVA test used to compare by analysis of variance the mean plaque index values corresponding to studied groups, highlights the significant difference between mean values corresponding to the groups and subgroups (p = 0.013, p<0.05). Significant difference exist also between the values corresponding to the ND and poorly controlled DM individuals, the significance level (p) corresponding to 95% confidence interval being 0.0451. Moreover, a statistically significant difference is record between the plaque index values within the two diabetes subgroups: good control versus poor control DM, p=0.003 (p<<0.05, CI=95%).

QH Index / Group	Mean	Std. Dev	Min	Max	Q25	Q50	Q75
Pre pubertal age: 6-10 years							
ND	3.176	0.500	2.500	4.133	2.830	3.058	3.50
Good control DM	3.132	0.736	2.000	4.000	2.660	3.500	3.50
Poor control DM	2.830	0.626	2.000	3.660	2.330	2.830	3.33
Pubertal age: 11-14 years							
ND	2.734	0.445	2.330	3.660	2.330	2.660	3.00
Good control DM	3.125	0.888	1.833	4.133	2.660	3.000	4.00
Poor control DM	3.076	0.884	1.833	4.133	2.330	3.080	4.00
Juvenile age: 15-18 years							
Martor	3.036	0.668	2.166	4.000	2.500	3.000	3.66
Good control DM	2.356	0.679	1.500	3.500	1.833	2.000	3.00
Poor control DM	3.925	1.207	1.833	5.000	3.660	4.133	5.00

Table 1. Statistical indicators of Quigley Heine Index for studied groups, according to age.

Quigley Heine Index can be properly evaluated in the studied groups taking into account the patient's age. The maximum standard deviation was found in the group of patients aged 15-18 years (juvenile period), significant differences being registered in this group between average values of nondiabetics and diabetics (table 1). Maximum values (QHI= 5) were recorded for the juvenile group (15-18 years old), in patients with poorly controlled IDDM. Considering the age intervals, comparative statistic studies of the oral hygiene parameter highlight the most significant differences among the juvenile age individuals from all studied groups (p<<0.05).

4.3.3 Periodontal status

Papillary Bleeding Index (PBI)

Bleeding index shows differences values in the two populations. Thus, the non diabetes group stands 0.5 minimum and 2.66 as maximum values, lower than those for patients with poorly controlled diabetes (PBI min = 1, max = 4.66). Large variations recorded among the bleeding index values in the group with poor metabolic control are also highlighted by the large standard deviation (SD = 0.97).

As displayed in figure 2, the average PBI in poorly controlled diabetes is 2,964, almost two times higher than in the non diabetic group (PBI = 1.56) and 1.75 times higher than in the well balanced diabetic disease group (PBI = 1.69), p<<0.05. Statistic analysis reveal no significant differences between PBI values of the systemically unaffected population and

diabetic subgroup with good metabolic control ($p = 0.58$), while significant differences are registered between the two subgroups of diabetics ($p = 0.000018$, $p << 0.05$).
Statistic analyses on PBI correlated to age stages highlights minimum values in the ND group within juvenile age ($PBI_{min}=0.50$) and maximum values ($PBI_{max}=4.66$) recorded in the prepubertal age group of patients with poorly controlled diabetes (table 2).

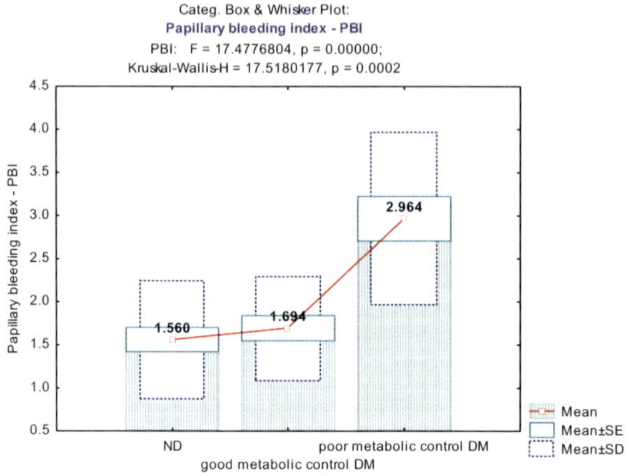

Fig. 2. Mean papillary bleeding index (PBI) in the non diabetes group, poorly controlled and good metabolic controlled diabetic children and adolescents.

Group \ PBI	Mean	Std. Dev	Min	Max	Q25	Q50	Q75
Pre pubertal age: 6-10 years							
ND	1.914	0.472	1.330	2.660	1.580	1.830	2.250
Good control DM	2.130	0.899	1.330	3.660	1.660	2.000	2.600
Poor control DM	3.039	1.187	2.000	4.660	2.165	2.748	3.913
Pubertal age: 11-14 years							
ND	1.235	0.593	0.660	2.330	0.660	1.330	1.500
Good control DM	2.650	0.850	1.330	3.660	2.600	2.660	3.000
Poor control DM	2.775	0.777	2.000	3.660	2.000	2.665	3.660
Juvenile age: 15-18 years							
ND	1.499	0.819	0.500	2.660	0.833	1.500	2.330
Good control DM	2.747	0.457	2.000	3.300	2.330	3.000	3.000
Poor control DM	3.132	1.260	1.000	4.000	3.000	3.660	4.000

Table 2. Statistics on papillary bleeding index (PBI) for the studied groups, according to age.

Statistic significant differences were recorded for the mean PBI values for all groups of patients divided per age groups (p<0.5). For prepubertal stage (6-10 years) mean PBI did not registered significant differences between ND and good metabolic control patients (p>0.5), while for pubertal stage significant differences were recorded across all studied groups (ND, good control and poor control DM). Considering the juvenile period (15-18 years), average PBI was higher in poor controlled diabetes compared to mean values of well metabolically balanced diabetics and of ND, the difference being statistically significant (p<0.5).

Clinical attachment loss

The highest incidence of increased clinical attachment loss along with the most elevated mean value were recorded in poorly controlled diabetics (CAL = 1.053 mm, figure 3).

Significant differences were recorded between the two subgroups of DM children and adolescents and between the groups of non diabetes and good metabolic control DM, respectively (p=0.002).

For a description of the lots included in the study based on loss of attachment, table 3 presents statistical indicators that define the characteristics of the groups in terms of this clinical indicator. For pre pubertal stage no real attachment loss was registered in all groups of patients enrolled in the study. The pubertal phase recorded a slight increase in the CAL levels, with maximum values up to 2mm, and 0.5mm as average. Quartile analysis (Q75) indicates that 75% of the children belonging to this age group presented mean CAL levels below 1 mm. Individuals aging between 15-18 years old recorded different values, with minimum CAL=0mm and peak CAL=4 mm, statistic analysis highlighting mean values below 2.3 mm for 75% of nondiabetics, while 75% of poor controlled SM subjects of this age group presented CAL up to 3.5 mm. Moreover, standard deviation was also higher for this age population compared to the others.

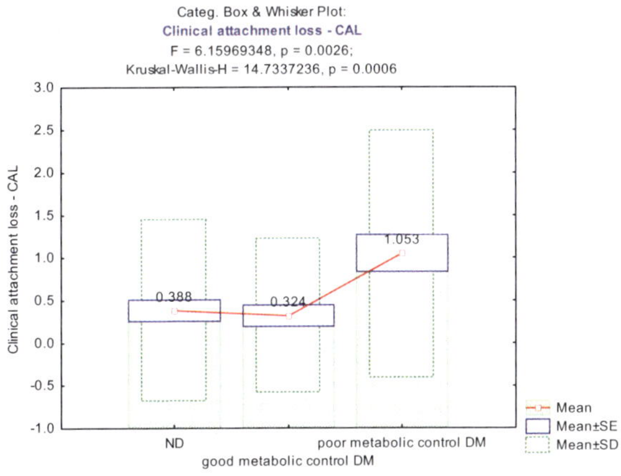

Fig. 3. Mean clinical attachment loss in the studied groups.

4.3.4 Analysis of serum and GCF inflammatory mediators

The inflammatory mediator profile in human whole blood and gingival fluid was characterized in more detail. Whole blood and crevicular fluid were collected from all subjects enrolled in the study, according to the previous mentioned protocol, and analyzed for IL-1β, IL-2, IL-10, and IFN-γ production. The degree of local and systemic inflammatory response was assessed by multiplex flow cytometry blood and gingival fluid cytokines level determinations. A significant interindividual variability in the amounts of inflammatory mediators secreted during the association of the periodontal breakdown with systemic alteration was observed for all the mediators tested.

Group \ CAL(mm)	Mean	Std. Dev.	Min	Max	Q25	Q50	Q75
Pre pubertal age: 6-10 years							
ND	0.000	0.000	0.000	0.000	0.000	0.000	0.0
Good control DM	0.000	0.000	0.000	0.000	0.000	0.000	0.0
Poor control DM	0.000	0.000	0.000	0.000	0.000	0.000	0.0
Pubertal age: 11-14 years							
ND	0.000	0.000	0.000	0.000	0.000	0.000	0.0
Good control DM	0.000	0.000	0.000	0.000	0.000	0.000	0.0
Poor control DM	0.500	0.786	0.000	2.000	0.000	0.000	1.0
Juvenile age: 15-18 years							
ND	1.033	1.545	0.000	4.000	0.000	0.000	2.3
Good control DM	0.786	1.280	0.000	3.000	0.000	0.000	2.5
Poor control DM	2.560	1.447	0.000	4.000	2.300	3.000	3.5

Table 3. Statistic indicators of clinical attachment loss (CAL-mm) for studied groups, according to age.

As shown in figure 4, diabetes mellitus elicited a significant increase ($p<0.05$) in local secretion of IL-1β.

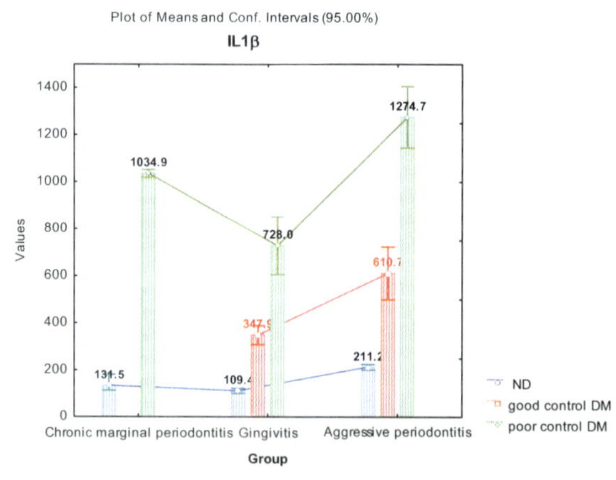

Fig. 4. Levels of gingival fluid IL-1β in the studied groups.

The lowest mean local interleukin 1β value was recorded in the systemically healthy population, the diabetic status associating a considerable increase in gingival fluid interleukin levels. In addition, systemically healthy patients with gingivitis recorded the lowest gingival fluid IL-1β level, a significant elevation of this mediator being associated to IDDM children and teenagers. Moreover, IL-1β, IL-2 and IFN-γ analysis according to the values of HbA_{1C}, revealed the existence of a statistic significant positive correlation betwen the measured parameters (Pearson test, r=0.73; 0.65 and 0.71 respectively), thus reflecting important elevations of cytokine levels induced by impaired metabolic balance of the diabetic young population.

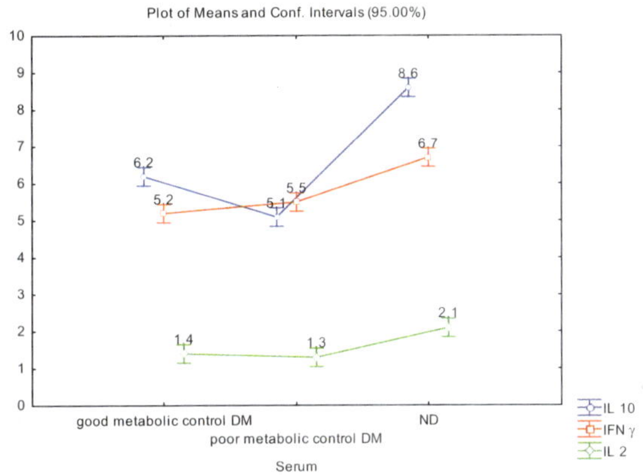

Fig. 5. Serum levels of IL-2, IL-10 and IFN-γ in the studied groups.

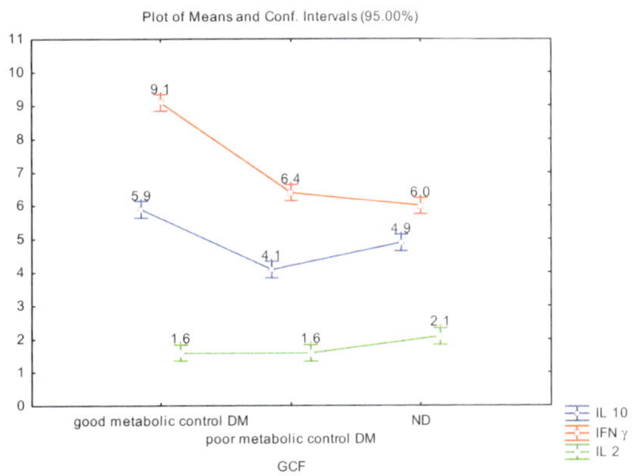

Fig. 6. GCF levels of IL-2, IL-10 and IFN-γ in the studied groups.

Serum IFN-γ in diabetic children recorded moderate values compared to that of ND, and significantly higher levels in gingival fluid (figure 5). While IL-10 gingival fluid secretion was enhanced in some diabetic subjects with good control of the metabolic disorder, the most common elevated levels were present in the serum of systemically unaffected group (figure 5 and 6). IL-10 registered a decreased average level of blood and GCF secretion in the diabetic population, with significantly differences between the two systemically affected subgroups. Considering IL-2 level, there is a very low secretion in diabetic patients with periodontal breakdown, both in blood and gingival fluid, probably determined by a local production of a blocking factor that induces this specific profile.

4.4 Discussions

Analysis of clinical parameters related to distribution, diagnosis and age highlights significant differences in the prevalence of severe periodontal breakdown between the two principal studied groups, with an 14.3% overall prevalence of chronic marginal periodontitis and aggressive periodontitis within systemically healthy individuals versus 28.5% in IDDM group. Moreover, the same proportion was maintained when considering the two diabetes subgroups, almost two times more subjects with poor controlled diabetes experiencing severe periodontal injury (40%) compared to good metabolically balanced age-matched diabetic individuals (19%). Thus, despite that the oral health status data showed gingivitis as the main periodontal alter in both groups, there were significant differences among diabetic subpopulations (81% versus 60% within good and poor controlled diabetics, respectively). This was followed by a 3.1 fold increased incidence of chronic superficial periodontitis within the diabetics (30%) compared to non-diabetic group (9.5%), and almost twice more prevalent aggressive periodontitis in IDDM children and teenagers (19% *vs.* 10%). Summarizing the results based on clinical diagnosis of periodontal injury related to age interval, the highest prevalence of gingivitis is specific for the prepubertal age, followed by an increase incidence of marginal superficial chronic periodontitis in pubertal stage and forms of aggressive periodontitis during juvenile age, among all studied groups. Considering the two main population groups, gingivitis is the main periodontal alter among systemically healthy subjects, the associated systemic disease eliciting an increase in the incidence of more severe periodontal breakdown.

Periodontal homeostasis breakdown along systemic alteration of type 1 DM was also assessed through evaluation of clinical parameters (PI, PBI, CAL) correlated with age, duration and metabolic control of diabetes mellitus (HbA1c values). Statistically significant differences were recorded both, between the mean PI values corresponding to the non diabetes group and poorly controlled DM individuals, and between the two diabetes subgroups ($p<<0.05$, CI=95%). Moreover, taking into consideration the age intervals, comparative statistic studies of the oral hygiene parameter highlight the most significant differences among the juvenile age individuals, for all studied groups ($p<<0.05$).

Papillary bleeding index in diabetic children and teenagers have significantly higher values, directly correlated to the age of systemic disease ($r=0.64$). Considering the patient's age, the most important statistical difference is registered along pubertal period, pointing out a significant difference between the mean PBI values in ND patients (PBI=1.23) versus good controlled diabetic group (PBI=2.65) ($p=0.007$, $p<<0.05$). Furthermore, mean BPI significantly differs in patients with poorly controlled diabetes than the average values in patients with good controlled diabetes and ND ($p<<0.05$), this pattern of overall changes in inflammatory periodontal parameter's levels persisting across all age groups (prepubertal, pubertal, juvenile). These results can be explained by increased activity of collagenases and vascular changes within diabetes that increase gums bleeding and thickening of the small vessels basal membrane of the gingiva.

Distribution of CAL values indicated the most elevated (between 1.5 - 4 mm) and highest mean level (CAL = 1.053 mm), in the group of subjects with poor controlled diabetes, about 2.7 and 3.25 times higher than that of ND (CAL = 0.388 mm) and good metabolic controlled IDDM (CAL = 0.324 mm), respectively. Reffering to age, the highest mean loss of attachment characterized the 15-18 years old poorly controlled IDDM subjects (CAL=2.56mm), 2.4 more elevated than in ND (CAL=1.03 mm) and 3.2 times higher than in good metabolically controlled diabetics (CAL=0.79mm) (table 3). In prepubertal stage, almost no one can question the loss of attachment (explained both by anatomic and physiologic characteristics of this phase and the very short period in which teeth are maintained on the arch). In addition, the disease's evolution is insufficient to elicit real periodontal breakdown of chronic marginal periodontitis type, most commonly, loss of attachment being rather related to diabetes time course.

Furthermore, HbA1c values correlated with clinical parameters of oral status indicated that poorly controlled diabetes (HbA1c >7%) is associated with elevated bleeding index. Comparison of the parameters that indicate the degree of periodontal disruption (PBI and CAL) with age of onset of systemic disease reveals that age of diabetes and its metabolic control can be important determinant indicators to evaluate DM as a risk factor for periodontal breakdown within children and adolescents.

Determination of gingival crevicular fluid with parallel serum levels of soluble inflammatory mediators is highly relevant for studying children and teenager periodontitis within systemic context, since this consistent oral fluid, which bathes the periodontal pocket, derives from gingival capillary beds and contains resident and emigrating inflammatory cells. Systemically healthy patients with the mild form of periodontal disease recorded the lowest IL-1β gingival fluid level, a significant increase of this mediator being associated to IDDM group. Moreover, in ND patients there was a dose–response relationship between the severity of periodontitis and gingival crevicular fluid IL-1β levels (two times higher mean values in systemically unaffected subjects with aggressive periodontitis), which suggested that periodontal disease may play a major role in elevating levels of this cytokine. Our results reveal an overall pattern of most prominent variability among poorly controlled diabetic children and teenagers, regardless of periodontal breakdown degree (gingivitis or aggressive periodontitis). Data from the literature are somehow conflicting, certain results on adult population mentioning the lack of correlation between production of IL-1β related cytokine, and HbA_{1c} levels in patients with type 2 diabetes and periodontitis (Engebretson et al., 2007). Our results recorded significant positive correlation (Pearson test, $r = 0.73$) between IL-1β and glycosylated hemoglobin levels in diabetic young individuals, translated also into increased interleukin levels directly related to the reduction in the degree of metabolic control of the systemic disorder. IFN-γ is an inflammatory cytokine associated with inflammation, tissue destruction, bone resorption and specific elevated production of collagenases, serum and local determinations of this important regulator of immune inflammatory response revealing different levels in diabetic individuals, higher when associated to a good metabolic control and more specific periodontal breakdown. Moderate IFN-γ serum levels were recorded in diabetic population compared to ND, the high expression of gingival fluid cytokines in severe periodontal alteration of these patients being probably a marker of continuous Th1 response against microbiologic challenge, especially bacterial pathogens colonized in gingival tissue. This can be explained by alterations in the oral microenvironment caused by much higher amounts of glucose and urea in gingival

fluid from DM individuals (data recorded by laboratory analysis of gingival fluid), that create a favorable environment for bacterial changes, with alteration of host immune response to periodontal pathogens, and suggests that Th1 mediated cytokine response may play a destructive role in the periodontium. The present results indicate that microbiological overlapping involves considerable efforts of the body, resulting in significant elevation of IFN-γ, but not of IL-2 which was very low both in blood and GCF diabetic individuals, suggesting the possible existence of a local factor that blocks the lymphocyte and macrophage secretion of this T lymphocytes factor of proliferation, mainly in diabetic patients with periodontal deterioration. The reasons for moderate IL-2 secretion are probably complex and may involve transcriptional or translational repression.
IL-10 registered decreased secretion in the diabetic population, both gingival fluid and serum values recording significantly higher differences between the two systemically affected subgroups. It is thus possible that reduction in IL-10 secretion within juvenile diabetic population could play an important role in switch of the oral tissue differentiation toward periodontal injuries.

4.5 Conclusion

Our study showed that DM modulates GCF expression of Il-1β, IL-10 and IFN-γ in patients with impaired periodontal territories. Very probably this is the result of immune system cells sensitization by endogenous ligands and bacterial products through various receptors, some of them recognized as important mediators of immune responses in inflammatory diseases. Applied statistic tests showed that the values of all studied clinical parameters referring to periodontal status in diabetic children and adolescents (plaque index, bleeding index, loss of attachment) are much higher than those of systemically healthy group. Thus, the present study clearly reinforce that children and adolescents are susceptible to destructive forms of periodontal disease, especially when the etiologic external factors (microbial flora) are associated with host-related systemic impairment, such as insulin dependent diabetes. In summary, our data support the notion that systemic alteration of IDDM type is associated with distinct patterns of GCF cytokine expression. Poor controlled young diabetic subjects were characterized by local higher IL-1β and decreased IL-10 and IFN-γ amounts, compared to systemically healthy subjects, suggesting that an imbalance between pro- and anti-inflammatory cytokines is associated with the possible switch of the biofilm-modulated periodontal status toward more specific breakdown. IL-1β, IL-10 and IFN-γ might be involved in controlling the inflammatory process at periodontally healthy and diseased sites, the present manuscript indicating that the interactions appeared to be different in subjects that were systemically healthy when compared with IDDM subjects. Moreover, the metabolic equilibrium of the systemic disease is significantly related to the gram negative species mediated cytokine translocation from the periodontal space into the circulation. Further studies of candidate biomarkers and of inflammatory shifts will be necessary to confirm these observations.

5. Acknowledgments

This work was supported by the University of Medicine and Pharmacy "Gr. T. Popa" Iasi and a Research Grant from the Romanian National Council of Scientific Research and Higher Education (CNCSIS), Nr. 1133. We thank D. Ungureanu and D. Haba of the

University of Medicine and Pharmacy Iasi for participating in planning of analyses, interpretation of data, and revisions of manuscript. Special thanks to M. Zlei and G. Grigore from the Division of Genetics and Immunology of Sf. Spiridon University Hospital for use and technical expertise with the multiplex flow cytometric analyses and C. Olteanu and G. Stefan for generous provision of samples for fluid cytokine analyses.

6. References

American Diabetes Association. (2006). Standards of medical care in diabetes, *Diabetes Care* 29 (Suppl. 1): S4–S42.

Armitage, GC. (1999). Development of a classification system for periodontal diseases and conditions, *Ann Periodontol.* 4(1):1-6.

Armitage, GC. (2000). Development of a classification system for periodontal diseases and conditions, *Northwest Dent.* 79(6):31-5.

Champagne, CM., Buchanan, W., Reddy, MS., Preisser, JS., Beck, JD.& Offenbacher, S. (2003). Potential for gingival crevice fluid measures as predictors of risk for periodontal diseases, *Periodontology* 2000. 31: 167-180.

Costa, FO., Cota, LOM., Costa, JE.& Pordeus, IA. (2007). Periodontal disease progression among young subjects with no preventive dental care: A 52-month follow-up study, *J Periodontol.* 78(2): 198-203.

De Pomereau, V., Dargent-Pare, C., Robert, JJ. & Brion, M. (1992). Periodontal status in insulin dependent diabetic adolescents, *J Clin Periodontol.* 19(9): 628-32.

Engebretson, S., Chertog, R., Nichols, A., Hey-Hadavi, J., Celenti, R. & Grbic, J. (2007). Plasma levels of tumour necrosis factor-alpha in patients with chronic periodontitis and type 2 diabetes. *J Clin Periodontol.* 34(1):18-24.

Iacopino, AM. (2001). Periodontitis and diabetes interrelationships: role of inflammation, *Ann Periodontol.* 6(1): 125-137.

Joo, SD. & Lee, JM. (2007). The comparison of inflammatory mediator expression in gingival tissues from human chronic periodontitis patients with and without type 2 diabetes mellitus, *J Korean Acad Periodontol.* 37(2 Suppl): 353-69.

Kinane, DF., Demuth, DR., Gorr, SU., Hajishengallis, GN. & Martin, MH. (2007). Human variability in innate immunity, *Periodontol 2000.* 45: 14-34.

Neubert, A., Hsia, Y., de Jong-van den Berg, LT., Janhsen, K., Glaeske, G., Furu, K., Kieler H., Nørgaard, M., Clavenna ,A. & Wong, IC. (2011). Comparison of anti-diabetic drug prescribing, in children and adolescents in seven European countries, *Br J Clin Pharmacol.*

Noda, D., Hamachi, T., Inoue, K. & Maeda, K. (2007). Relationship between the presence of periodontopathic bacteria and the expression of chemokine receptor mRNA in inflamed gingival tissues, *J Periodontal Res.* 42(6): 566-71.

Pihlstrom, BL., Michalowicz, BS. & Johnson, NW. (2005). Periodontal diseases, *Lancet.* 19: 1809-20.

Robertson, RP. & Harmon, JS. (2006). Diabetes, glucose toxicity, and oxidative stress: A case of double jeopardy for the pancreatic islet beta cell, *Free Rad. Biol. Med.* 41(2): 177-184.

Silness, J & Löe, H. (1964). Periodontal disease in pregnancy II. Correlation between oral hygiene and periodontal condition. Acta Odontol Scand 24: 121-135.

Simmons, RA. (2006). Developmental origins of diabetes: The role of oxidative stress, *Free Rad. Biol. Med.* 40(6): 917–922.

Tabholz, A., Soskolne, WA. & Shapira, L. (2010). Genetic and environmental risk factors for chronic periodontitis and aggressive periodontitis, *Periodontol 2000.* 53: 138-153.

Van Dyke, TE. (2009).The etiology and pathogenesis of periodontitis revisited - Guest editorial, *J Appl Oral Sci.* 17(1).

Part 4

Epidemiological Studies of Periodontal Disease

10

Epidemiology and Risk Factors of Periodontal Disease

Amin E. Hatem
Faculty of Dentistry, Tanta University
Egypt

1. Introduction

Historically, it was believed that all individuals are uniformly susceptible to developing periodontal disease and that accumulation of plaque, poor oral hygiene and perhaps occlusal trauma were sufficient to initiate periodontitis. However, during the past decades it has become accepted that periodontal disease is caused by specific bacterial infection and that individuals are neither uniformly susceptible to these infections nor to the damage caused by them. Study of the distribution of periodontal diseases and their risk factors on a global scale offers a unique investigational model that can assess causation between periodontal diseases and their suspected etiologic risk factors. An understanding of risk factors can lead to theories of causation that will allow clinicians to identify and target individuals susceptible to periodontal disease. This chapter aims to provide a comprehensive overview of the determinants and risk factors of periodontal diseases and how to predict the risk of their occurrence.

2. Goals of epidemiological studies of periodontal diseases

Epidemiology is the study of health and disease in populations and the effect of various biologic, demographic, environmental and lifestyles on these states. The essential features of epidemiology as a method of research, when compared to clinical research and case studies, are that 1) groups rather than individuals are the focus of study and 2) persons with and without a particular disease (e.g., periodontal diseases), and with and without the exposure of interest are included, rather than just patients.

The study of population groups rather than individuals allows for valid estimates while accounting for normal biological variation. Broadening a study to include those without disease, as well as those with it, provides a reference point against which to quantify risk. Epidemiologic studies are conducted to describe the health status of populations, elucidate the etiology of diseases, identify risk factors, forecast disease occurrence and assist in disease prevention and control.

3. Definitions of periodontal disease; Assessment in epidemiological studies

Epidemiology prerequisite is an accurate definition of periodontal disease. Unfortunately, in periodontal research, uniform criteria have not been yet established. Epidemiological studies have employed a wide array of symptoms including gingivitis, probing depths, clinical attachment level scores, and radiographically assessed alveolar bone loss in a particularly inconsistent manner. Considerable variation characterizes the threshold values employed for defining periodontal pockets as "deep" or "pathological," or the clinical attachment level and alveolar bone scores required for assuming that "true" loss of periodontal tissue support has, in fact, occurred. In addition, the number of "affected" tooth surfaces required for assigning an individual subject as a "case;" i.e., as suffering from periodontal disease, varies as well. These inconsistencies in the definitions inevitably affect the figures describing the distribution of the disease.

While the term "periodontal disease" may encompass all pathological conditions of periodontal tissues, gingivitis and periodontitis are used with different meanings. Gingivitis is an inflammatory lesion of marginal gingiva recognized in epidemiologic studies by color change and /or by bleeding on gentle probing within the gingival sulcus or pocket orifice. If loss or destruction of periodontal attachment or alveolar bone occur, the condition is characterized as periodontitis.

4. Measurement of periodontitis

The basic clinical measures for periodontitis are clinical attachment loss (CAL) and probing depth (PD). The standard protocol used today for measuring CAL and PD with a manual probe was first described long time ago and has not changed much since (Ramfjord, 1959). Various scaled indexes have been used in the past, but these were "composite" indexes which scored gingivitis and periodontitis on the same scale. Composite indexes are now considered invalid and have thus been discarded.

Although CAL, a measure of accumulated past disease at a site rather than current activity, remains a diagnostic "gold standard" for periodontitis, the absence of consensus on how best to incorporate CAL and PD into a case definition of periodontitis continues to hamper clinical and epidemiological research (Goodson, 1992). A case definition for periodontitis needs to establish 1) what depth of CAL at any one site constitutes evidence of disease processes; 2) how many such sites need to be present in a mouth to establish disease presence; and 3) how to include probing measurements and bleeding on probing (BOP) in the case definition. An approach like the Extent and Severity Index (Carlos et al., 2006), in which "extent" refers to the number of teeth in the mouth with CAL of ≥1 mm and "severity" is the mean CAL for those teeth, might be appropriate in some circumstances. Some consensus on age-related case definitions for "serious" and "moderate" disease would also assist research.

The inherent measurement problems have led researchers to look for markers of periodontitis which, if valid and reliable, would decrease our dependence upon clinical measures based on probing for diagnosing disease. As our understanding of periodontitis etiology has deepened, some markers have emerged as likely candidates. The most promising are the inflammatory cytokines that are expressed in gingival crevicular fluid (GCF) as part of the host response to inflammation, a number of which have been associated with active disease (Page, 1992). These cytokines include prostaglandin E2 (PGE2), tumor necrosis factor-alpha (TNF-α), IL-1 alpha (IL-1α), IL-1 beta (IL-1 β), and others. While it has been documented for some time that these and other constituents of GCF are associated with inflammatory response, actually quantifying these associations and determining the sensitivity of the measures is proving more difficult.

5. Periodontal disease trends

There is no globally accepted method for measurement of periodontal disease. Therefore, it is difficult to document changing patterns of periodontal disease over time periods. Nevertheless, during the last 40 years some evidence has accumulated of changes in the occurrence of gingivitis in developed countries. By repeating cross-sectional studies of the same age range using the same survey criteria, Anderson, 1981 reported a decline in gingivitis and improvement in dental cleanliness between 1963 and 1978 among 12-year-old children in England; and Cutress, 1986 reported a decline in prevalence of gingivitis between 1976 and 1982 in the 15- to 19-year age group in New Zealand from 98% of subjects and 51% of teeth to 79% of subjects and 34% of teeth.

By contrast, Curilovic et al. , 1977 found that, in Zurich, between 1957 and 1975, the prevalence of gingivitis in 7- to 17- year-old children was unchanged and its severity had increased. Moreover, between 1983 and 1993 gingival health and dental cleanliness in 5- to 15- year-old children in the United Kingdom deteriorated: the age-related subject prevalence of gingivitis increased from 19% to 53% in 1983 and from 26% to 63% in 1993 (O'Brien, 1994). In a Swedish study, Hugoson et al., 1995 carried out a series of three cross-sectional surveys in 1973, 1983 and 1993 to assess oral hygiene and gingivitis during deciduous, mixed and permanent dentition periods. On each occasion, they obtained random samples of approximately 100 subjects at each of the following age levels: 3, 5, 10, 15 and 20 years. Between 1973 and 1983, there was a substantial improvement in plaque, calculus and gingivitis levels, which were attributed to the introduction in 1974 of new dental health care programs based on prevention. However, between 1983 and 1993, the improvement in plaque levels and gingivitis was reversed, suggesting perhaps that the dramatic reduction in childhood caries between 1973 and 1983 had made children, parents and dental personnel complacent about dental health and oral hygiene. It has not so far been possible to demonstrate improvements in periodontitis in children and adolescents, but this is hardly surprising since it is unusual to find significant amounts of periodontal destruction in these age groups. One study, for instance, found no difference in the prevalence of marginal bone loss in a survey of bitewing radiographs from 2 cohorts of 16-year-old adolescents in 1975 and 1988 (Källestål et al., 1991). At both time periods, bone loss affected only 3.5% of subjects.

6. Determinants of periodontitis

Advances in research over recent years have led to a fundamental change in our understanding of the periodontal diseases. As recently as the mid-1960s, the prevailing model for the epidemiology of periodontal diseases included these precepts: 1) all individuals were considered more or less equally susceptible to severe periodontitis; 2) gingivitis usually progressed to periodontitis with consequent loss of bony support and eventually loss of teeth; and 3) susceptibility to periodontitis increased with age and was the main cause of tooth loss after age 35 (Kreshover & Russell, 1958; Russell, 1967). Advances in our understanding of periodontal diseases since that time have led to the concept of individual periodontal disease susceptibility and reevaluation of this old general susceptibility model.

A risk factor can be defined as an occurrence or characteristic that has been associated with the increased rate of a subsequently occurring disease. It is important to make the distinction that risk factors are associated with a disease but do not necessarily cause the disease. Risk factors may be modifiable or non-modifiable. Modifiable risk factors are usually environmental or behavioral in nature whereas non modifiable risk factors are usually intrinsic to the individual and therefore not easily changed. Non modifiable risk factors are also known as determinants. Evidence used to identify risk factors usually is derived from the following types of studies in order of increasing strength of evidence: case reports, case series, case-control study, cross-sectional studies, longitudinal cohort studies, and controlled clinical trials, also known as interventional studies. All of these studies can identify factors associated with a disease though they are not equal in strength. The longitudinal study may be capable of identifying a causal relationship. The interventional study gives the strongest evidence of a causal relationship and furthermore can provide evidence of the benefit of eliminating the risk factor. Associations identified through longitudinal and interventional studies are termed risk factors whereas associations, based on the observations of cross-sectional and case controlled studies are termed risk indicators. Thus the term risk factor denotes a greater weight of evidence supporting an association than does the term risk indicator (Thomas et al., 2005).

6.1 Modifiable risk factors

6.1.1 Smoking

Smoking behaviors have consistently been associated with attachment loss in most studies (Albandar, 2002). Smokers have a significantly higher risk of developing chronic periodontal disease (Grossi et al., 1994; Hyman & Ried, 2003; Tomar & Asma, 2000) and show a higher rate of periodontal destruction over time than non-smokers (Bergstrom et a., 2000; Elter et al., 1999). There is a dose-effect relationship between cigarette smoking and the severity of periodontal disease such that heavy smokers and those with a longer history of smoking show more severe tissue loss than light smokers (Tomar & Asma, 2000).

Generally, studies show that cigarette smoking is associated with a twofold to sevenfold increased risk of having attachment loss compared with nonsmokers, with a more pronounced risk in young smokers (Bergstrom et al., 2000; Bergstrom, 2003). The population risk due to cigarette smoking has been studied in large surveys and it is estimated that in the United States population, approximately 42% and 11% of periodontitis cases may be attributed to current and former cigarette smoking, respectively (Tomar & Asma, 2000). A survey in Brazilian adults estimated that 12% of periodontitis cases may be attributable to cigarette smoking (Susin et al., 2004). Cigar and pipe smoking have been shown to have detrimental effects on periodontal health similar to those attributed to cigarette smoking (Albandar et al., 2000).

6.1.2 Diabetes mellitus

Certain systemic diseases have been associated with an increased risk of attachment loss. Diabetes is a modifiable factor in the sense that though it cannot be cured, it can be controlled. Studies that have examined the relationship between diabetes and periodontitis are heterogeneous in design and aim. Thus, both positive and negative conclusions have been drawn with respect to the relationship between the two diseases. In general, no difference in impact has been determined between type 1 and type 2 diabetes mellitus.

Diabetic parameters examined include glycemic control, duration of disease, presence of other diabetes-associated complications and population studied. Periodontal parameters examined have included gingivitis, clinical attachment loss, and alveolar bone loss (Tomar & Asma, 2000). Studies have shown a relationship between poor glycemic control and periodontal disease parameters (Cutler et al., 1999; Guzman et al., 2003; Tervonen et al., 1994; Tsai et al., 2002). Finally, studies have been done which suggest that poorly controlled diabetics respond less successfully to periodontal therapy relative to well-controlled and non-diabetics (Westfelt et al., 1996; Tervonan & Karjalainen, 1997).

6.1.3 Dental plaque and oral hygiene

Population studies confirm the close relationship between dental plaque and gingivitis that was initially described by Löe et al., 1965 in non population-based studies. Throughout the globe, dental plaque growth and inflammation of gingival tissue are ubiquitous and strongly linked, irrespective of age, gender or racial/ethnic identification. It is clear from global epidemiology data that a less pronounced relationship appears to exist between dental plaque and severe periodontitis. Severe forms of human periodontitis frequently affect only a subset of population groups globally, even though plaque-induced gingivitis and slight to moderate forms of periodontitis are widespread within the same population groups (Albandar, 2002; Baelum & Scheutz, 2002; Gjermo et al., 2002; Sheiham & Netuveli, 2002).

While gingivitis parallels the level of oral hygiene in a population, it is by itself a poor predictor of subsequent periodontitis disease activity (Lang et a., 1990). Oral hygiene can favorably influence the ecology of the microbial flora in shallow-to moderate pockets, but it does not affect host response. Oral hygiene alone has little effect on subgingival microflora in deep pockets and personal oral hygiene practices among health professionals have been shown to be unrelated to periodontitis in these individuals (Merchant et al., 2002). The conclusion from older studies, mostly cross-sectional, in populations with poor oral hygiene is that plaque and supragingival calculus accumulations correlate poorly with severe periodontitis (Löe et al., 1992; Okamoto et al., 1988). Results from other well-controlled studies also concluded that the quantity of plaque accumulation was, at best, only weakly correlated with periodontitis (Grossi et al., 1995; Peretz et al., 1993).

Comprehensive oral hygiene programs are effective in preventing or reducing the level of gingival inflammation in children and adults. These programs, however, may not be viable in preventing aggressive periodontitis and it may be difficult to achieve a satisfactory level of oral hygiene in the general population to prevent chronic periodontitis and periodontal tissue loss effectively (Löe et al., 2000; Morris et al., 2001).

6.1.4 Specific microorganisms

Although there is sufficient evidence that accumulation and maturation of a plaque biofilm is necessary for the initiation and progression of periodontal diseases, studies show that bacterial species colonizing the gingival pocket play variable roles in the pathogenesis of these diseases and may therefore possess different levels of risk of periodontal tissue loss (Wolff et al., 1994) . Of all of the various microorganisms that colonize the mouth, there are three, Porphyromonas gingivalis (Pg), Tannerella forsythia (Tf), and Actinobacillus actinomycetemcomitans (Aa) have been implicated as etiologic agents in periodontitis.

The presence of periodontal pathogens, though necessary to cause disease, is not sufficient. Indeed the odds ratio of developing periodontal disease in an individual who harbors one of the putative periodontal pathogens is not high enough to consider them a risk factor (Ezzo

& Cutler, 2003). The presence of A. actinomycetemcomitans confers no additional risk of developing localized aggressive periodontitis in adults despite the fact that its presence is necessary for the disease to develop (Buchmann et al., 2000). It has been shown that Prevotella intermedia, P gingivalis, and Fusobacterium nucleatum may be risk indicators for periodontal disease in a diverse population, though they are not risk factors (Alpagot et al., 1996). Active infections with human cytomegalovirus and other herpesviruses have been proposed as possible risk factors for destructive periodontal diseases, including chronic periodontitis, aggressive periodontitis, and necrotizing periodontal diseases (Kamma & Slots, 2003). One study found that presence of herpesviruses in subgingival sites was associated with subgingival colonization of these sites with periodontopathic bacteria and with a threefold to fivefold increased risk of severe chronic periodontitis (Contreras et al., 1999).

While these organisms in the periodontal crevice are closely associated with periodontitis, an important finding is that supragingival plaque can serve as a natural reservoir for them (Sakellari et al., 2001). When the bacterial insult is strong enough to overwhelm host defense, bacteria in supragingival plaque migrate subgingivally to form a subgingival biofilm. Frequent professional supragingival cleaning, added to good personal oral hygiene, has been shown to have a beneficial effect on subgingival microbiota in moderately deep pockets (Hellstrom et al., 1996). These findings collectively form an evidence base for close control of supragingival plaque as part of periodontal therapy.

6.1.5 Psychological factors

Studies have demonstrated that individuals under psychological stress are more likely to develop clinical attachment loss and loss of alveolar bone (Hugoson et al., 2002; Pistorius et al., 2002; Wimmer et al., 2002). One possible link in this regard may be increases in production of IL-6 in response to increased psychological stress (Kiecolt- Glaser et al., 2003). Another study suggests that host response to P. gingivalis infection may be compromised in psychologically stressed individuals (Houri Haddad et al., 2003).

Despite existing evidence from case control and cross sectional studies, no longitudinal or interventional studies have been published that confirm psychological stress as a risk factor for periodontal disease. Perhaps the relationship is simply due to the fact that individuals under stress are less likely to perform regular good oral hygiene and prophylaxis (Croucher et al., 1997).

6.1.6 Obesity

Obesity is one of the most significant health risks of modern society, and is now recognized as a major health concern in both developed and developing countries (Doll et al., 2002). The prevalence of obesity is increasing at alarming rates, approaching epidemic proportions, particularly among children and young adults (Freidmn, 2000). Obesity itself has been recognized as a risk factor for numerous adult diseases, and may be a factor in the incidence of periodontitis.

Body mass index (BMI) (Elter et al., 2000; Grossi & Ho 2000), waist-to-hip circumference ratio (WHR) and body fat, (Saito et al., 1998; 2000, 2001) may be factors in the incidence of periodontal disease. Conditions associated with obesity, e.g. "the metabolic syndrome", a clustering of dyslipidemia and insulin resistance may exacerbate periodontitis (Grossi & Ho, 2000). Long-term interest in the role of nutrition and periodontal disease questions the role of nutrients in periodontal disease pathogenesis. Recently, an association between obesity and periodontal disease has been suggested (Amin, 2010). Furthermore, the results of the Third National Health and Nutrition Examination Survey conducted in the United States of America showed that waist to hip ratio, body mass index (BMI), fat free mass and log sum subcutaneous fat were significantly correlated to periodontitis, signifying that abnormal fat metabolism may be an important factor in the pathogenesis of periodontal diseases (wood et al., 2003). It has been proposed that the patterns of fat distribution and its relation to periodontal pathogenesis follow those observed with other obesity-related health problems, such as hypertension and type II diabetes, where visceral fat accumulation plays a key role in increasing susceptibility to these diseases (wood et al., 2003).

Obesity has been postulated to reduce blood flow to the periodontal tissues, promoting the development of periodontal disease (Shuldiner et al., 2001). Furthermore, obesity may enhance immunological or inflammatory disorders, which might be the reason obese subjects tend to exhibit escalating poor periodontal status relative to non-obese individuals (Nishida et al., 2005).

A proposed model linking obesity and periodontal infection suggested that insulin resistance mediates the relationship between them. Dietary free fatty acids contribute not only to obesity but also to insulin resistance by enhancing destruction of β cells of the pancreas (Saiti et al., 1999). Insulin resistance, in turn, contributes to a generalized hyperinflammatory state, including periodontal tissue, especially when triggered by oral pathogens. Furthermore, adipocytokines, which include tumor necrosis factor α (TNF-α) secreted by adipose tissues, appear to be directly related to periodontal destruction (Nishida et al., 2005). On the other hand, There is some evidence that cytokines such as interleukin-1 β (IL-1-β) and interferon γ and Gram negative lipopolysaccharides that are produced in high quantities in response to periodontal infection may interfere with lipid metabolism (wood et al., 2003). This may further enhance obesity and obesity-related health problems.

6.1.7 Socioeconomic status (SES)

Multitudes of disease conditions are associated with socioeconomic status, and cause/effect is plausible. Generally, those who are better educated, wealthier, and live in more desirable circumstances enjoy better health status than the less educated and poorer segments of society. Periodontal diseases are no different and have been related to lower SES (Astrom & Rise, 2001; Thomson & Locker , 2000). The ill effects of living in deprived circumstances can start early in life (Schou & Wight, 1994). Gingivitis and poor oral hygiene are clearly related to lower SES, but the relationship between periodontitis and SES is less direct. On the other hand, CAL of ≥4 mm and ≥7 mm in at least one site were both closely correlated with educational levels (Bethesda, 1987).

It is likely that the widely observed relation between SES levels and gingival health is a function of better oral hygiene among the better educated and a greater frequency of dental visits among the more dentally aware. While racial/ethnic differences in periodontal status have been demonstrated many times, it is thought unlikely that these represent true genetic differences. It is more likely that SES, a complex and multifaceted variable that can include a variety of cultural factors, is confounding these relationships.

6.2 Non-modifiable risk factors

6.2.1 Genetic factors

Although bacterial infection is the etiologic agent in periodontal disease, studies of identical twins suggest 50% of susceptibility to periodontal disease is due to host factors

(Michalowicz et al., 2000). Similarly, indigenous and relatively isolated populations have been shown to develop distinct periodontal disease that differ from group to group (Dowsett et al., 2001). Several gene polymorphisms have been investigated, some of which have been shown to be associated with an increased risk of periodontitis (Li et al., 2004; Noack et al., 2004). Various genetic risk factors, however, may explain only a part of the variance in the occurrence of periodontitis (Diehl et al., 1999). In addition, significant interactions seem to exist between genetic, environmental, and demographic factors (Albandar & Rams).

Most of the research relating to the strength of genetics as a determinant of disease has been laboratory and clinical studies rather than epidemiology, but that research should still be briefly reviewed here. The original 1997 report, using data from patients in private practices, found that a specific genotype of the polymorphic IL-1 gene cluster was associated with more severe periodontitis (Kornman et al., 1997). This relationship could be demonstrated only in non-smokers, which suggested right away that the genetic factor was not as strong a risk factor as smoking. The IL-1 gene cluster has received a lot of research attention since then. This is appropriate, given that the proinflammatory cytokine IL-1 is a key regulator of the host response to microbial infection, although IL-1 is unlikely to be the only genetic factor involved (Mark et al., 2000; McDevitt et al., 2000). IL-1 has been identified as a contributory cause of periodontitis in one epidemiological study (Thomson et al., 2001).

While there seems to be little doubt about a genetic component in periodontitis, the strength of that component is still being determined. At one end, a study among 169 twin pairs concluded that about half of the variance in periodontitis was attributable to heritability (Michalowicz et al., 2000). A combination of IL-1 genotyping and smoking history may provide a good risk profile for patients (McDevitt et al., 2000) and a smoking–genetic interaction may be a contributory factor in severity of periodontitis. The role of IL-1 in regulating host response to infection has been described as clearly present, but not essential (Cullinan et al., 2001). Further research, especially epidemiological studies of people with and without disease, will be necessary before the genetic contribution to the initiation and progression of periodontitis can be specified.

6.2.2 Aging

Ageing is associated with an increased incidence of periodontal disease (Grossi et al., 1994; Grossi et al., 1995). However it has been suggested that the increased level of periodontal destruction observed with aging is the result of cumulative destruction rather than a result of increased rates of destruction. The older assumption that periodontitis is a disease of aging is no longer tenable (Burt, 1994). The current view sees the greater periodontal destruction in the elderly as reflecting lifetime disease accumulation rather than an age-specific condition.

A relatively low prevalence of severe (as opposed to moderate) CAL among the elderly was first shown in Sweden and has since been demonstrated elsewhere (Hugoson & Jordan, 1982). Surveys of older people in the United States, Canada, and Australia have found that CAL or PD of 6 mm or more was prevalent in 15% to 30% of persons examined (Hunt et al., 1990; Locker & Leake, 1993). In all of these studies, CAL of 4 to 6 mm was common. Higher estimates of periodontal destruction came from a cross sectional New England study of community-living elderly people (Fox et al., 1994). All of these reports agree that CAL increases with age, but most did not find extensive loss of function in the affected teeth.

It can be hypothesized that the more susceptible members of the population are those in whom periodontitis begins in youth. If that is so, then the relatively low prevalence of severe CAL among many dentate elderly could be partly a survival phenomenon, meaning that those most susceptible to severe periodontitis have already lost teeth. The most rapid disease progression is seen in that relatively small number of persons in whom the disease starts young, and there is some evidence that these individuals have some genetic predisposition to periodontitis (Parkhill et al., 2000; Thomson et al., 2001). It is uncommon for elderly people with reasonably intact dentition to exhibit sudden bursts of periodontitis. Tooth retention, good oral hygiene, and periodontal health are closely associated, regardless of age (Abdellatif &, Burt, 1987).

6.2.3 Gender

Several studies also show an association between gender and attachment loss in adults, with men having higher prevalence and severity of periodontal destruction than women (Albandar, 2000; Morris et al., 2001). Data suggest that this finding may be related to gender-dependent genetic predisposing factors or other sociobehavioral factors (Reichert et al., 2002).

These gender differences have not been explored in detail, but are thought to be more related to poorer oral hygiene, less positive attitudes toward oral health, and dental-visit behavior among males than to any genetic factor. There are, of course, certain gender-related temporary syndromes related to hormonal conditions, such as pregnancy-associated gingivitis, as well as puberty-associated gingivitis which can affect children of both sexes (Albandar, 2005).

6.2.4 Ethnicity

The level of attachment loss is also influenced by race/ethnicity, although the exact role of this factor is not fully understood. Certain racial/ethnic groups, particularly subjects of African and Latin American background, have a higher risk of developing periodontal tissue loss than other groups. In the United States population, subjects of African or Mexican heritage have greater attachment loss than Caucasians (Albandar et al., 1999).

The association of periodontal disease with race/ethnicity is significantly attenuated when certain effects such as cigarette smoking and income are accounted for (Hyman & Reid, 2003). This effect modification suggests that certain racial/ethnic characteristics are indicators of or confounded by certain other effects. For instance, African Americans generally have lower socioeconomic status than Caucasians. Hence, the increased risk of periodontitis in certain racial/ethnic groups may be partly attributed to socioeconomic, behavioral, and other disparities (Poulton et al., 2002). On the other hand, there is evidence that increased risk may also be partly related to biologic/genetic predisposition (Albandar et al., 2002; Haubek et al., 2002).

7. Predicting the risk of periodontitis

Attempts to identify markers for future disease go back some years. The aim is to identify the presence of some easily measured entities that clinicians can readily test for in a patient that would predict with high reliability the risk for future disease. The presence of visible plaque and calculus, as one example of a hypothesized marker, was long assumed to predict future CAL or bone loss, but studies have shown that clinical measures of plaque and calculus by themselves do not predict future disease to any useful extent (Badersten et al., 1990; Persson et al., 1998). Models that have included the subgingival presence of specific pathogens such as Aa, Pg, and Tf with other indicators have shown a moderate degree of predictability (Timmerman et al., 2001; Tran et al., 2001).

Host response needs to be worked into the equation, and it is now recognized that smoking and genetic predisposition are major players in this regard. When smoking and IL-1 genotype status are included in a predictive model, none of the baseline clinical indicators added significantly to the model for subsequent tooth loss. The baseline clinical indicators performed much better in a model that included IL-1 genotype status in non-smokers (McGuire & Nunn, 1999).

Studies have investigated the role of psychosocial stress in terms of adverse life events or a history of clinical depression. Stress does seem to be associated with progressive periodontitis, whether assessed in a case-control study, cross-sectionally, or in a longitudinal design (Croucher et al., 1997; Elter et al., 1999; Genco et al., 1999). Since psychosocial distress is a well-documented risk factor for a number of different diseases, the identification of its predictive role in periodontitis strengthens the hypothesis that periodontitis is related to systemic diseases.

While risk prediction is still not a precise science in periodontology, enough advances in our knowledge of risk factors have been made to permit development of a risk calculator that is offered to practitioners to help assess a patient's risk of disease (Page et al., 2002). Refinement of risk prediction models in the future will give practitioners an ever improving evidence base upon which to select treatment.

8. Periodontal disease as a risk factor for other diseases

The possible role of periodontal infections as risk factors for systemic diseases has recently attracted special attention. Heart disease has been reported to be the condition most commonly found in Periodontitis patients (Umino & Nagao, 1993). DeStefano et al., 1993 reported that subjects with Periodontitis had a 25% increased risk for coronary heart disease (CHD) when compared to periodontitis-free individuals. Among men younger than 50 years of age at baseline, subjects with Periodontitis were 70% more likely to develop CHD than men without periodontal disease.

Loesche, 1994 reported that periodontal infections induce low-level bacteraemia, elevated white blood cell counts, and exposure of the host to endotoxins that may affect endothelial integrity, metabolism of plasma lipoproteins, platelet function and blood coagulation. Robert et al., 2002 concluded that, the accumulation of epidemiologic, in vitro, clinical and animal evidence suggests that periodontal infection may be a contributing risk factor for heart disease. However, legitimate concerns have arisen about the nature of this relationship.

Periodontal infections as a risk factor for pre-term low birth weight (PLBW) were discussed in a report by Offenbacher et al., 1996. The authors studied pregnancy outcome and a broad array of putative risk factors in 124 mothers and revealed that the adjusted odds ratio for PLBW for women with severe periodontal disease was 7.5. Interestingly, an attributable risk analysis indicated that as much as 18% of all PLBW cases could be due to periodontal infections. These data gain in credibility bearing in mind that experimental studies in rats have verified occurrence of PLBW among animals subjected to experimental Periodontitis (Collin et al., 1994a, 1994b).

9. References

Abdellatif, HM. & Burt, BA. (1987). An epidemiological investigation into the relative importance of age and oral hygiene status as determinants of periodontitis. *Journal of Dental Research,* Vol.66, pp. 13-18, ISSN 1544-0591

Albandar, JM.; Brunelle, JA. & Kingman, A. (1999). Destructive periodontal disease in adults 30 years of age and older in the United State. *Journal of Periodontology,* Vol.70, No.1, pp. 13-29, ISSN 0022-3492

Albandar, JM.; Streckfus, CF. & Adesanya, MR. (2000). Cigar, pipe, and cigarette smoking as risk factors for periodontal disease and tooth loss. *Journal of Periodontology,* Vol.71, No.12 pp. 1874-1881, ISSN 0022-3492

Albandar, JM. (2000). Global risk factors and risk indicators for periodontal diseases. *Periodontology 2000,* Vol. 29, pp. 177-206, ISSN 0906-6713

Albandar, JM. (2002). Global risk factors and risk indicators for periodontal diseases. *Periodontology 2000,* Vol. 29, pp. 177-206, ISSN 0906-6713

Albandar, JM. & Rams, TE. (2002). Risk factors for periodontitis in children and young persons. *Periodontology 2000,* Vol.29, pp. 207-222, ISSN 0906-6713

Albandar, JM.; DeNardin, AM. & Adesanya, MR. (2002). Associations of serum concentrations of IgG, IgA, IgM and interleukin-1beta with early-onset periodontitis classification and race. *Journal of Clinical Periodontology,* Vol.29, No.5, pp. 421-426, ISSN 0303-6979

Albandar, JM. (2005). Epidemiology and risk factors of periodontal disease. *Dental Clinics of North America,* Vol.49, pp. 517-532, ISSN 0011-8532

Alpagot, T.; Wolff, LF.; Smith, QT. & Trao, SD. (1996). Risk indicators for periodontal disease in a racially diverse urban population. *Journal of Clinical Periodontology,* Vol.23, pp. 982-988, ISSN 0303-6979

Amin, H. (2010). Relationship between overall and abdominal obesity and periodontal disease among young adults. *Eastern Mediterranean Health Journal,* Vol.6, No.4 pp. 4-8, ISSN 1020-3397

Anderson, RJ. (1981). The changes in the dental health of 12-yearold schoolchildren in two Somerset schools. A review after an interval of 15 years. *British Dental Journal,* Vol.150, pp. 218-221, ISSN 0007-0610

Astrom, AN. & Rise, J. (2001). Socio-economic differences in patterns of health and oral health behaviour in 25-yearold Norwegians. *Clinical Oral Investigation,* Vol.5, pp. 122-128, ISSN 1436-3771

Badersten, A.; Nilveus, R. & Egelberg, J. (1990). Scores of plaque,bleeding, suppuration and probing depth to predictprobing attachment loss. 5 years of observation followingnonsurgical periodontal therapy. *Journal of Clinical Periodontology,* Vol. 17, pp. 102-107, ISSN 0303-6979

Baelum, V. & Scheutz, F. (2002). Periodontal diseases in Africa. *Periodontology 2000,* Vol. 29, pp. 79-103, ISSN 0906-6713

Bergstrom, J.; Eliasson, S. & Dock, J (2000). A 10-year prospective study of tobacco smoking and periodontal health. *Journal of Periodontology,* Vol.71, No.8, pp. 1338-1347, ISSN 0022-3492

Bergstrom, J. (2003). Tobacco smoking and risk for periodontal disease. *Journal of Clinical Periodontology,* Vol. 30,No2, pp. 107-113, ISSN 0303-6979

Bethesda, MD. (1987). Oral Health of United States Adults. *National Institute of Dental Research,* NIH publication No. 87, 2868

Buchmann, R.; Muller, RE.; Heinecke, A. & Lange, DE. (2000). *Actinobacillus actinomycetemcomitans* in destructive periodontal disease. Three-year follow-up results. *Journal of Clinical Periodontology,* Vol.71, pp. 444-453, ISSN 0303-6979

Burt, BA. (1994). Periodontitis and aging: Reviewing recent evidence. *Journal of the American Dental Association,* Vol.125, pp. 273-279, ISSN 0002-8177

Carlos, JP.; Wolfe, MD. & Kingman, A (1986). The extent and severity index: A simple method for use in epidemiologic studies of periodontal disease. *Journal of Clinical Periodontology,* Vol.13, pp. 500-505, ISSN 0303-6979

Collins, JG.; Windley, HWr; Arnold, RR. & Offenbacher, S. (1994) a. Effects of a Porphyromonas gingivalis infection on inflammatory mediator response and pregnancy outcome in hamsters. *Infection and Immunity,* Vol.62, pp. 4356-4361, ISSN 1098-5522

Collins, JG.; Smith, MA; Arnold, RR. & Offenbacher, S. (1994) b. Effects of *Escherichia coli* and *Porphyromonas gingivalis* lipopolysaccharide on pregnancy outcome in the golden hamster. *Infection and Immunity,* Vol.62, pp. 4652-4655, ISSN 1098-5522

Contreras, A.; Umeda, M. & Chen, C. (1999). Relationship between herpesviruses and adult periodontitis and periodontopathic bacteria. *Journal of Periodontology,* Vol.70, No.5, pp. 478-484, ISSN 0022-3492

Croucher, R.; Marcenes, WS; Torres, MC.; Hughes, F. & Sheîham, A. (1997). The relationship between life-events and periodontitis. A case-control study. *Journal of Clinical Periodontology,* Vol.24, pp. 39-43, ISSN 0303-6979

Cullinan, MP.; Westerman, B. & Hamlet, SM. (2001). A longitudinal study of interleukin-1 gene polymorphisms and periodontal disease in a general adult population. *Journal of Clinical Periodontology,* Vol.28, pp. 1137-1144, ISSN 0303-6979

Curilovic, Z.; Mazor, Z. & Berchtold, H. (1977). Gingivitis in Zurich schoolchildren. A re-examination after 20 years. *Schweiz Monatsschr Zahnheikd,* Vol.87, pp. 801-808, ISSN 0906-6713

Cutler, CW.; Machen, RL.; Jorwani R. & Iacopino, AM. (2000). Heightened gingival inflammation and attachment loss in type 2 diabetics with hyperlipidemia. *Journal of Clinical Periodontology,* Vol.70, pp. 1313-1321, ISSN 0303-6979

Cutress, TW. (1986). Periodontal health and periodontal disease in young people: global epidemiology. *International Dental Journal,* Vol.36, pp. 146-151, ISSN 0020-6539

DeStefano, F.; Anda, RF.; Kahn, HS.; Williamson, DF. & Russell, CM. (1993). Dental disease and risk of coronary heart disease and mortality *British Medical Journal,* Vol. 306, pp. 688-691, ISSN 0959-8138

Diehl, SR.; Wang, Y. & Brooks, CN. (1999). Linkage disequilibrium of interleukin-1 genetic polymorphisms with early-onset periodontitis. *Journal of Periodontology,* Vol.70, No.4 pp. 418-430, ISSN 0022-3492

Doll, SG.; Paccaud, F & Bovert, B. (2002). Body mass index, abdominal adiposity and blood pressure: Consistency of their association across developing and developed countries. *International Journal of Obesity and Related Metabolic Disorders,* Vol.26, pp. 48-57, ISSN 0307-0565

Dowsett, SA.; Archila, I.; Segreto, VA. & Kowolik, MJ. (2001). Periodontal disease status of an indigenouspopulation of Guatemala, Central America. *Journal of Clinical Periodontology,* Vol.28, pp. 663-671, ISSN 0303-6979

Elter, JR.; Beck, JD. & Slade, GD (1999). Etiologic models for incident periodontal attachment loss in older adults. *Journal Clinical Periodontology,* Vol.26, No.2, pp. 113-23, ISSN 0303-6979

Elter, E.; Williams, R; Champagne, C.; Offenbacher, S. & Beck, J. (2000). Association of obesity and periodontitis. *Journal of Dental Research,* Vol.79 (abstract), pp. 625, ISSN 0022-0345

Ezzo, PJ. & Cutler, CW. (2003). Microorganisms as risk indicators for periodontal disease. *Periodontology 2000,* Vol.32, pp. 24-35, ISSN 0906-6713

Fox, CH.; Jette, AM.; McGuire & Feldman, HA. (1994). Periodontal disease among New England elders. *Journal of Periodontology,* Vol. 65, pp. 676-684

Freidmn, G. (2000). Obesity in the new mellenium. *Nature,* Vol.404, pp. 632-634, ISSN 0028-0836

Genco, R.; Ho, AW.; Grossi, SG.; Dunford, RG. & Tedesco, LA. (1999). Relationship of stress, distress and inadequate coping behaviors to periodontal disease. *Journal of Periodontology,* Vol. 80, pp. 1700-1703, ISSN 0022-3492

Genco, R.; Offenbacher, S. & Beck, J. (2002). Periodontal disease and cardiovascular disease. Epidemiology and possible mechanisms. *Journal of the American Dental Association,* Vol.133, No1, pp. 148-228, ISSN 0002-8177

Gjermo, P.; Rösing, CK; Susin, C. & Oppermann, R. (2002). Periodontal diseases in South and Central America. *Periodontology 2000,* Vol. 29, pp. 70-78, ISSN 0906-6713

Goodson, JM. (1992). Diagnosis of periodontitis by physical measurement: Interpretation from episodic disease hypothesis. *Journal of Periodontology,* Vol.63, (Suppl.), pp. 373-382, ISSN 0022-3492

Grossi, SG.; Zambon, JJ. & Ho, AW (1994). Assessment of risk for periodontal disease. Risk indicators for attachment loss *Journal of Periodontology,* Vol. 65, No.3 pp. 260-267, ISSN 0022-3492

Grossi, SG.; Genco, R. & Machtei, EE. (1995). Assessment of risk for periodontal disease. II. Risk indicators for alveolar bone loss. *Journal of Periodontology,* Vol.66, pp. 23-29, ISSN 0022-3492

Grossi, SG. & Ho, A. (2000). Obesity, insulin resistance and periodontal disease. *Journal of Dental Research,* Vol.79 (abstract), pp. 625, ISSN 0022-0345

Guzman, S.; Karima, M. ; Wang, HY & Van Dyke, TE. (2003). Association between interleukin-1 genotype and periodontal disease in a diabetic population. *Journal of Periodontology,* Vol.74, pp. 1183-1190, ISSN 0022-3492

Haubek, D.; Ennibi, OK. & Abdellaoui, L. (2002). Attachment loss in Moroccan early onset periodontitis patients and infection with the JP2-type of Actinobacillus actinomycetemcomitans. *Journal of Clinical Periodontology,* Vol.29, No.7, pp. 657-660, ISSN 0303-6979

Hellstrom, MK.; Ramberg, P; Krok, L. & Lindhe, J. (1996). The effect of supragingival plaque control on the subgingival microflora in human periodontitis. *Journal of Clinical Periodontology,* Vol.23, pp. 934-940, ISSN 0303-6979

Houri-Haddad, Y.; Itzchaki, O; Ben-Nathan, D. & Shapira, L. (2003). The effect of chronic emotional stress on the humoral immune response to Porphyromonas gingivalis in mice. *Journal of Periodontal Research,* Vol.38, pp. 204-209, ISSN 0022-3484

Hugoson, A.; Koch, G. ; Bergendal, T. & Thorstensson, H. (1995). Oral health of individuals aged 3–80 years in Jo¨nko¨ping, Sweden in 1973, 1983 and 1993. II. Review of clinical and radiographic findings. *Swedish Dental Journal,* Vol.19, pp. 243-260, ISSN 0347-9994

Hugoson, A.; Ljungquist, B. (2002). The relationship of some negative events and psychological factors to periodontal disease in an adult Swedish population 50 to 80 years, of age. *Journal of Clinical Periodontology,* Vol.29, pp. 247-253, ISSN 0303-6979

Hugoson, A. & Jordan, T. (2003). Frequency distribution of individuals aged 20-70 years according to severity of periodontal disease. *Community Dentistry and Oral Epidemiology,* Vol. 10, pp. 187-192, ISSN 0301- 5661

Hunt, RJ.; Levy, SM. & Beck, JD. (1990). The prevalence of periodontal attachment loss in an Iowa population aged 70 and older. *Journal of Public Health Dentistry,* Vol.50, pp. 251-256, ISSN 0022-4006

Hyman, JJ. & Reid, BC (2003). Epidemiologic risk factors for periodontal attachment loss among adults in the United States. *Journal of Clinical Periodontology,* Vol. 30, No.3,, pp. 230-237, ISSN 0303-6979

Källestål, C. & Matsson, L. (1991). Marginal bone loss in 16-year-old Swedish adolescents in 1975 and 1988. *Journal of Clinical Periodontology,* Vol.18, pp. 740-743, ISSN 0303-6979

Kamma, JJ. & Slots, J. (2003). Herpesviral-bacterial interactions in aggressive periodontitis. *Journal of Clinical Periodontology,* Vol.30, No.5, pp. 420-426, ISSN 0303-6979

Kiccolt-Glaser, JK.; Preacher, TKJ; MacCallum, RC.; Arkinson, C. & Glaser, R. (2003). Chronic stress and age-related increases in the proinflammatory cytokine Il-6. *Proceedings of the National Academy of Science USA,* Vol.100, pp. 9090-9095

Kornman, KS.; Crane, A. & Wang, HY. (1997). The interleukin-1 genotype as a severity factor in adult periodontal disease. *Journal of Clinical Periodontology,* Vol.24, pp. 72-77, ISSN 0303-6979

Kreshover, SJ. & Russell AL. (1958). Periodontal disease. *Journal of American Dental Association,* Vol.56, pp. 625-629, ISSN 0002-8177

Lang, NP.; Adler, R.; Joss, A. & Nyman, S. (1990). Absence of bleeding on probing. An indicator of periodontal stability. *Journal of Clinical Periodontology,* Vol.17, pp. 714-721, ISSN 0303-6979

Li, Y.; Xu, L. & Hasturk, H. (2004). Localized aggressive periodontitis is linked to human chromosome 1q25. *Human Genetics,* Vol.114, No.3, pp. 291-297, ISSN 1432-1203

Locker, D. & Leake, JL. (1993). Periodontal attachment loss in independently living older adults in Ontario, Canada. *Journal of Public Health Dentistry,* Vol.53, pp. 6-11, ISSN 0022-4006

Löe, H.; Theilade, E. & Jensen, SB. (1965). Experimental gingivitis in man. *Journal of Periodontology,* Vol.36, pp. 177-187, ISSN 0022-3492

Löe, H.; Anerud, A. & Boysen, H. (1992). The natural history of periodontal disease in man: Prevalence, severity, and extent of gingival recession. *Journal of Periodontology,* Vol.63, pp. 489-495, ISSN 0022-3492

Löe, H. (2000). Oral hygiene in the prevention of caries and periodontal disease. *International Dental Journal* , Vol.50, No.3, pp. 129-39, ISSN 0020-6539

Loesche, WJ. (1994). Periodontal disease as a risk factor for heart disease. *Compendium,* Vol.25, pp. 976-985, ISSN 1074-3197

Mark, LL.; Haffajee, AD. & Socransky, SS. (2000). Effect of the interleukin-1 genotype on monocyte IL-1beta expression in subjects with adult periodontitis. *Journal of Periodontal Research,* Vol. 35, pp. 172-177, ISSN 0022-3484

McDevitt, MJ.; Wang, HY. & Knobelman, C. (2000). Interleukin-1 genetic association with periodontitis in clinical practice. *Journal of Periodontology,* Vol.71, pp. 156-163, ISSN 0022-3492

McGuire, MK.; &Nunn, ME. (1999). Prognosis versus actual outcome. IV. The effectiveness of clinical parameters and IL-1 genotype in accurately predicting prognoses and tooth survival. *Journal of Periodontology,* Vol. 70, pp. 49-56, ISSN 0022-3492

Merchant, A.; Pitiphat, W.; Douglass, CW. ; Crohin, C. & Joshipura, K. (2002). Oral hygiene practices and periodontitis in health care professionals. *Journal of Periodontology,* Vol.73, pp. 531-535, ISSN 0022-3492

Michalowicz, BS.; Diehl, SR & Gunsolley, JC. (2000). Evidence of a substantial genetic basis for risk of adult periodontitis. *Journal of Clinical Periodontology,* Vol.71, pp. 1699-1707, ISSN 0303-6979

Morris, AL.; Steele, J. & White, DA. (2001). The oral cleanliness and periodontal health of UK adults in 1998. *Brittish Dental Journal,* Vol. 191, No.4, pp. 186-192, ISSN 0007-0610

Noack, b.; Gorgens, h & Hoffmann, T. (2004). Novel mutations in the cathepsin C gene in patients with pre-pubertal aggressive periodontitis and Papillon-Lefevre syndrome. *Journal of Dental Research,* Vol.83, No.5, pp. 368-370, ISSN 0022-0345

Nishida, N.; Tanaka, M & Hayashi, N. (2005). Determination of smoking and obesity as periodontitis risks using the classification and regression tree method. *Journal of Periodontology,* Vol.76, pp. 923-928, ISSN 0022-3492

O'Brien, m. (1994). *Children's dental health in the United Kingdom,* HMSO , London

Offenbacher, S.; Collins, JG.; Yalda, B. & Haradon, G. (1986). Periodontal health and periodontal disease in young people: global epidemiology. *International Dental Journal,* Vol.36, pp. 146-151, ISSN 0020-6539

Offenbacher, S.; Katz, V. & Fertik, G. (1996). Periodontal infection as a risk factor for preterm low birth weight. *Journal of Periodontology,* Vol.67, pp. 72-77, ISSN 0022-3492

Okamoto, H.; Yoneyama, T; Lindhe, J.; Haffajee, A. & Socransky, S. (1990). Methods of evaluating periodontal disease data in epidemiological research. *Journal of Clinical Periodontology,* Vol.15, pp. 430-439, ISSN 0303-6979

Page, RC. (1992). Host response tests for diagnosing periodontal diseases. *Journal of Periodontology,* Vol.63, (Suppl.), pp. 356-366, ISSN 0022-3492

Page, RC.; Krall, EA.; Martin, J.; Mancl, L. & Garcia, RI. (2002). Validity and accuracy of a risk calculator in predicting periodontal disease.. *Journal of the American Dental Association,* Vol. 133, pp. 569-576, ISSN 0002-8177

Parkhill, JM.; Hennig, BJ.; Chapple, IL; Heasman, PA & Taylor, JJ. (2000). Association of interleukin-1 gene polymorphisms with early-onset periodontitis. *Journal of Clinical Periodontology,* Vol.27, pp. 682-689, ISSN 0303-6979

Peretz, B.; Machtei, EE. & Bimstein, E. (1993). Changes in periodontal status of children and young adolescents: A one year longitudinal study. *Journal of Clinical Paediatric Dentistry,* Vol.18 pp. 3-6, ISSN 1053-4628

Persson, RE.; Persson, GR; Kiyak, HA. & Powell, LV. (1998). Powell LV. Oral
health and medical status in dentate low-income older persons. *Special Care Dentistry,* Vol. 18, pp. 70-71, ISSN 0275-1879

Pistorius, A.; Krahwinkel, T; Willerhausen, B. & Bockstegen, C. (2002). Relationship between stress factors and periodontal disease. *European Journal of Medical Research,* Vol.7, pp. 393-398, ISSN 0949-2321

Poulton, R.; Caspi, A. & Milne, BJ. (2002). Association between children's experience of socioeconomic disadvantage and adult health: a life-course study. *Lancet,* Vol. 360, No.9346 pp. 1640-1645, ISSN 0140-6736

Ramfjord, SP. (1959). Indices for prevalence and incidence of periodontal disease. *Journal of Periodontology,* Vol. 30, pp. 51-59, ISSN 0022-3492

Reichert, S.; Stein, SA. & Gautsch, A. (2002). Gender differences in HLA phenotype frequencies found in German patients with generalized aggressive periodontitis and chronic periodontitis. *Oral Microbiology and Immunology,* Vol.17, No.6, pp. 360-368, ISSN 0902-0055

Russell, AL. (1967). Epidemiology of periodontal disease. *International Dental Journal,* Vol.17, pp. 282-296, ISSN 0020-6539

Saito, T.; Shimazaki, Y & Sakamoto, M. (1998). Obesity and periodontitis. *New England Journal of Medicine,* Vol. 339, pp. 482-483, ISSN 0028-4793

Saito, T.; Shimazaki, Y & Yamashita, Y. (1999). Association between periodontitis and exercise capacity. *Periodontol insights,* Vol.6, pp. 9-12, ISSN 1195-2008

Saito, T.; Shimazaki, Y; Hideshima, A.; Tsuzuki, M. & Koga, T. (2000). Body mass index, abdominal adiposity and blood pressure: Relationship between upper body obesity and periodontitis. *Journal of Dental Research,* Vol.79 (abstract), pp. 625, ISSN 0022-0345

Saito, T.; Shimazaki, Y; Koga, T.; Tsuzuki, M. & Ohshima, A. (2001). Relationship between upper body obesity and periodontitis. *Journal of Dental Research,* Vol.80, pp. 1631-1636, ISSN 0022-0345

Sakellari, D.; Belibasakis, G; Chadjipadelis, T.; Arapostathis, K. & Konstantinidis, A. (2001). Supragingival and subgingival microbiota of adult patients with Down's syndrome. Changes after periodontal treatment. *Oral Microbiology and Immunology,* Vol.16, pp. 376-382, ISSN 0902-0055

Schou, L. & Wight, C. (1994). Does dental health education affect inequalities in dental health? *Community Dental Health,* Vol.11, pp. 97-100, ISSN 0265-539X

Sheiham, A. & Netuveli, GS. (2002). Periodontal diseases in Europe. *Periodontology 2000,* Vol.29, pp. 104-121, ISSN 0906-6713

Shuldiner, A.; Yang, R & Gong, D. (2001). Resistin, obesity and insulin resistance-the emerging role of the adipocytes as an endocrine organ. *New England journal of medicine,* Vol. 345, pp. 1345-1346, ISSN 0028-4793

Susin, C.; Oppermann, RV. & Haugejorden, O. (2004). Periodontal attachment loss attributable to cigarette smoking in an urban Brazilian population. *Journal Clinical Periodontology*, Vol.31, pp. 951-959, ISSN 0303-6979

Tervonen, T.; Oliver, RC. ; Wolff, LF.; Bereuter, J.; Anderson, L. & Aeppli, DM. (1994). Prevalence of periodontal pathogens with varying metabolic control of diabetes mellitus. *Journal of Clinical Periodontology*, Vol.21, pp. 375-379, ISSN 0303-6979

Tervonen, T. & Karjalainen K . (1997). Periodontal disease related to diabetic status. A pilot study of the response to periodontal therapy in type 1 diabetes. *Journal of Clinical Periodontology*, Vol. 24, pp. 505-510, ISSN 0303-6979

Thomas, E.; Van Dyke, DDS. & Sheilesh, D (2005). Risk factors for periodontitis. *Journal of the International Academy of Periodontology*, Vol.7 (January), pp. 3-7, ISSN 1466-2094

Thomson, WM. & Locker, D. (2000). Dental neglect and dental health among 26-year-olds in the Dunedin Multidisciplinary Health and Development Study. *Community Dentistry and Oral Epidemiology*, Vol.28, pp. 414-418, ISSN 0301- 5661

Thomson, WM.; Edwards, SJ. & Dobson-Le, DP. (2001). IL-1 genotype and adult periodontitis among young New Zealanders. *Journal of Dental Research*, Vol.80, pp. 1700-1703, ISSN 0022-0345

Timmerman, MF.; Van der Weijden, GA. & Abbas, F. (2000). Untreated periodontal disease in Indonesian adolescents. Longitudinal clinical data and prospective clinical and microbiological risk assessment. *Journal of Clinical Periodontology*, Vol. 27, pp. 932-942, ISSN 0303-6979

Timmerman, MF.; Van der Weijden, GA. & Arief, EM. (2001). Untreated periodontal disease in Indonesian adolescents. Subgingival microbiota in relation to experienced progression of periodontitis. *Journal of Clinical Periodontology*, Vol. 28, pp. 617-627, ISSN 0303-6979

Tomar, SL. & Asma, S (2000). Smoking-attributable periodontitis in the United States: findings from NHANES III. National Health and Nutrition Examination Survey. *Journal of Periodontology*, Vol.71, No.5,, pp. 743-751, ISSN 0022-3492

Tran, SD.; Rudney, JD.; Sparks, BS. & Hodges, JS. (2001). Persistent presence of Bacteroides forsythus as a risk factor for attachment loss in a population with low prevalence and severity of adult periodontitis. *Journal of Periodontology*, Vol. 72, pp. 1-10, ISSN 0022-3492

Tsai, C.; Hayes, C. & Taylor, GW. (2002). Glycemic control of type 2 diabetes and severe periodontal disease in the US adult population. *Community Dentistry and Oral Epidemiology*, Vol.301, pp. 182-192, ISSN 0301- 5661

Umino, M. & Nagao, M. (1993). Systemic diseases in elderly dental patients. *International Dental Journal*, Vol.43, pp. 213-218, ISSN 0020-6539

Westfelt, E.; Rylander, H; Blohme, G.; Jonasson, P. & Lindhe, J. (1996). The effect of periodontal therapy in diabetics. Results after 5 years. *Journal of Clinical Periodontology*, Vol.23, pp. 92-100, ISSN 0303-6979

Wimmer, G.; Janda, M; Wieselmann-Penkner, K. & Pertl, C. (2002). Coping with stress: its influence on periodontal disease. *Journal of Periodontology*, Vol.73, pp. 1343-1351, ISSN 0022-3492

Wolff, L.; Dahlen, G. & Aeppli, D. (1994). Bacteria as risk markers for periodontitis. *Journal of Periodontology*, Vol.65, No.5, pp. 498-510, ISSN 0022-3492

Wood, N.; Johnson, R & Streckfus, F. (2003). Comparison of body composition and periodontal disease using nutritional assessment techniques. *Journal of Clinical Periodontology*, Vol.30, pp. 321-327, ISSN 0303-6979

11

Epidemiology: It's Application in Periodontics

Surajit Mistry[1], Debabrata Kundu[1] and Premananda Bharati[2]
[1]*Department of Periodontics, Dr. R. Ahmed Dental College, Kolkata,*
[2]*Biological Anthropology Unit, Indian Statistical Institute, Kolkata, India*

1. Introduction

From immemorial time man has been interested in trying to cure and/or control of periodontal diseases. In view of the limitations of several theories (i.e., 'Focal infection theory', 'Theory of contagion' and 'Germ theory of disease'), scientific thought began to search the other factors or causes in the etiology of periodontal diseases namely social, economic, genetic, environmental and behavioral factors. Thus, a newer concept (Multi-factorial causation) of periodontal diseases has been evolved by investigators. Recently, evidence has also shed light on the relationship between systemic health and periodontal diseases, that is, possible adverse effects of periodontal disease on a wide range of organ systems (i.e., cardiovascular, endocrine, reproductive, respiratory). Hence, the application of epidemiology in the field of periodontics has utmost importance to measure prevalence, extent and severity of periodontal diseases, its relationship to other factors (age, oral hygiene, and nutrition), to assess the degree of association between periodontal diseases and systemic health and to improve treatment modalities for the prevention and control of periodontal diseases.

The word 'Epidemiology' (Epi- among, demos- people, logos- study) is derived from the term 'epidemic'. 'Epidemiology' is defined as the study of the distribution and determinants of health related states or events in population and the application of this study for the prevention and control of health problems (Last, 1983). Epidemiology is more often concerned with the well being of society as a whole rather than the well being of individual. Three most important components of epidemiology are study of disease frequency (incidence/prevalence), study of disease distribution (i.e., age, sex, race) and (3) Study of determinants (causative/risk factor) of disease. Etiologic (causative) agent is defined as the living/nonliving substances or forces which may initiate or exaggerate the disease process by its excessive presence or relative lack. Risk factor is a subjective determinant of some disease processes (periodontitis, cancer) when true disease causing agent is not fully established. In epidemiologic study, three types of causal relationship are identified between different variables and manifestation of disease (Brownson, 1998) as they are shown in Fig. 1. Variable is a characteristic that helps to measure changes of disease processes varies from person to person. It may be dependent/ uncontrolled variable (i.e., age, genetics) or independent variable that can be controlled or manipulated (i.e., smoking). The presence of risk factor does not imply that always disease will occur and in its absence, disease will not occur. In a disease, they are additive/synergistic, observable/identifiable, can be modified or non-modifiable. The basic aims of epidemiology are: (1) to explain distribution and magnitude of disease in population, (2) to identify causative/risk factors of disease, (3) to assess the risk in population (4) to study the complete course of disease, (5) to provide the data essential for treatment planning (6) implementation of programme for prevention and control of a disease and finally (7) to promote, protect and restore health of population. Dentist is concerned with the disease of a patient, where as, epidemiologist is concerned with the disease patterns in whole population and to determine preventive or control measures.

Causal Relationship

Sufficient Cause	Necessary Cause	Risk factor
(Any exposure/condition in presence of which disease will always occur. – eg, genetic abnormalities)	(Any exposure/condition that must be present for manifestation of a disease. Its presence does not always results in disease to occur– eg, Aggregatibacter actinomycetemcomitans is also found in healthy gingival sulcus)	(It has least causal relation)

Fig. 1. Different types of causal relationship between variables and disease.

2. Tools for measurement of epidemiology

Incidence is defined as the number of new cases of a disease occurring in a defined population during a given time period (Park, 2002). It is measured as number of new cases of a disease during specific time/ population at risk x 1000 (X/1000/year). Prevalence is the number of cases (old/new cases) of a disease within a specific point of time (point prevalence) or over a given period of time (period prevalence) in a designated population. Point prevalence is more commonly used. When population is stable, incidence and duration are not changing then the relationship between incidence (I) and prevalence (P) can be expressed as, $P = I \times D$ [D = mean duration]. As longer the disease process, prevalence will be increased (i.e., chronic periodontitis, tuberculosis) whereas in acute short lived cases, incidence rate will be higher than prevalence rate. Incidence and prevalence rate are used to assess the magnitude of communal health problems, to identify potential high risk population and useful for administrative and planning purposes. Usually two types of epidemiological methods (i.e., observational & experimental) are used in periodontics to assess different variables and control measures of diseases.

a. Observational studies-

I. Descriptive- eg, cross-sectional study and longitudinal study

II. Analytical- a) Case-control/Retrospective study

b) Cohort /Longitudinal/Follow-up study

b. Experimental studies-

I. Randomized control trial, II. Community trial, III. Field trial

Descriptive study: Descriptive study is the first phase of an epidemiological investigation. In periodontology, it is concerned with the occurrence and distribution of periodontal diseases in human populations and identifies the variables related with the disease. The variables most frequently examined in descriptive studies for periodontal diseases are time related, place related (urban/rural, geographical comparisons) and person related (age, sex, stress, social status, education etc.) characteristics. By comparing the distribution of periodontal diseases with the help of cross-sectional (prevalence assessment) and longitudinal design (incidence assessment) in different populations, it is possible to set hypotheses relating to disease etiology. The hypotheses can be accepted or rejected with the further application of analytical epidemiology. Cross-Sectional Study (i.e., also known as "prevalence study") is an observational study based on single examination of a cross section of population at given point of time. It provides gross idea about the defined population when sampling has been done correctly. Longitudinal Studies in which observations are repeated in the same population over a period of time by means of follow up examinations. Longitudinal studies are useful to study the natural course of disease and its future outcome, to identify the etiologic/risk factors and to find out the incidence rate which can not be achieved by cross-section study. Cross-sectional study is like a photograph whereas longitudinal study can be considered as a cine film.

Case-Control (retrospective) Study: It has three distinct features: i) exposure and disease have occurred before starting of study, ii) Study proceeds backward from effect to cause, and iii) control group is used to compare the study group.

Risk Factor (smoker)	Cases (periodontitis + ve)	Control (periodontitis -ve)
< 10 cigarette/day	33(a)	55 (b)
Non-smoker	2 (c)	27 (d)

Table 1. Frequency of periodontitis in smoker and non-smoker.

Frequency of exposure to cigarette for cases are (a/a+c) 94.2% and with control (b/b+d) 67.7%. If the frequency of smoking is higher in cases than control (non periodontitis), a association is said to be existed between smoking and periodontitis and vice versa. If 'p' value (statistical association) is less than 0.05, the association is regarded as statistically significant but does not imply causation. Exposure rate of 94.2% does not mean that all the smokers would develop periodontitis. In the case-control study, Odds ratio (measure of strength of the association between risk factor and disease) is the common end point. In Table 1, Odds ratio (ad/bc) is 8.1. It means that there is 8 times greater risk of smokers to develop periodontitis than non smokers. It is a key parameter in the analysis of case-control study which is rapid, in expensive and easy to carry out.

Cohort Study: It is a forward looking, observational study to obtain additional supportive evidence about the existence of association between suspected cause and disease. It is also called prospective, longitudinal, incidence study. In this study, cohorts are identified before appearance of disease, study groups are observed over a period, and study proceeds forward from cause to effect and establish a firm relationship between exposure and disease. Cohort is defined as a group of people who share a common characteristic or experience (age, exposure to drug) with in defined time period. It is indicated when association between exposure and outcome is already established by a case control study. In case control study, exposure and disease have already occurred when the study is initiated, where as in cohort study exposure had occur but disease has not. In general, both groups should be equally susceptible to disease, all the variables should be compared that influences disease frequency and all groups are followed under same condition over a period to determine the exposure.

Relative risk (Incidence among exposed / incidence among non-exposed) is exactly determined by cohort study because incidence rate in the case-control study is not accurate.

It is a direct and reliable measure of strength of association between exposure and outcome. If, it is 1 or less, indicates no association whereas >1 indicates positive association between cause and effect. It is '2' means, two times higher incidence rate of disease in exposed group than unexposed group and 100% increase in risk. 0.25 means less chance of disease in exposed person. Larger the relative risk, greater will be the strength of association between disease and the suspected factor which can be considered as a risk factor for the disease. Relative risk may alter as a result of bias (systematic error in the determination of association) that should be removed by matching (age, sex, etc.) in cohort study. The natural history of the disease is a key concept in epidemiology and is best established by cohort study.

Randomized control trial: To guard against different biased conditions (memory bias, observer bias), 'Single Blind Trial' (patient unaware), 'Double Blind Trial' (doctor and patient unaware about the group allocation and treatment received), and Triple Blind Trial (ideal, where doctor, participant and data analyzer unaware) are adopted. It is used in preventive and clinical trial, trial of etiological agent and evaluation of effectiveness of health services. In Fig.2, the strength of association increases in progressing toward the peak of the pyramid and simultaneously number of biases decrease. 2 or more systematic reviews (i.e., summary of multiple research studies investigated for same parameters) and meta-analysis (i.e., merging of statistical values of multiple studies into one analysis) provide strong causal relationship between risk factor and disease. The association is defined as the occurrence of two variables more often than would be expect by chance. Association does not always imply causal relationship. Correlation is the degree of association between characteristics or variables. Correlation coefficient ranges from -1 to +1. Correlation does not imply causation but causation always implies correlation. '1' indicates perfect association between two variables, '>0.75-1' implies high correlation, '0.75-0.4' for moderate correlation and < 0.4 indicates none or weak correlation. '0' means no association and '-1' indicates perfectly opposite relation.

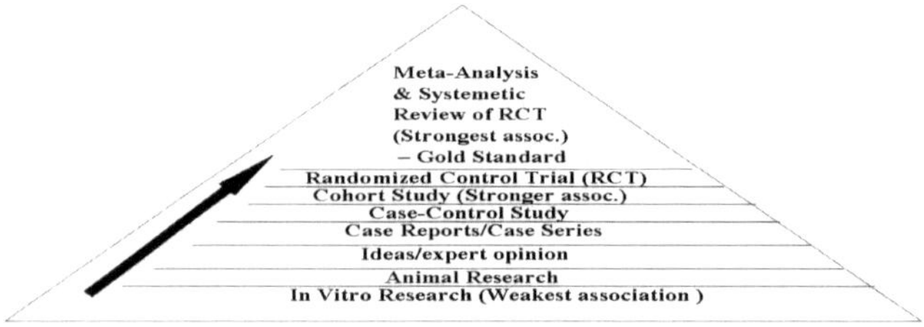
Meta-Analysis
& Systemetic
Review of RCT
(Strongest assoc.)
– Gold Standard
Randomized Control Trial (RCT)
Cohort Study (Stronger assoc.)
Case-Control Study
Case Reports/Case Series
Ideas/expert opinion
Animal Research
In Vitro Research (Weakest association)

Fig. 2. Strength of association increases toward the peak of the pyramid.

2.1 Sensitivity and specificity

A less accurate and inexpensive screening test is applied by observer on a group of healthy population for an unrecognized disease (ELISA for blood donor). Diagnostic test is applied in a single sick person (ELISA for suspected patient), which is more accurate and expensive. Validity refers to what extent the test accurately measures the variables. It has two components; sensitivity and specificity. Sensitivity is defined as the ability of a test to identify maximum true positive and minimum false negative results. 90% sensitivity means, 90% diseased patients screened by a test will give true positive and 10% a false negative results. Specificity is defined as the ability of a test to identify maximum true negative and minimum false positive cases or results. In fact, no screening/diagnostic test provides 100% specificity and 100% sensitivity. Sensitivity come in expense of specificity (inversely related). Two or more tests are required to enhance the sensitivity and specificity of the screening programme. Predictive value depends on sensitivity, specificity and prevalence. A highly sensitive test will be rarely false negative when someone has the disease. So clinician should choose it for screening during routine examination. As a highly specific test rarely gives false positive results, it is indicated when a positive results may harm to a person emotionally, physically or financially. Usually a highly sensitive test is done first to rule out non-diseased persons then a highly specific test is advocated to rule out false positive patients.

2.2 Statistical averages

Mean is simply the arithmetic mean of data. It is the most frequently used value for data analysis and presented along with the standard deviation. For the data 1, 2, 3, 4, the mean will be 2.5, but it is usually presented as 2.5 ± S.D [Standard Deviation]. 30 or more samples should preferably be analyzed to get acceptable value of SD. Greater variation of mean values and low sample size of a test provides higher value of standard deviation, which may hamper the test of significance. Median and mode have limited use in periodontology.

3. Concepts of prevention

Successful prevention of disease depends upon knowledge of causation, transmission, availability of prophylactic and therapeutic measures etc. It has four levels:

Primordial prevention: It is a type of primary prevention in present form. For example, many adult health problems (i.e., periodontitis, diabetes, cardiovascular disease) have their early origins in childhood when lifestyles are formed. Efforts are directed toward discouraging children from adopting harmful lifestyles (food, habits, smoking etc.) through proper education and motivation.

Primary prevention: Action taken to prevent the onset of a disease which removes the possibility that disease ever occurs. Intervention is taken during pre-pathogenesis phase of disease. Example- pit and fissure sealant application, plaque control instruction, daily tooth brushing and flossing, fluoridation/ defluridation of water, vaccination.

Secondary Prevention: Action which halts the process of disease at its incipient stage and prevents complications. Interventions are early diagnosis and treatment. In case of infectious disease, it provides secondary prevention to infected individual and primary prevention to community. Example- filling, oral prophylaxis by dentist, gingivectomy.

Tertiary prevention: Action taken to reduce or limits suffering, impairments and disabilities and to promotes rehabilitation. Intervention taken at let pathogenesis phase. Example- Root canal treatment, removable and fixed partial denture, extraction, dental implant retained removable and fixed prostheses.

4. Dental (periodontal) epidemiology

Dental epidemiology is the study of distribution and dynamics (time, pattern, etiologic agent) of dental diseases in human population. The periodontal disease epidemiology is one of the most important but complex part of dental epidemiology because pathologic changes in periodontal diseases involve both soft and hard tissues and there are so many subjective variation in objective measurement of periodontal indices like color change, pocket depth and swelling. In order to measure the incidence, prevalence and severity of periodontal diseases, its relationship to other factors and for assessment of treatment needs, special indices have been designed to provide objective measurement of identifiable features. It is a quantitative science and is measured by biostatistics. Using these indices and applying the appropriate statistical tests should allow the observer to make a valid comparison of periodontal disease conditions in respect to different variables and to measure the efficacy of therapeutic agents.

4.1 Indices used to assess gingival inflammation

4.1.1 Papillary Marginal Attachment Index

The first dental index, Papillary Marginal Attachment (PMA) Index was developed to count number of gingival unit affected with gingivitis that correlated with severity of gingival inflammation (Schour & Massler, 1948). The facial surface of gingiva around a tooth divided into three units: Mesial interdental papilla (P), Marginal gingiva (M), and Attached gingiva (A). Presence or absence of inflammation on each gingival unit recorded as 1 or 0 respectively. Summation of these three units of a tooth is considered as PMA score of the tooth and summation of score of all teeth and divided by number of teeth; is considered as PMA score of the person. Usually central incisor to second premolars was examined. In 1967, they added severity component for assessing gingivitis likewise- Papillary unit - 0-5, Marginal gingiva - 0-3, Attached gingiva - 0-3. It is used for epidemiological survey, in clinical trials and for patients' education.

4.1.2 Gingival Index

Gingival Index (GI) was developed to assess the severity and quality of gingival inflammation in individual or population (Loe & Silness, 1963). Only gingival tissue is assessed by this index. Blunt periodontal probe is used to assess and palpate the bleeding tendency by running the probe along the soft tissue wall of the entrance of gingival sulcus. Gingiva surrounding the tooth divided into 4 scoring units- Mesio-facial papilla, Facial marginal gingiva, Disto- facial papilla, Lingual marginal gingiva (to minimize examiners' variability in scoring, lingual gingiva were not subdivided). All 4 scoring units are examined by visual examination (dental mirror) and periodontal probe and scored from 0-3 for each of them. Gingival index may be used for selected or all teeth. The scoring criteria are 0 (normal), 1 (mild inflammation, slight color change, slight edema, no bleeding on palpation), 2 (moderate inflammation, redness, edema, bleeding on probing), and 3 (severe inflammation, marked redness & edema, tendency to spontaneous bleeding). The GI score of 4 units are totaled and then divided by 4 (surfaces) to yield the GI score of a tooth. The GI score per person is obtained by totaling all of the tooth scores and dividing by the number of teeth examined (Table 2).

Gingival index score	Degree of gingivitis
0.1-1	Mild
1.1-2	Moderate
2.1-3	Severe

Table 2. Degree of gingivitis in relation to gingival index score.

4.1.3 Modified Gingival Index

Modified Gingival Index (MGI) was introduced with two important changes in gingival index by eliminating sulcus probing, and by redefining the scoring system for mild inflammation to increase the sensitivity of lower values of scoring scale (Lobene et al., 1986). This non-invasive index allows for repeated evaluation of the sites without disturbing the plaque or irritating the gingiva. The scoring criteria are: 0 (Absence of inflammation), 1 (Mild inflammation, slight color change, little change in texture of a portion of papillary or marginal gingiva but not in entire gingiva), 2 (Mild inflammat- ion, change in texture involves entire papillary/marginal gingiva), 3 (Moderate inflam- mation, redness, edema, and/or hypertrophy of marginal or papillary gingiva), and 4 (Severe inflammation, marked redness, edema, and/or hypertrophy, spontaneous bleeding and ulceration). The score of 2 papillary and 2 marginal units are totaled and then divided by 4 (surfaces) to yield the MGI score of a tooth. The MGI score per person is obtained by totaling all of the tooth scores and dividing by the number of teeth examined. Either full or partial mouth assessment can be performed. It perhaps most widely used index in clinical trials of therapeutic agents. This index can not identify the gingivitis in absence of periodontitis because it does not involve pocket probing.

4.1.4 Periodontal Index

After realizing the true paucity of valid index in early 1950's for measuring the prevalence of advanced periodontal diseases; the 'Periodontal Index'(PI) was developed to determine the presence/absence of gingival inflammation, severity of inflammation, periodontal pocket formation and disturbance of masticatory function (Russell, 1956). It not only assesses all the gingival tissues encircling the tooth but also scores the supporting tissues. Mouth mirror, light source and explorer are used to assess tissue. The scoring criteria are: 0 (Absence of inflammation), 1 (Mild inflammation, slight color change, change in texture only a portion of papillary or marginal gingiva but not in entire gingiva), 2 (Mild inflammation involves entire papillary or marginal gingival unit), 4 (when radiograph is advised), 6 (Moderate inflammation, redness, edema, and/or hypertrophy of marginal or papillary gingival unit with pocket formation), and 8 (Severe inflammation, redness, edema, spontaneous bleeding and ulceration with advanced destruction and impairment of function). In doubtful condition, lower score should be considered. The periodontal index score per person is obtained by totaling all of the tooth scores and dividing by the number of teeth examined. It is an index with true biologic gradient because it measures both reversible and irreversible aspects of periodontal disease. It underestimates true level of periodontal destruction and early bone loss. As the number of teeth decrease, the chances of scoring bias will increase.

- 0.0-0.2 (Group PI score) – Clinically normal Reversible stage
- 0.3-0.9 (") – Simple gingivitis (")
- 0.7-1.9 - (") – Beginning of periodontal destruction – (")
- 1.6-5.0 - (") – Established periodontal destruction - Irreversible stages
- 3.8-8.0 - (") – Terminal disease (")

4.1.5 Gingivitis component of the Periodontal Disease Index

The periodontal disease index (PDI) was developed by Ramfjord SP in 1959, to which few criteria further added in 1967. The PDI is used to measure incidence and prevalence of periodontal disease. This index assesses gingivitis, gingival sulcus depth and plaque at all interproximal, facial and lingual surfaces on six selected teeth (i.e., Ramford's teeth # 16,21,24,36,41,44) because these teeth have been tested as reliable indicators for various regions of the mouth (Ramfjord, 1959, 1967). The calculus component assesses the presence and extent of calculus on facial and lingual surfaces of indexed teeth. Plaque and calculus component of PDI are not a part of PDI score rather helpful in a total assessment of periodontal status. The selection of indexed teeth may be altered in longitudinal studies and clinical trials, where all teeth or quadrants of teeth or the teeth appropriate for the objective of the study can be chosen. It can be used in large survey because it is quick and easy. The PDI is useful for comprehensive assessment of periodontal status in cross-sectional surveys, longitudinal studies and clinical trials of therapeutic or preventive procedures. The gingivitis index scoring criteria are: 0 (Absence of signs of gingivitis), 1 (Mild to moderate gingivitis, not extending around the tooth), 2 (Mild to moderate gingivitis extending all around the tooth), 3 (Severe gingivitis, marked redness and edema, tendency to bleed, and ulceration). The gingivitis scores per tooth are totaled and then divided by the number of teeth examined to yield the gingivitis score per person. Same measurement method follows for plaque and calculus score. The plaque, gingival sulcus depth and calculus index component will be discussed in separate section.

4.2 Indices used to assess gingival bleeding

4.2.1 Gingival index used by the National Institute of Dental Research (NIDR)

It was developed to assess gingival inflammation (Miller et al., 1987). It has two components: 1) Bleeding index, and 2) Calculus index. The mesio-buccal interproximal and mid-buccal gingiva on all teeth except molars and mesio-buccal interproximal and mid-buccal gingiva on mesial root of the molars are assessed. The sites are randomly determined as one half of the upper arch and contra-lateral side of the lowr arch. NIDR probe marked on 2, 4, 6, 8, 10 and 12 mm with alternating yellow color band are inserted 2mm into the gingival crevice in mid-buccal gingiva and gently drawn in a horizontal direction along the inner wall of the crevice to mesio-buccal interproximal direction. The score for bleeding index is 0 (no bleeding) and 1(bleeding present). The score of bleeding sites are totaled and then divided by the number of sites examined to yield the gingival bleeding index score of a person. Superficial gingival crevice palpation and interproximal cleaning aids are more suitable to assess gingivitis than indices that utilizes apical probing (i.e., useful for diagnosing periodontitis).

4.2.2 National Institute of Dental & Craniofacial Research (NICDR) protocol

The NICDR protocol was first used in The Third National Health and Nutrition Examination Survey (NHANES),1988-94 (NHANES III, 1997). Gingival assessment is one of the components of NIDCR protocol for assessment of periodontium. Similar technique as NIDR, has been used to assess the prevalence of gingivitis in NIDCR protocol but was slightly modified by adding mesio-facial site to the NIDR examination protocol, resulting three sites per tooth. As per NHANES III survey, gingival bleeding was more prevalent with 13-17 years age group (63%), then gradually decreases with increasing age. Adolescents have higher prevalence of gingivitis than pre-puberty and adult may be due to increasing sex hormone level that alters the composition of subgingival microflora and facilitates colonization of increasing level of Prevotella intermedia and Prevotella nigrescence (Nakagawa et al., 1994). Prevalence of gingivitis in males of any age group is higher than

female. It suggests that plaque control in puberty gingivitis is more important than rising level of hormone.
Several other indices are used to assess gingival bleeding such as Sulcus Bleeding Index (Mühlemann & Major, 1958), Bleeding Point Index (Lenox & Kopczyk, 1973), Ainamo's Gingival Bleeding Index (Ainamo & Bay, 1975), Carter's Gingival Bleeding Index (Carter & Barnes, 1974) and Eastman Interdental Bleeding Index (Caton & Polson, 1985).
The association between rate of plaque formation and gingivitis was observed in the classical study of 'experimental gingivitis in man' (Löe et al., 1965), which demonstrated the cause and effect relationship between plaque and gingivitis. 12 individuals (9-dental students, 1-instructor and 2-technicians) were asked to stop from all sorts of oral hygiene measures. Dental plaque increased quickly and all subjects developed gingivitis within 10-21days. It indicated that when brushing was omitted, the formation of plaque and development of gingivitis were closely parallel. Mean GI score increased from 0.27 to 1.05 at the end of 'no brushing period'. Gingivitis was resolved in all subjects within 1 week of reinstitution of tooth brushing. This evidence demonstrated the reversible nature of gingivitis and also showed a concomitant decrease in plaque and gingivitis. They concluded that bacterial plaque was essential in the production of gingivitis. Bleeding on probing can occur as early as 2 days after gingivitis begins in healthy mouth. If plaque and calculus are removed, gingival bleeding and ulceration will heal after 7-10days. If plaque accumulates further; bleeding return back within 2 days. Bleeding on probing from multiple sites in a single examination or from a particular site in subsequent examination is a good indicator of current inflammation at all stages of periodontal disease.

4.3 Indices used to assess periodontal destruction

Alveolar bone destruction is an important criterion for assessing severity of periodontal disease by using crevice measurement, radiographic evaluation of bone loss, assessment of gingival recession and tooth mobility. Radiograph only reveals interdental bone level and is not useful for buccal and lingual assessment of bone level or attachment loss.

4.3.1 Gingival sulcus measurement component of Ramfjord's PDI

This technique has been introduced for determining the gingival sulcus/pocket depth with a calibrated periodontal probe involves measuring the distance from cemento-enamel junction (CEJ) to the free gingival margin (First measurement score) and the distance from free gingival margin to the bottom of the gingival sulcus/pocket (Second measurement score). The subtraction of first measurement score from the second score yields the clinical attachment loss (Ramfjord, 1967). A) If the gingival margin is on the enamel, then the above calculation reveals the level of attachment. B) If the gingival margin is on the cementum, then the first measurement should be recorded as minus score and the second measurement as plus score. Then the clinical attachment level is measured by subtracting the first measurement score from the second score (i.e., addition of two scores). Ramfjord's PDI is still considered as the "gold standard" method for determining the status of periodontium. The first measurement is useful in assessing gingival recession or gain after therapy. In cross-section study, only 6 indexed teeth should be assessed. In longitudinal study and in clinical trial, other teeth can be included according to the objective of the study.

PDI criteria for epidemiologic surveys:
- When CAL = 0, Gingivitis score represents the PDI score of that tooth
- When CAL ≤ 3 in any of the two measured areas of tooth, PDI score of tooth = 4 (Gingivitis score is disregarded)
- When CAL > 3 - ≤ 6 in any of the two measured areas of tooth, PDI score of tooth = 5
- (Gingivitis score is disregarded)
- When CAL > 6 in any of the measured areas of tooth, PDI score of tooth = 6 (Gingivitis score is disregarded)

4.3.2 Extent and Severity Index (ESI)

This index was developed because of a lack of satisfaction with previous indices as PI and PDI do not provide the information about the extent of the periodontal disease (Carlos et al., 1986). PI was based on the concept that periodontal disease was slow growing continuous process. Later on, periodontal disease was viewed as chronic process with intermittent periods of activity and remission that affects individual tooth and sites around teeth at different rates within same mouth. The NIDR probe has been used to estimate percentage of sites affected by attachment loss >1mm (Extent- E) and mean attachment loss (LA) >1mm (Severity- S). 14 sites at upper arch and 14 sites at contra lateral half of lower arch were measured (Mesio-buccal interproximal and mid-buccal of all teeth except molars and Mesio-buccal interproximal and mid-buccal of mesial root of molars). Extent and severity index (ESI) described the distribution of the disease. NIDR includes the method of measurement of ESI but severity component is modified to > 3 mm of attachment loss. In epidemiological studies, measurements are rounded off to the next digit, so >1 mm is written as 2 mm. The percentage of sites examined that have LA > 1 mm represents the extent score, whereas; average LA/site among the diseased sites represents the severity score. ESI (20, 3.0) means 20% of sites had diseased and within diseased site average LA was 3mm. ESI measured for full mouth assessment or as much as sites/tooth.

4.4 Indices used to assess plaque accumulation

4.4.1 Plaque component of PDI (PII)

It is the first index attempted to assess the extent of plaque quantitatively covering the all four surface areas of Ramford's teeth (Ramfjord, 1959). Bismark brown disclosing agent was used. The PII scoring criteria are: 0 (absence of plaque), 1 (plaque covering <1/3 of gingival half of facial or lingual surface of a tooth), 2 (plaque covering >1/3 to 2/3 of gingival half of facial and lingual of the tooth), 3 (>2/3 of gingival half of facial and lingual of the tooth). The PII score per person is obtained by totaling all of the tooth scores and then dividing by the number of teeth examined. This index was modified by excluding interproximal area of tooth and restricting the scoring of plaque to the gingival half of the facial and lingual surface (Shick & Ash, 1961).

4.4.2 Oral Hygiene Index

The Oral Hygiene Index (OHI) is composed of the combined debris index and calculus index (Greene & Vermillion, 1960). The upper and the lower arches are divided separately into three segments (i.e., six sextants): i) the segment distal to the right canine, ii) segment distal to the left canine, and iii) the segment mesial to the right and left first premolars. Each segment is examined for debris or calculus. Debris includes plaque, materia alba and debris itself. From each segment, buccal and lingual surface of one tooth is used for calculating the individual index for that particular segment. The criteria used for assigning scores to the tooth surfaces for the OHI are described in the OHI-simplified section.

4.4.3 Oral Hygiene Index-Simplified (OHI -S)

Green & Vermillion in 1964 simplified the OHI by including only six teeth surfaces rather than twelve that were representative of all anterior and posterior segments of the mouth. This modification was called Oral Hygiene Index-Simplified (OHI -S). The tooth used for the calculation must have the greatest area covered by either debris or calculus. The method for scoring calculus is the same as that applied to debris. It has two components: debris index - simplified (DI-S) and calculus index – simplified (CI-S). The mouth mirror, and shephard's crook or sickle type explorer are used to examine facial surfaces of teeth # 11,16,26,31 and lingual surfaces of teeth # 36,46, by running the instrument from distal gingival crevice to mesial gingival crevice of a particular surface (½ of tooth circumference) subgingivally. In the absence of selected molars, second or third molar and in absence of selected anterior teeth, the teeth # 21 or 41 is substituted. At least two surfaces must have been examined for an individual score to be calculated. The CI-S score per person is obtained by totaling all of the buccal and lingual calculus scores and then dividing by the number of surface examined. The CI-S scoring criteria are: 0 (no calculus present), 1 (supragingival calculus covering ≤1/3 of exposed tooth surface), 2 (supragingival calculus covering >1/3 but ≤ 2/3 of exposed tooth surface or presence of flecks of subgingival calculus or both), 3 (subgingival calculus covering >2/3 of exposed tooth surface or continuous heavy band of subgingival calculus around the crevice of teeth or both). The debris score of all the buccal and lingual surfaces are totaled and then divided by the number of surface examined to yield the DI-S score of a person. The DI-S scoring criteria are: 0 (no debris or stain present), 1 (soft debris covering ≤ 1/3 of tooth surface or extrinsic stain regardless of area covered), 2 (soft debris covering >1/3 but ≤ 2/3 of exposed tooth surface), 3 (>2/3 surface area is involved). The average individual or group debris and calculus scores are combined to obtain the Simplified Oral Hygiene Index. It has been used extensively throughout the world because the criteria are objective and provide high level of reproducibility. The high degree of correlation (r=0.82) between the PI and the OHI-S helps to calculate the unknown score with regression analysis. The OHI-S is used in epidemiologic surveys, longitudinal studies and to evaluate the level of cleanliness of personal oral hygiene measures. The OHI-S score 0-1.2 of a person indicates good oral hygiene, 1.3-3.0 indicates fair oral hygiene and 3.1-6.0 indicates poor oral hygiene.

4.4.4 Plaque Index (PI)

It is unique among the indices because it ignores coronal extent of plaque and assesses only the thickness of plaque at the gingival area of the tooth using mouth mirror, and sickle type explorer or periodontal probe (Silness & Loe, 1964). As it is developed as a component parallel to the GI (Löe and Silness, 1963), it examines the same scoring units of the teeth (disto-facial/facial/ mesio-facial /lingual). Plaque index does not exclude or substitute a tooth with gingival restoration and crown. The scoring criteria are: 0 (no plaque at gingival area), 1 (a film of plaque on gingival margin and/or adjacent tooth surface, recognized only by running a probe across tooth surface), 2 (moderately soft deposits at margin and/or adjacent tooth surface that can be seen by naked eye), 3 (abundant soft matter at margin and adjoining surface). The assessment of plaque thickness is so subjective that to obtain accurate data, highly trained and experienced examiners are required.

4.4.5 Patient's Hygiene Performance Index

It is the first index to assess an individual's performance in removing debris after tooth brushing instruction. It records presence or absence of debris as 1 or 0 respectively using 6 surfaces of OHI-S teeth. It is more sensitive than OHI-S as it divides each tooth surface into 5areas: 3 longitudinal thirds and middle third horizontally into thirds. The scoring is done by using disclosing agent and is used for individual patient education.
Another plaque index was focused on gingival 1/3 of the tooth surface of the facial surfaces of all anterior teeth using basic fuschin disclosing agent (Quigley & Hein, 1962).

4.5 Indices used for calculus measurement

- Calculus component of Oral Hygiene Index-Simplified (Green & Vermillion, 1964).
- Calculus component of PDI (Ramfjord, 1959).
- NIDR Calculus Index- It measures the presence or absence of calculus on buccal and lingual surfaces of a tooth using NIDR probe (Miller et al., 1987). The scoring criteria are: 0 (absence of Calculus), 1 (supragingival calculus present), 2 (supra and subgingival calculus present). The calculus index score per person is obtained by totaling all of the teeth scores and then dividing by the number of teeth examined.

4.6 Indices for treatment needs

4.6.1 Gingival Plaque Index (GPI)

The Gingival plaque index (O'Leary et al., 1963) is a modification the PDI of Ramfjord to detect periodontitis at its initial stage so that treatment may be instituted promptly. It measures three components: Gingival status, periodontal status (crevice depth) and collectively materia alba, calculus and overhanging restoration (i.e., irritational index). For the assessment of gingival status, each arch was divided into anterior, left posterior, right posterior segments. Severest condition within each of the 6 segments determines the score of that segment, using the criteria: 0 (normal), 1 (mild to moderate inflammation partially encircled the tooth), 2 (mild/moderate inflammation completely encircled one/more tooth), 3 (marked inflammation, ulceration, spontaneous bleeding, recession and clefts). The gingival score per person is obtained by totaling all of the scores of the segments and then dividing by the number of segment examined.

4.6.2 Periodontal Treatment Need System (PTNS)

This index is considered the presence of gingivitis, plaque and calculus. It determines the presence/absence of periodontal pockets of ≥ 5 mm in each quadrant (Bellini & Gjermo, 1973).

4.6.3 Community Periodontal Index of Treatment Needs (CPITN)

Without knowing the response of the periodontal tissue to initial therapy, estimation of treatment needs may be subject to over/underestimation of what is clinically prudent.
World Health Organization appointed an expert committee to review the methods to assess periodontal status and treatment needs (Ainamo et al., 1982). The index that resulted after extensive field testing by the investigators from the World Health Organization (WHO) and

the International Dental Fedaration (FDI) was called Community Periodontal Index of Treatment Needs (CPITN). It is composed of the combined elements of GPI and PTNS to assess presence/absence of gingival bleeding on gentle probing, presence/absence of supra and/or subgingival calculus and subdivided the periodontal pocket into shallow and deep using WHO periodontal probe (i.e., 0.5mm ball tip and marking at 3.5mm, 5.5mm, 8.5mm and 11.5mm, black color coding between 3.5mm and 5.5mm). In epidemiological study, 10 index teeth are examined but only worst finding from index teeth is recorded per sextant resulting in six scores. It permits rapid examination to determine periodontal treatment needs. However, a great deal of useful information is lost when only the worst score per sextant is recorded. CPITN underestimates the number of pocket > 6 mm in older age group and overestimate the need for scaling in younger age group because the WHO probe has no marking below 3.5 mm (Gaengler et al., 1988).

CPITN score	Periodontal status	Treatment need
0	Healthy periodontium	No treatment
1	Bleeding observed by probing/spontaneous	Improvement of Oral hygiene
2	Calculus felt by probe; entire black area is visible	I+ professional scaling
3	Pocket depth 4-5mm; Gingival margin on the black band	I+ professional scaling
4	Pocket depth>6mm; Entire black band is invisible	I+II+ complex surgery

Table 3. Scoring criteria of community periodontal index of treatment needs (CPITN).

4.7 NIDCR protocol for periodontal disease assessment

It has three components: 1) gingival assessment (Described in the previous section -same as NIDR), 2) calculus assessment (at each site assessed for attachment loss, where calculus should be assessed using the scoring criteria of NIDR), and 3) assessment of periodontal destruction (NHANES III, 1997). The assessment of periodontal destruction includes: i) Loss of attachment, and ii) furcation involvement). The attachment loss is measured at facial and mesio-facial sites of teeth in two randomly selected quadrant using Ramfjord criteria by NIDR probe. Assessment of furcation involvement is done on eight selected teeth # 17,16,24,26,27,36,37,46,47, by using explorer no.17 for upper arch and cowhorn explorer no.3 for lower arch. Extent of furcation is assessed at mesial/facial/distal surface of maxillary molar, mesial/distal surface of maxillary premolar, buccal/lingual surface of mandibular molar. The criteria for scoring furcation involvement are: 0 (no furcation involvement), 1 (partially involved but not through and through involvement), 2 (complete through and through furcation involvement). For greater statistical reliability, combining two or more NHANES survey (2-year cycles) is strongly recommended.

4.8 Reliability of periodontal indices

The term reliability means the ability of an index to provide same results each time measuring a condition in the same subject repeatedly. Since, all measurements are subjected to error/bias (i.e., examination bias, observer bias, time bias) and variability (i.e., intra/inter-examiner), several indices should be used whenever possible. Because incorporation of unreliable indices in the prevalence estimates (from survey) which reveals significant difference in the comparative study results, become questionable when longitudinal study is performed. None of the periodontal indices are universally accepted. Recording of pocket depth (CAL is disregarded) in CPITN index may lead to underestimating disease severity among older population when gingival recession is prevalent. Therefore, the CPITN is not a reliable epidemiological index for periodontal study (Baelum et al., 1995).

4.9 Prevalence of gingivitis

A gingivitis case is a person with atleast mild inflammation in at least one of the examined gingival units (i.e., anatomic structure of gingiva such as interdental papillae, marginal gingiva or attached gingiva). Plaque induced gingivitis may be found in existing but non progressing attachment loss or stable periodontitis patient. Prevalence and severity of gingivitis increases with age, beginning at 5yrs of age, reaching highest at puberty (80-90%) then decreases but relatively high throughout the life (Stamm, 1986). Recently prevalence of gingivitis reported was less (80-85%) in India (Bhayya et al., 2010) compared to the studies conducted previously (99%). When gender wise prevalence of gingivitis was considered, males were showed poorer periodontal status (84% vs.78.3%) than the females ($p<0.01$) and the reason behind this can be attributed to the habits and consciousness of the females in doing better oral hygiene practices (Mehta et al., 2010). Even allowing for the differences in measurement techniques between the surveys, there appears to have been an improvement in gingival health in recent decades, which might be due to improvement in socio-economic status and education. In the NHANES III Survey, 50% of adults were found to have gingivitis. Whereas, in Sri Lankan tea workers, among whom both oral hygiene and the gingival condition were poorer at all ages, found 89 % cases were progressed beyond gingivitis to periodontitis (Loe et al., 1986). It suggests that higher prevalence and severity of gingivitis in developing countries was associated with extensive plaque and calculus deposits, low socio-economic status and education as compared to the peoples of developed countries. It has frequently been found that some gingival sites make the transition from being periodontally healthy to gingivitis may be due to genetic variability, stress, female sex hormones and higher dosages of oral contraceptives. The interproximal areas of teeth are most severely affected by gingivitis followed by buccal and lingual surface respectively. The interproximal and buccal surfaces of upper arch are more affected by gingivitis than lower arch and the relationship is reversed in the lingual surfaces (Löe et al., 1965). For facial surfaces, the areas most severely affected by gingivitis, in descending order, were the maxillary first and second molars, the mandibular anteriors, maxillary anteriors, maxillary premolars, mandibular first and second molars, and the mandibular premolars. Gingivitis most severely affected in the lingual surfaces, in descending order, were the mandibular first and second molars, mandibular premolars, mandibular anteriors, maxillary first and second molars, maxillary premolars, and the maxillary anteriors.

4.10 Incidence of periodontitis

Incidence of periodontal disease is not only means the onset of new disease in previously disease free adults in strict sense, but also refers to the development of new sites of periodontal lesions in diseased mouth and progression of existing attachment loss (i.e., progression of disease in already diseased sites). Incidence of periodontitis varies according to the case definition of the disease. The more severe the extent of attachment loss or bone loss that is taken as case definition, the lower will be the incidence of periodontitis (Oringer et al., 1998). Although some cross-sectional studies have confirmed in identifying age as a risk factor for progression of CAL (Papapanou & Wennstrom, 1990) but most of the longitudinal studies have shown progression of CAL is more closely related to the extent of baseline CAL than to age (Beck et al, 1990). A previous disease episode did not put a site at higher risk for a subsequent attack.

4.11 Prevalence of periodontitis

Among the basic clinical measures for periodontitis (bleeding on probing, presence of local factors, probing depth, bone loss), loss of clinical attachment (CAL), a measure of accumulated past disease at a site rather than current activity, remains a "gold standard" diagnostic method for periodontitis. The standard deviation of repeated CAL measurements of the same site by an experienced examiner with a manual probe is around 0.8 mm (Haffajee & Socransky, 1986). Accordingly, change in attachment level in a clinical study needs to be at least 2 mm (i.e., two to three times the standard deviation) to estimate the real change rather than measurement error. Therefore, CAL cut off limit of 1 mm, needs to be increased for the reasons of examiner reliability discussed above. Any prevalence information must be interpreted in light of the population studied and the periodontitis case definition (sites, extent) applied. The older belief was that susceptibility to periodontal diseases was virtually universal. Today, it is well documented that only 5% to 15% of any population suffers from severe generalized periodontitis, even though mild to moderate disease affects a majority of adults (Oliver et al., 1998). Periodontitis was regarded for years as primarily the outcome from bacterial infection. The concept has been changed and the host response is now seen as a key factor for development of periodontitis, which often modified by behavioral and environmental factors (Page et al., 1997). Body's immune system generate inflammatory response in an attempt to protect itself from pathogens but at the same time inflammatory mediators can lead to periodontal connective tissue and bone destruction. In India, prevalence of chronic periodontitis was increased steadily with age from 35% for 35-40 years age group to 85% for 80-90 years old (mean 21-30%), whereas prevalence of aggressive periodontitis was below 1% and the loss of attachment (3 mm or more) was 45-77% in 35-44 year age group and 55-96% in 65-74 year olds (Jacob, 2010). The general trend for loss of attachment observed was higher in rural than in urban Indians and was higher in males compared to females. The previous belief was that higher prevalence and severity of periodontitis existed among populations of developing nations than the developed nations, has not been confirmed by most studies (Baelum et al., 1997). Comparing the groups of Norwegian and Sri Lankan young adults, found strikingly similar rates of periodontal breakdown, despite the last group having much poorer oral hygiene conditions. Clear differences are only apparent in poorer oral hygiene and greater calculus accumulation in even a young age group in populations of developing countries (Loe et al., 1986). Thus, the prevalence and severity of the disease can be considered far more similar between different populations and are confined to small groups at high risk in each population. Prevalence of periodontitis is greater in patients with teeth present in one side of the arch than teeth present in the both side of the arch. Supra gingival calculus is most commonly found on the maxillary first molars followed by mandibular anteriors, and least on maxillary anteriors. Sub gingival calculus is commonly found, in the descending order, on the mandibular central and lateral incisors, maxillary first and second molars, maxillary anteriors and least commonly found on mandibular premolars and third molars. Supra gingival and sub gingival calculus (i.e., combined measurement) are most commonly found on the mandibular central and lateral incisors followed by the maxillary first molars and least commonly found on mandibular premolars and third molars. In general, severity of periodontitis follows the distribution pattern of subgingival and combined measurement of calculus; thus, incisors and molars are more severely involved than canine and premolar areas (least involvement).

4.12 Risk factors affecting prevalence and severity of periodontal diseases

According to current understanding of the pathogenesis of periodontal disease, it is essential to look at factors that may play a role in the initiation and progression of the disease. The risk factors that cannot be modified (e.g., age, sex, genetics) is often reffered to as determinant. The term risk indicator describes possible correlates of disease identified in case-control studies, and risk factor is best applied to those correlates confirmed in longitudinal (cohort) study and implies a modifiable condition.

4.12.1 Determinants of periodontitis

Age: The prevalence and severity of CAL is invariably related directly to age in cross-sectional surveys (Miller et al., 1987). But the older assumption that periodontitis is a disease of aging is no longer tenable. It is uncommon for elderly people with reasonably good periodontal health to exhibit sudden bursts of periodontitis (Page, 1984). The most rapid disease progression is seen in relatively small number of elderly persons in whom the disease starts at younger age, and there is some evidence that these individuals have some genetic susceptibility to periodontitis. It can be hypothesized that prevalence of the disease increases with age may be due to cumulative periodontal breakdown over time as a result of prolonged exposure to other risk factors (i.e., drug, altered food habits, lack of dexterity to maintain oral hygiene) rather than age related intrinsic deficiency which increases susceptibility to periodontal diseases (Genco, 1986). Although certain physiological changes in the periodontium occur with age but these changes alone are not responsible for periodontal breakdown in the elderly (Van der Velden, 1984). In contrast, age is an important factor for assessment of prognosis. The lesser extent of loss of attachment in younger patients should be considered more detrimental than greater extent of attachment loss in older age groups because younger patients have to be faced longer periods of exposure to offending agents. **Sex**: In one study, after adjusting age, oral hygiene and socio-economic status, males were found to have significantly greater extent of attachment loss and alveolar bone loss compared to females (Grossi, 1995). In another study, it was observed that males had consistently 10% higher prevalence of attachment loss than females (Miller et al., 1987). Increased prevalence and severity of periodontal disease in males are more likely due to less positive attitudes toward oral health, and dental-visit than to any genetic cause. However, the relationship observed between sex and the disease is not considered as strong and consistent. **Socioeconomic Status (SES):** The possible relationship between periodontal disease and socio-economic status was found in many studies (Locker & Leake, 1993). Generally, those who are better educated, rich, and live in more desirable circumstances enjoy better health status than the less educated and poor people. Gingival condition and poor oral hygiene are clearly related to lower SES, but the direct relationship between periodontitis and SES has been poorly established. It was found that the prevalence of CAL at all levels of severity was not closely related to household income (Miller et al., 1987). On the other hand, severe CAL (≥5 mm) in at least one site was closely correlated with educational levels due probably to better oral hygiene among the educated people (Miller et al., 1987). The racial/ethnic differences in periodontal status have been thought unlikely to represent true genetic differences. **Genetics:** The association between severe periodontitis and interleukin (IL)-1 specific genotype was found only in non-smokers (Kornman et al., 1997), suggested that the genetic factor was not as strong a risk factor as smoking. The strength of association between genetics and periodontitis is still being determined because IL-1 has been identified as a contributory cause of periodontitis among some patients only. However, a combination of IL-1 polymorphism and smoking may provide a good risk profile for patients (McDevitt et al., 2000); therefore, smoking–genetic interaction may be considered as a contributory factor in severity of periodontitis. Further research are needed before concluding remarks on genetic contribution in the initiation and progression of periodontitis, till then, restraining from smoking would be a higher priority than a search for genetic cause. **Race, Place, and History** of **previous periodontal diseases**: The advanced periodontal breakdown have been shown three times more prevalent in blacks than in the whites (Beck et al., 1990). Racial differences in education, socio-economic status and the distribution of genetic factors may also contribute to differences in the prevalence and severity of periodontal disease. Low prevalence of periodontitis-associated interleukin (IL)-1α/IL-1β composite genotype among Chinese suggesting their inherited resistance to develop severe and lower prevalence of periodontitis (Armitage et al., 2000). Prevalence and extent of periodontal disease is slightly more in rural areas but is not likely due to progression of current disease.

4.12.2 Risk factors

Plaque, Microbiota, and Oral Hygiene: In earlier studies, strong positive correlation has been found between poor oral hygiene and periodontal diseases (Greene & Vermillion, 1964). Bacteria that accumulate in dental plaque are primary causative agents of gingivitis. A study demonstrated the inverse relationship of meticulous oral hygiene practice (brushing frequency) with that of level of periodontal disease and tooth loss in patients with periodontal pocket (Merchant et al., 2002). But poor oral hygiene does not imply that all patients would be suffered from periodontitis rather the relationship is less straightforward. It has been shown that colonisation of virulent bacteria is necessary, but not sufficient to initiate the disease process. There is an interaction of bacterial factors with other favourable host and environmental factors which may dramatically modify the disease expression (Page et al., 1997). So poor oral hygiene is an important risk factor in susceptible persons and is of less important in individual with strong host resistance. Longitudinal data are available which dictates neglected dental care increases the prevalence and severity of periodontal disease. Frequent professional supragingival cleaning and good personal oral hygiene have been shown to have a beneficial effect on subgingival microbiota in shallow to moderately deep pockets (Westfelt, 1996). These finding form an evidence base for control of supragingival plaque as part of periodontal therapy. The resistance of host and other factors such as smoking and some systemic diseases are recently thought to overweigh the role of bacterial pathogens in the pathogenesis of periodontitis. Tissue destruction may be initiated and progressed by both direct and indirect effects of bacteria plus the effects of the altered host defence system. **Tobacco:** Smoking is clearly a risk factor for chronic periodontitis, independent of oral hygiene, age, or other factors but its role in gingivitis is unclear (Ismail et al., 1983). The risk of periodontitis attributed to smoker in the order of 2.5 to 6.0 or even higher compared to its nonuse and risk increases with increasing in frequency of exposure (Bergstrom & Preber, 1994). Exactly how it acts in the causal chain is still unclear. It has been stated that 90% of persons with refractory chronic periodontitis are smokers (Johnson & Slach, 2001). The healing following periodontal treatment is slower in smokers may be due to inhibition of growth and attachment of fibroblasts in the periodontal ligament and in slower reduction of white blood cells at diseased sites after therapy (Christan et al., 2002). Earlier studies showed no difference in prevalence of periodontal pathogens subgingivally (Preber et al., 1992), but more recent evidence suggests that smoking appears to promote a favorable habitat for pathogenic species in shallow pockets (Haffajee & Socransky, 2002). Decreased bleeding on probing in smokers might be due to suppression the vascular reaction by nicotine and compromising host response to infection. In experimental plaque-induced gingivitis, despite the rate of plaque accumulation being equal in smokers and non-smokers, the increase in gingival vascularity in smokers was only half of that seen in the non-smokers (Bergstrom et al., 1988). This is a masking effect on the signs of inflammation and should be considered while gingival bleeding is assessed. Some studies have confirmed that smoking suppresses hemorrhagic response (Bergstrom & Bostrom, 2002). However, others have found no difference in the extent of BOP between smokers and non-smokers despite the smokers having deeper pockets (van der Weijden et al., 2001). Recent studies suggest that inflamed sites in smokers have reduced vascular density and angiogenesis compared to inflamed sites in nonsmokers, thus impairing inflammatory response and wound healing (Rezavandi et al., 2002). Therefore, further study is needed on how smoking affects gingival bleeding. Smoking inhibits granulocyte function (chemotaxis, phagocytosis) and interactions between smoking and the IL-1 genotype-positive alleles in the progression of CAL, have also been indentified (Meisel et al., 2002). Smoking aggravates all tissue-destructive diseases (periodontitis), by stimulating the production of TNF-α and various tissue degrading cytokines (Fredriksson et al., 2002). Smoking has also been shown to be a stronger risk factor for periodontitis than insulin-dependent diabetes mellitus (Moore et al., 1999). The evidence is clear that smoking is a major risk factor for periodontitis. **Systemic factors:** One of the strongest systemic factor for high prevalence and extent of periodontal disease is uncontrolled diabetes mellitus. Both the Insulin and non-insulin dependent diabetics appear to be equal risk for periodontal disease. Not only poor glycemic control is the significant risk factor for periodontal disease but it has also been suggested that effective periodontal therapy in adjunct to systemic antibiotics can have a positive effect on the control of diabetes. A substantial body of evidence suggested a bidirectional relationship between both types of diabetes and periodontal disease (Taylor, 2001). Other diseases such as HIV infection, osteoporosis, and cardiovascular disease also showed an association with periodontal diseases but exactly what relationship exists is still unknown (Nunn, 2003). **Stress:** The psychological factors (financial strain, death of relative, negative life event, examinee, military life etc.) have been proposed as risk factor for periodontal disease. Psychological factors are thought to adversely affect the host immune response and disrupt homeostasis by releasing indigenous catecholamine and steroid hormone. In other way, emotional status of poor coping individual may lead to negligence in performing oral hygiene practices, dry mouth, changes in diet habits, increased smoking and bruxism, which making the individual more susceptible to oral diseases (Monteiro da Silva et al., 1998).

Several studies evaluated the effects of emotional stressors on periodontal health and reported significant increases in mean plaque score, subgingival calculus, bleeding on probing, pocket depth, attachment loss, bone loss, and tooth loss (Moss et al., 1996). Aggressive periodontitis and necrotizing ulcerative gingivitis (NUG) are the periodontal conditions most frequently associated with psychological stress. Significantly elevated cortisol level was observed in urine with NUG patients and that returned to normal after recovery (Cohen-Cole et al., 1983). Those individuals with more psychological stress were less responsive to periodontal therapy (Axtelius et al., 1998). The exact pathological link between stress and periodontal destruction, however, has not yet been established but are probably related to impaired immune function and altered oral health behaviors. In view of the successful treatment of NUG even in presence of the stressful condition or continued smoking (Cohen-Cole et al., 1983), the association is not sufficient to assume a causal relationship between these two conditions. It strongly suggests that stress has a limited role as an etiologic factor for periodontal disease. **Nutrition**: There are no nutritional deficiencies that by themselves can cause gingivitis or periodontal pockets. Most of the information regarding association between nutrition and periodontal diseases are primarily based on animal studies and few human reports that involved severe nutritional deficiencies (Pitiphat et al., 2002). Minor nutritional imbalance failed to show any effect on periodontal health. Validation of nutrition as a risk factor for periodontal disease requires longitudinal study designs to assess the timing between the deficiency and the onset of the disease. However, it is a difficult task to set an experimental design in human because nutritional requirement and food habit changes as one progresses from birth to elderly as well as due to ethical reasons. **Obesity:** Obesity may be considered as an unique form of malnutrition. A significant association was observed between higher body mass index and periodontal disease (attachment loss) that might be mediated via insulin resistance (Grossi et al., 2000). Relative risk increases 1.3 times with each 5% increment of body fat, after adjusting age, gender, oral hygiene status and smoking history (Siato et al., 1998). However, more researches are needed before obesity can be considered as risk factor for periodontitis. **Tooth factors:** Various abnormalities of tooth anatomy (enamel projection, enamel pearl, external root grooves) have been shown to be associated with furcation involvement. In addition, abnormal positioning of tooth (crowding, extreme labial or lingual positioning, open contact, occlusal discrepancy), overhanging restoration margin, subgingival crown margin have been implicated as strong predictor of periodontal breakdown (Nunn, 2003).

4.13 Risk assessment in periodontology - A new perspective

Recent research has demonstrated that some individuals or groups of individuals experience more severe form of periodontal disease than others. Therefore, the rationale for the risk assessment in periodontology is to target appropriate levels of prevention and care for high risk individuals (Stamm et al., 1991). The aim is to identify the presence of some easily measured entity by which clinicians would predict the risk of future disease with high reliability. The current understanding of periodontal diseases has put a further fundamental step in risk assessment for the disease (Page & Beck, 1997). A risk factor must be a part of the causal chain and criteria of identifying a risk factor are to be met only in longitudinal studies, by which the disease outcome can be compared to the baseline measures. The clinical measures of plaque and calculus do not predict the future disease to any useful extent (Badersten et al., 1990). The subgingival presence of specific periopathogens has shown a moderate degree of predictability. It is now recognized that host response, smoking and genetic predisposition (IL-1 genotype) have major role in this regard. The multiple predictors work better than any one single predictor (except smoking- universal predictor) for the risk assessment. However, enough advances in our knowledge about risk factors yet to be made to permit the development of a risk calculator to help assess a patient's risk of disease.

5. Aggressive periodontitis

The primary features of aggressive periodontitis include a history of rapid attachment and bone loss with familial aggregation. Secondary features include phagocyte abnormalities and a hyperresponsive macrophage phenotype. Localized aggressive periodontitis (LAgP) patients have interproximal attachment loss on at least two permanent first molars and incisors, with attachment loss on no more than two teeth other than first molars and incisors. Generalized aggressive periodontitis (GAgP) patients exhibit generalized interproximal attachment loss including at least three teeth that are not first molars and incisors (Armitage, 1999). The onset of these diseases is often circumpubertal. With time, the localized form appears to be self-limiting ('burn out' of the disease), or may progress to GAgP with increasing age (Gunsolley et al., 1995). The incidental attachment loss should be excluded before diagnosing a case of aggressive periodontitis, in which one or more teeth had greater than 3mm attachment loss, but were not met the criteria for AgP. Reported estimates of the prevalence of LAgP and GAgp in geographically diverse young populations were ranged from 0.1% to 15% (average < 1 %), and 0.03% to 0.59% (average 0.13%) respectively (Marazita et al., 1994). In NIDR survey of adolescent (14-17 years of age), it was estimated that 0.53% had LAgP and 0.13% had GAgP and 1.61% had incidental loss of attachment and the teeth most severely affected in descending order were first molar, second molar, incisors (Löe & Brown, 1991). They reported that males had slightly higher but statistically insignificant prevalence of LAgP and GAgP. In Afro-Americans, prevalence of LAgP in male was 2.9 times more than in female, whereas, among Whites, females were 2.5 times more prone to LAgP than the males (Löe & Brown, 1991). The findings of several studies have suggested the fairly equal distribution of the disease between genders (Saxby, 1984). When genders were examined among the races, then gender differences were much more evident. A study of aggressive periodontitis involving different ethnic groups estimated the prevalence of AgP in Afro-Americans was 0.8%, Whites 0.02% and Asians 0.2% (Saxén, 1980). In general, blacks are more susceptible to AgP than the Whites. The prevalence rate among gender is followed, in descending order, as black male, black female, white female and white male. The age group mostly affected by AgP is between puberty to 30 years of age. Not all patients infected with *Actinobacillus a0.ctinomycetemcomitans* (Aa) develop LAgP and not all patients with LAgP have detectable levels of Aa (Lang et al., 1999). To date, moreover, no single species is found in all cases of LAgP. A variety of functional neutrophil defects have been reported in 70-75% patients with LAgP. These include anomalies of chemotaxis, phagocytosis, bactericidal activity, superoxide production, FcγRIIIb (CD16) expression, leukotriene B4 generation, Ca^{2+} channel and second messenger activation, abnormally low number of chemoattractant receptors and an abnormally low amount of cell surface glycoprotein GP-110 (Van Dyke et al., 1990). Adherence receptors on neutrophils and monocytes, such as LFA-1 and Mac-1, are normal in LAgP patients. Neutrophilic chemotactic defect is genetic in origin which predisposes individual to LAgP and that is the cause why the disease run in family. Not all LAP patients have neutrophilic chemotactic defect and not all neutrophilic chemotactic defect patients have LAgP (Van Dyke et al., 1990). Therefore, other unidentifiable host factor likely to be involved in the pathogenesis of AgP. GAgP, can begin at any age and often affects the entire dentition. Individuals with GAgP exhibit marked periodontal inflammation and have heavy accumulations of plaque and calculus. Neutrophils from patients with GAgP frequently exhibit similar functional defects as observed in LAgP. The antibody response, and the clinical manifestations of aggressive periodontitis are modified by patients' genetic background as well as environmental factors such as smoking (Califano et al., 1996). The two forms of aggressive periodontitis can be considered to be different diseases unlike chronic periodontitis and appear to be associated with somewhat different subgingival bacterial profiles, difference in the number of affected teeth or pattern of damage and have separate genetic risk factors (Armitage, 2010). The '1999 World Workshop on the Classification of Periodontal Diseases' recommended deletion of age-dependent terms such as adult and juvenile periodontitis (Armitage, 1999). Nevertheless, age is still an important characteristic that can be useful in differentiating between chronic and aggressive forms of periodontitis. The loss of attachment in aggressive periodontitis (approximately 1–2 mm/year) patients progressed three or four times faster than in cases of chronic periodontitis (Average 0.2 mm/year), which serves as an important characteristic to distinguish clinically both the form of the disease (Baer, 1971). The mechanisms and regulation of bone loss associated with all forms of chronic or aggressive periodontitis appear biochemically, immunologically and histologically similar with respect to the molecular mediators and pathological processes. However, there are differences in the speed at which bone loss occurs (Bartold et al., 2010). There are no striking differences in risk factors between aggressive and chronic periodontitis, although the associated gene defects may be different (Stabholz et al., 2010). The general pattern of normal random migration and impaired chemotaxis in aggressive but not in chronic forms of periodontitis, could be due to a reduction of GP110 and f-Met-Leu-Phe surface receptors on neutrophils. The mode of inheritance of aggressive periodontitis is probably autosomal dominant among the African-American and Caucasian (Marazita et al., 1994). A strong familial influence has been observed on the prevalence of both the chronic and aggressive periodontitis. In the Japanese population, a polymorphism of the Fc-γRIIIb (CD16) was described in patients with both forms of periodontitis (Loos et al., 2003). Therefore, it can be suggested that no genetic risk factors or markers are able to distinguish between aggressive periodontitis and chronic periodontitis. The other environmental factors (smoking, oral hygiene, stress, obesity) have no uniqueness to either generalized aggressive periodontitis or chronic periodontitis. Oral hygiene, as assessed by plaque levels, is directly associated with disease severity in both entities, except in the localized form of aggressive periodontitis. Systemic diseases cannot be considered as risk factors for aggressive periodontitis. However, systemic diseases that can cause subtle perturbations in host susceptibility to infections (e.g. diabetes mellitus), can alter the clinical course of both chronic periodontitis and aggressive periodontitis.

6. References

Ainamo, J.; Barmes, D.; Beagrie, G.; Cutress, T.; Martin, J. & Sardo-Infirri, J. (1982). Development of the World Health Organisation (WHO) Community Periodontal Index of Treatment Needs (CPITN). *Int Dent J*, Vol.32, pp. 281-289.

Ainamo, J & Bay, I. (1975). Problems and proposals for recording gingivitis and plaque. *Int Dent J*, Vol.25, pp. 229-235.

Armitage, G. C. (1999). Development of a classification system for periodontal diseases and conditions. *Ann Periodontol*, Vol.4, pp. 1-6.

Armitage, G.C.; Wu, Y.; Wang, H.Y.; Sorrell, J.; di Giovine, F.S. & Duff, G.W. (2000). Low prevalence of a periodontitis-associated interleukin -1composite genotype in individuals of Chinese heritage. *J Periodontol*, Vol.71, pp. 164-171.

Armitage, G.C. (2010). Comparison of the microbiological features of chronic and aggressive periodontitis. *Periodontol 2000*, Vol.53, pp. 70–88.

Axtelius, B.; Soderfeldt, B.; Nilson, A.; Edwardson, S. & Attstrom, R. (1998). Therapy-resistant periodontitis, psychological characteristics. *J Clin Periodontol*, Vol. 25, pp. 482-491.

Badersten, A.; Nilveus, R. & Egelberg, J. (1990). Scores of plaque, bleeding, suppuration and probing depth to predict probing attachment loss. 5 years of observation following nonsurgical periodontal therapy. *J Clin Periodontol*, Vol. 17, pp. 102-107.

Baelum, V.; Luan, W.M.; Chen, X. & Fejerskov, O. (1997). Predictors of destructive periodontal disease incidence and progression in adult and elderly Chinese. *Community Dent Oral Epidemiol*, Vol. 25, pp. 265–272.

Baelum, V.; Manji, F.; Wanzala, P., et al. (1995). Relationship between CPITN and periodontal attachment loss in an adult population. *J Clin Periodontol*, Vol. 22: pp. 1-6.

Baer, P.N. (1971). The case for periodontosis as a clinical entity. *J Periodontol*, Vol. 42, pp. 516–520.

Bartold, P.M.; Cantley, M.D. & Haynes, D.R. (2010). Mechanisms and control of pathological bone loss in periodontitis. *Periodontol 2000*, Vol. 53, pp. 55–69.

Beck, J.D.; Koch, G.G.; Rozier, R.G. & Tudor, G.E. (1990). Prevalence and risk indicators for periodontal attachment loss in a population of older community-dwelling blacks and whites. *J Periodontol*, Vol. 61, pp. 521-528.

Bellini, H.T. & Gjermo, P. (1973). Application of the Periodontal Treatment Need System (PTNS) in a group of Norwegian industrial employees. *Community dent oral epidemiology*, Vol. 1, pp. 22-29.

Bergstrom, J. & Bostrom, L. (2001). Tobacco smoking and periodontal hemorrhagic responsiveness. *J Clin Periodontol*, Vol. 28, pp. 680-685.

Bergstrom, J.; Persson, L. & Preber, H. (1988) Influence of cigarette smoking on vascular reaction during experimental gingivitis. *Scand J Dent Res, Vol.* 96, pp. 34-39.

Bergstrom, J. & Preber, H. (1994). Tobacco use as a risk factor. *J Periodontol*, Vol. 65(Suppl.), pp. 545-550.

Bhayya, D.P.; Shyagali, R.T. & Mallikarjun, K. (2010). Study of oral hygiene status and prevalence of gingival diseases in 10-12 year school children in Maharashtra,India. *J Int Oral Health*, Vol. 2, No. 3, pp. 21-26.

Brownson, R.C. & Pettiti, D.B. eds. (1998) *Applied Epidemiology: Theory to Practice,* Oxford University Press, New york, USA.

Califano, J.V.; Gunsolley, J.C.; Nakashima, K.; Schenkein, H.A.; Wilson, M.E. & Tew, J.G. (1996). Influence of anti-Actinobacillus actinomycetemcomitans Y4 (serotype b) lipopolysaccharide on severity of generalized early-onset periodontitis. *Infect Immun*, Vol. 64, pp. 3908-3910.

Carlos, J.P.; Wolfe, M.D. & Kingman, A. (1986). The extent and severity index: A simple method for use in epidemiologic studies of periodontal disease. *J Clin Periodontol*, Vol. 13, pp. 500-505.

Carter, H.G. & Barnes, G.P. (1974). The Gingival Bleeding Index. *J Periodontol*, Vol. 45, No. 11, pp. 801-805.

Caton, J.G. & Polson, A.M. (1985). The interdental bleeding index: a simplified procedure for monitoring gingival health. *Comp Cont Educ Dent*, Vol. 6, pp. 88-92.

Christan, C.; Dietrich, T.; Hagewald, S.; Kage, A. & Bernimoulin, J.P. (2002). White blood cell count in generalized aggressive periodontitis after non-surgical therapy. *J Clin Periodontol*, Vol. 29, pp. 201-206.

Cohen-Cole, S.A.; Cogen, R.B.; Stevens, Jr. A.W.; Kirk, K.; Gaitan, E.; Bird, J.; Cooksey, R. & Freeman, A. (1983). Psychiatric, psychological, and endocrine correlates of acute necrotizing ulcerative gingivitis (trench mouth): a preliminary report. *Psychiatr Med*, Vol. 1, pp. 215-220.

Fredriksson, M.; Bergstrom, K. & Asman, B. (2002). IL-8 and TNF-α from peripheral neutrophils and acute-phase proteins in periodontitis. *J Clin Periodontol*, Vol. 29, pp. 123-128.

Gaengler, P.; Goebel, G.; Kurbad, A. & Kosa, W. (1988). Assessment of periodontal disease and dental caries in a population survey using the CPITN, GPM/T and DMF/T indices. *Community Dent Oral Epidemiol*, Vol. 16, No. 4, pp. 236–239.

Greene, J.C. & Vermillion, J.R. (1960). The oral hygiene index: A method for classifying oral hygiene status. *J Am Dent Assoc*, Vol. 61, pp. 29-35.

Greene, J.C. & Vermillion, J.R. (1964). The simplified oral hygiene index. *J Am Dent Assoc*, Vol. 68, pp. 7-13.

Grossi, S.G.; Genco, R.J.; Machtei, E.E., et al. (1995). Assessment of risk for periodontal disease. II. Risk indicators for alveolar bone loss. *J Periodontol*, Vol. 66, pp. 23-29.

Grossi, S.G. & Ho, A.W. (2000). Obesity, insulin resistance and periodontal disease (abstract). *J Dent Res*, Vol. 79(Spec Iss), pp. 625.

Gunsolley, J.C.; Califano, J.V.; Koertge, T.E.; Burmeister, J.A.; Cooper, L.C. & Schenkein, H.A. (1995). Longitudinal assessment of early onset periodontitis. *J Periodontol*, Vol. 66, pp. 321–328.

Haffajee, A.D. 7 Socransky, S.S. (1986) Attachment level changes in destructive periodontal diseases. *J Clin Periodontol*, Vol. 13, pp. 461-475.

Haffajee, A.D. & Socransky, S.S. (2001). Relationship of cigarette smoking to the subgingival microbiota. *J Clin Periodontol*, Vol. 28, pp. 377-388.

Jacob, P.S. (2010). Periodontitis in India and Bangladesh. Need for a population based approach in epidemiological surveys. A Literature review. *Bangladesh Journal of Medical Science*, Vol. 9, No. 3, pp. 124-130.

Johnson, G.K. & Slach, N.A. (2001) Impact of tobacco use on periodontal status. *J Dent Educ*, Vol. 65, pp. 313-321.

Kornman, K.S.; Crane, A.; Wang, H.Y., et al. (1997) The interleukin-1 genotype as a severity factor in adult periodontal disease. *J Clin Periodontol*, Vol. 24, pp. 72-77.

Lang, N.; Bartold, P.M.; Cullinan, M.; Jeffcoat, M.; Mombelli, A.; Murakami, S.; Page, R.; Papapanou, P.; Tonetti, M. & Van Dyke, T. (1999) Consensus report - aggressive periodontitis. *Ann Periodontol*, Vol. 4, pp. 53.

Last, J.M. (1983). *A Dictionary of Epidemiology: A handbook sponsored by the IEA*. Oxford University Press, New York.

Lenox, J.A. & Kopczyk, R.A. (1973) A clinical system for scoring a patient's oral hygiene performance. *J Am Dent Assoc*, Vol. 86, pp. 849-852.

Lobene, R.R.; Weatherford, T.; Ross, N.M.; Lamm, R.A. & Menaker, L. (1986). A modif-ied gingival index for use in clinical trials. *Clinical Preventive Dentistry*, Vol. 8, pp. 3–6.

Locker, D. & Leake, J.L. (1993). Periodontal attachment loss in independently living older adults in Ontario, Canada. *J Public Health Dent*, Vol. 53, pp. 6-11.

Löe, H.; Anerud, A.; Boysen, H. & Morrison, E. (1986). Natural history of periodontal disease in man. Rapid, moderate and no loss of attachment in Sri Lankan laborers 14 to 46 years of age. *J Clin Periodontol*, Vol. 13, pp. 431-445.

Löe, H. & Brown, L.J. (1991). Early onset periodontitis in the United States of America. *J Periodontol*, Vol. 62, pp. 608-616.

Loe, H. & Silness, J. (1963) Periodontal disease in pregnancy. *Acta Odontol Scand*, Vol. 21, pp. 533-551.

Loe, H.; Theilade, E. & Jensen, S.B. (1965) Experimental gingivitis in man. *J Periotloutol*, Vol. 36, pp. 177-187.

Loos, B.G.; Leppers-van de Straat, F.G.; van de Winkel, J.G. & van der Velden, U. (2003) Fc-gamma receptor polymorphisms in relation to periodontitis. *J Clin Periodontol*, Vol. 30, pp. 595–602.

Marazita, M.L.; Burmeister, J.A.; Gunsolley, J.C.; Koertge, T.E.; Lake, K. & Schenkein, H.A. (1994) Evidence for autosomal dominant inheritance and race-specific heterogeneity in earlyonset periodontitis. *J Periodontol*, Vol. 65, pp. 623-630.

McDevitt, M.J.; Wang, H.Y.; Knobelman, C., et al. (2000) Interleukin-1 genetic association with periodontitis in clinical practice. *J Periodontol*, Vol. 71, pp. 156-163.

Mehta, R.; Kundu, D.; Chakrabarty, S. & Bharati, P. (2010). Periodontal conditions and treatment in urban and rural population of West Bengal, India. *Asian Pacific Journal of Tropical Medicine*, pp. 152-157.

Meisel, P.; Siegemund, A.; Dombrowa, S.; Sawaf, H.; Fanghaenel, J. & Kocher, T. (2002). Smoking and polymorphisms of the interleukin-1 gene cluster (IL-1α, IL-1β, and IL-1RN) in patients with periodontal disease. *J Periodontol*, Vol. 73, pp. 27-32.

Merchant, A.; Pitiphat, W.; Douglass, C.W.; Crohin, C. & Joshipura, K. (2002) Oral hygiene practices and periodontitis in health care professionals. *J Periodontol*, Vol. 73, pp. 531-535.

Miller, A.K.; Brunelle, J.A.; Carlos, J.P.; Brown, L.J. & Loe, H. (1987). Oral Health of United States Adults; National Findings.: Bethesda, MD: U.S. Public Health Service, National Institute of Dental Research;. NIH publication number 87-2868.

Monteiro da Silva, A.M.; Newman, H.N.; Oakley, D.A. & O'Leary, R. (1998) Psychological factors, dental plaque levels and smoking in periodontitis patients. *J Clin Periodontol*, Vol. 25, pp. 517-523.

Moore, P.A.; Weyant, R.J.; Mongelluzzo, M.B., et al. (1999). Type 1 diabetes mellitus and oral health: Assessment of periodontal disease. *J Periodontol*, Vol. 70, pp. 409-417.

Moss, M.E.; Beck, J.D.; Kaplan, B.H.; Offenbacher, S.; Weintraub, J.A.; Koch, G.; Genco, R.J.; Machtei, E.E. & Tedesco, L.A. (1996) Exploratory case-control analysis of psycho-logical factors and adult periodontitis. *J Periodontol*, Vol. 67 (Suppl 10): pp. 1060-1069.

Muhlemann, H.R. & Mazor, Z.S. (1958) Gingivitis in Zurich school children. *Helv Odontol Acta,*Vol. 2, pp. 3.

Nakagawa, S.; Fujii, H.; Machida, Y.; Okud, K. (1994). A longitudinal study from prepuberty to puberty of gingivitis. Correlation between the occurrence of Prevotella intermedia and sex hormones. *J Clin Periodontol,* Vol. 21, pp. 658–665.

Nunn, M.E. (2003). Understanding the etiology of Periodontitis: an overview of periodontal risk factors. *Periodontol 2000,* Vol. 32, pp. 11-23.

O'Leary, T.J.; Gibson, W.A.; Shannon, I.L.; Schuessler, C.F. & Nabers, C.L. (1963) A screening examination for detection of gingival and periodontal breakdown and local irritants. *Periodontics,* Vol. 1, pp. 167-174.

Oliver, R.C.; Brown, L.J. & Löe, H. (1998). Periodontal diseases in the United States population. *J Periodontol,* Vol. 69, pp. 269-278.

Oringer, R.J.; Fiorellini, J.P.; Reasner, D.S. & Howell, T.H. (1998). The effect of different diagnostic thresholds on incidence of disease progression. *J Periodontol,* Vol. 69, pp. 872-878.

Page, R.C. & Beck, J.D. (1997). Risk assessment for periodontal diseases. *Int Dent J,* Vol. 47, pp. 61- 87.

Page, R.C.; Offenbacher, S.; Schroeder, H.E.; Seymour, G.J. & Kornman, K.S. (1997) Advances in the pathogenesis of periodontitis: Summary of developments, clinical implications and future directions. *Periodontol 2000,* Vol. 14, pp. 216-248.

Page, R.C. (1984). Periodontal diseases in the elderly: A critical evaluation of current information. *Gerodontol,* Vol. 3, pp. 63-70.

Papapanou, P.N. & Wennstrom, J.L. (1990). A 10-year retrospective study of periodontal disease progression. Clinical characteristics of subjects with pronounced and minimal disease development. *J Clin Periodontol,* Vol. 17, pp. 78-84.

Preber, H.; Bergstrom, J. & Linder, L.E. (1992). Occurrence of periopathogens in smoker and non-smoker patients. *J Clin Periodontol,* Vol. 19, No.9 Pt. 1, pp. 667-671.

Ramfjord, S.P. (1959). Indices for Prevalence and incidence of periodontal disease. *J Periodontol,* Vol. 30, pp. 51-59.

Ramfjord, S.P. (1967). The Periodontal Disease Index (PDI). *J Periodontol,* Vol. 38, pp.602.

Rezavandi, K.; Palmer, R.M.; Odell, E.W.; Scott, D.A. & Wilson, R.F. (2002) Expression of ICAM-1 and E-selectin in gingival tissues of smokers and non-smokers with periodontitis. *J Oral Pathol Med,* Vol. 31, pp. 59–64.

Russell, A.L. (1956) A system of classification and scoring for prevalence surveys of periodontal disease. *J Dent Res,* Vol. 35, pp. 350-359.

Ryder, M.I. (2010). Comparison of neutrophil functions in aggressive and chronic periodontitis. *Periodontol 2000,* Vol. 53, pp. 124–137.

Saxby, M.S. (1984). Sex ratio in juvenile periodontitis: the value of epidemiological studies. *Community Dent Health,* Vol. 1, pp. 29-32.

Saxén, L. (1980). Juvenile periodontitis. *J Clin Periodontol,* Vol. 7, pp. 1-19.

Schour, I. & Massler, M. (1948). Survey of gingival disease using the PMA index. *J Dent Res,* Vol. 27, pp. 733-734.

Shick, R.A. & Ash, M.M. Jr. (1961). Evaluation of the vertical method of toothbrushing. *J Periodontol,* Vol. 32, pp. 346-53.

Siato, T.; Shimazaki, Y. & Sakamoto, M. (1998). Obesity and periodontitis. *N Engl J Med,* Vol. 339, pp. 482-483.

Silness, P. & Loe, H. (1964). Periodontal disease in pregnancy. *Acta Odontol Scand*, Vol. 22, pp. 121-135.

Stabholz, A.; Soskolne, W.A.; Shapira, L. (2010). Genetic and environmental risk factors for chronic periodontitis and aggressive periodontitis. *Periodontol 2000*, Vol. 53, pp. 138–153.

Stamm, J.W.; Steward, P.W.; Bohannan, H.M.; Disney, J.A.; Graves, R.C. & Abernathy, J.R. (1991). Risk assessment for oral diseases. *Adv Dent Res*, Vol. 5, pp. 4-17.

Stamm, J.W. (1986). Epidemiology of gingivitis. *J Clin Periodontol*, Vol. 13, pp. 360-370.

Taylor, G.W. (2001). Bidirectional interrelationships between diabetes and periodontal diseases: an epidemiologic perspective. *Ann Periodontol*, Vol. 6, pp. 99-112.

Third National Health and Nutrition Examination Survey, 1988-94. (1997) Hyattsville, MD: Centers for Disease Control, Public use data file no. 7-0627.

Van der Velden. (1984). Effect of age on the periodontium. *J Clin Periodontol*, Vol. 11, pp. 281-294.

van der Weijden, G.A.; de Slegte, C.; Timmerman, M.F. & van der Velden, U. (2001) Periodontitis in smokers and non-smokers: Intra-oral distribution of pockets. *J Clin Periodontol*, Vol. 28, pp. 955-960.

Van Dyke, T.E.; Levine, M.J. & Genco, R.J. (1985). Neutrophil function and oral disease. *J Oral Pathol*, Vol. 14, pp. 95-120.

Van Dyke, T.E.; Warbington, M.; Gardner, M. & Offenbacher, S. (1990) Neutrophil surface protein markers as indicators of defective chemotaxis in LJP. *J Periodontol* Vol. 61, pp. 180-184.

Westfelt, E. (1996). Rationale of mechanical plaque control. *J Clin Periodontol*, Vol. 23, No. 3, pp. 263-267.

12

Periodontal Diseases in Greek Senior Citizens-Risk Indicators

Eleni Mamai-Homata[1], Vasileios Margaritis[1], Argy Polychronopoulou[1], Constantine Oulis[1] and Vassiliki Topitsoglou[2]
[1]Dental School, National and Kapodistrian University of Athens
[2]Dental School, Aristotle University of Thessaloniki
Greece

1. Introduction

Periodontal diseases are among the most common chronic diseases affecting people of all ages worldwide. However, their severe forms are more pronounced in older individuals primarily due to prolonged exposure to risk factors. One of the major risk factors of periodontal diseases is considered to be poor oral hygiene since the accumulation of dental plaque biofilms on clean tooth surfaces results in the development of an inflammatory process encompassing local gingival and periodontal tissues around teeth (Albandar, 2002). If the microbial film is not removed the local inflammation will persist and chronic gingivitis will be developed. Hence, dental plaque is considered today the primary etiologic factor of chronic gingivitis, while chronic periodontitis is now seen as resulting from a complex interplay of bacterial infection and host response, often modified by local factors within the mouth, systemic factors related to the host, and external (environmental) factors (Albandar, 2002).

For example, current preventive oral health practices, such as frequent tooth brushing and flossing as well as regular dental attendance, were found to be significantly associated with lower plaque, gingivitis and calculus scores (Lang et al., 1995). In addition, through these associations, the aforementioned preventive behaviors appeared to be indirectly related to shallower pocket depths and less attachment loss (Lang et al., 1995). Furthermore, socio-demographic variables like area of residence, gender, education and income are considered as risk indicators for periodontal diseases (Albandar, 2002; Locker & Leake 1992; Mamai-Homata et al., 2010)

Some of these, as well as other variables that have been associated with periodontal status may change overtime and therefore the prevalence and severity of periodontal diseases in a population may also change. Therefore, periodic surveys of the periodontal health status of the population and redetermination of the variables that may affect the initiation and/or progression of periodontal diseases are needed.

In Greece, a national oral health pathfinder survey was organized in 1985 by the dental department of the Ministry of Health, Welfare and Social Security in cooperation with the Regional Office for Europe of the World Health Organization. The purpose of that survey was to evaluate the oral health status and treatment needs of the population aged 7, 12 and 35-44 years-old and formulate measures for the prevention of dental caries and the elimination of periodontal diseases.

Twenty years later the Hellenic Dental Association in cooperation with the Dental Schools of Athens and Thessaloniki decided to carry out a second national oral health pathfinder survey in order to investigate trends in oral diseases epidemiology. In this survey the 65-74-years-old group was also included since the aging of the population in Greece (Karagiannaki, 2005), as in most industrialized countries (WHO, 1996), and the economic, social and health consequences of this demographic evolution made the investigation of the oral health of the elderly very important.

In this chapter, the oral hygiene behavior and dental attendance of Greek senior citizens aged 65-74-years-old will be analyzed, in relation to certain socio-demographic variables. Furthermore, their periodontal and oral hygiene status will be presented and the variations in these measures according to socio-demographic and behavioral parameters will be outlined.

2. Material and methods

A stratified cluster sample was selected according to WHO guidelines for national pathfinder surveys, which ensures the participation of a satisfactory size of people that may present different disease prevalence in the conditions that are being examined (WHO, 1997). The study covered two big cities (Athens and Thessaloniki), six counties (Achaia, Chania, Evros, Ioannina, Kastoria, Larissa) and three islands (Lesbos, Naxos and Kefallinia). Three communities of different socio-economic backgrounds were selected randomly within each of the big cities, while one urban and one rural community were selected randomly within each county or island. Therefore, the survey was conducted in 24 sites (15 urban and 9 rural) and 50 subjects were examined in each site. Samples of subjects aged 65-74 years were drawn from their homes and day centers for the elderly, according to WHO national pathfinder survey methodology for these age groups (WHO, 1997). The sample consisted of 1093 65-74-year-old senior citizens of Greek nationality, leaving in urban and rural areas. Three hundred and forty four (344) of the subjects examined (31.5%) were edentulous in both jaws and were excluded from the present study. Therefore, the final sample consisted of 749 dentate individuals aged 65-74 years.

Prior to the survey, a meeting was organized in Athens Dental School to train and calibrate the examiners. Inter- examiner reliability and agreement was assessed with an experienced investigator as gold standard. For the examined indices, levels of concordance were very good (kappa coefficient > 0.85). The examinations were carried out under artificial light (daray lamps) using dental mirrors and the WHO CPI periodontal probe. Cotton rolls and gauze were available for moisture control and removal of plaque when necessary.

The recorded variables were periodontal and oral hygiene status. The periodontal conditions were measured using the Community Periodontal Index (CPI) (WHO, 1997) and are presented according to the highest score recorded for each person (indicating the prevalence of conditions) and the mean number of sextants by score per person (indicating the severity or extent of the problem). The oral hygiene status was recorded by means of the simplified Oral Hygiene Index (OHI-S) (Green & Vermillion, 1964) and its scores were classified into three levels as described by Greene (Greene, 1967).

Socio-demographic (gender, area, education, monthly income) and behavioural (tooth brushing frequency, flossing frequency and reason for dental attendance) data reported to be associated with oral health were collected through a structured questionnaire that was completed face-to- face at the time of the clinical examination. The classification of education was based on the total number of years of education and was divided in four categories (6 years or less, 9 years, 12 years and more than 12 years). The economic status of the participants was recorded according to their monthly income and it was divided in two income categories (≤590 € and ≥591 €). Tooth brushing frequency was classified in four categories (never, <once a day, once a day and >once a day), while flossing frequency was classified in three categories (never, <once a day and ≥once a day). Finally, the surveyed population was divided in three categories according to the usual reason for dental attendance (pain, treatment, check-up).

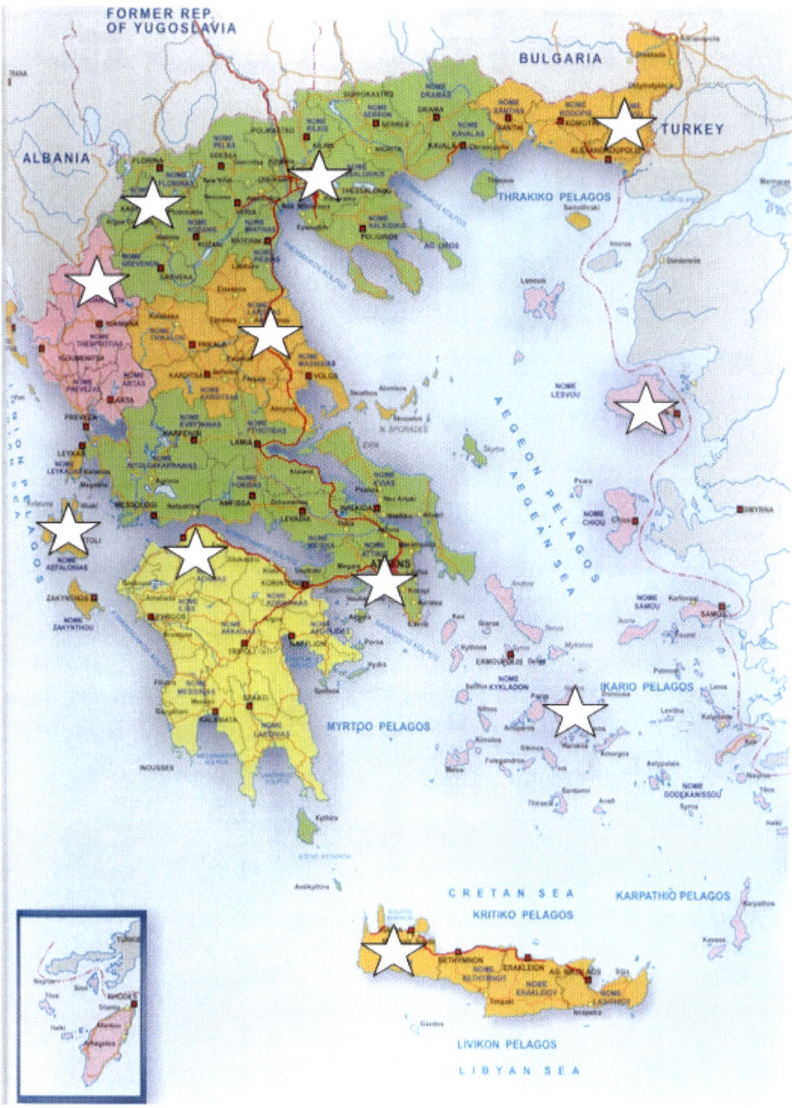

Fig. 1. Map of Greece. White stars represent the regions where the survey took place.

2.1 Data analysis

The outcome variables were oral health behaviours and attitude of the subjects (brushing frequency, flossing frequency and reason for dental visits), as well as CPI and OHI-s scores. The statistical analyses were conducted in three main stages. First, the prevalence of each dependent variable in the sample was calculated. Second, the potential effect of each socio-demographic factor (gender, area, education and monthly income) on the aforementioned variables was investigated univariately. Chi-square test was used to test the strength of associations between independent and categorical sample proportions. Mann-Whitney and Kruskall-Wallis tests were also conducted due to the non-Gaussian distribution of the mean number of sextants per CPI score.

Finally, the estimates of the relative risks of all outcome variables were reported by calculating the odds ratios (ORs) and the corresponding 95% confidence intervals (CIs), using ordinal and binary logistic regression analysis. The independent predictors were socio-demograhic and behavioural data. Significant confounders, as well as interactions were retained in the models. Deviance residuals were calculated in order to evaluate the model's goodness-of-fit. All reported probability values (p-values) were based on two-sided tests and compared to a significant level of 5%. The analysis of coded data was carried out using SPSS software version 19.0.

3. Results

3.1 Behavioural parameters

The reported tooth brushing frequency of Greek senior citizens according to their socio-demographic characteristics is presented in table 1. Regular tooth brushing (≥twice a day) was claimed by only 25.3% of the respondents, while most of them reported that they brushed their teeth once a day (33.0%). The percentages of those reporting that they never brushed their teeth (14.5%) or that they brushed their teeth less than once a day (27.2%) were relatively high.

The univariate analysis of the data (table 1) showed that women and those living in urban areas tended to brush teeth more often than men and those living in rural areas. Also, the educational level was found to positively affect the tooth brushing frequency of the surveyed population. However, when multivariate analysis was undertaken (table 2), only being a woman and having a high educational attainment increased the odds of having better tooth brushing habits.

Flossing frequency, as reported by the respondents is presented in table 3. Most subjects reported that they never used dental floss (92.5%), and only 3.1% that they used it once a day. Those living in urban areas used dental floss more frequently than those living in rural ones. The educational level as well as monthly income were found to positively affect the usage of dental floss. The results of the multiple regression modeling (table 4) showed that area of residence and education remained significant predictors of dental floss usage. Residents of urban areas and those with a high educational level were 8.5 times more likely to use dental floss regularly.

The distribution of participants according to the usual reason for dental attendance is shown in table 5. Most subjects (60.1%) reported visiting the dentist because of pain, 26.9% for treatment and only 13.0% for check-up. The percentage of people that attended the dentist because of pain was significantly higher amongst those living in rural areas and decreased significantly as their educational level and monthly income increased. Of all the statistically significant variables found in the initial univariate analyses, only high education was found to increase the likelihood of visiting the dentist for check-up in the multivariate model (table 6).

3.2 Clinical parameters

The mean DI-S, CI-S and OHI-S values in the overall sample were 1.06, 0.83 and 1.90 respectively. The classification of participants according to their OHI-S score showed that most subjects (43.0%) had good oral hygiene status (table 7). However, the percentage of those with poor oral hygiene was relatively high (21.3%). Women had better oral hygiene status than men. The percentage of people with poor oral hygiene status decreased significantly as their educational level and monthly income increased. Those with better oral hygiene habits (more frequent brushing and flossing) and those who used to visit the dentist for check-up had significantly better oral hygiene status. No significant differences were found between individuals living in rural or urban areas.

When all the socio-demographic and behavioural variables were introduced in multiple regression analysis to control for the effects of confounding factors gender, area, tooth brushing frequency and reason for dental attendance were found to strongly predict oral hygiene status (table 8). Being a woman, living in an urban area, brushing teeth at least once a day and visiting a dentist for check-up increased the odds of having better oral hygiene status.

Table 9 shows the distribution of the study population by CPI scores for each socio-demographic and behavioral characteristic. Since nine dentate subjects had a score X (excluded) in all sextants (the required two teeth were not present or were indicated for extraction), the final sample in the present analysis consisted of 740 individuals.

The percentage of subjects with healthy periodontium in the overall sample was 8.4%. The most frequently observed condition was shallow pockets of 4-5 mm (44.5%). Deep pockets of more than 6 mm were found in 15.4% of the subjects. Calculus with or without bleeding was present in the 23.5% of the population surveyed, while bleeding on probing was found in only 8.2% of the persons examined.

The univariate analysis of the data showed that women and those living in urban areas had better periodontal condition (table 9). Also, tooth brushing and flossing frequency were found to affect positively the periodontal health of the subjects examined. No significant differences were observed by education, monthly income and reason for visiting the dentist.

The ordinal logistic regression analysis (table 10) confirmed area, tooth brushing frequency and flossing frequency to be strong determinants for periodontal health in the surveyed population. Residents of rural areas experienced more periodontal diseases, while frequent daily tooth brushing and daily usage of dental floss resulted in lower CPI scores

The mean numbers of sextants by score per person are presented in table 11. On average there were 0.72 healthy sextants, 0.72 with bleeding on probing, 0.81 with calculus, 1.20 with shallow pockets and 0.25 with deep pockets, while a large proportion of sextants (2.36) were excluded due to tooth loss.

		Percent of participants who brush teeth			
Independent variables	**N**	**Never**	**<Once a day**	**Once a day**	**≥Twice a day**
Gender					
Women	320	9.4	19.7	36.6	34.4
Men	423	18.4	32.9	30.3	18.4
$X^2=42.404, p<0.0001$					
Area					
Rural	240	17.5	32.5	34.6	15.4
Urban	503	13.1	24.7	32.2	30.0
$X^2=19.796, p<0.0001$					
Education					
6 years or less	580	16.2	29.1	32.4	22.2
9 years	59	11.9	22.0	35.6	30.5
12 years	68	4.4	27.9	29.4	38.2
More than 12 years	31	12.9	0.0	41.9	45.2
$X^2=29.304, p<0.001$					
Monthly income (€)					
≤590	381	15.7	27.3	35.2	21.8
≥591	125	8.8	24.8	35.2	31.2
$X^2=6.919, p<0.075$					
Total	743	14.5	27.2	33.0	25.3

Table 1. Tooth brushing frequency of 65-74 year-old Greeks according to gender, area, education and monthly income.

Dependent variable	**Independent variables**	**Odds ratio**	**95% CI for Odds Ratio**	
Brushing frequency[a]	*Constant*	*0.717*		
	Gender (female vs male)	2.148	1.448	3.186
	Area (urban vs rural)	1.458	0.983	2.162
	Highest educational level	6.747	1.912	23.811
	Income ≥591€	1.106	0.689	1.776

[a] ≥1 time vs <1 time per day

Table 2. Odds ratios (OR) and 95% confidence intervals (CI) derived from multivariate binary logistic regression analysis with brushing frequency as the dependent variable in 65-74-year-old Greeks.

Independent variables	N	Percent of participants who used dental floss		
		Never	<Once a day	≥Once a day
Gender				
Women	317	90.5	6.3	3.2
Men	421	94.1	2.9	3.1
X^2=5.235, p<0.073				
Area				
Rural	237	96.6	3.0	0.4
Urban	501	90.6	5.0	4.4
X^2=10.299, p<0.006				
Education				
6 years or less	576	94.4	3.3	2.3
9 years	59	94.9	1.7	3.4
12 years	68	80.9	14.7	4.4
More than 12 years	30	76.7	6.7	16.7
X^2=40.850, p<0.0001				
Monthly income (€)				
≤590	379	94.4	4.0	2.6
≥591	125	86.4	6.4	7.2
X^2=6.920, p<0.031				
Total	738	92.5	4.3	3.1

Table 3. Flossing frequency of 65-74 year-old Greeks according to gender, area, education and monthly income.

Dependent variable	Independent variables	Odds ratio	95% CI for Odds Ratio	
Flossing frequency[a]	*Constant*	*0.004*		
	Gender (female vs male)	1.054	0.392	2.832
	Area (urban vs rural)	8.543	1.110	65.726
	Highest educational level	8.438	2.033	35.026
	Income ≥591€	1.220	0.392	3.798

[a] ≥1 time vs <1 time per day

Table 4. Odds ratios (OR) and 95% confidence intervals (CI) derived from multivariate binary logistic regression analysis with flossing frequency as the dependent variable in 65-74-year-old Greeks.

Independent variables	N	Percent of participants who attended the dentist for Pain	Treatment	Check-up
Gender				
Women	311	57.2	27.0	15.8
Men	414	62.3	26.8	10.9
X^2=4.036, p<0.133				
Area				
Rural	233	73.4	14.2	12.4
Urban	492	53.9	32.9	13.2
X^2=30.797, p<0.0001				
Education				
6 years or less	563	63.9	26.3	9.8
9 years	59	55.9	30.5	13.6
12 years	67	44.8	29.9	25.4
More than 12 years	31	38.7	22.6	38.7
X^2=35.932, p<0.0001				
Monthly income (€)				
≤590	368	64.4	23.9	11.7
≥591	124	46.0	28.2	25.8
X^2=18.098, p<0.0001				
Total	725	60.1	26.9	13.0

Table 5. Usual reason for dental attendance of 65-74 year-old Greeks according to gender, area, education and monthly income.

Dependent variable	Independent variables	Odds ratio	95% CI for Odds Ratio	
Reason of dental attendance[a]	*Constant*	*0.088*		
	Gender (female vs male)	1.674	0.983	2.850
	Area (urban vs rural)	1.023	0.574	1.821
	Highest educational level	4.469	1.819	10.979
	Income ≥591€	1.751	0.952	3.220

[a] check-up vs pain or treatment

Table 6. Odds ratios (OR) and 95% confidence intervals (CI) derived from multivariate binary logistic regression analysis with reason of dental attendance as the dependent variable in 65-74-year-old Greeks.

Independent variables	N	DI-S mean	CI-S mean	OHI-S mean (sd)	Percent of participants who have oral hygiene		
					Good score= 0.0-1.2	Fair score= 1.3-3.0	Poor score= 3.1-6.0
Gender							
Women	299	0.84	0.61	1.48 (1.35)	53.8	33.4	12.7
Men	378	1.23	0.99	2.23 (1.72)	34.4	37.6	28.0
X^2=33.946, p<0.0001							
Area							
Rural	234	0.99	0.81	1.90 (1.55)	40.6	37.6	21.8
Urban	443	1.09	0.82	1.89 (1.64)	44.2	34.8	21.0
X^2=0.886, p<0.649							
Education							
6 years or less	512	1.13	0.87	2.03 (1.61)	37.5	39.6	22.9
9 years	54	1.00	0.65	1.65 (1.56)	53.7	27.8	18.5
12 years	66	0.73	0.69	1.42 (1.48)	62.1	21.2	16.7
More than 12 years	33	0.61	0.55	1.09 (1.23)	69.7	24.2	6.1
X^2=29.412, p<0.0001							
Monthly income (€)							
≤590	345	1.04	0.81	1.93 (1.63)	41.2	38.0	20.9
≥591	115	0.87	0.64	1.51 (1.48)	55.7	`31.3	13.0
X^2=7.894, p<0.019							
Tooth brushing frequency							
<1 time per day	271	1.45	1.16	2.67 (1.74)	24.0	37.3	38.7
≥1 time per day	395	0.79	0.57	1.35 (1.24)	56.2	34.7	9.1
X^2=105.672, p<0.0001							
Flossing frequency							
<1 time per day	618	1.07	0.83	1.90 (1.57)	42.2	36.7	21.0
≥1 time per day	23	0.47	0.29	0.76 (1.18)	73.9	21.7	4.3
X^2=9.530, p<0.009							
Reason for dental attendance							
Pain or treatment	560	1.12	0.86	1.98 (1.63)	40.2	36.6	23.2
Check-up	90	0.62	0.55	1.16 (1.14)	65.6	30.0	4.4
X^2=25.628, p<0.0001							
Total	677	1.06	0.83	1.90 (1.61)	43.0	35.7	21.3

Table 7. Oral hygiene status of 65-74-year-old Greeks, measured by the simplified oral hygiene index, according to socio-demographic and behavioral parameters.

Dependent variable	Independent variables	Odds ratio	95% CI for Odds Ratio	
OHI-S score[a]	*Constant*	*0.379*		
	Gender (female vs male)	0.350	0.179	0.686
	Area (rural vs urban)	2.566	1.349	4.881
	Highest educational level	0.608	0.071	5.202
	Income ≥591€	0.604	0.285	1.283
	Tooth brushing frequency per day (≥1 time vs <1 time)	0.214	0.118	0.388
	Flossing per day (≥1 time vs <1 time)	0.499	0.062	4.038
	Reason for dental attendance (prevention vs pain or treatment)	0.249	0.071	0.868

[a] *OHI-S score= 3 represented the cut-off point*

Table 8. Odds ratios (OR) and 95% confidence intervals (CI) derived from multivariate binary logistic regression analysis with OHI-S score as the dependent variable in 65-74-year-old Greeks.

The statistical analysis of the data (table 11) showed that the mean number of healthy sextants was significantly greater in women, those with a high educational attainment, those that brushed and flossed teeth frequently and those who attended the dentist for check-up. On the other hand, residents of rural areas and individuals that used dental floss less than once a day had more sextants with shallow pockets, while men and those who brushed teeth less than once a day had more sextants with deep pockets. The mean number of excluded sextants (score X) was significantly greater in residents of urban areas, individuals with low level of education, those that brushed and flossed teeth less than once a day and those that used to visit the dentist because of pain or for treatment.

4. Discussion

The present study, which is part of the 2nd National Pathfinder Survey on the oral health of the Greek population, is the first nationwide reference on the periodontal and oral hygiene status of non-institutionalized Greek adults aged 65-74 years. Since the simplified pathfinder sampling methodology developed by WHO was used (WHO, 1997), the sample cannot be characterized as random, but it can be considered as illustrative of the whole population, as it ensures the participation of a satisfactory size of people living in representative urban and rural areas of Greece. Furthermore, the thorough training and calibration of the examiners ensures the reliable recording of the study parameters.

Independent variables	N	Percent of persons who have as highest score 0 Healthy	1 Bleeding	2 Calculus	3 Pockets 4-5 mm	4 Pockets ≥ 6 mm
Gender						
Women	322	10.6	9.6	21.1	47.8	10.9
Men	418	6.7	7.2	25.4	41.9	18.9
X^2=15.017, p<0.005						
Area						
Rural	257	4.7	5.1	11.3	63.0	16.0
Urban	483	10.4	9.9	30.0	34.6	15.1
X^2=66.991, p<0.0001						
Education						
6 years or less	564	6.9	8.0	23.6	45.6	16.0
9 years	60	10.0	10.0	31.7	36.7	11.7
12 years	68	10.3	10.3	16.2	50.0	13.2
More than 12 years	35	17.1	8.6	28.6	37.1	8.6
X^2=13.132, p<0.360						
Monthly income (€)						
≤590	377	8.0	9.5	20.2	46.2	16.2
≥591	127	11.0	9.4	26.0	40.9	12.6
X^2=3.887, p<0.422						
Tooth brushing frequency						
<1 time per day	303	3.3	5.6	23.8	46.5	20.8
≥1 time per day	425	11.8	10.4	24.0	43.1	10.8
X^2=33.349, p<0.0001						
Flossing frequency						
<1 time per day	679	7.4	7.8	24.6	46.5	13.7
≥1 time per day	23	26.1	26.1	21.7	17.4	8.7
X^2=23.254, p<0.0001						
Reason for dental attendance						
Pain or treatment	615	7.2	8.3	24.2	44.7	15.6
Check-up	96	15.6	9.4	21.9	40.6	12.5
X^2=8.331, p<0.080						
Total	740	8.4	8.2	23.5	44.5	15.4

Table 9. Periodontal conditions of 65-74 year-old Greeks measured by CPI according to socio-demographic and behavioral variables.

Dependent variables	Independent variables	Odds ratio	95% CI for Odds ratio	
CPI scores[a]	Gender (males vs females)	1.110	0.778	1.585
	Area (rural vs urban)	2.008	1.377	2.928
	Lowest educational level	1.384	0.638	3.002
	Income ≥591€	0.989	0.643	1.620
	Tooth brushing frequency per day (≥1 time vs <1 time)	0.558	0.387	0.805
	Flossing per day day (≥1 time vs <1 time)	0.288	0.123	0.668
	Reason for dental attendance (prevention vs pain or treatment)	0.885	0.548	1.495

[a] *CPI scores: 0= healthy; 1= bleeding, 2= calculus; 3= gingival pocket (4-5mm); 4= gingival pocket (>5mm).*

Table 10. Odds ratios (OR) and 95% confidence intervals (CI) derived from ordinal logistic regression analysis with CPI scores as the dependent variables in 65-74-year-old Greeks.

Periodontal health was assessed by means of the Community Periodontal Index (CPI) that measures the prevalence and severity or extent of periodontal diseases (WHO, 1997). The CPI recording system has attracted much criticism (Jenkins & Papapanou, 2001; Leroy et al., 2010) mainly because it does not measure tooth mobility or attachment loss and therefore increasingly underestimates periodontal disease extent and severity with increasing age. However, it is a simple, not time consuming index (Pilot & Miyazaki, 1994; Benigeri et al., 2000) that may provide useful data for planning and adjustment of preventive and treatment services in a population. It also constitutes the major source of descriptive epidemiological data on periodontal diseases in many countries, allowing international comparisons

Oral hygiene level was assessed using the simplified Oral Hygiene Index (OHI-S). A limitation of this index is that it scores the extent of plaque on the exposed tooth surface. Thus, it does not take into account the mass of plaque in the gingival margin that is considered more important in the pathogenesis of periodontal diseases. Yet, it is an easy to use index because its criteria are objective, the examination can be carried out quickly and a high level of reproducibility is possible with minimum training of the examiners. In addition, it has been widely used to evaluate the level of oral cleanliness in epidemiological studies.

Independent variables	Mean number of sextants with CPI score					
	0 Healthy	1 Bleeding	2 Calculus	3 Pockets 4-5 mm	4 Pockets ≥6 mm	X Excluded
Gender						
Women	0.87*	0.85*	0.63*	1.33	0.20*	2.23
Men	0.60*	0.60*	0.96*	1.12	0.29*	2.45
*Mann-Whitney U test, *p<0.05*						
Area						
Rural	0.59	0.73	0.50*	1.84*	0.22	2.11*
Urban	0.77	0.69	0.97*	0.91*	0.26	2.48*
*Mann-Whitney U test, *p<0.05*						
Education						
6 years or less	0.61*	0.68	0.82	1.24	0.24	2.47*
9 years	0.78*	0.86	1.03	1.05	0.22	2.03*
12 years	0.94*	0.88	0.60	1.37	0.34	1.88*
More than 12 years	1.87*	0.74	0.90	0.58	0.19	1.71*
*Kruskal-Wallis test, *p<0.05*						
Monthly income (€)						
≤590	0.78	0.72	0.64	1.33	0.22	2.41
≥591	0.91	0.68	0.86	0.92	0.29	2.31
Mann-Whitney U test, p>0.05						
Tooth brushing frequency						
<1 time per day	0.32*	0.51*	0.91	1.25	0.30*	2.72*
≥1 time per day	1.00*	0.85*	0.75	1.19	0.20*	2.08*
*Mann-Whitney U test, *p<0.05*						
Flossing frequency						
<1 time per day	0.67*	0.70	0.82	1.24*	0.25	2.39*
≥1 time per day	2.22*	1.35	0.83	0.61*	0.09	0.91*
*Mann-Whitney U test, *p<0.05*						
Reason for dental attendance						
Pain or treatment	0.56*	0.68	0.81	1.19	0.24	2.58*
Ceck-up	1.75*	0.98	0.80	1.27	0.31	0.92*
*Mann-Whitney U test, *p<0.05*						
Total	0.72	0.72	0.81	1.20	0.25	2.36

Table 11. Mean number of sextants per CPI score among 65-74 years-old Greeks according to socio-demographic and behavioral variables.

4.1 Behavioral parameters

The analysis of the data concerning the oral hygiene behavior of the surveyed population showed that regular tooth brushing (≥2 times per day) was reported by only one quarter of the dentate subjects, while less than one tenth of seniors used dental floss. Similar findings have been reported for the populations of Lithuania (Petersen et al., 2000) and China (Zhu et al., 2005). However, in most industrialized countries, the percentages of senior citizens claiming to use dental floss and brush teeth regularly or at least once a day were much higher (Chadwick et al.; Christensen et al., 2003; Davidson et al., 1997; Murtomaa et al., 1994; Payne & Locker, 1992; Whelton et al., 2007). In the present study, as in all other relevant studies (Chadwick et al.2011; Christensen et al.,2003; Payne & Locker, 1992; Whelton et al., 2007) flossing frequency was much lower than brushing frequency probably because flossing is a more complex activity requiring more time and a certain degree of manual dexterity.

In some surveys tooth brushing and/or flossing was reported as being less frequent in older age groups (Christensen et al., 2003; Davidson et al., 1997; Kelly et al., 2000; Payne & Locker, 1994; Petersen et al., 2000; Whelton et al., 2007; Zhu et al., 2005). Such a trend is confirmed by the comparison of the present results with those of Greek adults aged 35-44-years-old (Mamai-Homata et al., 2010). According to this comparison (figure 2) the percentage of senior citizens that brushed teeth regularly was about one-half of those aged 35-44-year-olds, while the percentage of those that used dental floss was less than one-third of the middle aged adults. It has been suggested that older age groups are less likely to have been exposed to preventive orientations early in life when socialization to self-care behaviors is thought to be most efficacious (Gift, 1988; Payne & Locker, 1992). Therefore, this may be a reason for the low levels of oral hygiene practices of the elderly.

The finding that those with a higher educational attainment brushed and flossed their teeth more often is consistent with those of other studies (Christensen et al., 2003; Davidson et al., 1997; Payne & Locker, 1994). Also, the observation that women were more likely to brush teeth at least once a day supports the view that the oral hygiene behavior of women is better than that of men (Chadwick et al.2011; Christensen et al., 2003; Davidson et al., 1997; Payne & Locker, 1992; Tada et al., 2004; Whelton et al., 2007). Finally, the correlation between flossing frequency and area of residence demonstrated in the present study supports earlier findings (Petersen et al., 2000) and indicates that people living in urban areas are better informed about the individual's role in the prevention of oral diseases.

The dental attendance of Greek seniors as measured by the reason for visiting a dentist indicates that their orientation towards prevention was weak. Only 13% reported that they attended the dentist for regular check-ups. Similar findings have been reported for the population of China (Zhu et al., 2005), while the percentage of those that used to visit a dentist for check-ups in Ireland was higher, but not satisfactory (Whelton et al., 2007). However, according to the latest report from the United Kingdom almost two thirds of dentate adults claimed that the usual reason they attended the dentist was for a regular check-up (Morris et al., 2009). The finding that dental visiting habits are influenced by education supports those of previous studies (Chen, 1986; Petersen, 1986).

The low number of seniors that used to go to the dentist for check-up is a worrying observation since it indicates that these people that are considered as high risk for root caries and oral cancer will have poor chances to detect early such conditions, as could have happened if they used to visit the dentist regularly.

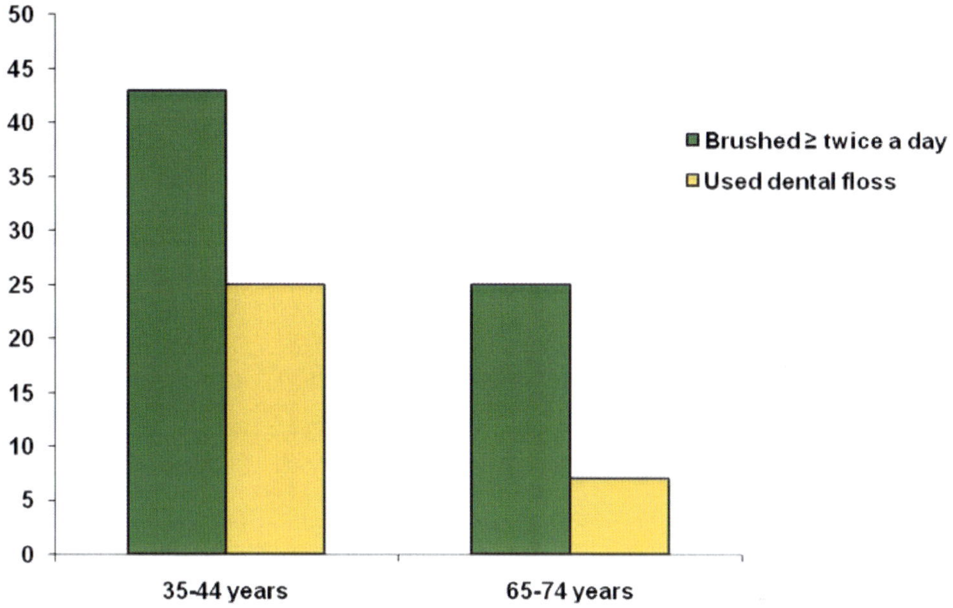

Fig. 2. Percentages of 35-44 and 65-74-year-old Greeks that brushed teeth ≥ twice a day and used dental floss.

4.2 Clinical parameters

The oral hygiene status of the Greek seniors cannot be considered as satisfactory, since more than half of the subjects had fair or poor oral hygiene scores. Comparison of these results with those of other countries is difficult since we didn't manage to find comparable recent data for non-institutionalized elderly. However, the mean OHI-S index is greater than that found among white Americans in the NHANNES I survey conducted in USA more than thirty years ago (Kelly & Harvey, 1979).

The results of the logistic regression analysis that gender, area of residence, tooth brushing frequency and reason for dental attendance are significantly correlated with oral hygiene level are in accordance with those of earlier studies (Christersson et al., 1992; Kelbauskas et al., 2003; Lang et al., 1995; Morris et al. 2001). The better oral hygiene status of women and those who brush teeth regularly is attributed to their better oral hygiene habits. Individuals that visit the dentist for check-ups are more likely to have professional tooth cleaning and oral hygiene instructions and therefore a better oral hygiene level. The poor oral hygiene status of people living in urban areas may be due to social inequalities.

The adult Dental Health Survey (ADHS) conducted in the United Kingdom in 1998 reported that 74% of adults claimed to clean their teeth at least twice daily and that 69% of them had visible plaque, compared with 79% who reported brushing only once per day (Kelly et al., 2000). In the present study 25.3% of seniors claimed to clean their teeth at least twice a day and 40% of them had fair or poor oral hygiene level, compared with 46% who reported brushing once per day. These findings indicate that both populations need oral hygiene instruction in order to improve their brushing techniques and achieve efficient plaque control.

The data of the study concerning the periodontal status of subjects examined have shown that only a few dentate participants had healthy periodontium and that the most frequently observed condition was shallow pocketing. These findings are in accordance with those observed in Croatia, Denmark, Germany, Ireland and Bulgaria (Artukovic et al., 2007; Krustrup et al., 2006; Schiffner et al., 2009; Whelton et al., 2007; Yolov, 2002), although in some other countries like France, Turkey, Hungary, China and Spain the most frequently observed condition in that age group was calculus (Bourgeois et al., 1999; Gokalp et al., 2010; Hermann, 2009; Hong-Ying et al., 2002; WHO, 2011).

Severe periodontal conditions (CPI scores 3 and 4) were found in 59.9% of the population. Comparison of these results with those reported for other European countries (figure 3) indicate that there are great differences across countries as regards the prevalence of periodontitis. They also indicate that the periodontal health status of the elderly in Greece is relatively poor, although better than that reported for Bulgaria, Croatia, Germany and Denmark. These differences could be attributed to different preventive regimes offered by the oral health systems of the countries, as well as to different exposures to risk factors of the populations like poor oral hygiene, tobacco-use and excessive consumption of alcohol that have been positively associated with periodontal diseases (Albandar, 2002; Tezal, 2001; Tomar & Asma, 2000). Also, some of the variations can be attributed to the fact that surveys are carried out by different examiners, under varying field conditions and with different sampling methods.

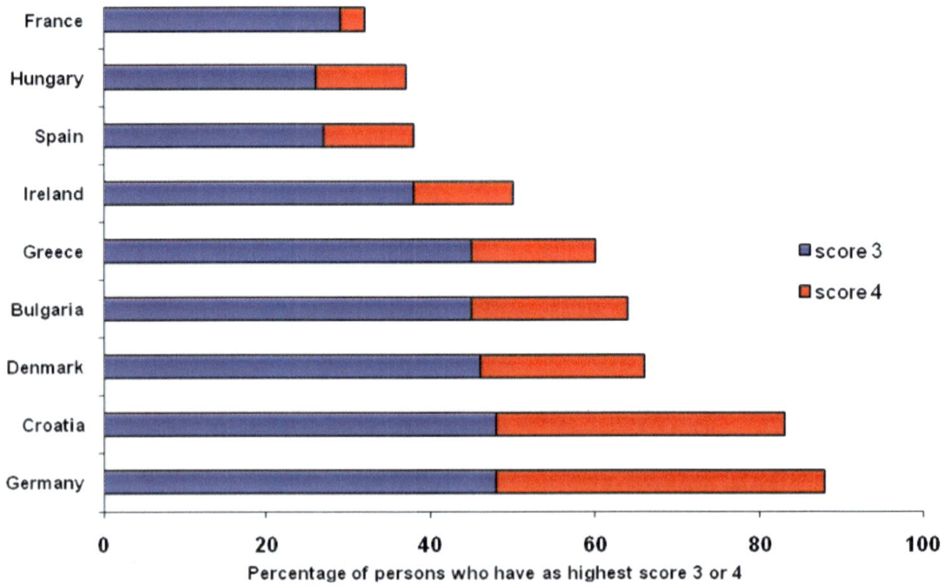

Fig. 3. Percent of persons with shallow or deep pockets (score 3 or 4) in European countries.

Of the independent variables considered in the present study, area of residence, as well as tooth brushing and flossing frequency were found to be the strongest determinants of periodontal diseases. These findings are consistent with those of other studies (Bourgeois et al., 1999; Marques, et al., 2000; Mengel et al., 1993). Given that the oral hygiene habits of the Greek seniors, as indicated from the present study, are far from been considered as satisfactory, improvement in oral hygiene practices should be an important public health issue.

The worse periodontal conditions of subjects living in rural areas may be explained by the fact that in rural areas of Greece, Public Health Centers provide preventive and restorative dental health services in children and adolescents up to 18-year-olds and treatment services in adults with acute dental problems. Therefore, adults living in rural areas are usually obliged to seek dental treatment in private dentists that practice mainly in urban areas, with a high cost and difficulties in accessing them. Such inefficiencies of the public health sector result in social inequalities that affect dental attendance and oral health.

The evaluation of the mean number of sextants affected per CPI score revealed that dentate elderly had on average 0.25 sextants with deep pockets indicating that the extent of severe periodontitis was relatively low. On the other hand, the average number of excluded sextants was high (2.36) suggesting a high prevalence of tooth loss. Similar findings have been reported for most other countries (Bourgeois et al., 1999; Hong-Ying et al., 2002; Kazeko & Yudina, 2004). The finding that frequent tooth brushing and flossing, as well as visiting the dentist for check-ups significantly affected the mean number of healthy and excluded sextants, emphasizes the role of good self-care practices on the maintenance of oral health.

5. Conclusions

Severe periodontal conditions (shallow and deep pocketing) were frequent among 65-74-year-old Greeks. However, the extent of deep pocketing was relatively low indicating that many of the elderly Greeks could retain their natural teeth in the future. On the other hand, their oral hygiene status cannot be considered as satisfactory in view of the fact that most of them had fair or poor level of oral hygiene. Their orientation towards prevention was weak since their oral hygiene habits were poor and their usual motive for visiting the dentist was pain or treatment. Socio-demographic factors and especially education significantly influenced the oral hygiene habits as well as the reason for dental attendance of the surveyed population. In turn, oral hygiene habits were significant predictors of periodontal and oral hygiene status. Residents of rural areas experienced more severe periodontal conditions and worse oral hygiene status.

These findings suggest that the periodontal health of Greek senior citizens could be greatly improved by preventive and oral health education efforts. Public health strategies should target the high-risk population groups, which according to the results of the study are the residents of rural areas and those with low educational attainment. Rural residents are mainly in need of preventive and treatment services since they experience more severe periodontal conditions and worse oral hygiene status. Individuals with low level of education are mainly in need of oral health education and oral hygiene instruction as they have worse oral self-care practices. Private dentists must also contribute to the improvement of the periodontal health of the population in spite of the fact that building patient's interest in effective oral hygiene procedures is time consuming (Krustrup &Petersen, 2006). Since this is the first national survey investigating the periodontal status of 65-74-year-old Greeks, it could serve as baseline for the surveillance of the periodontal health of the elderly.

6. Implications of the study: Future perspectives

As it has already been mentioned, periodic surveys of the periodontal health status of the elderly are needed in order to assess trends in periodontal diseases epidemiology in this population group. Since several covariates that have been associated with periodontal diseases may change overtime, the variables that may affect the initiation and/or progression of periodontal diseases should be also redefined. This redetermination is also necessary due to the demographic changes that have been occurred in Greece during the last decades. More specifically, the Greek population, in common with most industrialized countries, is rapidly ageing. Indicative of the magnitude of the demographic change that occurred over the last 25 years is that during the period 1974-99 the ratio of the population of 65 and over to the population between 15 and 64, decreased from about 5.2 to about 3.9 (Kariagiannaki, 2005). Therefore, it is necessary to develop specific oral health promotion strategies in order to manage the oral health problems of the senior citizens, such as periodontal diseases. Therefore, the results of the present survey could provide data which may contribute to a better understanding of the problem and a better planning of oral health care services for this specific age group.

Thus far, a relatively limited number of longitudinal studies have been conducted, in order to confirm whether previously reported risk factors, such as age, smoking and periodontal pathogens, are true risk factors and also to identify others that have not been included in studies conducted to date (e.g. blood pressure levels, serum levels of disease markers, nutritional factors) (Ogawa et al., 2002). Especially in Greece, since this is the first national survey investigating the periodontal status of 65-74-year-old Greeks, further research is required in order to confirm/identify more explanatory risk factors and to infer causal effects with the less possible bias.

According to the results of the present survey that support previous reports (Petersen, 2003; Pyle & Stoller, 2003), senior citizens are often at risk of periodontal diseases and also experience limited access to oral health care because of a variety of factors, such as place of residence, income, educational level and other individual as well as social factors. Consequently, disparities remain for access-limited groups despite oral health improvement for many Greeks. Thus, dental practitioners as well as dental public health policy makers should continue to work toward equity in oral health and focus not only on dental characteristics but also on the life characteristics of older adults, and on their quality of life issues (Chalmers, 2003).

7. Acknowledgements

This survey that is part of the National Program "Assessment and Promotion of the Oral Health of the Hellenic Population" has been carried out under the auspices of the Hellenic Dental Association in collaboration with the Dental Schools of Athens and Thessaloniki.

National surveys of oral health depend on the efforts of many different people and the authors would like to thank everybody who contributed to the survey and to the production of this chapter.

Therefore, we would like to thank and congratulate the survey examiners and interviewers for their energy and enthusiasm, and for being willing to adapt to the unfamiliar circumstances of carrying out dental examinations in people's own homes and day centers for the elderly.

We would also like to thank the coordinators of local dental societies as well as those who volunteered to be examined during the training of the survey dental team.
Finally, we would like to thank the people who agreed to participate in the survey. Without their willingness to contribute, the survey could not have been accomplished.
This survey was sponsored by a Colgate-Palmolive grant.

8. References

Albandar, J.M. (2002). Global risk factors and risk indicators for periodontal diseases. *Periodontology 2000*, Vol. 29, pp.177-206, ISSN, 0906-6713.

Artukovic, D.; Spalj, S.; Knezevic, A.; Plancak, D.; Panduric, V,; Anic-Milisevic, S.; Lauc, T. (2007). Prevalence of periodontal diseases in Zagreb population, Croatia, 14 years ago and today. *Collegium Antropologicum*, Vol. 31, No.2, pp.471-474, ISSN 0350-6134.

Benigeri, M.; Brodeur, J.M.; Payette, M.; Charbonneau, A.; Ismail, A.I. (2000). Community periodontal index of treatment needs and prevalence of periodontal conditions. *Journal of Clinical Periodontology*, Vol. 27, No 5 (May 2000), pp 308-312, on line ISSN: 1600-051X.

Bourgeois, D.M.; Doury, J. & Hescot, P. (1999). Periodontal conditions in 65-74 year old adults in France, 1995. *International Dental Journal*, Vol. 49, No 3 (June 1999), pp. 182-186, ISSN: 0020-6539. Chadwick, B.; White, D.; Lader, D & Pitts, N. (2011). Service considerations-a report from the Adult

Dental Health Survey 2009, NHS, 9.07.2011. Available from http://www.ic.nhs.uk/statistics-and-data-collections/primary-care/dentistry/adult-dental-health-survey-2009--summary-report-and-thematic-series.

Chalmers, J.M. (2003). Oral health promotion for our ageing Australian population. *Australian Dental Journal*, Vol. 48, No 1 (March 2003), pp 2-9, on line ISSN: 1834-7819.

Chen, M.S. (1986). A Sociodemographic Analysis of Preventive Dental Behavior among White American Families. *Health Education & Behavior*, Vol. 13, No. 2 (Summer 1986), pp. 105-115, Print ISSN: 1090-1981.

Christensen, L.B.; Petersen, P.E.; Krustrup, U. & Kjoller, M (2003). Self-reported oral hygiene practices among adults in Denmark. *Community Dental Health*, Vol.20, No.4, (December 2003), pp.229-235. ISSN: 0265 539X.

Christersson, L.A.; Grossi, S.G.; Dunford, R.G.; Machtei, E.E. & Genco, R.J. (1992). Dental Plaque and Calculus: Risk Indicators for Their Formation. *Journal of Dental Research*, Vol. 71, No. 7, (July 1992), pp. 1425-1430, print ISSN: 0022-0345.

Davidson, P.L.; Rams, T.E. & Andersen R.M. (1997). Socio-behavioral determinants of oral hygiene practices among USA ethnic and age groups. *Advances in Dental Research*, Vol.11, No.2, (May 1997), pp.245-253, print ISSN: 0895-9374.

Gift, H. (1988). Issues of aging and oral health promotion. *Gerodontics*, Vol. 4, No 5 (October 1988), pp.194-206, ISSN: 0109-565x.

Gokalp, S.; Dogan B.G.; Tekcicek, M.; Berberoglu, A.; Unluer, S. (2010). National survey of oral health status of children and adults in Turkey. *Community Dental Health*, Vol.27, No 1 (March 2010), pp. 12-17, ISSN: 0265 539X.

Greene, J.C.; Vermillion, J.R. (1964). The simplified oral hygiene index. *Journal of the American Dental Association*, Vol. 68, pp 7-13, Print ISSN: 0002-8177.

Greene JC (1967). The oral hygiene index-development and uses. *Journal of Periodontology*, Vol. 38 (suppl), pp. 625-637.

Hermann, P.; Gera, I.; Borbely, J.; Fejerdy, P.; Madlena, M. (2009). Periodontal health of an adult population in Hungary: findings of a national survey. *Journal of Clinical Periodontology*, Vol. 36, No 6 (June 2009), pp. 449-457, on line ISSN: 1600-051X.

Hong-Ying, W.; Petersen, P.E.; Jin-You, B. & Bo-Xue, Z. (2002). The second national survey of oral health status of children and adults in China. *International Dental Journal*, Vol. 52, No 4 (August 2002), pp. 283-290, ,ISSN: 0020-6539.

Jenkins, W.M.M. & Papapanou P.N. (2001). Epidemiology of periodontal disease in children and adolescents. *Periodontology 2000*, Vol. 26, No.1, (June 2001), pp.16-32, ISSN 0906-6713.

Karagiannaki, E. (2005). Changes in the living arrangements of elderly people in Greece: 1974-1999. *Centre for Analysis of Social Exclusion, London School of Economics*, 9.07.2011. Available from
http: //sticerd.lse.ac.uk/dps/case/cp/CASEpaper104.pdf.

Kazeko, L. & Yudina N. (2004). Periodontal Status in Population of Belarus. *Stomatologija, Baltic Dental and Maxillofacial Journal*, Vol. 6, pp. 111-114.

Kelbauskas, E; Kelbauskiene, S. & Paipaliene, P. (2003). Factors influencing the health of periodontal tissue and intensity of dental caries. *Stomatologija, Baltic Dental and Maxillofacial Journal*, Vol. 5, pp. 144-148.

Kelly, J.E. & Harvey, C.R. Basic data on dental examination findings of persons 1-74 years: United Slates - 1971-1974, Hyattsville, Maryland; National Center for Health Statistics. 1979; DHEW publication No. (PHS) 79-1662. (Vital and Health Statistics; Series 11; No.214).

Kelly, M.; Steele, J.; Nuttall, N.; Bradnock, G.; Morris, J.; Pine, C.; Pitts, N.; Treasure, E. & White, D. (2000). Adult Dental Health Survey-Oral Health in the United Kingdom 1998. The Stationery Office.9.07.2011. Available from http: //www. statistics. gov.uk/ downloads/ theme_health/ AdltDentlHlth98_v3.pdf.

Krustrup, U. & Petersen, P.E. (2006). Periodontal conditions in 35-44 and 65-74-year-old adults in Denmark. *Acta Odontologica Scandinavica* Vol. 64, No 2 (April 2006), pp. 65-73, ISSN 0001-6357.

Lang, W.P.; Ronis, D.L.; Farghaly, M.M. (1995). Preventive Behaviors as Correlates of Periodontal

Health Status. *Journal of Public Health Dentistry*, Vol.55, No.1 (January 1995), pp.10-17, on line ISSN: 1752-7325.

Leroy, R.; Eaton, K.A. & Savage, A. (2010). Methodological issues in epidemiological studies of periodontitis – How can it be improved? *BMC Oral Health*, Vol. 10, No 8. Available from
http:// www.biomedcentral.com/1472-6831/10/8 doi: 10.1186/1472-6831-10-8, ISSN 1472-6831.

Locker, D. & Leake, J.L. (1993). Risk Indicators and Risk Markers for Periodontal Disease Experience in Older Adults living independently in Ontario, Canada. *Journal of Dental Research*, Vol. 72 No. 1, (January 1993), pp. 9-17, print ISSN: 0022-0345.

Mamai-Homata, E.; Polychronopoulou, A; Topitsoglou, V; Oulis, C. & Athanassouli T, (2010). Periodontal diseases in Greek adults between 1985 and 2005-Risk indicators. *International Dental Journal*, Vol. 60, No 4 (August 2010), pp. 293-299, ISSN: 0020-6539.

Marques, M.D.; Teixeira-Pinto, A.; da Costa-Pereira, A. & Eriksen, H.M. (2000). Prevalence and determinants of periodontal disease in Portuguese adults: results from a multifactorial approach. *Acta Odontologica Scandinavica*, Vol. 58, No 5 (October 2000), pp.201-206, ISSN 0001-6357.

Mengel, R.; Koch, H. & Pfeifer, C.; Flores-de-Jacoby L. (1993). Periodontal health of the population in eastern Germany (former GDR). *Journal of Clinical Periodontology*, Vol. 20, No. 10 (November 1993), pp. 752-755, , on line ISSN: 1600-051X.

Morris, A.J.; Steele, J. & White, D.A. (2001). The oral cleanliness and periodontal health of UK adults in 1998. *British Dental Journal*, Vol. 191, No. 4 (August 2001), pp. 186-192, ISSN: 0007-0610.

Morris, J.; Chenery, V.; Douglas, G. & Treasure, E. (2011). Service considerations-a report from the Adult Dental Health Survey 2009, NHS, 9.07.2011. Available from http://www.ic.nhs.uk/statistics-and-data-collections/primary care/dentistry/adult-dental-health-survey-2009--summary-report-and-thematic-series.

Murtomaa, H. & Metsaniitty, M. (1994). Trends in toothbrushing and utilization of dental services in Finland. *Community Dentistry and Oral Epidemiology*, Vol. 22, No 4 (August 1994), pp. 231-234, on line ISSN: 1600-0528

Ogawa, H.; Yoshihara, A.; Hirotomi, T.; Ando, Y. & Miyazaki, H. (2002). Risk factors for periodontal disease progression among elderly people. *Journal of Clinical Periodontology*, Vol. 29, No.7 (July 2002), pp. 592-597, on line ISSN: 1600-051X.

Payne, B.J. & Locker, D. (1992). Oral self-care behaviours in older dentate adults. *Community Dentistry and Oral Epidemiology*, Vol. 20, No.6, (December 1992), pp.376-380, on line ISSN: 1600-0528.

Payne, B.J. & Locker, D. (1994). Preventive oral health behaviors in a multi-cultural population: the North York Oral Health Promotion Survey. *Journal of the Canadian Dental Association*, Vol. 20, No 2 (February 1994), pp. 129-130, 133-139, ISSN: 0008-3372.

Petersen, P.E. (1986). Dental Health Behaviour among 25-44-year-old Danes. *Scandinavian Journal of Primary Health Care*, Vol. 4, No 1 (February 1986), pp. 51-57, ISSN: 0281-3432.

Petersen, P.E. (2003). The World Oral Health Report 2003: continuous improvement of oral health in the 21st century-the approach of the WHO Global Oral Health Programme. *Community Dentistry and Oral Epidemiology*, Vol. 31, (Suppl. 1), pp. 3-24, on line ISSN: 1600-0528.

Petersen, P.E.; Aleksejuniene, J.; Christensen, L.B.; Eriksen H.M. & Kalo, I. (2000). Oral health behavior and attitudes of adults in Lithuania. *Acta Odontologica Scandinavica*, Vol.58, No.6 (December 2000), pp. 243-248, ISSN 0001-6357.

Pilot, T. & Miyazaki, H. (1994). Global results: 15 years of CPITN epidemiology. *International Dental Journal*, Vol. 44, No 5 (October 1994), pp. 553-560, ISSN 0020-6539.

Pyle, M. & Stoller,E. (2003). Oral Health Disparities Among the Elderly: Interdisciplinary Challenges for the Future. *Journal of Dental Education*, Vol.67, No 12, pp. 1327-1336, print ISSN: 0022-0337.

Schiffner, U.; Hoffmann, T.; Kerschbaum T. & Micheelis W. (2009). Oral health in German children, adolescents, adults and senior citizens in 2005. *Community Dental Health*, Vol. 26, No 1 (March 2009), pp. 18-22, ISSN: 0265 539X.

Tada, A. & Hanada N. (2004). Sexual differences in oral health behaviour and factors associated with oral health behaviour in Japanese young adults. *Public Health* Vol. 118, No. 2 (March 2004), pp 104-109.

Tezal, M.; Grossi, S.G.; Ho, A.W. & Genco, R.J. (2001). The effect of alcohol consumption on periodontal disease. *Journal of Periodontology*, Vol. 72, No. 2 (February 2001), pp.183-189.

Tomar, S.L. & Asma, S. (2000). Smoking-attributable periodontitis in the United States: findings from NHANES III. National Health and Nutrition Examination Survey. *Journal of Periodontology*, Vol.71, No 5 (May 2000),pp. 743-751.

Whelton, H.; Crowley, E.; O'Mullane, D.; Woods, N.; McGrath, C.; Kelleher, V.; Guiney, H.; Byrtek, M.(2007). Oral Health of Irish Adults 2000 - 2002. 9.07.2011. Available from http://www.dohc.ie/publications/pdf/oral_health02.pdf?direct=1.

World Health Organization. Global Oral Data Bank. Periodontal country profiles. 7.06.2011. Available from http://www.dent.niigata-u.ac.jp/prevent/perio/perio.html.

World Health Organization (1996). Population ageing: a public health Challenge. Geneva, World Health Organization, 1996 (WHO Fact Sheet No. 135).

World Health Organization (1997). Oral Health Surveys. Basic methods. 4th ed. Geneva: 1997.

Yolov, T. (2002). Periodontal condition and treatment needs (CPITN) in the Bulgarian population aged over 60 years. *International Dental Journal*, Vol. 52, No 4 (August 2002), pp. 255-260, ISSN 0020-6539.

Zhu, L.; Petersen; P.E.; Wang, H.Y.; Bian, J-Y & Zhang, B-X (2005). Oral health knowledge, attitudes and behaviour of adults in China. *International Dental Journal*, Vol.55, No.4, (August 2005), pp.231-241, ISSN 0020-6539.

13

Periodontal Diseases in Anthropology

Hisashi Fujita
*Department of Anthropology,
Niigata College of Nursing,
Japan*

1. Introduction

Dental caries and periodontal disease are two of the most common human diseases along with the common cold. Signs of dental caries have been seen even in early hominids (Australopithecus). It is well known that many signs of dental caries and periodontal disease were also seen in the Krapina Neanderthals and the archaic homo sapiens Kabwe man (also called "Broken Hill Man": human from 300,000-130,000 years ago) (Fig. 1). Dental caries and periodontal disease are not diseases that appeared in the modern era, so-called "modern diseases" or "diseases of civilization." Instead, they are ancient diseases with a long history of afflicting mankind. Therefore, the study of dental caries and periodontal disease in ancient people can be a major key to unlock information on their daily lives and behavioural patterns. Such a study on ancient human skeletal remains can provide information on dietary habits and lifestyles in various stages of human evolution, including diet, subsistence and oral hygiene.

Dental caries is considered to be the disease with the most case reports in dental paleopathology. The reason is that dental caries occurs in teeth which have the hardest tissue in the human body. Therefore, even if ancient human skeletal remains are excavated in poorly preserved conditions, dental caries can be distinguished relatively easily and data can be accumulated easily for statistical analysis. Studies of dental caries date back to the Meiji and Taisho era in Japan. Today, studies on dental caries are still being actively conducted by (including myself) Sakura; 1964; Sakura, 1989; Yukinari, 1975; Turner, 1979; Inoue et al., 1981; Fujita et al., 1994; Fujita, 1995; Fujita & Suzuki; 1995; Fujita and Hirano,1999; Fujita, 2002; Oyamada et al., 2004; Temple, 2007a, 2007b; Temple and Larsen, 2007; Oyamada et al., 2010). Since there are many studies on dental caries in ancient human skeletal remains from various countries, this chapter will use the results of recent studies as reference (Garcin et al., 2010; Meller et al., 2009). What about the other prevalent disease, periodontal disease? Unfortunately, there are almost no comprehensive studies on periodontal disease in anthropology (Fujita, 1999; Reich et al., 2011; Meller et al., 2009; Silvestoros et al., 2006). Although teeth are made of the hardest material in the body, alveolar bones are fragile. Periodontal disease occurs in this fragile type of bone. Thus, an examination of alveolar bone is not always easy in ancient human skeletal remains that were buried in the soil for many years and a statistical study can be difficult to perform.

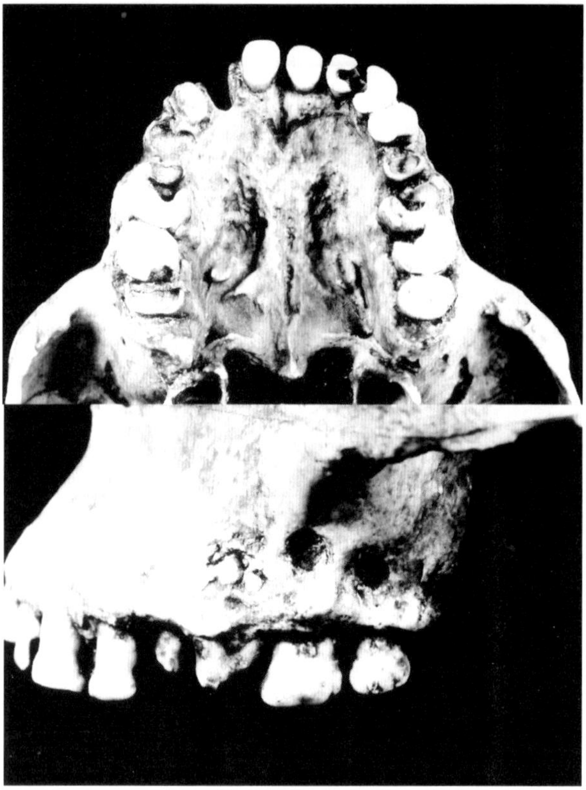

Fig. 1. Signs of dental caries and periodontal disease in the Kabwe man. Surprisingly, a fossilized man from over 100,000 years ago had advanced periodontal disease and dental caries as shown.

As is commonly known, humans underwent evolutionary development from Australopithecine, Homo erectus, Neanderthal man, to modern human (Cro-Magnon man and onward). Unfortunately, fossilized human bones earlier than those of Neanderthal man have not been found in Japan. Even modern human bones from the Pleistocene epoch are rare. Therefore, human skeletal remains from the Jomon period and onward are the remains that can be analyzed and statistically examined as a collection or "group." This chapter will examine how periodontal disease and dental caries have changed in Japanese people from the Jomon period onward.

2. High prevalence of dental caries in Jomon people

In my study of the Jomon people, the surprising result was the high incidence of dental caries, although it was lower than that of the general modern population. When the prevalence of dental caries among the Jomon people was compared to those from similar societies of hunters and gatherers, the Jomon people generally had a higher prevalence of dental caries. Table 1 shows the prevalence of dental caries among people from similar stages of hunter and gatherer societies as the Jomon people.

The prevalence of dental caries was much larger in the Jomon people than even the present day Inuits of Greenland or Aboriginal people of Australia. The Jomon prevalence of dental caries was very high, unlike any other hunter and gatherer societies in the world. Most of the hunters and gatherers who do not farm have a very low prevalence of dental caries. With the transition of their economy from hunting and gathering to farming, the incidence of dental caries is known to increase sharply. In Japan, the prevalence of dental caries increased sharply in the Yayoi people who adopted agriculture. The high prevalence of dental caries in the Jomon people is thought to demonstrate the intake of large amounts of cariogenic starchy foods prepared in a way to further facilitate dental caries' occurrence.

In recent years, we have examined dental caries in excavated human skeletal remains from approximately BP 2100 and AD 400-700 in the Korean peninsula and found low prevalence of dental caries (Fujita and Choi, 2008; Fujita et al., 2011). These people had knowledge of agriculture, but their prevalence of dental caries was similar to, or even less than, those of the Jomon people of Japan. This result has drawn much interest for the following reasons: it indicates that the spread of agriculture was not necessarily the same on the Korean peninsula or the Japanese islands. In addition, people who lived in geographical conditions more suited for hunting and gathering very likely practiced these activities for subsistence even if they knew about agriculture.

Groups	Age	Economic level	Caries rate (%)
Jomon (Japan)	15,000-2,300 yrs BP	hunting-gathering	8.2
Jomon (Hokkaido)	15,000-2,300 yrs BP	hunting-gathering	2.6
Yayoi (Doigahama, Japan)	2,000 yrs BP	agriculture	19.7
Yayoi (Mitsu, Japan)	2,000 yrs BP	agriculture	16.2
Kofun (Japan)	ca. AD 1700-1400 yrs	agriculture	8.3
Muromachi (Japan)	ca. AD 1400 yrs	agriculture	14.6
Edo (Japan)	AD 1603-1868 yrs	agriculture	12.1
Old Copper (USA)	7,600 yrs BP	hunting-gathering	0.4
SJO-68 (USA)	3,000 yrs BP	hunting-gathering	2.4
Australian Aborigine (Australia)	Modern	hunting-gathering	4.6
Inuits (Denmark)	Modern	hunting-gathering	2.2
Inuits (USA)	Modern	hunting-gathering & trade	1.9

Caries rate (%): 100 (carious teeth/ teeth present)

Table 1. Comparison of the prevalence of dental caries among various groups. Many hunters and gatherers of the world have low prevalence of dental caries, but the Jomon people had a very high prevalence rate. The dental caries prevalence increased in Yayoi individuals from the Northern Kyushu site, but decreased in Japanese people in subsequent periods. The prevalence has not increased dramatically up to the modern period.

3. Close association between dental caries and periodontal disease

3.1 Elderly-type dental caries in modern times

The title of this book is "Periodontal Diseases," but the focus of the above section was dental caries. The reason is that dental caries and periodontal disease have a close association in ancient people. Therefore, it seemed inappropriate to discuss either one as a disease independent of the other. This section will discuss dental caries and periodontal disease in Japanese people from the Jomon period. In this process, the reader will gain an understanding of the close association between dental caries and periodontal disease in ancient people.

Dental caries in the Jomon people can be compared with that in modern day people in a few ways. I focused on the sites where dental caries occurred. The preferred sites for dental caries are occlusal and interproximal areas in modern day people. The Jomon people were more susceptible to dental caries in the interproximal and buccal cervical areas, and root areas (Fig. 2). Occlusal dental caries were rare.

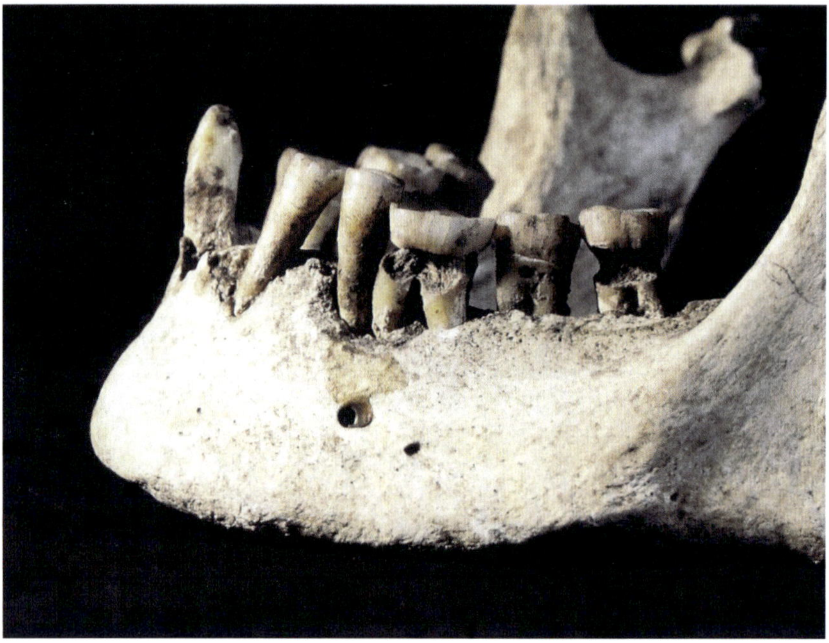

Fig. 2. Dental caries that developed in the root areas in Jomon people.The figure shows a typical pattern of cervical root dental caries in Jomon people.

The pattern of carious sites in the Jomon people is very similar to that found in the modern day elderly. The direct cause is the exposure of cervical and root areas due to gingival recession and alveolar bone loss. Crowns are covered by enamel, but cervical and root areas are composed of cementum. Therefore, these areas are structurally weaker against the invasion of dental caries. Figure 3 is an oral image of a man in his 70s who presented to the Department of Oral Surgery of the Tokyo Metropolitan Geriatric Hospital. His gingiva was inflamed and his alveolar bone was receded. He clearly had periodontal disease. Unlike the

Jomon people, this patient did not have buccal dental caries, probably due to the effects of brushing teeth. However, the occurrence of root dental caries due to alveolar bone loss was determined to be almost the same as in the Jomon people. Therefore, the pattern of dental caries in the Jomon people was similar to the elderly-type dental caries in modern times.

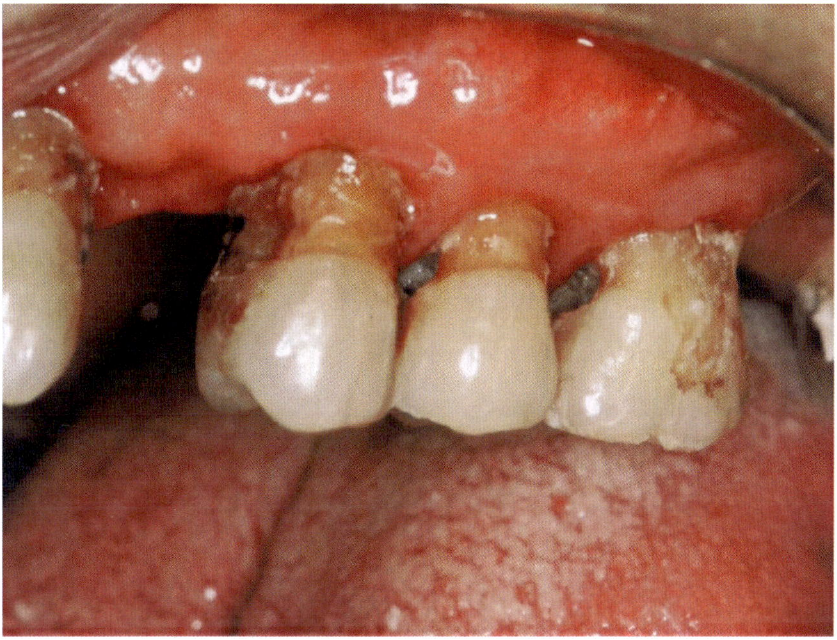

Fig. 3. Root dental caries in a modern day 70 year old person The root dental caries shown are very similar to dental caries in Jomon people. The labial and buccal surfaces of the cervical root areas were dental caries-free, probably because of brushing teeth.

Interestingly, researchers from various countries also obtained similar results on carious sites in ancient man. Moore and Corbett, and Whittaker et al. studied the dental caries in ancient English man (Moore and Corbett, 1973; Whittaker et al., 1981). Lunt et al. studied dental caries from prehistoric times and medieval Scotland (Lunt, 1974). All of these researchers indicated that there were high incidences of cervical and root dental caries. Below I raise two factors explaining the aforementioned results.

4. Decreasing attrition levels with changing time periods

4.1 Dental attrition level and close association with the incidence of dental caries

The progress of attrition was incomparably fast in people in ancient times and the Middle Ages relative to modern day people. If dental caries in the occlusal pits and fissures was slight, the progression of attrition could have been faster than that of such dental caries. Therefore, it is speculated that dental caries itself could have disappeared in many cases. This phenomenon is seen in modern day Nigeria. Kubota et al. conducted follow-up surveys among Nigerians with dental diseases. Class I dental caries in 11 first and second molars and class II dental caries in 2 second molars from the 1986 survey had disappeared in the 1991 survey and were healthy and sound (Kubota et al., 1993).

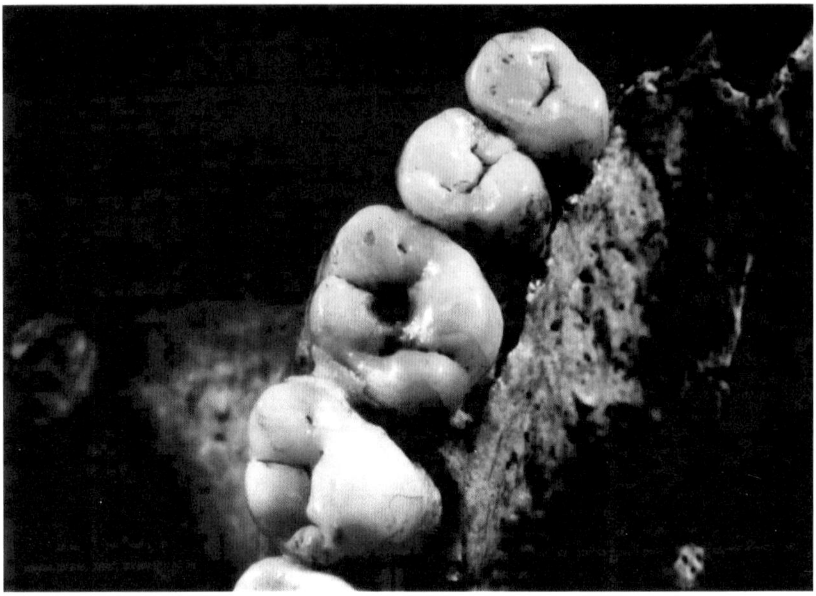

Fig. 4. Occlusal dental caries in Jomon people.This type of dental caries was rarely encountered in Jomon people except in young individuals. The absence of such dental caries is thought to be closely associated with marked attrition levels in Jomon people.

Figure 4 shows occlusal dental caries in the Jomon people. Although the prevalence of occlusal dental caries was low in the Jomon period, it certainly did exist. Cusps and fissures were well preserved on this individual's occlusal surfaces. An anthropologist who is familiar with the bones and teeth of ancient skeletal remains can easily determine that the individual was rather young. That is, such an individual with well preserved cusps and fissures could have occlusal dental caries.

The Jomon people were eating food that was much harder than the food modern day people eat, therefore, their dental attrition was considerable. Occlusal dental caries is speculated not to have occurred in an individual with occlusal surfaces, such as those shown in Figure 4. In other words, occlusal dental caries should have occurred in young people, but it would not be found in individuals beyond a certain age as dental attrition progressed with aging. If attrition was very considerable, slight occlusal dental caries could have disappeared due to dental attrition as in the aforementioned Nigerian cases.

Factors other than diet likely also contributed to marked dental attrition in the Jomon people. As shown in Figure 5, dental attrition of the anterior teeth could have occurred due to use of teeth for hide tanning, just as with the Inuit people. It is speculated that teeth were used as "tools." There was pulp exposure in this individual. Even if the Jomon people ate hard food, factors other than diet must be considered to explain the extreme dental attrition to this extent. Since teeth are the hardest structures in the body, they were likely "important tools" for ancient people.

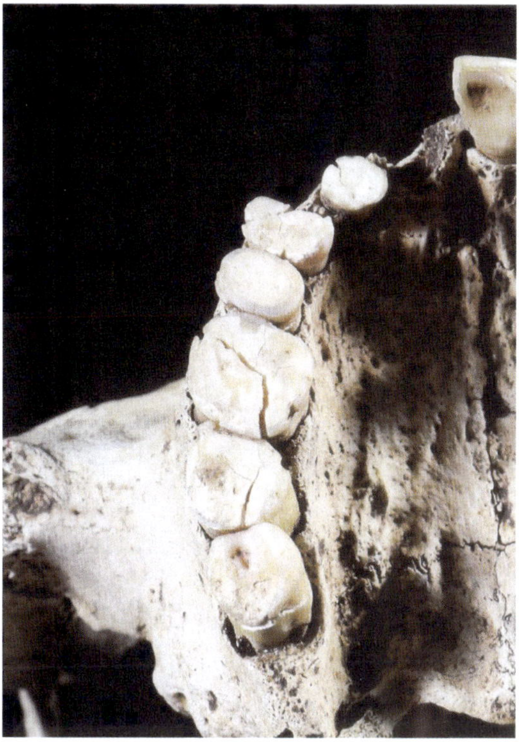

Fig. 5. Teeth with marked attrition in Jomon people. The occlusal surfaces were flattened and dental caries were probably difficult to develop on such surfaces.

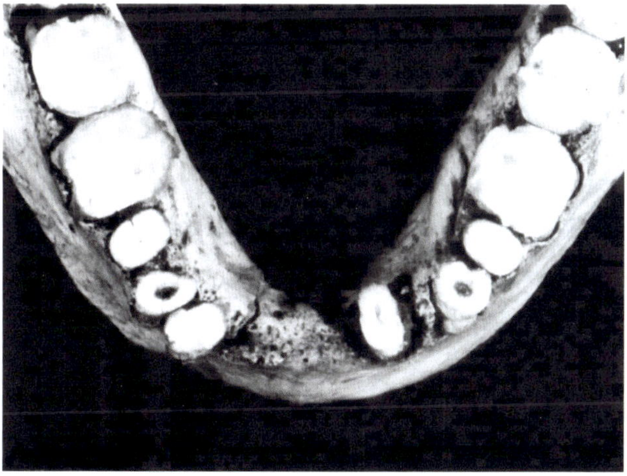

Fig. 6. Anterior teeth with pulp exposure in Jomon people. The pulp exposure could have been caused by some type of tasks performed using teeth. In the modern era, Inuits are known to use their teeth for hide tanning.

Our study has shown that the level of dental attrition clearly decreased as time approached closer to the present (Fujita, 1993; Fujita and Ogura, 2009). In Japan, dental attrition was most severe in the Jomon people and decreased in the order of Kofun, Kamakura, Muromachi and Edo people, thus, dental attrition decreased as the time periods approached the present. As a result, Edo people developed dental caries that caused large cavities on the occlusal surfaces, such as shown in Figure 6. Dental caries causing this type of large cavity on the occlusal surface was not seen in the Jomon period because of marked dental attrition.

5. High incidence of periodontal disease in ancient people

The second reason for the high incidence of root dental caries is periodontal disease, which is speculated to have also occurred at a very high frequency during the Jomon period. Periodontal disease and dental caries have a close association. When alveolar bones were examined in people from the Jomon period to the Edo period, many individuals had considerably advanced bone resorption. As in modern day people, bone resorption due to periodontal disease was seen in ancient people.

The incidence of periodontal disease is closely associated with aging. Thus, the following paragraph will briefly describe aging and lifespan of the Jomon people.

The average lifespan of the Jomon people has been estimated to be less than 15 years for both males and females. This short average lifespan was due to the remarkably high infant mortality prevalence which reduced the overall average lifespan of people in the Jomon period. In anthropology, when studying a group with an extremely short lifespan, focus is placed on the average life expectancy of the 15 year old survivors. Fifteen is an age at which a person gains some degree of resistance to diseases. In the Jomon individuals who survived the first 15 years of life, the average life expectancy was considered to be approximately 15 years. That is, an average lifespan of such individuals was approximately 30 years (Kobayashi, 1967). Even if there were some individuals with a lifespan longer than 30 years, the alveolar bone resorption in the Jomon people is speculated to have progressed 20-30 years faster than in modern day people. This notion suggested that the Jomon people physiologically aged considerably faster due to various physical stresses that modern day people are not subject to. It also suggested that periodontal disease was very common in the time period without special measures for disease prevention and treatment. As previously mentioned, the average lifespan was less than 15 years in the Jomon people. It was approximately 15 years in the Muromachi period and approximately 20 years in the Edo period. According to Japanese government statistics of the Taisho period, it was 42 years for both men and women. That is, the average lifespan of Japanese people remained almost unchanged from the Jomon period to the Edo period, even though the Jomon people lived several thousand years ago on what is now the Japanese islands. Lifespan increased dramatically in more recent times, only in the decades after World War II, and Japan has now become the country with the longest lifespan in the world. This longevity is thought to be the result of improved nutrition and medical advancement. It can easily be speculated that people from a time with much shorter lifespans had poor nutrition, hygiene and medical care, just as with the people in modern developing countries, and that they lived in societies with high rates of infant mortality. As mentioned earlier, these people had various physical stresses, the prevalence of their physiological aging was fast and they developed periodontal disease at a young age.

6. Evidence of periodontal disease in ancient human skeletal remains

It is very difficult to obtain strong evidence of periodontal disease in ancient human skeletal remains. In general, periodontal disease is studied in such remains by (1) obtaining findings of horizontal and vertical resorption of the alveolar bone or osteoporosis-like findings, and (2) measuring the degree of alveolar bone loss with a calliper. These methods are effective and will naturally continue to be used in the future. However, they have several problems, for example, even if the individual had periodontal disease, when the teeth were lost in the affected area, bony tissue would have gradually filled those tooth sockets in the alveolar bone. Thus, there would have been no evidence of such tooth sockets or inflammatory lesions after 1-2 years. In this type of case, we can only observe the form of the individual at the time of death through the skeletal remains. It is difficult for us to determine whether or not tooth loss in this type of an area was caused by periodontal disease. In addition, alveolar bone loss gradually advances due to aging, even without inflammatory lesions such as periodontal disease. Therefore, even if the alveolar bone loss can be measured by a calliper, we cannot necessarily attribute it to periodontal disease.

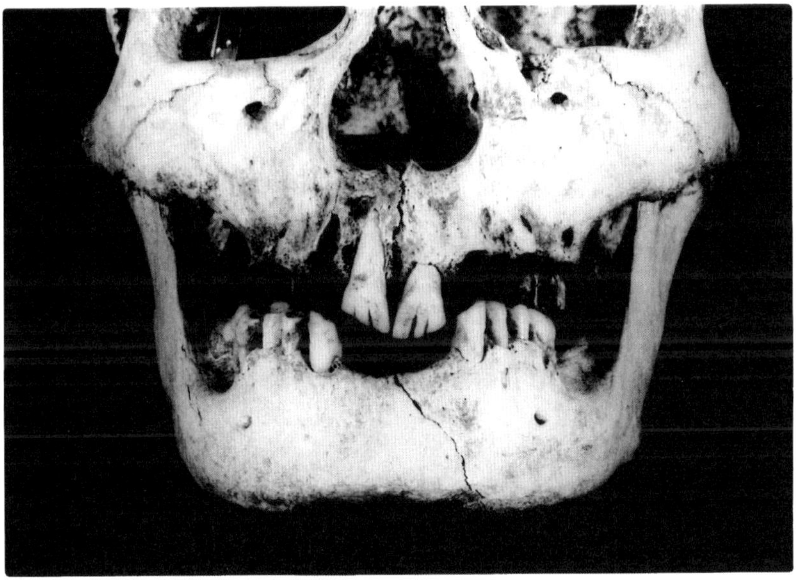

Fig. 7. Ritual tooth ablation in Jomon people. Mandibular four incisors were extracted. Maxillary incisors forked: "Sajyo kenshi" in Japan.

For the above reasons, I examined the absence or presence of dental caries and the state of tooth loss in 76 Jomon individuals in whom maxillary and mandibular alveolar bones remained complete (Fujita, 1999). The advantages of this method were elimination of bias due to the observed number of tooth types, comparisons of the same number of teeth in the maxillae and mandibles, and similar examinations performed with individuals as a unit. I compared teeth from the first premolar or second premolar to the second molar because the Jomon people often extracted their anterior teeth (incisors, canines and sometimes first premolars) as their custom (Fig.6).

	Tooth number comparison	No. of missing teeth in maxilla	No. of missing teeth in mandible	No. of Observed teeth1)	Significance2)
Whole Jomon	4-7	67	34	1216	***
Whole Jomon	5-7	45	26	912	*

1)maxilla and mandible teeth were pooled
2)* : $P<0.05$; *** : $P<0.001$

Table 2. Comparison of the number of lost teeth between the maxillae and mandibles in Jomon people. The number of lost teeth was significantly greater in the maxillae than mandibles.

	Tooth number comparison	No. of missing teeth in maxilla	No. of missing teeth in mandible	No. of Observed teeth1)	Significance2)
Whole Jomon	4-7	41	64	1216	*
Whole Jomon	5-7	34	59	912	**

1) maxilla and mandible teeth were pooled
2)* : $P<0.05$; ** : $P<0.01$

Table 3. Comparison of the number of carious teeth between the maxillae and mandibles in Jomon people. The number of carious teeth was significantly greater in the mandibles than maxillae. When Table 2 was also considered, periodontal disease is suggested to be the cause of lost maxillary teeth in Jomon people.

In addition, third molars were also excluded because they were sometimes missing or unerupted. I was able to obtain very interesting results. When the Jomon people were analyzed as a group or by individual, the number of missing teeth was significantly greater in the maxilla than mandible (Tables 2 and 3).
However, the number of carious teeth was higher in the mandible than the maxilla. These results showed that the phenomena occurring in the maxilla were exactly the opposite of those in the mandible. That is, the results are thought to indicate that the majority of maxillary teeth lost in Jomon people were due to periodontal disease. In another study, I found that Edo people also had a higher prevalence of tooth loss in the maxilla than the mandible. In modern people, the survival prevalence of the first premolars is slightly higher in the mandible than maxilla. The prevalence of the second premolars is similar in both jaws. The prevalence of the first molars and second molars is higher in the maxilla than in the mandible. Then why were teeth in the maxilla more easily lost than in the mandible in Jomon and Edo people? The maxilla consists of mainly cancellous bone and the mandible consists of mainly compact cortical bone. The maxilla is thought be more susceptible to tooth loss because it has weaker alveolar bone supporting the teeth compared to the mandible. As periodontal disease advances, the maxilla is presumed to lose the ability to support teeth at an earlier stage than the mandible. Nowadays anyone can visit a dental clinic and receive scientific dental care, but since people in past eras could not receive such modern scientific dental care, there were likely various differences in the conditions of periodontal disease between these people and modern people. In other words, modern dental treatments can be the reason for the high survival prevalence of maxillary teeth in modern people.

When one takes into consideration that dental caries and periodontal disease are the two major causes of tooth loss, periodontal disease is strongly suggested to be the cause of maxillary tooth loss. In ancient people in Japan (here "ancient" is used to mean antiquity), periodontal disease occurred in even the younger generations. The mechanism involved alveolar bone loss leading to exposed roots which developed dental caries.

As explained above, dental caries and periodontal disease in ancient skeletal remains are closely intertwined, and neither can be considered without the other. In ancient people with short average lifespans, their periodontal disease advanced from a relatively young age with dental caries development accompanying this advancement. Moreover, these people had multiple root dental caries - the elderly-type dental caries in modern times.

I recently conducted a study on the number of remaining teeth in Edo individuals (Fujita, 2011). According to the Japanese survey of dental diseases conducted in 1999, the number of teeth present (number of remaining teeth) was 25.22-28.55 teeth in individuals aged 20-49 years. From our examination of Edo individuals, the number of teeth present was 29.5 teeth in the early middle age males, 30 teeth in the early middle age females, 26.67 teeth in the late middle age males and 27.08 teeth in the late middle age females. These numbers were relatively high compared to those in the 1999 survey. It was unexpected that the Edo individuals had so many remaining teeth. The notion that "people of long past ages lost more teeth more quickly" is clearly untrue in people of Edo-period Japan. In our study, three males were estimated to be elderly and had no, or very few, remaining teeth. Two of them were edentulous in both jaws. Thus, the results showed that although remaining teeth were well-retained in the early and late middle age groups, the number of missing teeth increased rapidly and the remaining teeth were few in the elderly group. In general, the high number of remaining teeth can be explained by the low incidence of dental caries and periodontal disease, two of the main causes of tooth loss. In the case of the Edo people, one needs to also consider the difference in dental treatments between the Edo period and the present. Tooth extraction is performed relatively easily in modern day people as a part of dental treatment. In contrast, extraction could not be performed so easily in Edo people, even if they had dental caries or periodontal disease, and such teeth were often left untreated. Therefore, the number of remaining teeth could have been greater than expected in the Edo people. However, periodontal disease progressed to a severe level in elderly individuals over 50 years and tooth loss probably dramatically increased.

7. Site of dental caries closely associated with periodontal disease

Figure 7 is a plot of carious sites in Japan from the Jomon period to modern times. This figure indicates a few very interesting facts.

First, the percentage of dental caries on the occlusal surface is almost the same among people in modern times, the Kamakura period and the Edo period. The percentages are low for the Jomon and Kofun periods. As indicated previously in Figure 6, the occurrence of occlusal dental caries is thought to have been inhibited in the Jomon and Kamakura periods when attrition was considerable. In the Edo people, the attrition level was low and dental caries often developed on the occlusal surfaces. The incidence of periodontal disease was likely higher than that of occlusal dental caries and the percentage of root dental caries is speculated to have become high. There was generally high incidence of interproximal root dental caries in all time periods. It can be seen that interproximal root dental caries is the most characteristic dental caries of Japanese people throughout all aforementioned time periods. The incidence of dental caries was low for lingual surfaces and lingual root areas in all time periods, and the cleaning action of the tongue is thought to be the reason. This tendency for higher incidence of root dental caries than occlusal dental caries was also seen in the human skeletal remains (AD 300-700) from the Yean-ri site in South Korea. The cause was obviously alveolar bone loss due to periodontitis leading to the exposure of roots and invasion of dental caries in those areas. Therefore, periodontal disease is not a modern disease, but existed with humans from ancient times. Our ancestors were also plagued by this disease.

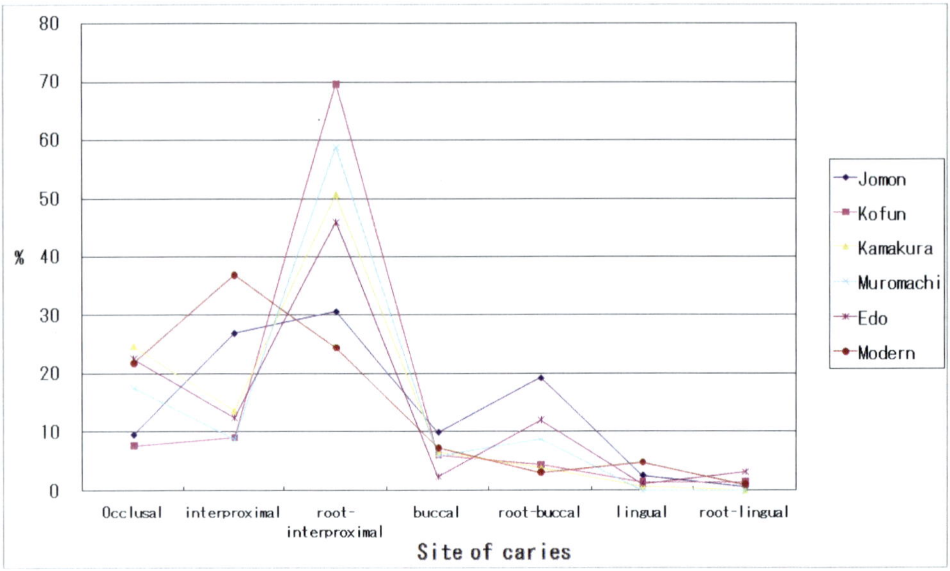

Fig. 8. Sites for dental caries' occurrences by time period. Multiple cervical root dental caries occurred in ancient people. The causes were likely root surface exposure due to periodontitis and lack of teeth brushing. Except in modern day people, the incidence of dental caries tended to be high in the interproximal cervical root areas.

8. Association of wedge-shaped defects with periodontal disease and teeth brushing

The major etiological theories of wedge-shaped defects involve loss of cervical enamel due to occlusal forces, bruxism, and teeth brushing. However, a clear theory has not been established regarding the cause of these lesions. Some researchers think that the cause is microfractures at the cervical regions due to occlusal forces, but are these microfractures really the cause? A wedge-shaped defect is often considered a geriatric problem in modern society. Ancient people ate harder foods than modern day people and the teeth of ancient people were subjected to stronger occlusal forces. As a result, their dental attrition was considerable. Thus, studies on ancient people can be important in understanding the cause of wedge-shaped defect. I have examined the absence or presence of wedge-shaped defects and the dental attrition level in ancient human skeletal remains from the Jomon period to the Edo period. These materials were from a total of 8002 individuals: 297 Jomon individuals, 60 Kofun individuals, 124 Kamakura individuals, 42 from Muromachi individuals and 105 Edo individuals. The level of attrition was determined by the method of

Fujita (1993). The number of individuals was insufficient for some time periods, so individuals of different ages and sexes were pooled together. The attrition levels were marked and the occlusal forces were speculated to be strong in the Jomon people who were hunters and gatherers in Japan. However, wedge-shaped defects were not observed in the cervical areas of the examined Jomon individuals (Fig.9). In subsequent periods (Yayoi, Kofun, Kamakura and Muromachi), attrition decreased perhaps because their food became softer. Wedge-shaped defects were not observed in any of these periods. It was found only in Edo skeletal remains (Fig.10). This result indicated that the origin of wedge-shaped defects in Japan was in the Edo period. In Japan, the practice of brushing teeth is thought to have begun with the introduction of Buddhism to Japan in AD 538, however, it is still unknown whether teeth brushing was performed on a regular basis. In the Edo period, teeth brushing was prevalent even among common people and tooth brushes (*fusayouji*) were used. In one theory, microfractures occur in the cervical regions due to strong occlusal forces. Based on this theory, there must be some signs of wedge-shaped defects in individuals with strong occlusal forces, such as in the Jomon individuals who had severe attrition exposing pulp. That is, our findings indicate the invalidity of this theory which states that occlusal forces produce abfractions and cause wedge-shaped defects. Instead, it is thought that periodontal disease occurred and the root surfaces became exposed. Subsequently, wedge-shaped defects are thought to have occurred due to the use of coarse abrasive powder or improper brushing of teeth. That is, a phenomenon similar to modern day incorrect brushing of teeth occurred in the Edo individuals. In Japan, the historical origin of wedge-shaped defects dates back at least as early as the Edo period, and periodontal disease and teeth brushing were strongly suggested to be the cause (Fujita, 2011).

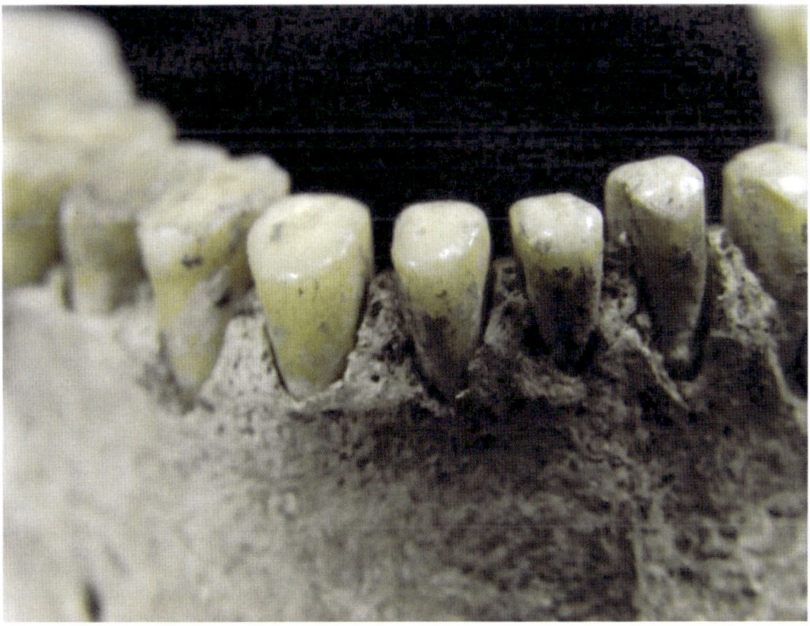

Fig. 9. There is no evidence of wedge-shaped defects despite the severe dental attrition of Jomon people.

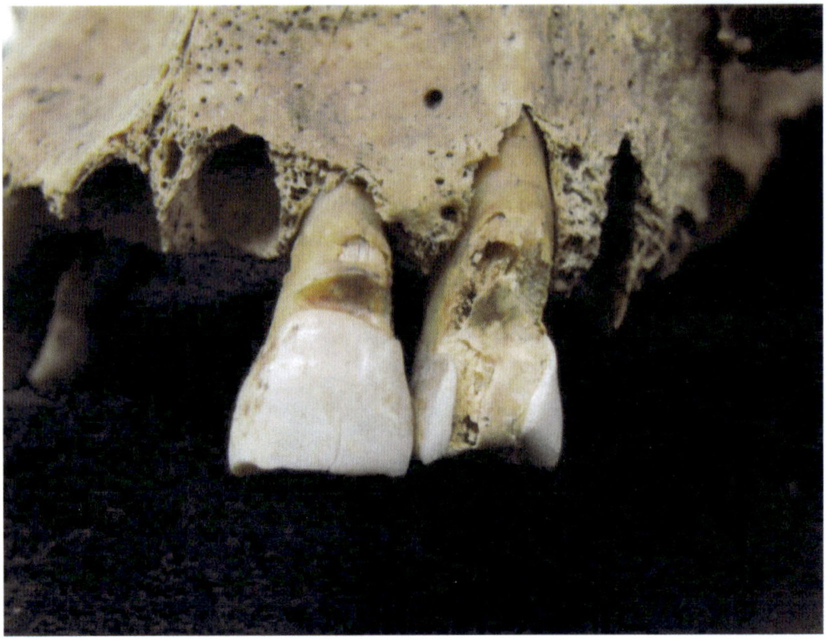

Fig. 10. Wedge-shaped defect in Edo people. The wedge-shaped defect probably developed because of teeth brushing of the root areas which were exposed due to periodontitis.

9. Conclusion

Dental caries and periodontal disease in ancient skeletal remains should not be treated as merely ancient objects or viewed from a single perspective. It is important to consider various factors, including environmental factors, which people of that time faced: average lifespan, diet, attrition, aging and teeth brushing habits. In other words, dental caries and periodontal disease in ancient skeletal remains can provide valuable information about the environmental and hygiene conditions of that time. Although teeth are small structures in the body, much information can be obtained from them. It is not an exaggeration to say that a thrill of dental paleopathology is being able to obtain such a wealth of information. Time periods are indeed borderless. Most readers of this book are likely dental and medical associated professionals, but no one actually knows what field of study will be useful to one's own research area. Therefore, it is important to be open to other areas of research so that one can obtain ideas useful to one's research. I will be happy if results of anthropologists who handle ancient remains can be utilized to create a new vision of 21st century dental hygiene and public health. Much about the present and the future can be learned from our ancestors and I hope that the information in this chapter can help open the door to such information.

10. References

Fujita, H. (1993). Degree of dental attrition of the Kanenokuma Yayoi population. *Anthropological Science*, Vol. 103, No. 3, pp. 291-300, ISSN 0918-7960

Fujita, H., Suzuki, T., Ishiyama, N., Hirano, H. & Watanabe, I. (1994). Distribution of dental caries cavities in the Neolithic Joon population of Japan. *Japanese Journal of Oral Biology*, Vol. 36, No. 5, pp. 558-561, ISSN 0385-0137

Fujita, H. (1995). Geographical and chronological differences in dental caries in the Neolithic Jomon period of Japan. *Anthropological Science*, Vol. 103, No.1, pp. 23-37, ISSN 0918-7960

Fujita, H. & Suzuki, T. (1995). Dental caries in the Jomon peoples. *Koukogaku Zasshi*, Vol. 80, No. 3, PP. 95-107, ISSN 0003-8075 (in Japanese)

Fujita, H. & Hirano, H. (1999). Dental caries in older adults in the Edo period, Japan. *Japanese Journal of Gerodontology*. Vol.13, No.3, pp. 175-182, ISSN 0914-3866 (in Japanese with English summary)

Fujita, H. (1999). Periodontal diseases in the Jomon peoples. *The Journal of the Archaeological Society of Waseda University*, No. 107, pp.65-76, 0452-2516 (in Japanese)

Fujita, H. (2002). Historical change of dental carious lesions from prehistoric to modern times in Japan. *Japanese Journal of Oral Biology*, Vol.44, No.2, PP. 87-95, ISSN 0385-0137

Fujita, H. & Ogura, M. (2009). Degree of dental attrition with sex and aging among Jomon and Edo people in Japan. *Journal of Oral Biosciences*, Vol. 51, No. 3, pp. 165-171, ISSN 1349-0079

Fujita, H. (2011). The origin of wedge-shaped defect in Japan. *Japanese Journal of Gerodontology*, Vol. 26, No. 3, ISSN 0914-3866 (in press) (in Japanese)

Garcin, V., Veleminsky, P., Trefny, P., Alduc-Le Bagousse, A., Lifebvre, A. & Bruzek, J. (2010). Dental health and lifestyle in four early mediaeval juvenile populations: comparisons between urban and rural individuals and between coastal and inland settlement. *Homo*, Vol. 61, No. 6, pp. 421-439, ISSN 0018-442X

Haraga, S., Hamasaki, T., Ansai, T., Kakuta, S., Akifusa, S., Yoshida, A., Hanada, N., Miyazaki, H. & Takehara, T. (2006). Distribution and site characteristics of dental caries in paddy rice-cultivating Yayoi people of ancient Japan. *Journal of Dental Health*, Vol.56, pp. 71-78, ISSN 0023-2831

Inoue, N., Ching, H. K., Ito, G. & Kamegai, T. (1981). Dental diseases in Japanese skeletal remains. II: Later Jomon period. *Journal of the Anthropological Society of Nippon*, Vol. 89, No.3, pp. 363-378, ISSN 0003-5505

Inoue, N., Kuo, C. H., Ito, G. & Kamegai, T. (1981). Dental diseases in Japanese skeletal remains. III: Kofun period. *Journal of the Anthropological Society of Nippon*, Vol. 89, pp. 419-426, ISSN 0003-5505

Kobayashi, K. (1967). Trend in the length of life based on human skeleton from prehistoric to modern times in Japan. *Journal of the Faculty of Science, the University of Tokyo*, Vol. 3, No. 2, pp. 107-162.

Kubota, K, Hollist, N. O., Olusile, A. O., Yonemitsu, M., Minakuchi, S., Watanabe, H., Ohnishi, M., Ohsawa, K., Ono, Y. Ajaji-Obe, S. O. & Grillo, T. A. I. (1993). The time-related social and economic factors of dental health from a longitudinal dental survey in Nigeria. *Journal of the Japanese Society for Mastication Science and Health Promotion*, Vol. 3, No. 1, pp. 27-35, ISSN 0917-8090

Lunt, D. A. (1974). The prevalence of dental caries in the permanent dentition of Scottish prehistoric and mediaeval populations. *Archives of Oral Biology*, Vol.19, pp.431-437, ISSN 0003-9969

Meller, C., Urzua, I., Moncada, G. & von Ohle, C. (2009). Prevalence of oral pathologic findings in an ancient pre-Columbian archaeological site in the Atacama Desert. *Oral Diseases*, Vol. 15, No. 4, pp. 287-294, ISSN 1354-523X

Minagawa, M. (ed.) (1993). The degree of gourmet inspected from the skeletal remains in Jomon people. Asahi Shimbun, ISBN 402-2740-14-0,Tokyo

Moore, W. J. & Corbett, M. E. (1973). The distribution of dental caries in ancient British populations. II. Iron age, Romano-British and mediaeval periods. *Caries Research*, Vol. 7, pp. 139-153, ISSN 0008-6568

Moore, W. J. & Corbett, M. E. (1976). The distribution of dental caries in ancient British populations. III The 17th century. *Caries Research*, Vol. 10, pp. 401-414, ISSN 0008-6568

Nishida, M. (1980). Foods and subsistence in the Jomon period. *Anthropology Quarterly*, Uzankaku Press, ISSN 0387-3072, Tokyo, Japan.

Ono, A. (1957). Anthropological studies on the teeth of the Yayoi-age men from Mitsu, Kanzaki-gun, Saga-prefecture. *Jinruigaku Kenkyu*, Vol. 4, pp. 423-462 (in Japanese with English summary)

Oyamada, J., Kitagawa, Y., Manabe, Y. & Rokutanda, A. (2004). Dental pathology in the samurai and commoners of early modern Japan. *Anthropological Science*, Vol. 112, pp. 235-246, ISSN 0918-7960

Oyamada, J., Igawa, K., Kitagawa, Y., Manabe, Y., Kato, K. Matsushita, T. & Rokutanda, A. (2007). Low AMTL ratios in medieval Japanese dentition excavated from the Yuigahama-minami site in Kamakura. *Anthropological Science*, Vol. 115, pp. 47-53, ISSN 0918-7960

Reich, K. M., Huber, C. D., Lipping, W. R., Ulm, C., Watzek, G. & Tangle, S. (2010). Atrophy of residual alveolar ridge following tooth loss in an historical population. *Oral Diseases*, Vol . 17, No. 1, pp. 33-44, ISSN 1354-523X

Robinson, J. T. (1952). Some hominid features of the ape-mandentition. *Journal of Dental Association, Series Africa*, Vol. 7, pp.102-107

Sakura, H. (1964). Historical change in the frequency of dental caries among the Japanese people. *Journal of the Anthropological Society of Nippon* Vol. 71, No. 4, pp. 153-177, ISSN 0003-5505 (in Japanese with English summary)

Sakura, H. (1989). Low incidence of dental caries among a rural population in the early modern age unearthed from the Oterayama site. *Bulletin of National Science Museum,* Tokyo. *Series D*, Vol. 11, pp.1-5.

Sanui, Y. (1960). Anthropological researches on the teeth of the prehistoric Yayoi-ancient excavated from the Doigahama site, Yamaguchi-prefecture. *Jinruigaku Kenkyu*, Vol. 7, pp. 861-884. (in Japanese with English summary)

Silverstros, S. S., Mamalis, A. A., Sklavounou, A. D., Tzerbos, F. X. & Rontogianni, D. D. (2006). Eosinophilic granuloma masquerading as aggressive periodontitis. *Journal of Periodontology*, Vol. 77, No. 5, pp. 917-921, ISSN 0022-3492

Suzuki, K. (1989). Japanese archaeology for studying. Yuhikaku Press, ISBN 4-641-18076-8, Tokyo, Japan

Turner, C. G. II (1979). Dental anthropological indications of agriculture among the Jomon people of central Japan. *American Journal of Physical Anthropology*, Vol. 51, pp. 619-636, ISSN 1096-8644

Watanabe, H. & Grillo, A. I. (1990) Five-year follow-up caries study among Nigerian children. *Community Dentistry and Oral Epidemiology*, Vol. 18, No. 4, pp. 197-199, 1990

Whittaker, D. K., Molleson, T., Bennett, R. B., Edwards, I., Jenkins, P. R. & Llewelyn, J. K. (1981). The prevalence and distribution of dental caries in a Romano-British population. *Archives Oral Biology*.Vol. 26, pp. 237-245, ISSN 0003-9969

Yukinari, M. (1975) Dental caries of the Jomon population in Japan. *Niigata Medical Journal*, Vol. 89, pp. 68-75, ISSN 0029-0440 (in Japanese with English summary).

Part 5

Treatment of Periodontal Disease

14

Laser Radiation as an Adjunct to Nonsurgical Treatment of Periodontal Disease

Juan Antonio García Núñez[1], Alicia Herrero Sánchez[1], Ana Isabel García Kass[1] and Clara Gómez Hernández[2]
[1]*Faculty of Odontology, Universidad Complutense of Madrid (UCM),*
[2]*Instituto Fisica-Quimica Rocasolano,*
Consejo Superior de Investigaciones Científicas (CSIC), Madrid,
Spain

1. Introduction

It is well known that biofilm and calculus responsible for periodontal disease can be of different nature depending on their supra or subgingival location, and that the physical or chemical methods used for their elimination, achieve different results in both places (Davies et al., 1998). Since the use of laser confocal microscope and the study of biofilms in their natural state, it has been observed that the behaviour of bacteria is quite different to the observed in traditional cultures. In their natural state, the bacterial colonies are constituted by several microcolonies included in a matrix, which has canals through which flow fluids transporting nutrients, metabolic wastes, enzymes, oxygen and other products enabling the presence of different environments (Costerton et al. 1987).

The biofilms adhered on the internal and external walls of the periodontal pocket, the free biofilm and the possibility of a bacterial penetration through the epithelium to the underlying connective tissue can cause a gingival inflammatory reaction. This inflammation may progress with vasodilation, cellular migration and release of mediators, thus increasing the inflammatory response and perpetuating the disease. This situation makes microorganisms more resistant to drugs, which frequently are unable to reach the colonies protected by the matrix and by the presence of resistent bacteria (Donlan & Costerton, 2002). The inflammatory phenomena triggered by the bacteria and their waste products attracts macrophages that produce, among others, interleukin 1 (IL-1) and tumor necrosis factor alfa (TNF-α), which have the ability to activate osteoclasts and produce bone resorption. TNF-α activates the adhesion molecules of the endothelial cells of the vessels, favouring the adhesion of monocytes and diapedesis. It also stimulates the arrival of T lymphocytes, which contribute with receptor activator of nuclear factor kappa B ligand (RANKL) to the bone, consequently favouring the bone loss (Kong et al., 1999). But this process is more complex as it needs some proteins such as nuclear factor kappa B (NF-kB), receptor activator of nuclear factor kappa B (RANK), RANKL and osteoprotegerin (OPG), among others, which may change the answer of the osteoclast precursors and therefore modify the osseous destruction. The NF-kB plays a basic role as activator of immunoglobulins during the infectious process (Gilmore, 2006). So, as IL-1 and TNF-α favour the synthesis of RANK-L and thus the activation of RANK, it allows the differentiation of the preosteoclast into osteoclast. But this process may be hindered when OPG (a soluble protein expressed in numerous tissues and in osteoblastic cells) appears (Aubin & Bonnelye, 2000), blocking the union between RANK and RANKL, stopping the process of bone destruction (Fig. 1). OPG is a tumor necrosis factor receptor -like molecule, which is produced by gingival fibroblasts, ligament and epithelial cells (Sakata et al., 1999), that can be modulated by several inflammatory cytokines.

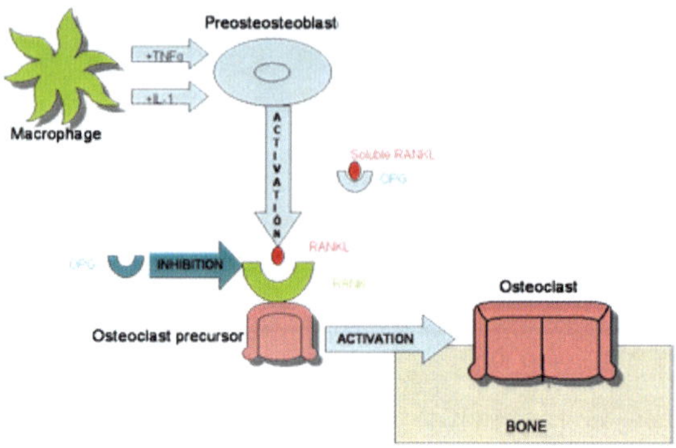

Fig. 1. Activation by RANKL and inhibition by OPG of bone resorption.

These proteins can be detected at the periodontal pocket and are related to the degree of evolution of the periodontal disease (Bostanci et al., 2007). Its monitoring allows us with much more precision than the clinic to detect the possible biological effects over the periodontal status, once applied the treatment.

Searching for effective techniques for the elimination of the biofilm and reduction of the inflammation, the mechanical treatment is still considered the gold standard. Using scaling and root planing (SRP), ultrasonic scalers and adequate hygiene techniques, acceptable results can be achieved, but these treatments alone are unable to eliminate completely all the bacteria due to radicular morphologic factors, deep pockets with a difficult access (Adriaens & Adriaens, 2004), bacterial invasion of adjacent gingival tissues and fast variation of the bacterial colonies (Costerton et al., 1999). Nowadays, antibiotics are used as complementary elements but its use should be restricted to the minimum due to the frequent development of resistances, and to the difficulty of maintaining stable and effective levels during a long period of time (Socransky & Haffajee, 2002). For this reason it becomes necessary the additional research of substances or techniques that can modify the pH, the oxygen concentration or the nutrient disposition of the dental plaque in order to modify the microflora of the biofilm. We also need to find systems able to interfere with the bacterial genetic signals and to modify the inflammatory response in the periodontal tissues.

An alternative to be considered is the use of laser technology. Several studies guarantee its beneficial effects such as sulcular and/or pocket debridement, reduction of subgingival bacterial load and decrease of inflammation (Ando et al., 1996; Folwaczny et al., 2002; Schwarz et al., 2008). Recently, in the periodontal field, it has also been introduced the photodynamic therapy (Chan & Lai, 2003; Maisch et al., 2007). Nowadays, the use of lasers within the periodontal pocket has become a promising field in the periodontal therapy.

2. Lasers employed in periodontics

Currently, different equipments of laser radiation (Er:YAG, Er,Cr:YSGG, Nd:YAG, diode, CO_2), are available in Periodontics, each one with particular features and diverse effects, making necessary the selection of the most suitable for each type of application (Table 1). Some of these lasers are effective in eliminating the residual calculus and detoxifying the radicular cementum (Er:YAG) (Aoki et al., 2004; Ishikawa et al., 2004; Schwarz et al., 2008); on the contrary others are unable to eliminate the calculus but can act over the soft tissues reducing the inflammation, as they modify the tissue oxidation systems and the cytokines which mediate in inflammation (Nd:YAG, diode) (Gómez et al., 2011). Although these effects over the tissues are difficult to evaluate clinically, they are guaranteed by molecular biology techniques. The results seem to be variable, but the investigation should help us to select the wavelength of the radiation, pulse duration, energy/power applied, pulse shape, repetition rate, time of exposure, sequence, type of wave, continuous (cw) or pulsed, type of applicator (cutout or rigid fiberglass), and other factors which can provide the desired objectives.

	Biostimulation	**Photodynamic**	**Photocoagulation**	**Photovaporization**	**Photoablation**
diode 635 nm	**	**			
diode 650 nm	**	**			
diode 675 nm	**	**			
diode 690 nm	**	**			
diode 810 nm	**$_a$		**		
diode 980 nm	**$_a$		**	*	
Nd:YAG 1,064 nm/cw	*$_a$		**	*	
Nd:YAG 1,064 nm/pulsed					**
Er,Cr:YSGG 2,790 nm					**
Er:YAG 2,940 nm					**
CO_2 10,600 nm				**	

a= at low-level laser power

Table 1. Periodontal laser systems and tissue interaction.

The therapeutic application of laser radiation can be clinically useful only if the appropriate instrumentation is available. Since the laser has been introduced into medicine, and so into dental discipline, a number of different applicators have been developed for day-to-day clinical use. The types of applicators most used in Periodontics are shown next. For instance, those with rigid fiberglass are set over handpieces. They should be used sliding them almost parallel to the radicular surface (Fig. 2), with a 20° angle in a coronoapical sense, as the perpendicular application produces damage in the cementum. Due to their size, the applicators with cutout fiberglass (Fig. 3) allow intrasulcular insertion and can reach deep areas. The displacement is also done in a coronoapical sense, outlining the whole radicular surface following the depth of the periodontal pockets, in the same manner as in a periodontal probing. Other rigid and thin applicators should be used with spiral or circular movements instead of coronoapically, in order to optimize results.

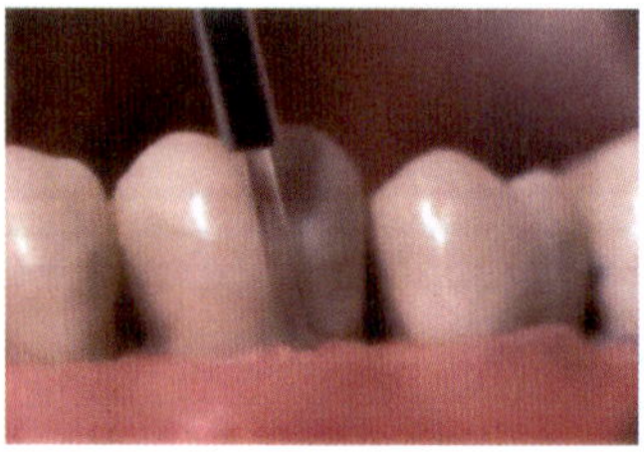

Fig. 2. Application of rigid fiberglass.

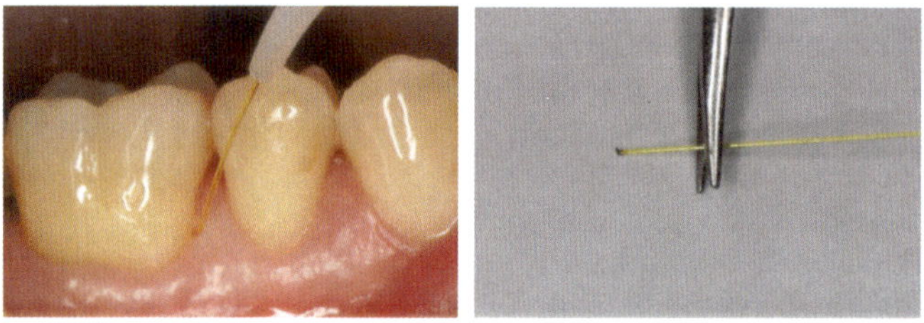

Fig. 3. A) Application with cutout fiberglass. B) Cutout fiberglass.

In Periodontics we need treatments to eliminate the plaque and calculus, and to eliminate and/or reduce the gingival inflammatory phenomena. We have to operate therefore over the soft and hard dental tissues. For this reason, the basic effects of periodontal lasers over these soft and hard tissues are presented next, in order to show the possibilities of this technology applied alone, and mainly in combination with SRP.

3. Lasers on dental soft tissues

The earliest clinical studies mentioning the application of lasers in the non-surgical treatment of periodontitis began in the early 1990s using a Nd:YAG laser with the development of flexible optical fibres. Since then, many studies have been carried out to evaluate the possible advantages of the use of lasers (Nd:YAG, diode (GaAlAs, InGaAsP), Er:YAG, Er,Cr:YSGG and CO_2) with wavelengths ranging from 635 to 10,600 nm. Recently, systematic reviews have compiled different clinical and microbiological effects of different types of laser radiation used as monotherapy or adjunctive therapy compared with SRP. However, less information to demonstrate the anti-inflammatory effect of the laser radiation is available from the literature.

3.1 Nd:YAG laser radiation

The Nd:YAG laser is nowadays the most important solid-state laser. The essential advantages of the Nd:YAG laser are its simple and compact construction and its high average power output. The neodymium (Nd+) ion, implanted into various host crystals, is the source of the laser radiation. Among the many crystals which have been investigated, one material stands out: $Y_3Al_5O_{12}$, yttrium-aluminium-garnet, a crystal with a garnet structure, which enables a laser emission at 1,064 nm, in the near-infrared spectral region. This allows its transmission through 200 to 400 micron of diameter optical fibre, making easier its use and reaching even the internal side of the periodontal pocket (Fig. 3). Unlike other infrared lasers with a strong absorption by water, such as Er:YAG or CO_2, the wavelength of Nd:YAG laser presents a poor absorption by water, thus increasing scattering and infiltration of its energy into the biological tissues. The photothermal effects of Nd:YAG laser are useful in soft tissue surgeries. Thanks to its great penetration depth and thermogenesis properties, this type of laser produces a thick coagulation layer in the irradiated area, presenting a great haemostatic capacity, being efficient for the ablation of potentially haemorrhagic soft tissues (Perry et al., 1997, Romanos, 1994).

There is little evidence to support the efficacy of Nd:YAG laser treatment as an adjunct to nonsurgical periodontal treatment in adults with periodontal inflammation. In the last decade, there are barely clinical studies published analyzing the clinical evolution and the inflammatory mediator levels in the gingival crevicular fluid (GCF) after irradiation with Nd:YAG laser in the affected sites in patients with chronic periodontitis. The results obtained in four clinical studies, performed by three different research groups, should be emphasized (Gómez et al., 2011; Miyazaki et al., 2003; Qadri et al., 2010, 2011). The overheating of the irradiated tissues and the consequent damage of the oral hard and soft tissues, could explain the limited support to this kind of laser radiation from the scientific community (Miserendino et al., 1994). For this reason, to avoid thermal damage, the irradiation parameters employed in these clinical studies were selected according to the results obtained in previous *in vitro* investigations, where potential morphological alterations of root surface irradiation were assessed under standardized conditions (Bader, 2000; Gómez et al., 2009).

Concerning the evolution of the clinical parameters, the application of Nd:YAG laser both as monotherapy or as an adjuvant to scaling and root planing, did not offer significant advantages versus the treatment with ultrasonic devices, both at 8 (Gómez et al., 2011) (Fig. 4) and at 12 weeks (Miyazaki et al., 2003).

Nevertheless, Qadri et al., in their split mouth trial, found better clinical results in the test side (SRP + Nd:YAG) than in the control side (SRP) during the long term follow up (up to 20 months) (Qadri et al., 2011).

When analyzing the inflammatory mediators, Miyazaki, in a 12 weeks study, found a non statistically significant decrease of IL-1β in Nd:YAG group used as monotherapy in comparison with ultrasonic devices for the non surgical treatment of chronic periodontitis (Miyazaki et al., 2003). On the contrary, Gómez did find in a short term study (4 and 8 weeks) significant decreases both in IL-1β as in TNF-α when using Nd:YAG as an adjuvant to SRP versus SRP alone (Fig. 5). In this same study, the total antioxidant status (TAS) of the gingival fluid, gradually increased until the eighth week after the treatment with SRP + Nd:YAG, while it remained stable when the treatment consisted of SRP, being these differences statistically significant (Gómez et al., 2011). The total antioxidant capacity of the gingival fluid decreases in periodontitis as a consequence of the inflammatory lesion, and it recovers after non surgical therapy (Brock et al., 2004; Chapple et al., 2007; Tsai et al., 2005). Thus, Gómez observed that the total antioxidant capacity of GCF was influenced by the reduction of periodontal inflammation after successful non-surgical therapy complemented by Nd:YAG radiation (Gómez et al., 2011). Finally, in the study of Qadri in which the long-term effects of a single application of a water-cooled pulsed Nd:YAG in combination with SRP were investigated, the authors found less bone loss and a lower GCF volume than in the control group (SRP alone), and thus the severity of periodontal inflammation seemed to be reduced (Qadri et al., 2011).

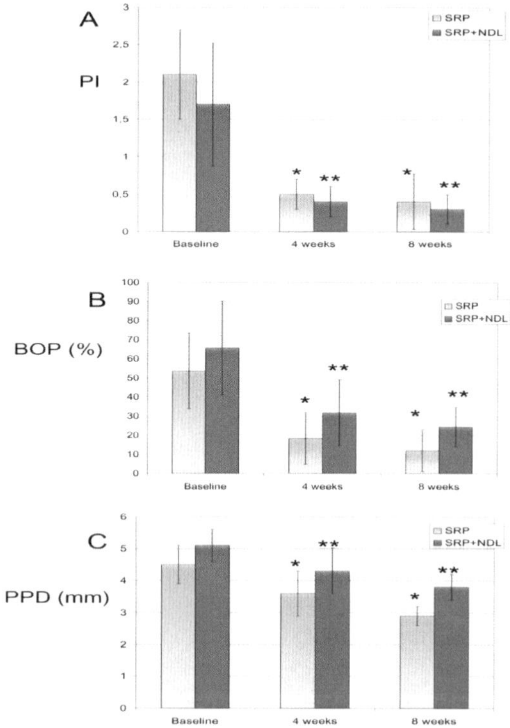

Fig. 4. *A)* Plaque Index (PI), B) Bleeding on Probing (BOP) and C) Probing Pocket Depth (PPD): Mean Scores (± SD), (n=30 patients) at baseline, 4 and 8 weeks post-therapy. (*) Significance of differences compared to baseline within SRP group at different points of time by a non-parametric Wilcoxon test ($p<0.05$). (**) Significance of differences compared to baseline within SRP+NDL group at different points of time by a non-parametric Wilcoxon test ($p<0.05$). (Gómez et al., 2011)

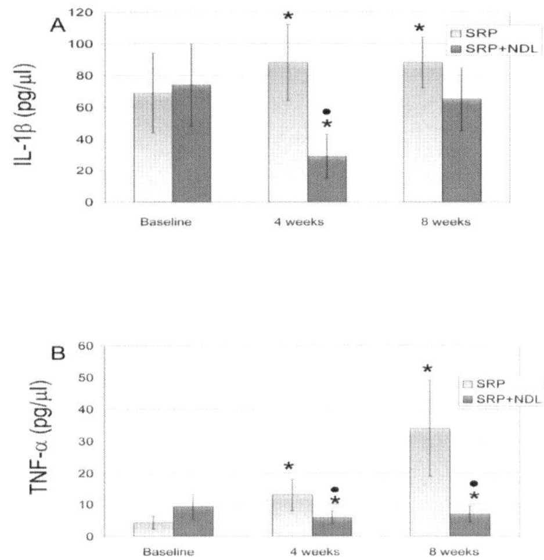

Fig. 5. A) Interleukin 1β (IL-1β) and B) Tumour Necrosis Factor α (TNF-α): Mean Scores (± SD), (n= 30 patients) at baseline, 4 and 8 weeks post-therapy. (*) Significance of differences compared to baseline within the groups at different points of time by a non-parametric Wilcoxon test ($p<0.05$). (•) Significance of differences compared to baseline between the groups at different points of time by a non-parametric Mann-Whitney test ($p<0.05$). (Gómez et al., 2011)

3.2 Fluorescence-controlled Er: YAG laser radiation

In erbium lasers, erbium ions (Er^{3+}) are implanted in the solid-state materials yttrium aluminium garnet (YAG, $Y_3Al_5O_{12}$). Its pulsed infrared radiation, at 2,940 nm, is characterized by being highly absorbed by water, therefore it is particularly indicated for a precise and located ablation of the biological tissues with a high water content. Theoretically, the absorption coefficient of water for the Er:YAG laser is 10,000 cm^{-1}, and thus 15 and 2,000 times higher than for CO_2 and Nd:YAG lasers, respectively. This high absorption coefficient results in extremely small optical penetration depths and therefore in tissue ablation with minimal thermal damage. Additionally, the OH groups, as components of the hydroxyapatite, show their higher absorption around 2,800 nm, explaining thereby its ablation capacity over the enamel, dentin and bone, so this type of laser is indicated both for soft and hard tissues. The energy transport from the laser system to the patient is done by an articulated arm or by a flexible waveguide made of zirconium fluoride or crystalline sapphire. A variety of new applicators are continuously extending the potential dental uses.
Based on the results of *in vitro* studies, Watanabe performed the first clinical application of an Er:YAG laser for debridement in 1996 (Watanabe et al., 1996). Nowadays, after the investigation carried out in the clinical field with this type of laser radiation, it seems that Er:YAG laser emerges as the most adequate laser system as an alternative or adjuvant tool of SRP. This is due to the lower thermal damage generated on the hard tissues (Schwarz et al., 2008). Although the *in vitro* capability of calculus and plaque removal of Er:YAG laser has been displayed, clinical studies have shown divergent clinical outcomes in the initial treatment of chronic periodontitis. Crespi (Crespi et al., 2007) reported a significant reduction in clinical parameters at 6 months in the Er:YAG group compared to the group

treated by SRP with ultrasonic scalers, while a recent study has found that adjunctive use of Er:YAG laser to conventional SRP did not reveal a more effective result than SRP alone in the short term of 6 months (Rotundo et al., 2010).

A new Er:YAG laser equipment introduced to improve the results is a device that allows the control of Er:YAG laser radiation by incorporating a feedback system that selectively detects subgingival calculus (Fig. 2). Few clinical studies have evaluated the treatment outcomes after laser debridement by using fluorescence controlled Er:YAG radiation. In the split-mouth study of Sculean it was observed that fluorescence-controlled Er:YAG radiation led to clinical improvement at 3 and 6 months, similar to ultrasonic debridement (Sculean et al., 2004). Tomasi evaluated the clinical and microbiological outcomes after a feedback-controlled Er:YAG laser and ultrasonic device debridement during periodontal supportive therapy (Tomasi et al., 2006). They observed that mean PPD reduction and CAL (clinical attachment level) gain were significantly higher in the laser group after 1 month of healing. However, both treatments resulted in a significant reduction of subgingival microflora, although no significant differences were observed between groups at each time point investigated. Derdilopoulou compared the microbiological effects of SRP, Er:YAG laser with feedback, sonic and ultrasonic scalers in patients with chronic periodontitis over a period of 6 months. The treatment methods employed resulted in a comparable reduction of the evaluated periodontopathogens, where Er:YAG laser did not demonstrate to be superior (Derdilopoulou et al., 2007). Finally, more encouraging were the results obtained by Domínguez, when Er:YAG laser was employed as an adjuvant to SRP. Though no statistically significant differences were observed between both groups in any of the investigated clinical parameters (Domínguez et al., 2010) (Fig. 6), the cytokine levels in the GCF were reduced with the feedback-controlled Er:YAG laser radiation (Fig. 7). Since the outcome in the SRP+ Er:YAG group was only slightly better than in the SRP group, previous mechanical subgingival debridement is necessary. Despite the above described advantage of using this laser prototype, no additional effect of the Er:YAG laser therapy was found on the local (GCF) total antioxidant capacity.

Finally, in a study reported by Schwarz, immunohistochemical characterization of wound healing following non-surgical periodontal treatment revealed that fluorescence-controlled Er:YAG laser radiation was effective in controlling disease progression, and may support the formation of a new connective tissue attachment (Schwarz et al., 2007).

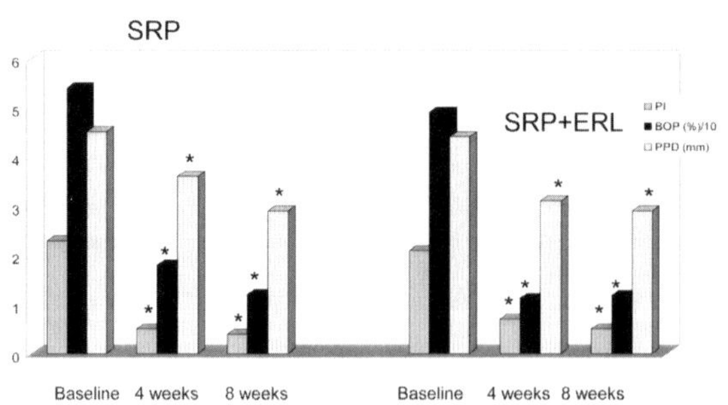

Fig. 6. Plaque Index (PI), Bleeding on probing (BOP) and Probing Pocket Depth (PPD): Mean Scores (± SD), (n=30 patients) at baseline, 4 and 8 weeks. (*) Significance of differences compared to baseline within the groups at different time points by Wilcoxon test ($p<0.05$). (**) Significance of differences compared to baseline between the groups at different time points by Mann-Whitney test ($p<0.05$). (Domínguez et al., 2010)

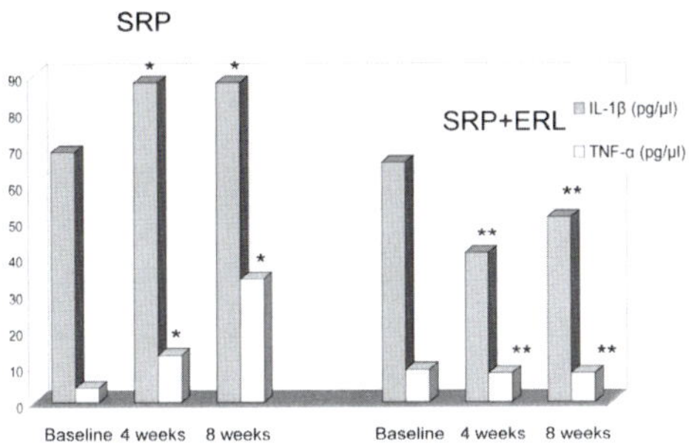

Fig. 7. Interleukin1β (IL-1β) and Tumour Necrosis Factor α (TNF-α): Mean Scores (± SD), (n=30 patients) at baseline, 4 and 8 weeks. (*) Significance of differences compared to baseline within the groups at different time points by Wilcoxon test ($p<0.05$). (**) Significance of differences compared to baseline between the groups at different time points by Mann Whitney test ($p<0.05$). (Domínguez et al, 2010)

3.3 Photodynamic therapy (PDT)

Photodynamic therapy basically involves three nontoxic ingredients: visible harmless light, a nontoxic photosensitizer (i.e. a photoactivable substance) and oxygen (Fig 8). It is based on the principle that the photosensitizer binds to the target cells and can be activated by light of a suitable wavelength. Following activation of the photosensitizer, singlet oxygen and other reactive agents that are extremely toxic to certain cells and bacteria are produced. This singlet oxygen might cause toxic effects on the microorganisms: damage of the membrane lipids, destruction of protein and ion channels, elimination of critical metabolic enzymes, cell agglutination and inhibition of exogenous virulence factors such as lipopolysaccharide, collagenase and protease. Photosensitizers for PDT are selected for their ability to rapidly penetrate bacterial biofilms and to selectively stain and kill the prokaryotic cells under illumination while avoiding damage to human tissues (Konopla & Goslinski, 2007).

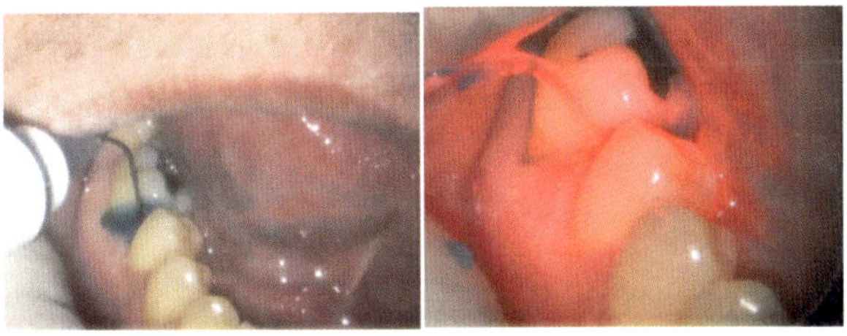

Fig. 8. A) Periodontal pocket irrigation with methylene blue, B) Subsequent photosensitizer activation with diode laser at 670 nm.

Several studies have reported the use of PDT therapy as an adjunct to nonsurgical treatment for initial and supportive therapy of chronic periodontitis. In view of the published results, the adjunctive use of photodynamic therapy to SRP may result, on a short-term basis (up to 3 or 6 months), in higher reductions in bleeding on probing with PPD reductions and CAL gains comparable to those obtained after SRP alone (Chondros et al., 2009; Christodoulides et al., 2008; Ge et al., 2011; Polansky et al., 2009). The higher improvement in mean full-mouth bleeding scores (FMBS) might be attributed in part to the additional photobiomodulation effect mediated by the low-level laser irradiation during photodynamic therapy (Qadri et al., 2005).

Photodynamic therapy has been introduced as an important novel disinfection therapy in the field of dentistry. Taking into account the microbiological improvement of PDT, some research groups did not find additional benefit of SRP+PDT above SRP at any follow-up evaluation (Chistodoulides et al. 2008; Polansky et al., 2009; Yilmaz et al., 2002). Chondros (Chondros et al., 2009) found a significant reduction in *F. nucleatum* and *E. nodatum* in the group receiving the combined treatment (SRP+PDT) at the 3-month evaluation.

A recent study of 10 patients in supportive periodontal therapy with 70 residual pockets (PPD≥5mm) and a parallel group design, has confirmed positive effects of repeated adjunctive PDT to SRP treatment on those residual pockets treated, such as greater PPD reductions, CAL gains and decreased BOP percentages after 6 months post-therapy (Lulic et al., 2009). These positive results could be related with the study protocol: SRP of the residual pockets followed by immediate PDT application, repeating this sequence of treatment five times in 2 weeks.

The presence of BOP is considered an objective indicator of gingival inflammation (Chaves et al., 1993; Lang et al. 1990). The published results of SRP+PDT treatment generally show a tendency to reduce BOP or FMBS, and thus a tendency to reduce inflammation. It should be pointed out that there are hardly any studies in the literature relating PDT and proinflammatory cytokines, with the exception of de Oliveira´s. These authors investigated cytokine levels in GCF of patients with aggressive periodontitis after PDT or SRP. The results showed that both treatment modalities significantly reduced TNF-α and RANKL levels following treatment (de Oliveira et al., 2009). Recently, histological examinations of periodontal tissues of rats treated 1 month before with toluidine blue-mediated PDT, revealed a remarkable reduction of inflammatory reactions (reduced infiltration of inflammatory cells, mainly lymphocytes), greater than in periodontal tissues conventionally treated (Qin et al., 2008). In addition, after the application of a single *in vitro* PDT treatment, an inactivation of host destructive cytokines (which impair periodontal restoration) was seen by means of a cytokine inactivation assay that measured E-selectin expression in response to IL-1β and TNF-α (Braham et al., 2009).

Although the results published in the literature seem to indicate that the adjunctive use of PDT may improve some outcomes, randomized controlled clinical studies, evaluating the clinical, microbiological and immunological potential benefits of photodynamic therapy in the treatment of periodontitis, are still limited. The main drawbacks may be related to the rather limited number of patients, the short-term duration of studies (i.e. 3 or 6 months) and the fact that the most effective protocol of PDT has not yet been established.

Finally, we should point out that in few years PDT has progressed greatly in the biomedical field. Nowadays, numerous research groups are working in this field investigating its application. New photosensitizers are being developed searching its faster removal from healthy tissues, acting at lower doses and being able to absorb longer wavelengths. This would allow higher light penetration, requiring lower doses of photosensitizer, while new sources of irradiation are also being developed.

3.4 New research lines: Phototherapy/biostimulation

The variety of biological effects which laser radiation may produce in the oral tissues are not yet completely understood. Among the many physiological ones, it is important to recognize benefitial biostimulant effects of laser radiation in cells of the oral tissues during laser therapy, such as the contribution to a faster healing during the reparation process of the periodontium, which may not take place during the conventional mechanical therapy. These biostimulant effects have been associated with the use of low level laser radiation (Peplow et al., 2010). According to the first law of photochemistry, the biological effect observed after the application of laser radiation of low energetic level, can only be a result of the presence of a photoacceptor molecule, able to absorb the photonic energy emitted (Karu, 2007). Additionally, there are no photothermal nor photoacoustic mechanisms associated to this effect, so no heating is observed macroscopically. One target identified in laser phototherapy is a highly specialized enzyme, cytocrome C oxidase, which plays a crucial role in cellular bioenergy (Karu, 2007). Some studies indicate that after laser irradiation at 633 nm, an increment of both the mitochondrial membrane potential and the proton gradient occurs, causing changes in the optical properties of mitochondria, thus increasing the rate of exchange of adenosine diphosphate/adenosin triphosphate (ADP/ATP) (Alexandratou et al., 2002). Moreover, it has been proposed that laser irradiation reduces the catalytic center of cytocrome C oxidase, originating more available electrons for the reduction of dioxygen (Byrnes et al., 2005). The upregulation of ATP following low level laser therapy is also coupled with transient increases of the reactive oxygen species (ROS), participating afterwards in transduction of intercellular signals (Tafur & Mills, 2008). It has been observed that the modulation of cellular metabolism and transduction of signals alter the gene expression (Snyder et al., 2002), the cellular proliferation (Moore et al., 2005), the mitochondrial membrane potential (Alenxandratou et al., 2002), the generation of transient reactive oxygen species (Lubart et al., 2005), the level of calcium ion (Tong et al., 2000) the gradient of protons and the oxygen consumption.

The efficacy of low-level laser therapy in periodontal disease is still controversial. Ribeiro (Ribeiro et al., 2008) corroborated that the use of diode laser as an adjunct to SRP 4 times in the first two days of treatment did not provide any apparent clinical benefit in teeth with shallow to moderate pockets. Lai (Lai et al., 2009) also observed that phototherapy used as a complement of non surgical periodontal therapy eight times in the first three months of treatment did not improve healing response as assessed by both clinical and radiographic parameters. In the study of Yilmaz, laser used as a monotherapy did not affect the inflammatory response more than oral hygiene instructions (Yilmaz et al, 2002). The group treated with subgingival debridement plus low level laser therapy obtained the same results as that treated only with subgingival debridement, thus demonstrating that mechanical subgingival debridement is always necessary. However, other studies verify the efficacy of phototherapy. For example, Qadri (Qadri et al, 2005) observed significantly higher reductions in PPD, PI, GI, GCF and MMP-8 in the laser treated sites. Therefore, the use of a low level laser radiation as an adjunct to the periodontal treatment showed a positive influence on inflammation and healing. Pejčic (Pejčic et al., 2010) confirmed that low level laser radiation at 670 nm may be successfully used as an adjunctive treatment method, which, together with conventional periodontal therapy, achieves better long term results (up to 6 months after treatment). Thus the PI, GI and BOP decreased, demonstrating that the number of laser applications is of great importance in order to obtain the best results in the irradiated tissue, achieving a considerable antiinflammatory effect after the fifth application. In addition, Kreisler (Kreisler et al., 2005) when using a 809 nm GaAlAs semiconductor laser operated at 1 W power output as an adjunct to SRP, observed a significant improvement concerning the tooth mobility, PPD and CAL, not finding significant differences in PI, GI, BOP and GCF volume.

A higher number of well-designed long term randomized controlled clinical trials over a longer period of time may be required in order to evaluate the adjunctive use of low-level diode laser radiation during non-surgical periodontal therapy and to clarify controversy.

4. Lasers on dental hard tissues

Until the beginning of the 1990s, the use of laser systems in periodontal therapy was limited to soft tissue procedures, such as gingivectomy and frenectomy, as application to periodontal hard tissues had previously been shown to be clinically unpromising (Cohen & Ammons, 2002; Pick & Colvard, 1993). In the last decades, laser therapy has been proposed as an alternative or an adjunct to conventional non-surgical therapy, due to its capability to obtain tissue ablation and haemostasia, bactericidal effect against periodontal pathogens and detoxification of root surface (Aoki et al., 2004; Folwaczny et al., 2002; Ishikawa et al., 2004; Schwarz et al., 2008).
CO_2 and Nd:YAG lasers can produce carbonization and major thermal side effects when used on hard tissues such as root surface and bone (Israel et al., 1997; Wilder-Smith et al., 1995) (Fig. 10). The CO_2 irradiation is well absorbed by water, and by the main mineral components of hard tissues, especially phosphate ions (-PO4) of the hydroxyapatite (Koort & Frentzen, 1995). Since ablation is basically produced by heat generation, unlike other laser systems such as Er:YAG laser, carbonization occurs easily on the irradiated surface (Sasaki et al., 2002). When used with relatively low energy output in a pulsed and/or defocused mode, CO_2 lasers have been used to achieve root conditioning, detoxification, and bactericidal effects on contaminated root surfaces (Coffelt et al., 1997). However, at low energy outputs in a continuous mode, it is unable to remove subgingival calculus and when used with high energy outputs, especially in a cw mode, it is inappropriate for calculus removal due to major thermal side effects, such as carbonization, melting and cracking on the cementum and dentin (Misra et al., 1999).

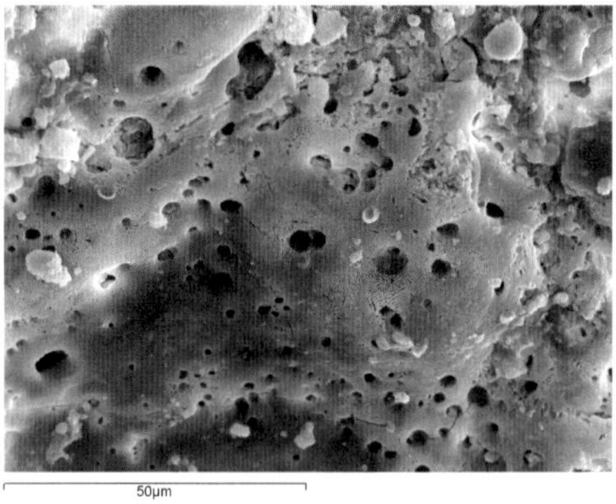

Fig. 9. Scanning electron microscope obtained image of a radicular surface treated with Nd:YAG (1,5 W, 10 Hz).

Nd:YAG laser presents low absorption by water, which produces scattering of its energy and thus a great penetration into the tissues. *In vitro* and *in vivo* studies have shown that this laser is inefficient to successfully achieve root surface debridement, due to its poor ability to remove calculus. Nd:YAG should be employed as an adjunct to conventional mechanical treatments, rather than as a primary instrument in the treatment of periodontal pockets (Liu et al., 1999). The same as CO_2 laser, Nd:YAG produces different root surface alterations, induced by heat generation during irradiation (Fig. 9) (Cobb, 1996; Gómez et al., 2006; 2009). Nevertheless, several *in vitro* studies have demonstrated the ability of these lasers to create a compatible surface for soft tissue attachment (Israel et al. 1997; Wilder-Smith et al., 1995).

In 1989 Hibst and Keller (Hibst & Keller, 1989; Keller & Hibst, 1989) reported the possibility of dental hard tissue ablation by Er:YAG laser irradiation, which is highly absorbed by water. Since then, numerous studies on hard tissue treatment using the Er:YAG laser have indicated the ability of this laser to ablate dental hard tissses and carious lesions without producing major thermal side effects.

The absorption of Er:YAG laser in water is the highest because its 2,940 nm emission wavelength matches with the large absorption band for water. Additionally, as part of the apatite component, OH^- groups show a relatively high absorption at 2,940 nm. As the Er:YAG laser is well absorbed by all biological tissues that contain water molecules, it is indicated not only for the treatment of soft tissues but also for ablation of hard tissues.

In vitro studies have shown that the Er:YAG laser application is effective in eliminating subgingival calculus, with similar results when compared with ultrasonic instrumentation (Aoki et al., 2000; Folwaczny et al., 2000; Herrero et al. 2010). However, some authors showed a greater amount of residual calculus in the areas treated with the Er:YAG laser (Eberhard et al. 2003). Factors such as the quantity and quality of the initial calculus (texture, thickness and water content) and root anatomy, together with the individualized instrumentation technique, may influence the results independently of the mode of implementation (Herrero et al., 2010). Due to their similar composition, calculus and cementum have similar ablation thresholds; therefore, it would be impossible to carry out selective and effective removal of calculus with the use of Er:YAG laser application without causing root damage (Aoki et al., 1994).

Different energy settings have been reported to be more efficient for calculus removal without damaging the root cementum. Most of the studies suggest the use of energies between 100-160 mJ (Crespi et al., 2006; Folwaczny et al., 2000; Frentzen et al., 2002). Higher energies may damage the radicular surface and lower energies are unable to eliminate the calculus effectively (García et al., 2001). Folwaczny et al. reported that the angulation tip to the root surface has a strong influence on the amount of root substance removed during Er:YAG laser irradiation (Folwaczny et al, 2000). Moreover, the use of water coolant minimizes heat generation by cooling the irradiated area and absorbing excessive laser energy. In addition, a water spray facilitates hard tissue ablation by eliminating the target moist (Burkes et al., 1992). A secondary effect of calculus removal is the elimination of cementum and subsequent dentinal tubular exposure (Fig. 10). Even though the amount of cementum on the root surface is highly variable and depends on factors such as patient age and previous periodontal treatment, *in vitro* studies have described that the number and diameter of exposed dentinal tubules was significantly higher in areas treated with laser than with ultrasonic scalers (Gómez et al., 2009; Herrero et al., 2010; Theodoro et al., 2003).

The last generation of Er:YAG laser includes a calculus detection device based on the signal of the fluorescence emitted from the mineralized tissues (feedback system). Preliminar *in vitro* and clinical studies show that the Er:YAG laser debridement, when performed with automatic calculus detection, allows an efficient calculus removal similar to the obtained with ultrasonic scaling, without the partial ablation of subjacent cementum observed with the Er:YAG laser prototypes without feedback system, thus resulting in almost no dentinal tubule exposure (Herrero et al., 2010; Krause et al. 2003; Schwarz et al.,2006).

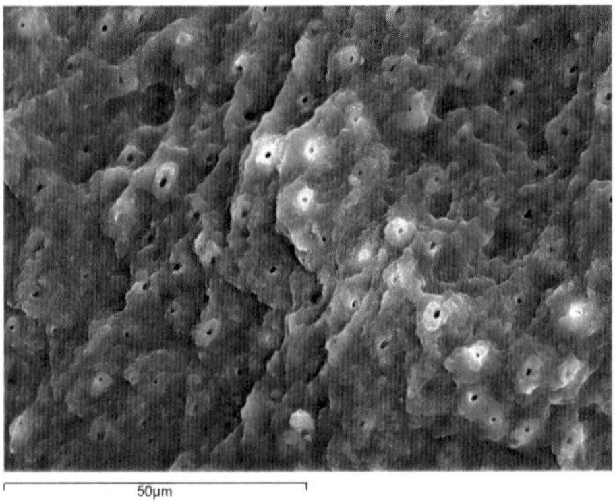

Fig. 10. Scanning electron microscope obtained image of a radicular surface treated with Er:YAG (120 mJ/pulse, 10 Hz).

The Er:YAG laser does not cause carbonization or melting of the irradiated root surface, but it has been demonstrated that the surface presents micro-irregularities, is slightly rougher and chalky, probably due to the mechanical ablation effect (Aoki et al., 1994; Aoki et al., 2000; Crespi et al., 2006; Folwaczny et al., 2000; Herrero et al., 2010). Some craters may be formed as a result of directing the laser beam too perpendicularly to the root surface or by using a non beveled tip, which hampers uniform radiation (Folwaczny et al. 2000; 2002). There is no clear indication in the literature of which is the ideal root surface to improve healing. It is well accepted that a rough surface does not negatively affect periodontal healing (Kathiblou & Ghoddsi, 1983). According to several authors (Eberhard et al., 2003; Folwaczny et al., 2000), the surface treated with Er.YAG laser is similar to the one observed after EDTA (Lasho et al., 1983) or citric acid conditioning (Wen et al., 1992), which for many years have been used as root conditioners improving the results of periodontal treatment (Schwarz et al., 2003a). On the contrary, the presence of a rough root surface may favour plaque retention and, therefore, limit the results of cause-related periodontal therapy (Adriaens & Adriaens, 2004).

5. Lasers for the treatment of periimplantitis

Bacterial colonization in the implant surface is considered the main aethiological factor of implant failure (Becker et al., 1990). The bacterial presence in the implant surface may cause inflammation of the peri-implant mucous membrane, and, if not treated, it may progress apically, resulting in periimplantitis and bone resorption. Therefore, removal of bacterial plaque is the main objective in the therapy of periimplant infections (Mombelli & Lang, 1994). However, the debridement of implant surfaces is difficult to achieve, particularly in the rough ones. Different mechanical and chemical methods have been proposed (Augthum et al., 1998; Ericsson et al., 1996) in order to reach this objective. Recent in vitro studies suggest the use of specific devices, made of materials with lower hardness than titanium (plastic scalers, rubber cups) for the mechanical debridement (Matarasso et al., 1996). As mechanical methods are inefficient when used alone, chemical agents, such as local or systemic antimicrobials, have also been used (Ericsson et al., 1996; Norowski & Bumgardner, 2009).

Different laser systems have also been proposed for the debridement of implant surfaces (Kreisler et al., 2002a; Kreisler et al., 2002b). Recent *in vitro* studies show that, due the radiation features, only CO_2, diode and Er:YAG lasers are adequate for implants surface debridement. This is because their wavelengths are scarcely absorbed by titanium, increasing slightly the implant temperature during irradiation (Kreisler et al., 2002a; Oyster et al., 1995; Romanos et al., 2000). Nevertheless, Nd:YAG laser produces an important thermal damage in the titanium surface (Kreisler et al., 2002a; Romanos et al., 2000). Additionally, only CO_2 and Er:YAG have demonstrated bactericidal effects in *in vitro* studies, so both systems could be useful in the decontamination and detoxification of the implant surface (Kreisler et al., 2002c). As CO_2 as well as diode lasers are not effective for calculus removal in radicular surfaces nor in titanium implants, they should only be employed as adjuvants of the mechanical procedures (Moritz et al., 1998; Schwarz et al., 2003b). However, recent studies show that non surgical instrumentation of implants with Er:YAG laser, when using a specific applicator, is effective in calculus and subgingival plaque removal, without producing thermal damage to the implant surface (Schwarz et al., 2003b). The results of this study indicate that Er:YAG laser radiation does not damage titanium surfaces and subsequently does not influence the attachment rate of cultured human osteoblast-like cells (SAOS-2). Results of a preliminar clinical study by the same author, showed that non surgical treatment of periimplantitis with Er:YAG at 100 mJ/pulse and 10 Hz produces a significant reduction of PPD and CAL gain (Schwarz et al., 2005).

Recently, 940 and 980 nm diode lasers have created a great expectation, due to their excellent incision, excision and coagulation properties over the soft tissues, allowing subsequently to proceed in low energy conditions (low-level laser therapy, described previously in the above section), decreasing simultaneously the inflammatory process and achieving a faster healing of tissues (Romanos et al., 2009). The use of lasers in the treatment of periimplantitis is promising, but more studies evaluating its real efficacy are necessary.

6. Conclusions

We have to take into account that laser treatments are in continuous evolution; possibly in the next years our scope will be to have equipments combining different photonic properties allowing us to choose the most adequate system for each necessity. Although there has been a great progress in the last years, most of the studies are difficult to be evaluated clinically, due to their short duration (2 to 3 months). More long term systematic studies are necessary to evaluate the clinical and biological effects of each type of laser, the time and application mode, unique/multiple doses and application frequency. It will also be essential to know the appropriate energies of each kind of laser, deepening in its knowledge, as its application comfort, the silence, the anesthesia reduction and other advantages make them attractive for society and professionals.

7. Acknowledgments

All work described in the present chapter related with our experimental results was supported by an Intramural Project 200880I215 of the Spanish CSIC and a Grant from the Eugenio Rodríguez Pascual Foundation.

8. References

Adriaens, P.A. & Adriaens, LM. (2004). Effects of nonsurgical periodontal therapy on hard and soft tissues. *Periodontology 2000*, Vol.36, No.1, (October 2004), pp. 121–145, ISSN 0906-6713,

Alexandratou, E.; Yova, D., Handris, P., Kletsas, D. & Loukas, S. (2002). Human fibroblast alterations induced by low power laser irradiation at the single cell level using confocal microscopy. *Photochemical and Photobiological Sciences*, Vol.1, No.8, (August 2008), pp. 547-552, ISSN 1474-905x

Ando, Y.; Aoki, A., Watanabe, H. & Ishikawa, I. (1996). Bactericidal effect of erbium YAG laser on periodontopathic bacteria. *Lasers in Surgery and Medicine*, Vol.19, No.2, (January 1996), pp. 190-200, ISSN 0196-8092

Aoki, A.; Ando, Y., Watanabe, H. & Ishikawa, I. (1994). *In vitro* studies on laser scaling of subgingival calculus with an erbium:YAG laser. *Journal of Periodontology*, Vol.65, No.12, (December 1994), pp. 1097-1106, ISSN 0022-3492

Aoki, A.; Miura, M., Akiyama, F., Nakagawa, N., Tanaka, J., Oda, S., Watanabe, H., & Ishikawa, I. (2000). *In vitro* evaluation of Er.YAG laser scaling of subgingival calculus in comparison with ultrasonic scaling. *Journal of Periodontal Research*, Vol. 35, No. 5 (October 2000), pp. 266-277, ISSN 0022-3484

Aoki, A.; Sasaki, K.M., Watanabe, H. & Ishikawa, I. (2004). Lasers in nonsurgical periodontal therapy. *Periodontology 2000*, Vol.36, No.1, (October 2004), pp. 59-97, ISSN 0906-6713

Aubin J.E. & Bonnelye E. (2000). Osteoprotegerin and its ligand: a new paradigm for the regulation of osteoclastogenesis and bone resorption. *Osteoporosis International*, Vol. 11, No. 11 (November 2000), pp. 905-913, ISSN 0937-941X

Augthun M.; Tinschert J & Huber A. (1998). In vitro studies on the effect of cleaning methods on different implant surfaces. *Journal of Periodontology*, Vol.69, No.8, (August 1998), pp. 857-864, ISSN 0022-3484

Bader, H.I. (2000). Use of laser in periodontic. *Dental Clinics of North America*, Vol.44, No.4, (October 2000), pp. 779-791, ISSN 0011-8532

Becker, W.; Becker, B.E., Newman, M.G. & Nyman, S. (1990). Clinical and microbiologic findings that may contribute to dental implant failure. *The International Journal of Oral & Maxillofacial Implants*, Vol.5, No.1, (Spring 1990), pp. 31-38, ISSN 0882-2786

Bostanci, N.; Ilgenli, T., Emingil, G., Afacan, B., Han, B., Töz, H., Atilla, G., Hughes, F.J., Belibasakis G. N. (2007). Gingival crevicular levels of RANKL and OPG in periodontal diseases: implications of their relative ratio. *Journal of Clinical Periodontology*, Vol.34, No.5,(May, 2007), pp. 370-376, ISSN 0303-6979

Braham, P.; Herron, C., Street, C. & Darveau, R. (2009). Antimicrobial photodynamic therapy may promote periodontal healing through multiple mechanisms. *Journal of Periodontology*, Vol.80, No.11, (November 2009), pp. 1790-1798, ISSN 0022-3492

Brock, G.R.; Butterworth, C.J., Matthews, J.B. & Chapple I.L. (2004). Local and systemic total antioxidant capacity in periodontitis and health. *Journal of Clinical Periodontology*, Vol.31, No. 7, (July 2004), pp. 515-521 (July 2004), ISSN 0303-6979

Burkes, E.J.; Jr, Hoke, J., Gomes, E. & Wolbarsht, M. (1992). Wet versus dry enamel ablation by Er.YAG laser. *Journal of Prosthetic Dentistry*, Vol.67, No.6, (June 1992), pp. 847-851, ISSN 0022-3913

Byrnes K.R.; Wu, X., Waynant, R.W., Ilev, I.K. & Anders, J.J. (2005). Low power laser irradiation alters gene expression of olfactory ensheathing cells in vitro. *Lasers in Surgery and Medicine*, Vol.37, No.2, (August 2005), pp. 161-171, ISSN 0196-8092

Chan, Y., & Lai, C.H. (2003). Bactericidal effects of different laser wavelengths on periodontopathic germs in photodynamic therapy. *Lasers in Medical Science*, Vol.18, No.1, (March 2003), pp. 51–55, ISSN: 0268-8921

Chapple, I.L.; Brock, G.R., Milward, M.R., Ling, N. & Matthews, J.B. (2007). Compromised GCF total antioxidant capacity in periodontitis: cause or effect?. *Journal of Clinical Periodontology*, Vol.34, No.2,(February 2007), pp. 103-110, ISSN 0303-6979

Chaves, E.S.; Wood, R.C., Jones, A.A., Newbold, D.A., Manwell, M.A. & Kornman, K.S. (1993). Relationship of "bleeding on probing" and "gingival index bleeding" as clinical parameters of gingival inflammation. *Journal of Clinical Periodontology*, Vol.20, No.2, (February 2003), pp. 139-143, ISSN 0303-6979.

Chondros, P.; Nikolidakis, D., Christodoulides, N., Rössler, R., Gutknecht, N. & Sculean, A. (2009). Photodynamic therapy as adjunct to non-surgical periodontal treatment in patients on periodontal maintenance: a randomized controlled clinical trial. *Lasers in Medical Science*, Vol. 24, No. 5, (September 2009), pp. 681-688, ISSN 0268-8921

Christodoulides, N.; Nikolidakis, D., Chondros, P., Becker, J., Schwarz, F., Rössler R, & Sculean, A. (2008). Photodynamic therapy as an adjunct to non-surgical periodontal treatment: a randomized controlled clinical trial. *Journal of Periodontology*, Vol. 79, No.9, (September 2008), pp. 1638-1644, ISSN 0022-3492

Cobb, C.M. (1996). Non-surgical pocket therapy: mechanical. *Annals of Periodontology*, Vol.1, No.1, (November 1996), pp. 443-490, ISSN 1553-0841

Coffelt, D.W.; Cobb, C.M., MacNeill, S., Rapley, J.W. & Killoy, W.J. (1997). Determination of energy density threshold for laser ablation of bacteria. An *in vitro* study. *Journal of Clinical Periodontology*, Vol.24, No.1, (January 1997), pp. 1-7, ISSN 0303-6979

Cohen, RE. & Ammons, W.F. (2002). Lasers in periodontics (Academy report). AAP (The American Academy of Periodontology). The Research, Science and Therapy Committee of the American Academy of Periodontology. *Journal of Periodontology*, Vol.73, No.10, (October 2002), pp. 1231-1239, ISSN 0022-3492

Costerton, J.W.; Cheng, K.J., Geesey, G.G., Ladd, T.I., Nickel, J.C., Dasgupta, M. & Marcie TJ. (1987). Bacterial biofilms in nature and disease. *Annual Review of Microbiology*, Vol.41, (October 1987), pp. 435-464, ISSN: 0066-4227

Costerton, J.W.; Stewart, P.S. & Greenberg, E.P. (1999). Bacterial biofilms: A common cause of persistent infection. *Science*, Vol.284, No.5418, (May 1999), pp. 1318-1322. ISSN 0036-8075

Crespi, R.; Barone, A. & Covani, U. (2006). Er:YAG laser scaling of diseased root surfaces: a histologic study. *Journal of Periodontology*, Vol.77, No.2, (February 2006), pp. 218-222, ISSN 1553-0841

Crespi, R.; Cappare, P., Toscanelli, I., Gherlone, E. & Romanos, G.E. (2007). Effects of Er:YAG laser compared to ultrasonic scaler in periodontal treatment: a 2-year follow-up split-mouth clinical study. *Journal of Periodontolology*, Vol.78, No.7, (July 2007), pp. 1195-1200, ISSN 0022-3492

Davies, D.G.; Parsek, M.R., Pearson, J.P., Iglewski, B.H., Costerton, J.W. & Greenberg, E.P. (1998). The involvement of cell-to cell in the development of bacterial biofilm. *Science*, Vol.280, No.5361, (April 1998), pp. 295-298, ISSN 0036-8075

Derdilopoulou, F.V.; Nonhoff, J., Neumann, K. & Kielbassa, A.M. (2007). Microbiological findings after periodontal therapy using curetters, Er:YAG, laser, sonic, and ultrasonic scalers. *Journal of Clinical Periodontolology* Vol.34, No.7 (July 2007), pp. 588-598, ISSN 0303-6979

Domínguez, A.; Gómez, C., García-Kass, A.I. & García-Núñez, J.A. (2010). IL-1□, TNF-□, Total antioxidative status and microbiological findings in chronic periodontitis treated with fluorescence-controlled Er:YAG laser radiation. *Lasers in Surgery and Medicine,* Vol.42, No.7, (January 2010), pp. 24-31, ISSN 0196-8092

Donlan, R.M. & Costerton J.W. (2002). Biofilms: survival mechanisms of clinical relevant microorganisms. *Clinical Microbiology Reviews* Vol.15, No.2, (April 2002), pp. 167-193. ISSN: 0983-8512

Eberhard, J.; Ehlers, H., Falk, W., Açil, Y., Albers, H.K. & Jepsen, S. (2003). Efficacy of subgingival calculus removal with Er:YAG laser compared to mechanical debridement: an *in situ* study. *Journal of Clinical Periodontology,* Vol.30, No.6, (June 2003), pp. 511-518, ISSN 0303-6979

Ericsson, I.; Persson, L.G., Berglundh, T., Edlund, T. & Lindhe, J. (1996). The effect of antimicrobial therapy on periimplantitis lesions. An experimental study in the dog. *Clinical Oral Implants Research,* Vol.7, No.4, (December 1996), pp. 320-328, ISSN 0905-7161

Folwaczny, M.; Mehl, A., Haffner, C., Benz, C. & Hickel, R. (2000). Root substance removal with Er:YAG laser radiation at different parameters using a new delivery system. *Journal of Periodontology,* Vol.71, No.2, (February 2000), pp. 147-155, ISSN 1553-0841

Folwaczny, M.; Mehl, A., Aggstaller, H. & Kickel, R. (2002). Antimicrobial effects of 2.94 micron Er:YAG laser radiation on root surfaces: an *in vitro* study. *Journal of Clinical Periodontology,* Vol. 29, No. 1, (January 2002), pp. 73-78, ISSN 0303-6979.

Frentzen, M.; Braun, A. & Aniol, D. (2002). Er:YAG laser scaling of diseased root surfaces. *Journal of Periodontology,* Vol. 73, No. 5, (May 2002), pp. 524-530, ISSN 1553-0841

García, J.A.; Sanz, M., Aranda, J.J., Herrero, A. (2001). Remoción del cálculo subgingival con láser Er:YAG versus ultrasonidos: estudio *in vitro* con MEB. *Avances en Odontoestomatología,* Vol.17, No. 6, (July-August, 2001), pp. 273-285, ISSN 0213-1285

Ge, L.; Shu, R., Li, Y., Li, C., Luo, L., Song, Z., Xie, Y. & Liu, D. (2011). Adjunctive effect of photodynamic therapy to scaling and root planing in the treatment of chronic periodontitis. *Photomedicine and Laser Surgery,* Vol.29, No.1, (January 2011), pp. 33-37, ISSN 1549-5418

Gilmore, T.D. (2006). Introduction to NF-κβ: players, pathways, perspectives. *Oncogene,* Vol.25, No.51, (October 2006), pp. 6680-6684, ISSN 0950-9232

Gómez, C.; Costela, A., García-Moreno, I. & García, J.A. (2006). In vitro evaluation of Nd:YAG laser radiation at three different wavelenghts (1064, 532 and different wavelengths (1064, 532 and 355 nm) on calculus removal in comparison with ultrasonic scaling. *Photomedicine and Laser Surgery,* Vol.24, No.3, (June 2006), pp. 366-376, ISSN 1549-5418

Gómez, C.; Bisheimer, M., Costela, A., García-Moreno, I., García A. & García, J.A. (2009). Evaluation of the effects of Er:YAG and Nd:YAG lasers and ultrasonic instrumentation on root surfaces. *Photomedicine and Laser Surgery,* Vol.27, No.1, (February 2009), pp. 43-48, ISSN 1549-5418.

Gómez, C.; Domínguez, A., García-Kass, A. & García-Nuñez, J.A. (2011). Adjunctive Nd:YAG laser application in chronic periodontitis: clinical, immunological and microbiological aspects. *Lasers in Medical Science*, Vol. 26, No.4 (July 2011) pp 453-463. ISSN 0268-8921

Herrero, A.; García-Kass, A.I., Gómez, C, Sanz, M. & García, J.A. (2010). Effects of two kinds of Er:YAG laser system on root surface in comparison to ultrasonic scaling: an *in vitro* study. *Photomedicine and Laser Surgery*, Vol.28, No.4, (August 2010), pp.497-504, ISSN 1549-5418

Hibst, R. & Keller, U. (1989). Experimental studies of the application of the Er:YAG laser on dental hard substances. I. Measurement of the ablation rate. *Lasers in Surgery and Medicine*, Vol.9, No.4, (January 1989), pp. 338-344, ISSN 0196-8092

Ishikawa, I.; Aoki, A. & Takasaki, A.A. (2004). Potential applications of Erbium:YAG laser in periodontics. *Journal of Periodontal Research*, Vol.39, No.4, (August 2004), pp. 275-285, ISSN 0022-3484

Israel, M.; Cobb, C.M., Rossmann, J.A. & Spencer, P. (1997). The effects of CO_2, Nd:YAG and Er:YAG lasers with and with-out surface coolant on tooth root surfaces. An *in vitro* study. *Journal of Clinical Periodontology*, Vol.24, No.9, (September 1997), pp. 595-602, ISSN 0303-6979

Karu T. (2007). *Ten lectures on basic science of laser phototherapy*. Prima Books AB, ISBN 9789197647809, Grangesberg, Sweden.

Kathiblou, F.A. & Ghoddsi A. (1983). Root surface smoothness or roughness in periodontal treatment. *Journal of Periodontology*, Vol. 54, No.6, (June 1983), pp. 365-367, ISSN 1553-0841.

Keller, U. & Hibst, R. (1989). Experimental studies of the application of the Er:YAG laser on dental hard substances. II. Light microscopic and SEM investigations. *Lasers in Surgery and Medicine*, Vol. 9, No.4, (January 1989), pp. 345-351, ISSN 0196-8092

Kong, Y-Y.; Yoshida H, Sarosi I, Tan H-L, Timms E, Capparelli C, Morony S, Oliveira-dos-Santos, A.J., Van, G., Itie, A., Khoo, W., Wakeham, A., Dunstan, C.R., Lacey, D.L., Mak, T.W., Boyle, W.J. & Penninger, J.M. (1999). OPGL is a key regulator of osteoclastogenesis, lymphocyte development and lymph-node organogenesis. *Nature*, Vol. 397, No. 6717, (January 1999), pp. 315-323, ISSN 0028-0836

Konopka, K. & Goslinski, T. (2007). Photodynamic therapy in dentistry. *Journal of Dental Research*, Vol. 86, No.8, (August 2007), pp. 694-707, ISSN 0022-0345

Koort, H.J. & Frentzen, M. (1995). Laser effects on dental hard tissue, In: Lasers in Dentistry, Miserendino LJ, Pick RM, Editors, pp. 57-70, Quintessence, ISBN 0867152826, Chicago

Krause, F.; Braun, A. & Frentzen, M. (2003). The possibility of detecting subgingival calculus by laser-fluorescence *in vitro*. *Lasers in Medical Science*, Vol.18, No .1, (March 2003), pp. 32-35, ISSN 0268-8921

Kreisler, M.; Al Haj, H., Götz, H., Duschner, H. & d´Hoedt, B. (2002a). Effect of simulated CO_2 and GaAlAS laser surface decontamination on temperature changes in Ti-plasma sprayed dental implants. *Lasers in Surgery and Medicine*, Vol.30, No.3, (March 2002), pp. 233-239, ISSN 0196-8092

Kreisler, M.; Götz, H. & Duschner, H. (2002b). Effect of Nd:YAG, Ho:YAG, Er:YAG, CO_j and GaAlAs laser irradiation on surface properties of endosseous dental implants. *International Journal of Oral & Maxillofacial Implants*, Vol.17, No.2, (March-April 2002), pp. 202-211, ISSN 0901-5027

Kreisler, M.; Kohnen, W., Marinello, C., Götz, H., Duschner, H., Jansen, B. & d´Hoedt, B. (2002c). Bactericidal effect of the Er:YAG laser on dental implant surfaces: an in vitro study. *Journal of Periodontology*, Vol.73, No.11, (November 2002), pp. 1292-1298, ISSN 1553-0841

Kreisler, M.; Al Haj, H. & d´Hoedt, B. (2005). Clinical efficacy of semiconductor laser application as an adjunct to conventional scaling and root planing. *Lasers in Surgery and Medicine*, Vol. 37, No.5, (December 2005), pp. 350-355, ISSN 0196-8092

Lai, S.M.L.; Zee, K.Y., Lai, M.K. & Corbet, E.F. (2009). Clinical and radiographic investigation of the adjunctive effects of a low-power He-Ne laser in the treatment of moderate to advanced periodontal disease: a pilot study. *Photomedicine and Laser Surgery*, Vol. 27, No.2, (April 2009), pp. 287-293, ISSN 1549-5418

Lang, N.P.; Adler, R., Joss, A. & Nyman, S. (1990). Absence of bleeding on probing. An indicator of periodontal stability. *Journal of Clinical Periodontology*, Vol.17, No.10, (November 1990), pp. 714-721, ISSN 0303-6979

Lasho, D.J.; O´Leary, T.J. & Kafrawy, A.H. (1983). A scanning electron microscopic study of the effects of various agents on instrumented periodontally involved root surfaces. *Journal of Periodontology*, Vol.54, No.4, (April 1983), pp. 210-220, ISSN 1553-0841

Liu, C.M.; Hour, L.T., Wong, M.Y. & Lan, W.H. (1999). Comparison of Nd:YAG laser versus scaling and root planing in periodontal therapy. *Journal of Periodontology*, Vol.70, No.11, (November 1999), pp. 1276-1282, ISSN 1276-1282

Lubart, R.; Eichler, M., Lavi, R., Friedman, H. & Shainberg, A. (2005). Low-energy laser irradiation promotes cellular redox activity. *Photomedicine and Laser Surgery*, Vol. 23, No.1, (February 2005), pp.3-9, ISSN 1549-5418

Lulic, M.; Leiggener Görög, I., Salvi, G.E., Ramseier, C.A., Mattheos, N. & Lang N.P. (2009). One-year outcomes of repeated adjunctive photodynamic therapy during periodontal maintenance: a proof-of-principle randomized-controlled clinical trial. *Journal of Clinical Periodontology*, Vol.36, No.8, (August 2009), pp. 661-666, ISSN 0303-6979.

Maisch, T. (2007). Anti-microbial photodynamic therapy: useful in the future? *Lasers in Medical Sciences*, vol. 22, No.2, (June 2007), pp. 83–91, ISSN 0268-8921

Matarasso, S.; Quaremba, G, Coraggio, F., Vaia, E., Cafiero, C. & Lang, N.P. (1996). Maintenance of implants: an in vitro study of titanium implant surface modifications, subsequent to the application of different prophylaxis procedures. *Clinical Oral Implants Research*, Vol.7, No.1, (March 1996), pp. 64-72, ISSN 0905-7161

Miserendino, L.J.; Levy, G.C., Abt, E. & Rizoiu, I.M. (1994). Histologic effects of a thermally cooled Nd:YAG laser on the dental pulp and supporting structures of rabbit teeth. *Oral Surgery, Oral Medicine, Oral Pathology*, Vol.78, No.1, (July 1994), pp. 93-100, ISSN 0030-4220.

Misra, V.; Mehrotra, K.K., Dixit, J. & Maitra, S.C. (1999). Effect of a carbon dioxide laser on periodontally envolved root surfaces. *Journal of Periodontology*, Vol.70, No.9, (September 1999), pp. 1046-1052, ISSN 0905-7161

Miyazaki, A.; Yamaguchi, T., Nishikata, J., Okuda, K., Suda, S., Orima, K., Kobayashi, T., Yamazaki, K., Yoshikawa, E. & Yoshie, H. (2003). Effects of Nd: YAG and CO_2 laser treatment and ultrasonic scaling on periodontal pockets of chronic periodontitis patients. *Journal of Periodontology*, Vol.74, No.2, (February 2003), pp. 175-180, ISSN 0022-3492

Mombelli, A. & Lang, N.P. (1994). Microbial aspects of implant dentistry. *Periodontology 2000*, Vol.4, No.1, (February 1994), pp. 74-80, ISSN 0906-6713

Moore, P.; Ridgway, T.D., Higbee, R.G., Howard, E.W. & Lucroy, M.D. (2005). Effect of wavelength on low-intensity laser irradiation-stimulated cell proliferation in vitro. *Lasers in Surgery and Medicine*, Vol.36, No.1, (January 2005), pp. 8-12, ISSN 0196-8092

Moritz, A.; Schoop, U, Goharkhay, K., Schauer, P., Doertbudak, O., Wernisch, J. & Sperr W. (1998). Treatment of periodontal pockets with a diode laser. *Lasers in Surgery and Medicine*, Vol. 22, No. 5, (June 1998), pp. 302-311, ISSN 0196-8092

Norowski, P.A. Jr. & Bumgardner, J.D. (2009). Biomaterial and antibiotic strategies for peri-implantitis: a review. *Journal of Biomedical Materials Reserch Part B: Applied Biomaterials*, Vol. 88, No.2, (February 2009), pp. 530-543, ISSN 1552-4973

de Oliveira, R.R.; Schwartz-Filho, H.O., Novaes, A.B., Garlet, G.P., de Souza, R.F., Taba, M., Scombatti de Souza, S.L., & Ribeiro, F.J. (2009). Antimicrobial photodynamic therapy in the non-surgical treatment of aggressive periodontitis: cytokine profile in gingival crevicular fluid, preliminary results. *Journal of Periodontology*, Vol. 80, No.1, (January 2009), pp. 98-105, ISSN 0022-3492

Oyster, D.K.; Parker, W.B., Gher, M.E. (1995). CO_2 lasers and temperature changes of titanium implants. *Journal of Periodontology*, Vol. 66. No. 12. (December 1995), pp. 1017-1024, ISSN 0905-7161

Pejčic, A.; Kojovic, D., Kesic, L. & Obradovic, R. (2010). The effects of low level laser irradiation on gingival inflammation. *Photomedicine and Laser Surgery*, Vol.28, No.1, (February 2010), pp. 69-74, ISSN 1549-5418

Peplow, P.V.; Chung, T.Y. & Baxter G.D. (2010). Laser photobiomodulation of wound healing: a review of experimental studies in mouse and rat animal models. *Photomedicine and Laser Surgery*, Vol.28, No.3, (June 2010), pp.291-325, ISSN1549-5418

Perry, D.A.; Goodis, H.E. & White, J.M. (1997). In vitro study of the effects of Nd:YAG laser probe parameters on bovine oral soft tissue excision. *Lasers in Surgery and Medicine*, Vol.20, No.1, (January 1997), pp. 39-46, ISSN 0196-8092

Pick, R.M. & Colvard, M.D. (1993) Current status of lasers in soft tissue dental surgery. *Journal of Periodontology*, Vol. 64, No.7, (July 1993), pp. 589-602, ISSN 0905-7161

Polansky, R.; Haas, M., Heschl, A. & Wimmer, G. (2009). Clinical effectiveness of photodynamic therapy in the treatment of periodontitis. *Journal of Clinical Periodontology*, Vol. 36, No. 7, (July 2007), pp.575-580, ISSN 0303-6979

Qadri, T.; Miranda, L., Tunér, J. & Gustafsson, A. (2005). The short term effects of low-level lasers as adjunct therapy in the treatment of periodontal inflammation. *Journal of Clinical Periodontology*, Vol. 32, No.7, (July 2005), pp. 714-719, ISSN 0303-6079

Qadri, T.; Poddani, P., Javed F, Tunér, J. & Gustafsson, A. (2010). A short-term evaluation of nd:YAG laser as an adjunct to scaling and root planning in the treatment of periodontal inflammation. *Journal of Periodontology*, Vol.81, No.8, (August 2010), pp. 1161-1166, ISSN 0022-3492

Qadri, T.; Javed, F., Poddani, P., Tunér, J. & Gustafsson, A. (2011). Long-term effects of a single application of a wáter-cooled pulsed Nd:YAG laser in supplement to scaling and root planing in patients with periodontal inflammation. *Lasers in Medical Science*, DOI 10.1007/s10103-010-0807-8, ISSN 0268-8921

Qin, Y.L.; Luan, X.L., Bi, L.J., Sheng, Y.Q., Zhou, C.N. & Zhang, Z.G. (2008). Comparison of toluidine blue-mediated photodynamic therapy and conventional scaling treatment for periodontitis in rats. *Journal of Periodontal Research*, Vol.43,No.2, (April 2008), pp. 162-167, ISSN 0022-3484

Ribeiro I.W.J.; Sbrana, M.C., Esper, L.A. & Almeida, A.L.P.F. (2008). Evaluation of the effect of the GaAlAs laser on subgingival scaling and root planing. *Photomedicine and Laser Surgery*, Vol.26, No.4, ((August 2008), pp. 387-391, ISSN 1549-5418

Romanos, G.E. (1994). Clinical applications of the Nd:YAG laser in oral soft tissue surgery and periodontology. *Journal of Clinical Laser Medicine and Surgery*, Vol.12, No.2, (April 1994), 103-108, ISSN 1044-5471

Romanos, G.E.; Everts, H. & Nentwing, G.H. (2000). Effects of diode and Nd:YAG laser irradiation on titanium discs: a scanning electron microscope examination. *Journal of Periodontology*, Vol. 71, No.5, (May 2000), pp. 810-815, ISSN 0905-7161

Romanos, G.E.; Gutknecht, N., Dieter, S., Shwarz, F., Crespi, R. & Sculean, A. (2009). Laser wavelengths and oral implantology. *Laser in Medical Science*, Vol.24, No.6 (November 2009), pp 961-970, ISSN 0268-8921.

Rotundo, R.; Nieri, M., Cairo, F., Franceschi, D., Mervelt, J., Bonaccini, D., Esposito, M. & Pini-Prato, G. (2010). Lack of adjunctive benefit of Er:YAG laser in non-surgical periodontal treatment: a randomized split-mouth clinical trial. *Journal of Clinical Periodontology*, Vol. 37, No. 6, (June 2010), pp.526-533, ISSN 0303-6979

Sakata, M.; Shiba, H., Komatsuzawa, H., Fujita, T., Ohta, K., Sugai, M., Suginata, H., & Kurihana, H. (1999). Expression of osteoprotegerin (osteoclastogenesis inhibitory factor) in cultures of human dental mesenchymal cells and epithelial cells. *Journal of Bone and Mineral Research*, Vol.14, No.9, (September 1999), pp.1486-1492, ISSN 0884-0431.

Sasaki, K.M.; Aoki, A., Masuno, H., Ichinose, S., Yamada, S. & Ishikawa I. (2002). Compositional analisis of root cementum and dentin after Er:YAG laser irradiation compared with CO_2 lased and intact roots using Fourier transformed infrared spectroscopy. *Journal of Periodontal Research*, Vol. 37, No. 1, (February 2002), pp. 50-59, ISSN 0022-3484

Schwarz, F.; Aoki, A., Sculean, A., Georg, T., Scherbaum, W. & Becker, J. (2003a). *In vivo* effects of an Er:YAG laser, an ultrasonic system and scaling and root planing on the biocompatibility of periodontally diseased root surfaces in cultures of human PDL fibroblasts. *Lasers in Surgery and Medicine*, Vol. 33, No. 2, (August 2003) pp. 140-147, ISSN 0196-8092

Schwarz, F.; Rothamel, D., Sculean, A., Georg, T., Scherbaum, W. & Becker, J. (2003b). Effects of an Er:YAG laser and the Vector® ultrasonic system on the biocompatibility of titanium implants in cultures of human osteoblast-like cells. *Clinical Oral Implants Research*, Vol.14, No.6, (December 2003), pp. 784-792, ISSN 0905-7161

Schwarz, F.; Sculean, A., Rothamel, D., Schwenzer, K., Georg, T. & Becker, J. (2005). Clinical evaluation of an Er:YAG laser for non-surgical treatment of peri-implantitis: a pilot study. *Clinical Oral Implants Research*, Vol. 16, No. 1, (February 2005), pp. 44-52, ISSN 0905-7161

Schwarz, F.; Bieling, K., Venghaus, S., Sculean, A., Jepsen, S. & Becker, J. (2006). Influence of fluorescence-controlled Er:YAG laser radiation, the Vector system and hard instruments on periodontally diseased root surfaces in vivo. *Journal of Clinical Periodontology*, Vol.33, No.3, (March 2006), pp. 200-208, ISSN 0303-6979

Schwarz, F.; Jepsen, S., Herten, M., Aoki, A., Sculean, A. & Becker, J. (2007). Immunohistochemical characterization of periodontal wound healing following nonsurgical treatment with fluorescence controlled Er:YAG laser radiation in dogs. *Lasers in Surgery and Medicine*, Vol. 39, No. 5, (June 2007), pp. 428-440, ISSN 0196-8092

Schwarz, F.; Aoki, A., Becker, J. & Sculean, A. (2008). Laser application in non-surgical periodontal therapy: a systematic review. *Journal of Clinical Periodontology*, Vol.35, No.(suppl s8), (September 2008), pp. 29-44, ISSN 0303-6979

Sculean, A.; Schwarz, F., Berakdar, M., Romanos, G.E., Arweiler, N.B. & Becker, J. (2004). Periodontal treatment with an Er:YAG laser compared to ultrasonic instrumentation: a pilot study. *Journal of Periodontology*, Vol. 75, No. 7, (July 2004), pp. 966-973, ISSN 0022-3492

Snyder, S.K.; Byrnes, K.R., Borke, R.C., Sanchez, A. & Anders J.J. (2002). Quantification of calcitonin gene-related peptide mRNA and neuronal cell death in facial motor nuclei following axotomy and 633nm low power laser treatment. *Lasers in Surgery and Medicine*, Vol.31, No. 3, (September 2002), pp. 216-222, ISSN 0196-8092

Socransky, S.S. & Haffajee, A.D. (2002). Dental biofilms: difficult therapeutic targets. *Periodontology 2000*, Vol.28, No. 1, (January 2002), pp. 12–55, ISSN 0906-9713

Tafur, J. & Mills, P.J. (2008). Low-intensity light therapy: Exploring the role of redox mechanisms. *Photomedicine and Laser Surgery*, Vol.26, No.4, (August 2008), pp. 323-328, ISSN 1549-5418

Theodoro, L.H.; Haypek, P., Bachmann, L.M., Garcia, V.G., Sampaio, J.E., Zezell, D.M., Eduardo, Cde. P. (2003). Effect of Er:YAG and Diode laser irradiation on the root surface: morphological and thermal analysis. *Journal of Periodontology*, Vol. 74, No. 6, (June 2003), pp. 838-843, ISSN 0905-7161

Tomasi, C.; Schander, K., Dahlén, G. & Wennström, J.L. (2006). Short-term clinical and microbiologic effects of pockets debridement with an Er:YAG laser during periodontal maintenance. *Journal of Periodontology*, Vol.77, No.1, (January 2006), pp.111-118, ISSN 0022-3492

Tong, M.; Liu, Y.F., Zhao, X.N., Yan, C.Z., Hu, Z.R. & Zhang ZH. (2000). Effects of different wavelengths of low level laser irradiation on murine immunological activity and intracellular Ca2+ in human lymphocytes and cultured cortical neurogliocytes. *Lasers in Medical Science*, Vol.15, No.3, (September 2000), pp. 201-206, ISSN 0268-8921

Tsai, C.C.; Chen, H.S., Chen, S.L., Ho, Y.P., Ho, K.Y., Wu, Y.M. & Hung, C.C. (2005). Lipid peroxidation: a possible role in the induction and progression of chronic periodontitis. *Journal of Periodontal Research*, Vol.40, No.5, (October 2005), pp. 378-384, ISSN 0022-3484

Watanabe, H.; Ishikawa, I., Suzuki, M. & Hasegawa, K. (1996). Clinical assessments of the Erbium:YAG laser for soft tissue surgery and scaling. *Journal of Clinical Laser Medicine and Surgery*, Vol.14, No.2, (April 1996), pp. 67-75, ISSN 1044-5471

Wen, C.R.; Caffesse, R.G., Morrison, E.G., Nasjleti, C.E. & Parikh, U.K. (1992). *In vitro* effects of citric acid application techniques on dentin surfaces. *Journal of Periodontology*, Vol. 63, No. 11, (November 1992), pp. 883-889, ISSN 0905-7161.

Wilder-Smith, P.; Arrastia, A.M., Schell, M.J., Liaw, L.H., Grill, G. & Berns, M.W. (1995). Effect of Nd:YAG laser irradiation and root planing on the root surface: structural and termal effects. *Journal of Periodontology*, Vol. 66, No. 12, (December 1995), pp. 1032-1039, ISSN 0905-7161

Yilmaz, S.; Kuru, B., Kuru, L., Noyan, U., Argun, D. & Kadir, T. (2002). Effect of gallium arsenide diode laser on human periodontal disease: a microbiological and clinical study. *Laser in Surgery and Medicine*, Vol. 30, No.1, (January 2002), pp. 60-66, ISSN 0196-8092

15

Present and Future Non-Surgical Therapeutic Strategies for the Management of Periodontal Diseases

Renata S. Leite[1,3] and Keith L. Kirkwood[2,3]
[1]*Department of Stomatology and*
[2]*Craniofacial Biology, College of Dental Medicine,*
[3]*Center for Oral Health Research, Medical University of South Carolina,*
Charleston, SC,
USA

1. Introduction

Periodontal disease is a chronic bacterial infection of the periodontium affecting the tissues surrounding and supporting the teeth. Periodontal disease progression is associated with subgingival bacterial colonization and biofilm formation principal to chronic inflammation of soft tissues, degradation of collagen fibers supporting the tooth to the gingiva and alveolar bone, as well as resorption of the alveolar bone itself. Since the fundamental role of microorganisms in its etiology was systematically demonstrated some forty years ago, research efforts have long focused on identifying the pathogenic microorganisms and their virulence factors (Socransky and Haffajee, 1994). The search for these putative microorganisms was driven, in part, by knowledge indicating that colonization of the oral cavity and presence of dental biofilm is normally associated with health, similarly to the colonization of the colon. To treat periodontal diseases as an infectious disease, numerous therapeutic strategies aimed at eradication of periodontal pathogens have been studied over the years, including local and systemic delivery of antimicrobial and antibiotic agents. This review will cover an update on chemotherapeutic agents used adjunctively to treat and manage periodontal diseases.

In the current paradigm of periodontal disease, specific periodontal pathogens are necessary for disease initiation; however, the extent and severity of tissue destruction are largely dependent on the nature of the host-microbial interactions. These interactions are dynamic, since both the microbial composition of the dental biofilm and the competency of host immune responses can vary, in the same individual, over time. This concept was developed in parallel to the advances on the understanding of the immune response, and research on periodontal disease has been emphasizing mechanisms of host-microbial interactions to understand the disease process, as well as for the development of novel therapeutic strategies. For the past two decades, the host response to the bacterial challenge originating from the dental biofilm has been considered to play a major role on both initiation of the disease and on the tissue destruction associated with its progress (Kirkwood, et al., 2007). The importance of host-microbial interactions is reinforced by epidemiological data indicating different susceptibilities to periodontal disease among individuals, in spite of the long-term presence of oral biofilm (Baelum and Fejerskov, 1986, Baelum, et al., 1988, Loe, et al., 1986). Other studies demonstrating increased susceptibility and greater severity of periodontal disease in individuals with impaired immune response due to systemic conditions also indicate the significance of the host response to the bacterial challenge (Feller and Lemmer, 2008, Mealey, 1998). Both past and future directions of host-modulatory agents will be addressed here to provide the dental practitioner with a broader prospective of chemotherapeutic agents used to manage periodontal diseases.

2. Antibiotics

Contemporary periodontal therapies aim at mechanical removal of bacterial deposits to maintain a healthy sulcus or produce an environment suitable for new attachment. The inability of mechanical treatment to produce a desirable root surface in all cases coupled with the nature and complexity of the subgingival biofilm has fueled the search for adjunctive treatment regimens that increase the likelihood to successfully manage periodontal diseases.

While more than 700 bacterial species may be present in the gingival sulcus, it is clear that only a subset of bacterial species are consistently found to be associated with diseased sites. These findings make the prospect of targeted antibiotic therapy an attractive goal. The literature on antimicrobial periodontal therapy has been thoroughly reviewed (Ellen and McCulloch, 1996, Goodson, 1994, van Winkelhoff, et al., 1996).

2.1 Systemic antibiotics

Adjunctive systemic antibiotic therapies have indicated beneficial effects for patients with periodontal diseases., The optimal timing of antimicrobial drug administration is still a subject of discussion, as the literature is controversial whether it should be administered during the initial non-surgical phase (Loesche, et al., 1992), or during a subsequent surgical phase (Herrera, et al., 2008). Although not directly confirmed yet by a clinical trial, it seems preferable, from a general health point of view, to let patients benefit early from the positive systemic effects of successful periodontal therapy. Table 1 provides an overview of some orally active systemic antibiotics commonly used in clinical periodontics.

Caution should be noted that none of these antibiotics is to be used as a monotherapy to treat periodontal diseases. Systemic antibiotics reach the periodontal tissues by transudation from the serum then cross the crevicular and junctional epithelia to enter the gingival sulcus. The concentration of the antibiotic in this site may be inadequate for the desired antimicrobial effect without mechanical disruption of the plaque biofilm. In addition to any effect produced in the sulcus, a systemically administered antibiotic will produce antimicrobial effects in other areas of the oral cavity. This additional effect will reduce bacterial counts on the tongue and other mucosal surfaces, thus potentially aiding to delay re-colonization of subgingival sites. Research however, indicates that antibiotics are detectable in the sulcus and the range of their concentrations in the gingival crevicular fluid is known to be in therapeutic range treatment efficacy. Table 2 provides information to facilitate the clinician's decision to the most reasonable choice of antibiotic, dose and duration of administration.

Many studies have been completed and published describing the effect of systemic antibiotic therapy on periodontal disease. Several different treatment regimens have been employed successfully to manage periodontal diseases (Slots and Ting, 2002). Considering a number of studies, it can be stated generally that systemic antibiotic therapy has little effect on supragingival plaque accumulation with a possible exception in one study where doxycycline significantly decreased plaque accumulation at a twelve-week evaluation compared to placebo (Ng and Bissada, 1998).

Antibiotic Class	Agent	Effect	Target Organisms	Limitation
Penicillin	Amoxicillin	Bacteriocidal	Gram + and Gram -	Penicillinase sensitive Patient hypersensitivity
	Augmentin	Bacteriocidal	Narrower spectrum than Amoxicillin	More expensive than Amoxicillin
Tetracycline	Tetracycline	Bacteriostatic	Gram + > Gram -	Bacterial resistance
	Minocycline	Bacteriostatic	Gram + > Gram -	
	Doxycycline	Bacteriostatic	Gram + > Gram -	
Quinolone	Ciprofloxacin	Bacteriocidal	Gram - rods	Nausea, GI discomfort
Macrolide	Azithromycin	Bacteriostatic OR Bacteriocidal depending on concentration		
Lincomycin	Clindamycin	Bacteriocidal	Anaerobic bacteria	
Nitroimidazole	Metronidazole	Bacteriocidal to Gram -	Gram -; esp. *P. gingivalis* and *P. intermedia*	Not good choice for *A. Actinomycetemcomitans* infections

Table 1. Systemic antibiotic choices.

Single Agent	Regimen	Dosage/Duration
Amoxicillin	500 mg	Three times per day X 8 days
Azithromycin	500 mg	Once daily X 4-7 days
Ciprofloxacin	500 mg	Twice daily X 8 days
Clindamycin	300 mg	Three times daily X 10 days
Doxycycline or Minocycline	100-200 mg	Once daily X 21 days
Metronidazole	500 mg	Three times daily X 8 days
Combination Therapy		
Metronidazole + Amoxicillin	250 mg of each	Three times daily X 8 days
Metronidazole + Ciprofloxacin	500 mg of each	Twice daily X 8 days

Table 2. Systemic antibiotic dosing regimens.

Except for the combination of metronidazole with amoxicillin, systemic antibiotic treatment produces no clinically significant effects on periodontal pocket depth reduction compared with controls (Winkel, et al., 2001) ((Cionca, et al., 2009). A seven-day regimen of systemic metronidazole significantly reduced the percentage of sites with bleeding compared to controls (Watts, et al., 1986). Others have reported a 12-month reduction in bleeding after treatment with a metronidazole-amoxicillin combination compared to a placebo treatment (Lopez, et al., 2000). With respect to clinical attachment levels, systemic metronidazole and combinations of metronidazole with other antibiotics has shown improvement in several studies. Several investigators found significant improvement of attachment levels at sites initially 4-6 mm in depth with a seven-day treatment with metronidazole (Elter, et al., 1997, Loesche, et al., 1992, Loesche, et al., 1984). Winkel et al. showed that the combination of metronidazole and amoxicillin for 7 to 14 days produced a significant increase in the percentage of sites showing improved attachment levels compared to control sites (Winkel, et al., 2001). A combination of metronidazole and clindamycin for three weeks also produced improved attachment levels. (Gomi, et al., 2007, Sigusch, et al., 2001).

Some data to date supports a clinical benefit from the use of azithromycin as a systemic approach in combination with mechanical routines. In one limited study, seventeen subjects receiving azithromycin (500 mg), three days before full-mouth scaling and root planing produced greater clinical improvement than in seventeen subjects treated with full-mouth scaling and root planing alone (Gomi, et al., 2007). Dastoor et al. studied thirty patients who reported smoking more than one pack per day and presented with periodontitis. A comparison was made between the response to treatment with periodontal surgery and 500 mg Azithromycin per day for three days and treatment with periodontal surgery only. The addition of Azithromycin did not enhance improvements seen in both groups for attachment gain, depth reduction and reduction of bleeding on probing. However, the adjunctive use of Azithromycin was associated with a lower gingival index at two weeks and what the authors saw as more rapid wound healing. The addition of Azithromycin also produced reductions of red-complex bacteria that were maintained to three months (Dastoor, et al., 2007).

It is important to remember that the systemic antibiotic therapy is not intended as a monotherapy but is always best as an adjunctive therapy combined with traditional mechanical therapy and patient plaque control.

2.2 Local antibiotic therapy

After considering the risk to benefit ratio of systemic antibiotic administration as an adjunct treatment of periodontal diseases, interest in antibiotic therapy applied locally was developed. Historically, the first such local antibiotic therapy for periodontal disease was the Actisite™(no longer commercially available) fiber system. Actisite™ was supplied as hollow, nonabsorbable fibers filled with tetracycline (12.7 mg/9 inch fiber). The fiber was inserted into the pocket, wrapped repeatedly circumferentially around the tooth keeping the fiber in the pocket. Often a periodontal dressing was placed to aid maintaining the fiber in the pocket. The fiber was retained for ten days until operator removal. During this ten-day period drug concentrations of more than 1300 µg/ml of tetracycline were achieved and maintained. When the fiber was removed the soft tissue was often distended allowing temporary improved access and visibility of the root surfaces for any additional root planing or calculus removal. Following removal of the fiber the soft tissues generally showed shrinkage and pocket reduction and reduction of the inflammatory response were commonly seen. The Actisite™ system, while very effective, was tedious to use and required the second visit for removal of the fiber. These issues fueled the development of an absorbable system (Table 3).

Antimicrobial Agent	Delivery Form	Drawback	GCF Concentration	Time to Absorption	Brand Name
Tetracycline 12.7 mg per 9 inches of fiber	Hollow fibers	2nd procedure for fiber removal	>1300 ug/ml for 10 days	Not absorbable	Actisite No longer commercially available
10% Doxycycline	Fluid; multi-site depending on volume of site; in syringe	Often pulls out when removing syringe	250 ug/ml still noted at 7 days	21 days	Atridox
25% Metronidazole Gel	Fluid; multi-site depending on volume of site; in syringe	May require multiple applications for desirable results	More than 120 mg/ml of sulcus fluid in the first few hours	Concentration decreases rapidly after the first few hours (Knoll-Kohler, 1999)	Elyzol
2% Minocycline Spheres	Solid; in unit doses applied with syringe	Unit doses may not be sufficient for every site volume	Therapeutic drug levels for 14 days	14 days	Arestin

Table 3. Local antibiotic delivery systems.

The first resorbable local antibiotic system was Atridox™(Atrix Laboratories). In this system, longer half-lived doxycycline replaced tetracycline supplied at a concentration of 42.5 mg per unit of material. Atridox™ improved the local antibiotic routines by allowing placement of the material to the depth of most pockets and in a manner that allowed it to conform to the shape of the pocket unlike the solid fibers of Actisite™. Depending on the size of the pocket, more than one site could be treated with a single unit of Atridox™.

Further development of absorbable local antibiotic systems led to Arestin™ (OraPharma) that uses minocycline in a microsphere configuration, each sphere measuring 20-60 microns in diameter. The antibiotic maintains therapeutic drug levels and remains in the pocket for 14 days. This configuration of the material allows placement to the depths of most pockets and while the material cannot conform to the shape of the pocket as well as the Atridox™ gel it is still better than the solid Actisite™ fibers.

Another material, not available in the United States, is Elyzol™(Colgate), a metronidazole gel system. This material is supplied as 25% metronidazole in a glyceryl mono-oleate and sesame oil base. The concentration of Metronidazole in this system is 250 mg/g of material that is applied as a gel using a syringe method.

Overall efficacy of local antibiotic therapies has been evaluated using meta-analysis of fifty articles, each reporting studies of at least six months follow-up (Bonito, et al., 2005). The meta-analysis considered studies of the addition of local adjuncts and found such additions provide generally favorable but minimal differences. The clinical effects of these various systems have been reported in several publications. Table 4 summarizes several studies of various local adjunctive materials. The overall treatment effect is somewhat variable and while found to be statistically significant has led many to be suspect of the general clinical benefit.

Agent	Subjects	Depth Change with S/RP Only	Depth Change with S/RP + Agent	Sites With At Least 2 mm Attachment Gain with S/RP + Agent
Tetracycline Fibers (Goodson, et al., 1991)	107	0.67	1.02 (fiber only)	Not reported
Doxycycline gel (Garrett, et al., 1999)	411	1.08	1.30 (drug only)	38% (drug only)
Doxycycline gel (Wennstrom, et al., 2001)	105	1.3	1.5	52%
Doxycycline gel (Machion, et al., 2006)	48	1.5 - 2.19	1.63-2.29	34.4% vs. 18.1% S/RP only
Minocycline spheres (Williams, et al., 2001)	728	1.08	1.32	42%
Minocycline spheres (Goodson, et al., 2007)	127	1.01	1.38	Not reported; reports attachment gain of 1.16 with agent, 0.8 S/RP only
Metronidazole gel (Ainamo, et al., 1992)	206	1.3	1.5 (drug only)	Not reported
Azithromycin gel (Pradeep, et al., 2008)	80	2.13	2.53	Not reported; reports greater gain at all time points with agent

Table 4. Local Antibiotic System Studies.

3. Antiseptics

The use of chemical agents with anti-plaque or anti-gingivitis action as adjuncts to oral hygiene seems to be of limited value, since mouthrinses do not appreciably penetrate into the gingival crevice, but they are of specific benefit when used as adjuncts to control gingival inflammation, especially in acute situations and during periods of interrupted hygiene (Ciancio, 1989). The challenge with chemical plaque control is to develop an active anti-plaque agent that does not disturb the natural flora of the oral cavity. The American Dental Association (ADA) Seal of Acceptance is seen as a standard for oral health care products. The ADA Seal Program ensures that professional and consumer dental products meet rigorous ADA criteria for safety and effectiveness. Guidelines have been established for the control of gingivitis and supragingival plaque (http://www.ada.org/ada/seal/index.asp). These guidelines describe the clinical, biological, and laboratory studies necessary to evaluate safety and effectiveness and are subject to revision at any time. Importantly, they do not describe criteria for evaluating the management of periodontitis or other periodontal diseases. All claims of efficacy, including all health benefit claims, (e.g. gingivitis reduction), and all claims which imply a health benefit (e.g. plaque reduction) must be documented. There will be two Seal statements to be used with an Accepted product, depending on whether or not the product's mechanism of action is related to plaque reduction.

Oral antiseptics have evolved from short-lived effects (soon after rinsing) as with the first generation antimicrobials (Table 5) to the second generation, which have the antimicrobial effect that lasts for a time period after the mouthrinse has been expectorated (Table 6).

Anti-microbial	**Commercial Name**	**ADA Seal of Acceptance**	**Active ingredients**	**Alcohol content**	**Mechanism of Action**	**Efficacy published by the manufacturer**
Phenolic Compounds	Listerine (Johnson & Johnson)	Yes	Essential oils: Thymol (0.06%) Eucalyptol (0.09%) Methyl salicylate (0.06%) Menthol (0.04%)	26.9%	Appears to be related to alteration of the bacterial cell wall	52% plaque reduction 36% gingivitis reduction (www.listerine.com)
Sanguinarine	Viadent (Colgate)	No	0.03% Sanguinarine extract	5.5%	Alteration of bacterial cell surfaces so that aggregation and attachment is reduced	28% plaque reduction 24% gingivitis reduction (www.colgateprofessional.com/products/Viadent-Advanced-Care-Oral-Rinse/details)
Quaternary Ammonium Compounds	Cepacol and Scope (Procter & Gamble)	No	Cepacol: 0.05% CPC Scope: 0.045% CPC + 0.005% domiphen bromide	Cepacol 14% Scope 18.9%	Related to increased bacterial cell wall permeability, which favors lysis, decreased cell metabolism and a decreased ability for bacteria to attach to tooth surfaces.	15.8% plaque reduction 15.4% gingivitis reduction (www.cepacol.com/products/mouthwash.asp) and (www.pg.com/product_card/prod_card_main_scope.html)

Table 5. First generation antimicrobials.

On the downside, it is also recognized that oral hygiene products may have the potential for producing harm in the mouth, some of which are more serious and long lasting than others. These types of harm range from production of a cosmetic nuisance, such as staining occurring as a result of the use of cationic antiseptics like chlorhexidine and cetylpyridinium chloride, to more permanent damage to the dental hard tissues through possible erosive and abrasive effects of low-pH mouthrinses and toothpastes respectively. Of serious concern is controversially the ability to produce carcinogenic changes to the oral mucosa through the use of alcoholic mouthrinses. Recently, the potential harm of oral hygiene products to oral and systemic health was fully reviewed with reference to present-day evidence (Addy, 2008).

Antimicrobial	Cetylpyridinium chloride	Chlorhexidine
Commercial Name	Crest Pro-Health (Procter & Gamble)	Peridex (3M Espe) Periogard (Colgate)
ADA Seal of Acceptance	No	Yes
Active ingredients	0.07% CPC	0.12% Chlorhexidine gluconate (solutions.3m.com/wps/portal/3M/en_US/preventive-care/home/products/home-care-therapies/peridex/) and (www.colgateprofessional.com/products/Colgate-Periogard-Rinse-Rx-only/details)
Mechanism of Action	Bactericidal agent interacts with the bacterial membrane. The cellular pressure disrupts the cell membrane and effectively kills the bacteria.	Positively charged chlorhexidine molecule binds to negatively charged microbial cell wall, altering osmotic equilibrium, causing potassium and phosphorous leakage, precipitation of cytoplasmic contents and consequent cell death.
Efficacy published by the manufacturer	Similar to Listerine (www.dentalcare.com/soap/products/index.htm)	Certain aerobic and anaerobic bacteria reduction from 54 - 97% through six months use (solutions.3m.com/wps/portal/3M/en_US/preventive-care/home/products/home-care-therapies/peridex/) - 29% gingivitis reduction - 54% plaque reduction (www.colgateprofessional.com/products/Colgate-Periogard-Rinse-Rx-only/details)

Table 6. Second generation antimicrobials.

3.1 Phenolic compounds

Among the first generation antimicrobials, the phenolic compounds, such as Listerine® and its clones, are the only ones that have the ADA Seal of Acceptance to prevent and reduce supragingival plaque accumulation and gingivitis. Short-term studies have shown plaque and gingivitis reduction averaging 35% (Fornell, et al., 1975) and long-term studies have shown plaque reduction between 13.8 and 56.3% and gingivitis reduction between 14 and

35.9% (DePaola, et al., 1989, Gordon, et al., 1985). Possible adverse effects reported in the literature include a burning sensation, bitter taste and possible staining of teeth.

3.2 Chlorhexidine

Chlorhexidine gluconate (0.12%), such as Peridex® and Periogard®, is sold in the United States by prescription only. It was the first antimicrobial shown to inhibit plaque formation and the development of chronic gingivitis (Loe and Schiott, 1970). Chlorhexidine is effective against gram-positive and negative bacteria and yeast. It has very low toxicity, since it is poorly absorbed from the GI tract and 90% is excreted in the feces. Chlorhexidine 0.12% is indicated for short-term (less than 2 months), intermittent short-term (alternating on and off every 1 to 2 months) and long-term (greater than 3 months to indefinitely) use (Table 7). Of all the products included here, chlorhexidine appears to be the most effective agent for reduction of both plaque and gingivitis with short-term reductions averaging 60% (Flotra, et al., 1972). Long-term reductions in plaque averaged between 45-61% and in gingivitis, 27-67% (Ciancio, 1989). Adverse effects reported may include staining of teeth, reversible desquamation, poor taste and alteration of taste and an increase in supragingival calculus (Flotra, et al., 1972, Overholser, et al., 1990).

Short-term indication (less than 2 months)	**Intermittent short-term indications (alternating on and off every 1 to 2 months)**	**Long-term indications (greater then 3 months to indefinitely)**
Gingivitis	Gingivitis	Patients with reduced resistance to bacterial plaque: AIDS, leukemia, kidney disease, bone marrow transplants, agranulocytosis, thrombocytopenia
Following periodontal and oral surgery	Periodontal maintenance	Physically handicapped patients: rheumatoid arthritis, scleroderma, disturbance of muscles and/or motor capacity and coordination
During initial periodontal therapy	Physically and /or mentally handicapped	Patients treated with: cytotoxic drugs, immunosuppressive drugs, and radiation therapy.
Treatment of candidiasis	Extensive prosthetic reconstruction	

Table 7. Chlorhexidine 0.12% Indications.

3.3 Other antimicrobial mouthrinses

Several other agents have been evaluated for their effect on bacterial plaque and gingivitis, but results are inferior to those of chlorhexidine and phenolic compounds (see Table 8). Pires et al. (Pires, et al., 2007) have concluded that a mouthwash containing a combination of Triclosan/Gatrez and sodium bicarbonate has an *in-vitro* antimicrobial activity superior to that of a placebo, but still inferior to that of chlorhexidine.

Anti-microbial	Commercial Name	ADA Seal of Acceptance	Active ingredients	Mechanism of Action	Efficacy
Oxygenating agents	Peroxyl (Colgate)	No	Hydrogen Peroxyde	Anti-inflammatory properties reduce bleeding on probing, a major sign of inflammation; bacterial load is not necessarily reduced; bubbling action cleans and alleviates discomfort to promote healing.	Long-term studies do not support effectiveness. Short-term studies offer contradictory findings.
Chlorine Dioxide	RetarDEX (Periproducts) Oxyfresh	No	1% chlorine dioxide	Stable, free radical and an oxidant with algicidal, bactericidal, cysticidal, fungicidal, sporicidal, and viricidal properties.	Minimal plaque reduction, but has shown decreases involatile sulfur compounds and halitosis.
Zinc Chloride	Breath Rx	No	-Zinc chloride -Phenolic oils (Thymol and Eucalyptus oil)	Zinc has an affinity to sulfur and odorizes sulphydryl groups with zinc ions forming stable mercaptides with the substrate, the precursors, and/or the volatile sulfur compounds directly.	BreathRx is a scientific bad breath treatment specially designed to help treat both the causes of bad breath and the symptoms.
Triclosan	Not available in the US	N/A	Triclosan	A low toxicity, non-ionic phenolic derivative with a wide spectrum of antimicrobial and anti-inflammatory activities (Kim, et al., 2005).	*In vitro* studies show antimicrobial activity superior to that of a placebo, but inferior to that of chlorhexidine (Pires, et al., 2007)

Table 8. Other antimicrobial mouthrinses.

Antiseptics compared	Methodology	Results	References
Listerine Viadent Peridex Placebo	31 volunteers with healthy gingiva ceased all oral hygiene procedures but rinsing with the designated mouthrinse for 21 days	Peridex was superior in its ability to maintain optimal gingival health during the entire time of mouthrinse use.	Siegrist et al. (Siegrist, et al., 1986)
Listerine Peridex Placebo	Double blind, controlled clinical trial. After a baseline complete dental prophylaxis,124 healthy adults used the mouthrinse as a supplement to regular oral hygiene for 6 months.	Both Listerine and Peridex significantly inhibited development of plaque by 36.1% and 50.3%, respectively, and the development of gingivitis by 35.9% and 3.0.5% respectively, compared to placebo.	Overholser et al. (Overholser, et al., 1990)
Chlorhexidine 0.12% Hydrogen Peroxide 1% Placebo	32 subjects ceased oral hygiene procedures, but rinsed, twice a day, with the designated mouthrinse for 21 days.	The chlorhexidine group showed 95% reduction in gingivitis incidence, 100% reduction in BOP, and 80% reduction in plaque scores compared to placebo.	Gusberti et al. (Gusberti, et al., 1988)

Table 9. Comparison studies.

4. Anti-inflammatory strategies

It is well established that periodontal disease is an infectious disease and that the host immune and inflammatory response to the microbial challenge mediates tissue destruction (Offenbacher, 1996). Considering that the primary etiology of the disease are bacteria in the plaque and their products, mechanical and chemical approaches to reduce the presence of periodontopathogens in the plaque have been largely used in the treatment of periodontal patients over the years (Greenwell, 2001). Most recently, the better understanding of the participation of host immune-inflammatory mediators in the disease progression has increased the investigation of the use of modulating agents as an adjunctive therapy to the periodontal treatment. Inhibition or blockade of proteolytic enzymes, pro-inflammatory mediators and of osteoclast activity has been the focus of these agents which has lead to encouraging results in pre-clinical and clinical studies (Reddy, et al., 2003). More specifically, three types of host-modulatory agents have been investigated for the management of periodontitis including anti-proteinases (MMP inhibitors), anti-inflammatory agents, and anti-resorptive agents.

4.1 MMP Inhibitors

One important group of proteolytic enzymes present in the periodontal tissues is formed by the matrix metalloproteinases (MMPs), which include collagenases, gelatinases and metalloelastases. MMPs are produced by many periodontal tissues and are responsible for remodeling the extracellular matrix (Birkedal-Hansen, 1993). In 1985, tetracyclines were found to have anti-collagenolytic activity and proposed as a host modulating agent for periodontal treatment (Golub, et al., 1985). Initial studies demonstrated that doxycycline was the most potent tetracycline in inhibition of collagenolytic activities (Burns, et al., 1989). This property of doxycycline provided the pharmacological rationale for the use of a low or subantimicrobial dose of doxycycline (SDD) that was shown to be efficient in inhibiting mammalian collagenase activity without developing antibiotic resistance (Golub, et al., 1990).

Several clinical studies have been conducted assessing the benefits of the SDD as an adjunctive therapy to scaling and root planing (SRP) in the treatment of the periodontal disease. Reddy et al. recently presented a meta-analysis (Reddy, et al., 2003) of 6 selected clinical studies comparing long-term systemic SDD (20mg bid doxycycline) to placebo control in periodontal patients. A statistically significant adjunctive benefit on clinical attachment levels (CAL) and probing depth was found when SDD was used in combination with SRP, in both 4 to 6mm and ≥ 7mm pocket depth categories. Bleeding on probing (BOP) was not assessed in the meta-analysis but, in general, SDD did not improve this parameter when compared to placebo. No significant adverse effects were reported in any of the studies.

4.2 Non-steroid anti-inflammatory drugs

The non-steroidal anti-inflammatory drugs (NSAIDs) represent the next major pharmacological class of agents that has been well studied as inhibitors of the host response in periodontal disease. These agents are well known for the ability to prevent prostanoid formation. In this process, arachidonic acid liberated from membrane phospholipids of cells after tissue damage or stimulus is metabolically transformed via cyclooxygenase or

lipoxygenase pathways in compounds with potent biological activities (Offenbacher, 1996). The cyclooxygenase enzymes are recognized to have two isoforms: cyclooxygenase 1 (COX1) which is a constitutive enzyme present in most of cells and cyclooxygenase 2 (COX2) which is inducible and is present in cells involved in inflammatory processes (DeWitt, et al., 1993). The cyclooxygenase pathway produces prostaglandins, prostacyclin and thromboxane, called prostanoids. Some prostanoids have proinflammatory properties and have been associated with destructive process in inflammatory diseases. In periodontal diseases, Prostaglandin E_2 (PGE_2) has been extensively correlated to inflammation and bone resorption (Offenbacher, 1996). Its levels in gingival tissues and in the gingival crevicular fluid (GCF) have been shown to be significantly elevated in periodontally diseased patients compared to healthy patients (Dewhirst, et al., 1983, Offenbacher, et al., 1981).
Selective NSAIDs are capable of inhibiting COX-2 without affecting constitutive isoform COX-1. Some studies have indicated that COX-2 inhibitors retain bone sparing effects (Bezerra, et al., 2000, Holzhausen, et al., 2002, Holzhausen, et al., 2005, Shimizu, et al., 1998) without inducing adverse effects associated with COX-1 suppression, such as gastro-duodenal problems and renal toxicity (Hawkey, 1993, Lindsley and Warady, 1990). Several adjunctive periodontal clinical trials have been conducted with NSAIDs. In a systematic review (Reddy, et al., 2003), ten clinical studies in which therapeutic outcomes of NSAIDs were expressed in clinical attachment level (CAL) or alveolar crestal height as measured by subtraction radiography were selected. In these studies a variety of different NSAIDs were systemically or locally administered, including flurbiprofen, meclofenamate, ibuprofen, ketorolac, naproxen and aspirin. Although the heterogeneity of data did not permit a meta-analysis, limited quantitative analysis tended to show a significant benefit related to alveolar bone maintenance when NSAIDs were combined with conventional therapy. Notably, none of these studies found significantly less attachment loss after NSAIDs adjunctive therapy when compared to SRP alone.

4.3 Anti-bone resorptive therapeutics

Alveolar bone destruction is the hallmark feature of periodontal disease. The use of bone-sparing drugs that inhibit alveolar bone resorption is another field in host-modulation therapy. Bisphosphonates are a class of agents that binds to hydoxyapatite in bone matrix to prevent matrix dissolution by interfering with osteoclast function through a variety of direct and indirect mechanisms (Rogers, et al., 2000). The principal therapeutic purpose of bisphosphonates is in the prevention and treatment of osteoporosis and also in treatment of Paget's disease and metastatic bone disease (Fleisch, 1997). In periodontics, their use was proposed initially for diagnostic and therapeutic use. As therapeutic agents, bisphosphonates were shown to reduce alveolar bone loss and increase mineral density but not to improve clinical conditions in animal periodontitis models (Brunsvold, et al., 1992, Reddy, et al., 1995). Five studies that assessed the effect of bisphosphonates as an adjunctive agent to SRP in human periodontal treatment were found to date (El-Shinnawi and El-Tantawy, 2003, Jeffcoat, et al., 2007, Lane, et al., 2005, Rocha, et al., 2004, Rocha, et al., 2001). Alendronate was the bisphosphonate used in four studies during a period of 6 months. One study used risedronate during 12 months (El-Shinnawi and El-Tantawy, 2003). All the studies presented significant clinical improvement when compared to placebo, including: probing depth reduction, clinical attachement gain, bleeding on probing reduction, alveolar bone gain and increase in bone mineral density. These results encourage the use of

bisphosphonates as an adjunctive agent to periodontal therapy. Additional studies need to be implemented to confirm the benefits of these drugs.
However, there can be significant dental related adverse effects associated with the use of bisphosphonates therapeutics. High-dose, long-term use of bisphosphonates has been reported to be associated with osteonecrosis of the jaw (ONJ) (Marx, 2003, Ruggiero, et al., 2004). Data from multiple sources indicates that patients with prior dental problems may have a higher risk of ONJ. However, as more data is being reported, it still remains controversial that bisphosphonates indeed are causative for ONJ. Since bisphosphonates are potent osteoclast inhibitors, their long-term use may suppress bone turnover and compromise healing of even physiologic micro-injuries within bone (Odvina, et al., 2005). Despite the encouraging therapeutic results, further long-term studies are warranted to determine the relative risk-benefit ratio of bisphosphonate therapy.

5. Future host modulatory approaches

A variety of treatment strategies have been developed to target the host response to LPS-mediated tissue destruction. MMP inhibitors such as low dose formulations of doxycycline have been used in combination with scaling and root planing (Caton, et al., 2001) or surgical therapy (Gapski, et al., 2004). In addition, high-risk patient populations such as diabetics or patients with recurrent periodontal disease have benefited from systemic MMP administration (Chang, et al., 1996, Golub, et al., 2001, Novak, et al., 2002). Encouraging results have been shown using soluble antagonists of TNF and IL-1 delivered locally to periodontal tissues in nonhuman primates (Assuma, et al., 1998, Graves, et al., 1998).

5.1 Novel host modulators

Host response modulation is key therapeutic target used to control periodontal inflammation leading to tissue and bone destruction. Bone loss as a consequence of bacterial-induced inflammation due to subgingival plaque in the periodontal pocket is controlled by the expression of cytokines that direct the biological process of osteoclast differentiation. Several inflammatory cytokines, including interleukin (IL)-1, IL-6 and other cytokines enhance the expression of receptor activator of nuclear factor kappa-B ligand (RANKL) which induced osteoclast formation and leads to bone resorption. RANK is the receptor located on osteoclast precursor cells that respond to RANKL to initiate formation of mature osteoclasts. To balance the effects of RANKL, osteoprotegerin (OPG) acts as a decoy receptor to bind RANKL and inhibits osteoclast development. In periodontal disease, the roles of RANKL, RANK, and OPG in the alveolar bone resorption have been extensively investigated. Based on pre-clinical animal studies and on preliminary human clinical studies, the OPG/RANKL/RANK axis is a new target for the treatment of destructive periodontal disease and other bone resorption related diseases (Cochran, 2008). However, further studies are necessary to determine the most efficacious therapeutic approach based upon molecular interactions in the periodontal environment.
All immune cells within periodontal tissues generate innate immune cytokines require intracellular signaling to transduce extracellular cues into biochemical information required for inflammatory cytokine gene expression. Cytokines and bacterial components activate many signal transduction pathways. With this concept in mind, new strategies for preventing cell activation via targeting signal transduction pathways could abolish both cell

activation by cytokines or other stimuli and production of proinflammatory cytokines. Signal transduction pathways closely involved in inflammation include the mitogen-activated protein kinase (MAPK) pathway, phosphatidylinositol-3 protein (PI3-kinase) pathway, janus kinase-signal transducer and activator of transcription (Jak-STAT), and nuclear factor kappa B (NF-kB). Thus, small molecule inhibitor compounds have emerged as the new therapeutic strategies that are being explored are aimed at inhibiting signal transduction pathways involved in inflammation. Pharmacological inhibitors of NF-kB and p38 mitogen activating protein (MAP) kinase pathways are actively being developed to manage inflammatory bone diseases (Adams, et al., 2001, Kumar, et al., 2001). p38 inhibitors have already shown promise in preclinical models of periodontal diseases (Kirkwood, et al., 2007, Rogers, et al., 2007). Using this novel strategy, inflammatory mediators including proinflammatory cytokines (IL-1, TNF, IL-6), MMPs and others would be inhibited at the level of cell signaling pathways required for transcription factor activation necessary for inflammatory gene expression or mRNA stability. These therapies may provide the next wave of adjuvant chemotherapeutics that may be used to manage chronic periodontitis.

6. Future directions

Most therapeutics has relied on systemic delivery. Thus, it may be difficult to potentially use systemic therapeutics for periodontal disease due to the long-term chronic nature of the periodontal inflammation and destruction. The future may be the adjunctive use of locally delivered therapeutics, and the need for new targets of therapeutics for periodontal disease. Also, the need for new in situ delivery systems with the ability to locally deliver therapeutics to the periodontal lesion bypassing systemic issues of toxicity.

7. Acknowledgment

This work was supported by P20RR017696 and R01DE018290 from the National Institutes of Health.

8. References

Adams, J. L., A. M. Badger, S. Kumar, and J. C. Lee. 'P38 Map Kinase: Molecular Target for the Inhibition of Pro-Inflammatory Cytokines', *Prog Med Chem* Vol. 38, 1-60, 2001.

Addy, M. 'Oral Hygiene Products: Potential for Harm to Oral and Systemic Health?', *Periodontol 2000* Vol. 48, No. 1, 54-65, 2008.

Ainamo, J., T. Lie, B. H. Ellingsen, B. F. Hansen, L. A. Johansson, T. Karring, J. Kisch, K. Paunio, and K. Stoltze. 'Clinical Responses to Subgingival Application of a Metronidazole 25% Gel Compared to the Effect of Subgingival Scaling in Adult Periodontitis', *J Clin Periodontol* Vol. 19, No. 9 Pt 2, 723-9, 1992.

Assuma, R., T. Oates, D. Cochran, S. Amar, and D. T. Graves. 'Il-1 and Tnf Antagonists Inhibit the Inflammatory Response and Bone Loss in Experimental Periodontitis', *J Immunol* Vol. 160, No. 1, 403-9, 1998.

Baelum, V., and O. Fejerskov. 'Tooth Loss as Related to Dental Caries and Periodontal Breakdown in Adult Tanzanians', *Community Dent Oral Epidemiol* Vol. 14, No. 6, 353-7, 1986.

Baelum, V., L. Wen-Min, O. Fejerskov, and C. Xia. 'Tooth Mortality and Periodontal Conditions in 60-80-Year-Old Chinese', *Scand J Dent Res* Vol. 96, No. 2, 99-107, 1988.

Bezerra, M. M., V. de Lima, V. B. Alencar, I. B. Vieira, G. A. Brito, R. A. Ribeiro, and F. A. Rocha. 'Selective Cyclooxygenase-2 Inhibition Prevents Alveolar Bone Loss in Experimental Periodontitis in Rats', *J Periodontol* Vol. 71, No. 6, 1009-14, 2000.

Birkedal-Hansen, H. 'Role of Cytokines and Inflammatory Mediators in Tissue Destruction', *J Periodontal Res* Vol. 28, No. 6 Pt 2, 500-10, 1993.

Bonito, A. J., L. Lux, and K. N. Lohr. 'Impact of Local Adjuncts to Scaling and Root Planing in Periodontal Disease Therapy: A Systematic Review', *J Periodontol* Vol. 76, No. 8, 1227-36, 2005.

Brunsvold, M. A., E. S. Chaves, K. S. Kornman, T. B. Aufdemorte, and R. Wood. 'Effects of a Bisphosphonate on Experimental Periodontitis in Monkeys', *J Periodontol* Vol. 63, No. 10, 825-30, 1992.

Burns, F. R., M. S. Stack, R. D. Gray, and C. A. Paterson. 'Inhibition of Purified Collagenase from Alkali-Burned Rabbit Corneas', *Invest Ophthalmol Vis Sci* Vol. 30, No. 7, 1569-75, 1989.

Caton, J. G., S. G. Ciancio, T. M. Blieden, M. Bradshaw, R. J. Crout, A. F. Hefti, J. M. Massaro, A. M. Polson, J. Thomas, and C. Walker. 'Subantimicrobial Dose Doxycycline as an Adjunct to Scaling and Root Planing: Post-Treatment Effects', *J Clin Periodontol* Vol. 28, No. 8, 782-9, 2001.

Chang, K. M., M. E. Ryan, L. M. Golub, N. S. Ramamurthy, and T. F. McNamara. 'Local and Systemic Factors in Periodontal Disease Increase Matrix-Degrading Enzyme Activities in Rat Gingiva: Effect of Micocycline Therapy', *Res Commun Mol Pathol Pharmacol* Vol. 91, No. 3, 303-18, 1996.

Ciancio, Sebastian. 'Non-Surgical Periodontal Treatment', *Procedings of the World Workshop in Cinical Periodontics* Vol. II, II1-II12, 1989.

Cionca, N., C. Giannopoulou, G. Ugolotti, and A. Mombelli. 'Amoxicillin and Metronidazole as an Adjunct to Full-Mouth Scaling and Root Planing of Chronic Periodontitis', *J Periodontol* Vol. 80, No. 3, 364-71, 2009.

Cochran, D. L. 'Inflammation and Bone Loss in Periodontal Disease', *J Periodontol* Vol. 79, No. 8 Suppl, 1569-76, 2008.

Dastoor, S. F., S. Travan, R. F. Neiva, L. A. Rayburn, W. V. Giannobile, and H. L. Wang. 'Effect of Adjunctive Systemic Azithromycin with Periodontal Surgery in the Treatment of Chronic Periodontitis in Smokers: A Pilot Study', *J Periodontol* Vol. 78, No. 10, 1887-96, 2007.

DePaola, L. G., C. D. Overholser, T. F. Meiller, G. E. Minah, and C. Niehaus. 'Chemotherapeutic Inhibition of Supragingival Dental Plaque and Gingivitis Development', *J Clin Periodontol* Vol. 16, No. 5, 311-5, 1989.

Dewhirst, F. E., D. E. Moss, S. Offenbacher, and J. M. Goodson. 'Levels of Prostaglandin E2, Thromboxane, and Prostacyclin in Periodontal Tissues', *J Periodontal Res* Vol. 18, No. 2, 156-63, 1983.

DeWitt, D. L., E. A. Meade, and W. L. Smith. 'Pgh Synthase Isoenzyme Selectivity: The Potential for Safer Nonsteroidal Antiinflammatory Drugs', *Am J Med* Vol. 95, No. 2A, 40S-44S, 1993.

El-Shinnawi, U. M., and S. I. El-Tantawy. 'The Effect of Alendronate Sodium on Alveolar Bone Loss in Periodontitis (Clinical Trial)', *J Int Acad Periodontol* Vol. 5, No. 1, 5-10, 2003.

Ellen, R. P., and C. A. McCulloch. 'Evidence Versus Empiricism: Rational Use of Systemic Antimicrobial Agents for Treatment of Periodontitis', *Periodontol 2000* Vol. 10, 29-44, 1996.

Elter, J. R., H. P. Lawrence, S. Offenbacher, and J. D. Beck. 'Meta-Analysis of the Effect of Systemic Metronidazole as an Adjunct to Scaling and Root Planing for Adult Periodontitis', *J Periodontal Res* Vol. 32, No. 6, 487-96, 1997.

Feller, L., and J. Lemmer. 'Necrotizing Periodontal Diseases in Hiv-Seropositive Subjects: Pathogenic Mechanisms', *J Int Acad Periodontol* Vol. 10, No. 1, 10-5, 2008.

Fleisch, H. A. 'Bisphosphonates: Preclinical Aspects and Use in Osteoporosis', *Ann Med* Vol. 29, No. 1, 55-62, 1997.

Flotra, L., P. Gjermo, G. Rolla, and J. Waerhaug. 'A 4-Month Study on the Effect of Chlorhexidine Mouth Washes on 50 Soldiers', *Scand J Dent Res* Vol. 80, No. 1, 10-7, 1972.

Fornell, J., Y. Sundin, and J. Lindhe. 'Effect of Listerine on Dental Plaque and Gingivitis', *Scand J Dent Res* Vol. 83, No. 1, 18-25, 1975.

Gapski, R., J. L. Barr, D. P. Sarment, M. G. Layher, S. S. Socransky, and W. V. Giannobile. 'Effect of Systemic Matrix Metalloproteinase Inhibition on Periodontal Wound Repair: A Proof of Concept Trial', *J Periodontol* Vol. 75, No. 3, 441-52, 2004.

Garrett, S., L. Johnson, C. H. Drisko, D. F. Adams, C. Bandt, B. Beiswanger, G. Bogle, K. Donly, W. W. Hallmon, E. B. Hancock, P. Hanes, C. E. Hawley, R. Kiger, W. Killoy, J. T. Mellonig, A. Polson, F. J. Raab, M. Ryder, N. H. Stoller, H. L. Wang, L. E. Wolinsky, G. H. Evans, C. Q. Harrold, R. M. Arnold, G. L. Southard, and et al. 'Two Multi-Center Studies Evaluating Locally Delivered Doxycycline Hyclate, Placebo Control, Oral Hygiene, and Scaling and Root Planing in the Treatment of Periodontitis', *J Periodontol* Vol. 70, No. 5, 490-503, 1999.

Golub, L. M., S. Ciancio, N. S. Ramamamurthy, M. Leung, and T. F. McNamara. 'Low-Dose Doxycycline Therapy: Effect on Gingival and Crevicular Fluid Collagenase Activity in Humans', *J Periodontal Res* Vol. 25, No. 6, 321-30, 1990.

Golub, L. M., J. M. Goodson, H. M. Lee, A. M. Vidal, T. F. McNamara, and N. S. Ramamurthy. 'Tetracyclines Inhibit Tissue Collagenases. Effects of Ingested Low-Dose and Local Delivery Systems', *J Periodontol* Vol. 56, No. 11 Suppl, 93-7, 1985.

Golub, L. M., T. F. McNamara, M. E. Ryan, B. Kohut, T. Blieden, G. Payonk, T. Sipos, and H. J. Baron. 'Adjunctive Treatment with Subantimicrobial Doses of Doxycycline: Effects on Gingival Fluid Collagenase Activity and Attachment Loss in Adult Periodontitis', *J Clin Periodontol* Vol. 28, No. 2, 146-56, 2001.

Gomi, K., A. Yashima, T. Nagano, M. Kanazashi, N. Maeda, and T. Arai. 'Effects of Full-Mouth Scaling and Root Planing in Conjunction with Systemically Administered Azithromycin', *J Periodontol* Vol. 78, No. 3, 422-9, 2007.

Goodson, J. M. 'Antimicrobial Strategies for Treatment of Periodontal Diseases', *Periodontol 2000* Vol. 5, 142-68, 1994.

Goodson, J. M., M. A. Cugini, R. L. Kent, G. C. Armitage, C. M. Cobb, D. Fine, M. E. Fritz, E. Green, M. J. Imoberdorf, W. J. Killoy, and et al. 'Multicenter Evaluation of Tetracycline Fiber Therapy: Ii. Clinical Response', *J Periodontal Res* Vol. 26, No. 4, 371-9, 1991.

Goodson, J. M., J. C. Gunsolley, S. G. Grossi, P. S. Bland, J. Otomo-Corgel, F. Doherty, and J. Comiskey. 'Minocycline Hcl Microspheres Reduce Red-Complex Bacteria in Periodontal Disease Therapy', *J Periodontol* Vol. 78, No. 8, 1568-79, 2007.

Gordon, J. M., I. B. Lamster, and M. C. Seiger. 'Efficacy of Listerine Antiseptic in Inhibiting the Development of Plaque and Gingivitis', *J Clin Periodontol* Vol. 12, No. 8, 697-704, 1985.

Graves, D. T., A. J. Delima, R. Assuma, S. Amar, T. Oates, and D. Cochran. 'Interleukin-1 and Tumor Necrosis Factor Antagonists Inhibit the Progression of Inflammatory Cell Infiltration toward Alveolar Bone in Experimental Periodontitis', *J Periodontol* Vol. 69, No. 12, 1419-25, 1998.

Greenwell, H. 'Position Paper: Guidelines for Periodontal Therapy', *J Periodontol* Vol. 72, No. 11, 1624-8, 2001.

Gusberti, F. A., P. Sampathkumar, B. E. Siegrist, and N. P. Lang. 'Microbiological and Clinical Effects of Chlorhexidine Digluconate and Hydrogen Peroxide Mouthrinses on Developing Plaque and Gingivitis', *J Clin Periodontol* Vol. 15, No. 1, 60-7, 1988.

Hawkey, C. J. 'Gastroduodenal Problems Associated with Non-Steroidal, Anti-Inflammatory Drugs (Nsaids)', *Scand J Gastroenterol Suppl* Vol. 200, 94-5, 1993.

Herrera, D., B. Alonso, R. Leon, S. Roldan, and M. Sanz. 'Antimicrobial Therapy in Periodontitis: The Use of Systemic Antimicrobials against the Subgingival Biofilm', *J Clin Periodontol* Vol. 35, No. 8 Suppl, 45-66, 2008.

Holzhausen, M., C. Rossa Junior, E. Marcantonio Junior, P. O. Nassar, D. M. Spolidorio, and L. C. Spolidorio. 'Effect of Selective Cyclooxygenase-2 Inhibition on the Development of Ligature-Induced Periodontitis in Rats', *J Periodontol* Vol. 73, No. 9, 1030-6, 2002.

Holzhausen, M., D. M. Spolidorio, M. N. Muscara, J. Hebling, and L. C. Spolidorio. 'Protective Effects of Etoricoxib, a Selective Inhibitor of Cyclooxygenase-2, in Experimental Periodontitis in Rats', *J Periodontal Res* Vol. 40, No. 3, 208-11, 2005.

Jeffcoat, M. K., G. Cizza, W. J. Shih, R. Genco, and A. Lombardi. 'Efficacy of Bisphosphonates for the Control of Alveolar Bone Loss in Periodontitis', *J Int Acad Periodontol* Vol. 9, No. 3, 70-6, 2007.

Kim, Y. J., C. Rossa, Jr., and K. L. Kirkwood. 'Prostaglandin Production by Human Gingival Fibroblasts Inhibited by Triclosan in the Presence of Cetylpyridinium Chloride', *J Periodontol* Vol. 76, No. 10, 1735-42, 2005.

Kirkwood, K. L., J. A. Cirelli, J. E. Rogers, and W. V. Giannobile. 'Novel Host Response Therapeutic Approaches to Treat Periodontal Diseases', *Periodontol 2000* Vol. 43, 294-315, 2007.

Knoll-Kohler, E. 'Metronidazole Dental Gel as an Alternative to Scaling and Root Planing in the Treatment of Localized Adult Periodontitis. Is Its Efficacy Proved?', *Eur J Oral Sci* Vol. 107, No. 6, 415-21, 1999.

Kumar, S., B. J. Votta, D. J. Rieman, A. M. Badger, M. Gowen, and J. C. Lee. 'Il-1- and Tnf-Induced Bone Resorption Is Mediated by P38 Mitogen Activated Protein Kinase', *J Cell Physiol* Vol. 187, No. 3, 294-303, 2001.

Lane, N., G. C. Armitage, P. Loomer, S. Hsieh, S. Majumdar, H. Y. Wang, M. Jeffcoat, and T. Munoz. 'Bisphosphonate Therapy Improves the Outcome of Conventional Periodontal Treatment: Results of a 12-Month, Randomized, Placebo-Controlled Study', *J Periodontol* Vol. 76, No. 7, 1113-22, 2005.

Lindsley, C. B., and B. A. Warady. 'Nonsteroidal Antiinflammatory Drugs. Renal Toxicity. Review of Pediatric Issues', *Clin Pediatr (Phila)* Vol. 29, No. 1, 10-3, 1990.

Loe, H., A. Anerud, H. Boysen, and E. Morrison. 'Natural History of Periodontal Disease in Man. Rapid, Moderate and No Loss of Attachment in Sri Lankan Laborers 14 to 46 Years of Age', *J Clin Periodontol* Vol. 13, No. 5, 431-45, 1986.

Loe, H., and C. R. Schiott. 'The Effect of Mouthrinses and Topical Application of Chlorhexidine on the Development of Dental Plaque and Gingivitis in Man', *J Periodontal Res* Vol. 5, No. 2, 79-83, 1970.

Loesche, W. J., J. R. Giordano, P. Hujoel, J. Schwarcz, and B. A. Smith. 'Metronidazole in Periodontitis: Reduced Need for Surgery', *J Clin Periodontol* Vol. 19, No. 2, 103-12, 1992.

Loesche, W. J., S. A. Syed, E. C. Morrison, G. A. Kerry, T. Higgins, and J. Stoll. 'Metronidazole in Periodontitis. I. Clinical and Bacteriological Results after 15 to 30 Weeks', *J Periodontol* Vol. 55, No. 6, 325-35, 1984.

Lopez, N. J., J. A. Gamonal, and B. Martinez. 'Repeated Metronidazole and Amoxicillin Treatment of Periodontitis. A Follow-up Study', *J Periodontol* Vol. 71, No. 1, 79-89, 2000.

Machion, L., D. C. Andia, G. Lecio, F. H. Nociti, Jr., M. Z. Casati, A. W. Sallum, and E. A. Sallum. 'Locally Delivered Doxycycline as an Adjunctive Therapy to Scaling and Root Planing in the Treatment of Smokers: A 2-Year Follow-Up', *J Periodontol* Vol. 77, No. 4, 606-13, 2006.

Marx, R. E. 'Pamidronate (Aredia) and Zoledronate (Zometa) Induced Avascular Necrosis of the Jaws: A Growing Epidemic', *J Oral Maxillofac Surg* Vol. 61, No. 9, 1115-7, 2003.

Mealey, B. L. 'Impact of Advances in Diabetes Care on Dental Treatment of the Diabetic Patient', *Compend Contin Educ Dent* Vol. 19, No. 1, 41-4, 46-8, 50 passim; quiz 60, 1998.

Ng, V. W., and N. F. Bissada. 'Clinical Evaluation of Systemic Doxycycline and Ibuprofen Administration as an Adjunctive Treatment for Adult Periodontitis', *J Periodontol* Vol. 69, No. 7, 772-6, 1998.

Novak, M. J., L. P. Johns, R. C. Miller, and M. H. Bradshaw. 'Adjunctive Benefits of Subantimicrobial Dose Doxycycline in the Management of Severe, Generalized, Chronic Periodontitis', *J Periodontol* Vol. 73, No. 7, 762-9, 2002.

Odvina, C. V., J. E. Zerwekh, D. S. Rao, N. Maalouf, F. A. Gottschalk, and C. Y. Pak. 'Severely Suppressed Bone Turnover: A Potential Complication of Alendronate Therapy', *J Clin Endocrinol Metab* Vol. 90, No. 3, 1294-301, 2005.

Offenbacher, S. 'Periodontal Diseases: Pathogenesis', *Ann Periodontol* Vol. 1, No. 1, 821-78, 1996.

Offenbacher, S., D. H. Farr, and J. M. Goodson. 'Measurement of Prostaglandin E in Crevicular Fluid', *J Clin Periodontol* Vol. 8, No. 4, 359-67, 1981.

Overholser, C. D., T. F. Meiller, L. G. DePaola, G. E. Minah, and C. Niehaus. 'Comparative Effects of 2 Chemotherapeutic Mouthrinses on the Development of Supragingival Dental Plaque and Gingivitis', *J Clin Periodontol* Vol. 17, No. 8, 575-9, 1990.

Pires, J.R., C.J. Rossa, and A.C. Pizzolitto. 'In Vitro Antimicrobial Efficiency of a Mouthwash Containing Triclosan/Gantrez and Sodium Bicarbonate', *Braz Oral REs* Vol. 21, No. 4, 342-7, 2007.

Pradeep, A. R., S. V. Sagar, and H. Daisy. 'Clinical and Microbiologic Effects of Subgingivally Delivered 0.5% Azithromycin in the Treatment of Chronic Periodontitis', *J Periodontol* Vol. 79, No. 11, 2125-35, 2008.

Reddy, M. S., N. C. Geurs, and J. C. Gunsolley. 'Periodontal Host Modulation with Antiproteinase, Anti-Inflammatory, and Bone-Sparing Agents. A Systematic Review', *Ann Periodontol* Vol. 8, No. 1, 12-37, 2003.

Reddy, M. S., T. W. Weatherford, 3rd, C. A. Smith, B. D. West, M. K. Jeffcoat, and T. M. Jacks. 'Alendronate Treatment of Naturally-Occurring Periodontitis in Beagle Dogs', *J Periodontol* Vol. 66, No. 3, 211-7, 1995.

Rocha, M. L., J. M. Malacara, F. J. Sanchez-Marin, C. J. Vazquez de la Torre, and M. E. Fajardo. 'Effect of Alendronate on Periodontal Disease in Postmenopausal Women: A Randomized Placebo-Controlled Trial', *J Periodontol* Vol. 75, No. 12, 1579-85, 2004.

Rocha, M., L. E. Nava, C. Vazquez de la Torre, F. Sanchez-Marin, M. E. Garay-Sevilla, and J. M. Malacara. 'Clinical and Radiological Improvement of Periodontal Disease in Patients with Type 2 Diabetes Mellitus Treated with Alendronate: A Randomized, Placebo-Controlled Trial', *J Periodontol* Vol. 72, No. 2, 204-9, 2001.

Rogers, J. E., F. Li, D. D. Coatney, J. Otremba, J. M. Kriegl, T. A. Protter, L. S. Higgins, S. Medicherla, and K. L. Kirkwood. 'A P38 Mitogen-Activated Protein Kinase Inhibitor Arrests Active Alveolar Bone Loss in a Rat Periodontitis Model', *J Periodontol* Vol. 78, No. 10, 1992-8, 2007.

Rogers, M. J., S. Gordon, H. L. Benford, F. P. Coxon, S. P. Luckman, J. Monkkonen, and J. C. Frith. 'Cellular and Molecular Mechanisms of Action of Bisphosphonates', *Cancer* Vol. 88, No. 12 Suppl, 2961-78, 2000.

Ruggiero, S. L., B. Mehrotra, T. J. Rosenberg, and S. L. Engroff. 'Osteonecrosis of the Jaws Associated with the Use of Bisphosphonates: A Review of 63 Cases', *J Oral Maxillofac Surg* Vol. 62, No. 5, 527-34, 2004.

Shimizu, N., Y. Ozawa, M. Yamaguchi, T. Goseki, K. Ohzeki, and Y. Abiko. 'Induction of Cox-2 Expression by Mechanical Tension Force in Human Periodontal Ligament Cells', *J Periodontol* Vol. 69, No. 6, 670-7, 1998.

Siegrist, BE., FA. Gusberti, MC Brecx, Weber HP, and NP Lang. 'Efficacy of Supervised Rinsing with Chlorhexidine Digluconate in Comparison to Phenolic and Plant Alkaloid Compounds', *J Periodontal Res* Vol. 21 (suppl. 16), No. 60, 1986.

Sigusch, B., M. Beier, G. Klinger, W. Pfister, and E. Glockmann. 'A 2-Step Non-Surgical Procedure and Systemic Antibiotics in the Treatment of Rapidly Progressive Periodontitis', *J Periodontol* Vol. 72, No. 3, 275-83, 2001.

Slots, J., and M. Ting. 'Systemic Antibiotics in the Treatment of Periodontal Disease', *Periodontol 2000* Vol. 28, 106-76, 2002.

Socransky, S. S., and A. D. Haffajee. 'Evidence of Bacterial Etiology: A Historical Perspective', *Periodontol 2000* Vol. 5, 7-25, 1994.

van Winkelhoff, A. J., T. E. Rams, and J. Slots. 'Systemic Antibiotic Therapy in Periodontics', *Periodontol 2000* Vol. 10, 45-78, 1996.

Watts, T., R. Palmer, and P. Floyd. 'Metronidazole: A Double-Blind Trial in Untreated Human Periodontal Disease', *J Clin Periodontol* Vol. 13, No. 10, 939-43, 1986.

Wennstrom, J. L., H. N. Newman, S. R. MacNeill, W. J. Killoy, G. S. Griffiths, D. G. Gillam, L. Krok, I. G. Needleman, G. Weiss, and S. Garrett. 'Utilisation of Locally Delivered Doxycycline in Non-Surgical Treatment of Chronic Periodontitis. A Comparative Multi-Centre Trial of 2 Treatment Approaches', *J Clin Periodontol* Vol. 28, No. 8, 753-61, 2001.

Williams, R. C., D. W. Paquette, S. Offenbacher, D. F. Adams, G. C. Armitage, K. Bray, J. Caton, D. L. Cochran, C. H. Drisko, J. P. Fiorellini, W. V. Giannobile, S. Grossi, D. M. Guerrero, G. K. Johnson, I. B. Lamster, I. Magnusson, R. J. Oringer, G. R. Persson, T. E. Van Dyke, L. F. Wolff, E. A. Santucci, B. E. Rodda, and J. Lessem. 'Treatment of Periodontitis by Local Administration of Minocycline Microspheres: A Controlled Trial', *J Periodontol* Vol. 72, No. 11, 1535-44, 2001.

Winkel, E. G., A. J. Van Winkelhoff, M. F. Timmerman, U. Van der Velden, and G. A. Van der Weijden. 'Amoxicillin Plus Metronidazole in the Treatment of Adult Periodontitis Patients. A Double-Blind Placebo-Controlled Study', *J Clin Periodontol* Vol. 28, No. 4, 296-305, 2001.

Part 6

Periodontium and Aging

16

Effects of Human Ageing on Periodontal Tissues

Eduardo Hebling
Department of Community Dentistry, Piracicaba Dental School, University of Campinas, Piracicaba, Brazil

1. Introduction

Aging and death are two natural consequences to which the human individuals are subject after their birth. Improvement in both social living conditions and health care has led to a greater life span in the world [1], resulting in an increase in periodontal disease expectancy among the dentate elderly [2]. Although moderate loss of both alveolar bone and periodontal attachment is common in the elderly, severe periodontitis, defined as periodontal attachment loss of 6 mm or more and radiographic bone loss of 50% or more involving at least one tooth, is not a natural consequence of ageing. Some loss of periodontal attachment and alveolar bone may be expected in older persons, but age alone in healthy adults does not lead to a critical loss of periodontal support [3].

Human ageing induces histophysiological and clinical alterations in oral tissues [4]. These alterations must be understood to differentiate pathological conditions from the altered physiology of oral tissues resulting from ageing [5]. Some studies in humans and animals have demonstrated that alterations in periodontium dynamics occur with age [6,7].

In spite of the fact that the periodontal disease severity is known to be associated with age, functional changes in periodontal tissue cells during the ageing process have not been well characterized [8]. It is important to define how cellular ageing affects the progression of periodontal diseases associated with ageing [6]. The understanding of the influence of human aging in the dynamic of the inflammatory process in patients with periodontal disease may help in the treatment planning of these patients.

2. Age-dependent changes of the periodontal tissues

The tissues that support the teeth are called the periodontium, which consists of gingiva, periodontal ligament, cementum, and alveolar bone. Anatomical and functional changes in periodontal tissues have been reported as being associated with the ageing process [9].

Gingiva, a tissue exposed to the oral cavity, is histologically composed by epithelium and connective tissues. Changes in the human oral epithelium caused by ageing are related to a thinning of the epithelium and diminished keratinization. Conflicting results have been reported regarding the shape of the retepegs. A flattening of retepegs and an increase in the height of the epithelial ridges associated with ageing were both demonstrated. In a morphological 3-dimensional study of the epithelium-connective tissue interface, connective tissue ridges were observed to be more prevalent in young individuals whereas connective tissue papillae were predominant in old individuals. The change from ridges to papillae involves the formation of epithelial cross-ridges with advanced age [9].

Furthermore, it has been shown that the number of cellular elements decreases as age increases. The fibroblasts are the main cells in the synthesis of periodontal connective tissue. There are phenotypic subpopulations of fibroblasts with different functions in the synthesis and maintenance of extracellular matrix constituents [10]. *In vivo* and *in vitro* studies have shown functional and structural alterations in fibroblasts associated with ageing [6, 11-13].

Gingival fibroblasts (GF) may be constantly affected by oral bacteria and their products, such as the lipopolysaccharides (LPS), present in their cell walls. The LPS induces GF to release some inflammatory cytokines such as prostaglandin E_2 (PGE_2), interleukin (IL)-1 β, and plasminogen activator (PA) [6, 14]. The influence of these inflammatory mediators on both GF and periodontal ligament fibroblasts (PLF) might account for the severity of periodontal disease [6].

Quantitative differences in protein synthesis were found in young and old gingival fibroblasts *in vitro*. The collagen production decreased more than 5-fold as a function of increasing donor age [15]. Old fibroblasts also presented an increased rate of collagen intracellular phagocytosis, which can affect the balance between synthesis and degradation of collagen in the connective tissue [12]. The ageing process in GF causes an increase in DNA structure metilation of collagen alpha 1 gene, followed by a reduction in mRNA levels and collagen type I synthesis [13]. Alterations in the composition of extracellular matrix proteoglycans secreted by GF *in vitro* were also observed. The proteoglycans secreted by old fibroblasts might increase the rates of heparan sulfate and reduce chondroitin sulfate when compared to those secreted by young fibroblasts [16].

The periodontal ligament, which is a soft connective tissue, anchors the tooth into the alveolar bone and functions as a cushion between hard tissues to mitigate the occlusal force. It is basically constituted by fibroblasts, cementoblasts, osteoblasts, osteoclasts, Malassez epithelial rests and collagen matrix (Sharpey´s fibers). The periodontal ligament cells are involved in the repair of alveolar bone, cementum and periodontal ligament itself, being able to differentiate into osteblasts, cementoblasts and fibroblasts [17]. With age, the fiber and cellular contents decrease and the structure of the periodontal ligament becomes irregular. Periodontal ligament fibroblasts (PLF) are constantly subject to mechanical stress caused by occlusal forces. Cultured PLF were observed to produce a large amount of PGE_2, IL-1β, and PA in response to mechanical stress [6].

The ageing process might induce a significant reduction in chemotaxy, motility, and proliferation rate of periodontal ligament cells. The chemotaxy and differentiation of osteoclasts from the periodontal ligament induced by devitalized osseous matrix might be influenced by donor's age. A reduction in osteoblast chemotaxy and lower rate of osteoclast differentiation in the cells of elderly donors were observed [18].

The cells of the periodontal ligament from the elderly showed lower rates of chemotaxy and proliferation than those of the periodontal ligament from young patients [19]. The reduced ability of senescent cells to express the *c-fos* ligant might be associated with the low rates of chemotaxy and proliferation of these cells [20]. The expression of osteocalcin in fibroblasts from the periodontal ligament is either reduced or ceased in senescent fibroblasts. This reduction may be directly related to the cell's difficulty in progressing in the cellular cycle (G1-S) and accomplishing cell respiration [21].

Cementum is a calcified connective tissue covering the roots of teeth. Its formation is a continuous process which occurs throughout the life of humans and animals. With age, the cementum increases in width. It has been demonstrated that there is a tendency towards greater cemental apposition in the apical region of the teeth. Collagen fibers are embedded in the cementum during its formation [9]. Ageing and death of cells are common characteristics of the life cycle of the cementocytes. This might be due to a rapid reduction in the accessibility of nutritive substances and poor elimination of waste products of the cementocytes. In general, cementum is cellular-except at the root apices and in the furcation areas of multirooted teeth. With age, cementum becomes acellular. Although remodeling of cementum occurs infrequently, resorption at the cementum surface followed by cementum apposition is often observed and, with age, this might result in irregular cementum surfaces [9, 22].

Both the alveolar bone and the periodontal ligament serve as support to the teeth. It is well known that bone formation steadily declines with age, leading to a significant reduction in bone mass [23]. The alveolar bone has high plasticity and under physiological conditions it is preserved by the equilibrium between osteoblastic and osteoclastic activities. These cells are directly or indirectly influenced by the parathyroid hormone (PTH), vitamin D metabolites, calcitonin, estrogen, plasmatic concentration of calcium and phosphate, neurotransmitters, growth factors, and local cytokines [24].

The reduction in bone formation might be due to a decrease in osteoblast-proliferating precursors or to decreased synthesis and secretion of essential bone matrix proteins [6, 23]. The extracellular matrix surrounding osteoblasts has been shown to play an important role in bone metabolism. A possible dysfunction of this matrix might occur concomitantly with the ageing process [6].

Oxygen-free radicals have been reported to cause cellular damage and, consequently, contribute to the ageing process [25, 26]. In an *in vitro* study, oxygen radical-treated fibronectin (FN) was found to inhibit bone nodule formation by osteoblasts when compared to intact FN. This finding suggested that intact FN plays an important role in osteoblast activity and that FN damaged by oxygen radicals during the ageing process might be related to less bone formation [6].

3. Systemic ageing and periodontium

Some alterations in the organism endocrine profile influence the osseous metabolism with age. Vitamin D deficiency is a common phenomenon in persons living in elderly homes [27]. The low levels of calcium resulting from vitamin D deficiency associated with renal insufficiency might lead to secondary hyperparathyroidism [28]. The high levels of PTH resulting from secondary hyperparathyroidism act in the mobilization of osseous calcium, which might cause mineralization problems, bone fractures, and a reduction in osseous density [29]. With regard to the periodontium, osteopenia and osteoporosis are considered important risk factors for alveolar bone loss in the presence of periodontal diseases [30, 31].

Female patients with osteoporosis or osteopenia presented greater levels of alveolar bone loss, when compared to patients with normal mineral osseous density [32, 33]. Estrogen hormonal reposition therapy in patients with osteoporosis might reduce gingival inflammation and alveolar bone loss in relation to patients with untreated osteoporosis [34, 35]. In a randomized double-blind study, patients with osteoporosis treated with estrogen reposition showed an increase in alveolar bone levels, when compared to the placebo group [36].

The supplement ingestion of calcium (1000-1200 mg/day) and vitamin D (400-600 IU/day) in elderly patients with osteoporosis has been tested. After 5 years of treatment, the results showed a reduction in tooth loss in patients who ingested calcium and vitamin D, when compared to the placebo group [37]. Studies evaluating periodontal status and hormonal reposition therapies, indicated for prevention and treatment of osteoporosis, have reported the reduction in alveolar bone loss and tooth loss as secondary benefits. It is worth emphasizing that some risks in hormonal reposition therapy have been recently reported; for example, an increase in the incidence of breast cancer, thromboembolic diseases, and myocardial infarction has been found [38].

4. Immunosenescence and periodontal cells interaction

Immunosenescence refers to the gradual deterioration of the immune system caused by natural aging. It involves the host's capacity to respond to infections and the development of long-term immune memory. This is not a random deteriorative phenomenon; rather it appears to repeat inversely an evolutionary pattern. Most of the parameters affected by immunosenescence appear to be under genetic control. Immunosenescence can also be sometimes envisaged as the result of the continuous challenge of the unavoidable exposure of the organism to a variety of antigens such as viruses and bacteria [39].

Aging is a complex, continuous, and slow process that gradually involves most if not all organs of the organism, causing their abnormal functioning of in both qualitative and quantitative terms, as well as morphological or structural changes. So, senescence is not represented by a pre-established moment, but consists of a long-lasting preparation of the organism for a morpho-functional involution, which itself is a normal part of the biological cycle [40]. In this context, periodontal tissues also are included.

The immune system also undergoes age-related modifications leading to structural changes in the lymphoid organs, and functional impairment of some types of immunocompetent cells. The most evident changes in the immune system occur in the thymus, a specialized organ of the immune system. The thymus is a primary lymphoid organ, but also an endocrine gland, responsible for T-cell production and maturation [41].

The thymus is the largest and most active during the neonatal and pre-adolescent periods. By the early teens, the thymus begins to atrophy and thymic stroma is replaced by adipose tissue. Nevertheless, residual T lymphopoiesis continues throughout adult life. Thymus involution in humans is observed until the age of 70 years [42]. The consequences of thymic involution in the peripheral pool of T-cells are still a matter of controversy. Thus, whereas some authors report no significant decline in the total number of T-cells, but considerable shifts in the ratios of activated/memory T-cells [41], others claim that the age-related changes in the thymus and T-cells are quantitative, not qualitative [43]. In any case, it remains to be clarified whether changes in the immune system with age have something to do with survival [44], although the stage of being elderly is associated with an increase in infections, tumors, and other diseases related to a decline in the immune function [45].

T-lymphocytes are considered thymus-dependent cells of fundamental importance in the immune response. Reductions in peripheral blood T-lymphocytes, mitotic agents, anti-CD3, and monoclonal antibodies are the main alterations in the senescent phenotypes of T-lymphocytes. The proliferative phase alterations in T-lymphocytes may be induced by the reduced secretion of interleukin-2 (IL-2) and reduced expression of its high-affinity receptors. The reduced expression patterns of IL-2 and IL-2R in peripheral monocytes of elderly patients have been reported as influencing the proliferative response of T-lymphocytes [46]. IL-2 is produced by helper T-cells and plays an important role in the proliferation and differentiation of virgin T-cells into effector T-cells (this term is used frequently for populations of T-cells with cytolytic activities and for T-helper cells, which secrete cytokines and activate directly other immune cells, to distinguish them from another class of T-cells known as regulatory T-cells) [47].

Ageing-related immunological alterations in the leukocyte subpopulations [48] and B-lymphocyte subpopulations [49] have been reported. The reduction in the peripheral blood population of B-lymphocytes is associated with the decrease in the production of high-specificity antibodies as well as in the avidity of antigen-antibody legation [50]. In establishment of long-term memory of immune response, the maturation of antigen-induced $CD4^+$ T-cells, which are postthymic human cell, results in the terminally differentiated $CD45RA^+$. An increase in $CD45RA^+$ memory cell circulation in relation to $CD45RO^+$ virgin cells disturbing the response to new antigens has been noted. Other changes in immune senescence include a decline in macrophage, neutrophil, and natural killer function with ageing [51].

A more rapid and severe development of gingivitis as well as changes in inflammatory response induced by gingivitis in elderly patients have been reported [52]. A greater presence of alpha 2-macroglobulin, IgG3, and B-lymphocytes in the crevicular fluid, and a reduction in polymorphonuclear leukocytes (PMN) have also been observed in the elderly [53].

Periodontal ligament cells from the elderly showed an increase in the production of plasminogen activator (PA) [54], prostaglandin E2 (PGE2), interleukin-1β (IL-1β) [6, 54] and interleukin-6 (IL-6) [55] when compared to younger cells.

Lipopolysaccharide (LPS), responsible for bacterial cytotoxicity, is a component of the gram negative bacterial cell wall. It induces the activation of transcription factors in lymphocytes, promoting regions of DNA which activate genes that contribute to the adaptive response and secretion of pro-inflammatory cytokines [56].

PA is a serine protease that acts in the activation of plasmatic plasminogen into plasmin and it is secreted by many cell types, including periodontal fibroblasts. The activity of PA and the expression of tissue plasminogen activator (tPA) mRNA in fibroblasts from the periodontal ligament *in vitro* submitted to mechanical tension were evaluated. The cells from elderly individuals presented greater activity of PA and greater expression of tPA mRNA when compared to those from young individuals [7]. The action of PA is involved in physiological and pathological mechanisms of periodontium, including host-microbiota interaction, PMN migration, and proliferation and migration of both epithelial cells and fibroblasts [57]. Analysis of PA distribution in the periodontium showed that, in healthy periodontium, PA is expressed in the superficial cells of the junctional epithelium. However, in patients with periodontitis, PA is expressed in all the epithelium lining of the periodontal pocket. The alteration in the pattern of PA distribution, according to periodontal status, suggests that PA is involved in the periodontal homeostasis [58].

The levels of tPA and the plasminogen activator inhibitor-2 (PAI-2) are greater in gingival crevicular fluid of patients with periodontitis than in periodontally healthy patients [59]. Patients with high levels of alveolar bone loss presented higher levels of tPA and PAI-2 than those with low levels of alveolar bone loss. A greater release of PA induced by ageing might affect the gingival fibroblasts and the periodontal ligament, and aggravate the inflammation process and the degradation of the extracellular matrix from periodontal tissues in the elderly [7, 53].

Fibroblasts from old mice (20 months) demonstrated a significant increase in the synthesis of PGE2 and IL-1β when compared to the fibroblasts from young mice (6 weeks) [54, 60]. An increase in the production of PGE2 and Cox 2 mRNA stimulated by LPS and mechanical stress, respectively, was also observed in periodontal ligament cells from elderly donors [61, 62]. PGE2 is produced by the metabolism of arachidonic acid through the cyclooxygenase (COX) pathway and has a recognized role in the inflammatory process, through vascular dilatation, increased in vascular permeability, and sensibilization of nociceptors to the stimulus of histamine and bradykinin. PGE2 may have an indirect effect on alveolar bone resorption by the sensibility of osteoclasts to the action of other cytokines involved in this process [63]. In patients with periodontitis, high levels of PGE2 were observed to be related to the severity of periodontal disease and the increase in alveolar bone loss [64, 65]. The greater production of PGE2 by old periodontal ligament cells might account for the greater rate of alveolar bone resorption in elderly patients [54, 66].

In vitro studies have demonstrated an increase in the synthesis of IL-1β and in the expression of IL-1β mRNA in fibroblasts from human elderly donors and in fibroblasts of old mice, stimulated by mechanical stress [60, 66]. Human gingival fibroblasts from elderly donors presented greater production of IL-6 by the stimulus of LPS from Campylobacter rectus when compared to young donors [55]. IL-1β is the most active cytokine in the process of bone resorption, being 15 times more potent than IL-1α and 1000 times more potent than TNF-β [67]. Patients with severe periodontal disease (periodontal pocket >6mm) presented with a rate of IL-1β twice times higher than that observed for patients with moderate (<4mm) and intermediate (4-6 mm) periodontal disease [67]. In the same way, another study demonstrated that patients with periodontal bone loss had more IL-1β in the gingival fluid when compared to periodontal patients without bone loss ($P<0.0001$) [68]. The levels of IL-1α, IL-1β, plaque accumulation, gingival fluid, and gingival inflammation in young adults (20-22 years) and elderly (61-65 years) were compared with experimental periodontal disease. Levels of IL-1β in the gingival fluid were significantly higher in elderly, with a progressive increase until the 21st day of oral hygiene suspension, while levels of IL-1α were similar for both groups. In the elderly there was also an increase in plaque accumulation, gingival fluid, and clinical signs of inflammation [69].

The pattern of IL-1β and IL-6 secretion in periodontal disease in menopausal patients was analyzed [34]. The results demonstrated that menopausal patients that were not in hormone reposition therapy presented higher rates of IL-1β ($p < 0.0004$) and IL-6 ($p>0.05$) than patients under hormonal treatment. IL-6 has an important role in the osseous lyses in periodontitis. It acts stimulating the growth and proliferation of osteoclast precursors and there is evidence that it is an extracellular messenger signaling osteoblast resorption for the osteoclast [55]. A greater concentration of IL-1β e IL-8 in patients with estrogen deficiency compared to untreated patients without estrogen deficiency was also observed [70]. The hypothesis that the greater liberation of IL-1β by older periodontal ligament cells may represent an important factor for the greater rate of alveolar bone resorption in elderly patients has been proposed [54, 60, 66].

Periodontal ligament fibroblasts also express osteoblastic phenotypes, such as the production of bone-like matrix proteins, high alkaline phosphatase activity, and the formation of calcified nodules [71]. In addition, human periodontal ligament cells express and secrete osteoprotegerin (OPG) [72] and receptor activator of NF-kappa B ligand (RANKL) such as osteoblasts, suggesting that the periodontal ligament plays a role in alveolar bone metabolism [73].

RANKL, a member of tumor necrosis factor (TNF) ligand family, is expressed on osteoblast/stromal cell membranes. This ligand binds to the receptor activator of NF-kappa B (RANK), which is a receptor on the membrane of osteoclasts and mononuclear pre-osteoclasts, and induces osteoclast differentiation and activity [74, 75]. In contrast, OPG is known to inhibit osteoclast differentiation and activity by interrupting the interaction between RANKL and its receptor, RANK, by binding to RANKL as a decoy receptor with higher affinity than RANK [76].

RANKL expressed on gingival or synovial fibroblasts may direct macrophages present in connective tissue and monocytes recruited from blood to differentiate into osteoclasts, which leads to bone destruction in periodontitis or arthritis. RANKL is expressed also on activated T-cells [73, 75]. RANKL promoted the survival of mature dendritic cells and enhances the ability of these cells to stimulate T-cell proliferation in a mixed leukocyte reaction. In addition, RANKL induced the production of proinflammatory cytokines (IL-1 and IL-6) and cytokines that direct differentiation of T- cells, such as IL-12 and IL-15 from dendritic cells [77].

In periodontitis, LPS, which is a combination of lipid and polysaccharide, is a component of the outer membrane of gram-negative bacteria [56]. It has been reported that toll-like-receptor-4 (TLR4), a protein that in humans is encoded by the TLR4 gene and it detect lipopolysaccharide from Gram-negative bacteria, is essential for the response to LPS [78]. Human periodontal ligament fibroblasts express TLR4, suggesting that LPS directly acts on these cells. LPS interacts with endotoxin and CD14 (endotoxin receptor) to present LPS to TLR-4, which activates inflammatory gene expression through NF-kappa-B. CD14 is a critical receptor for LPS because monoclonal antibodies directed against CD14 can inhibit the biological effects induced both *in vitro* and *in vivo* by LPS [79].

LPS induces inflammatory cytokines, such as interleukin-1 beta (IL-1β) and tumor necrosis factor-alpha (TNF-α), in macrophages and neutrophilic leukocytes that infiltrate areas infected with bacteria, and in periodontal ligament fibroblasts [80]. These cytokines are thought to play an important role in the pathogenesis of periodontitis because they cause inflammation and destruction of periodontal tissue and resorption of alveolar bone by various biological mechanisms. IL-1 and TNF-a induce bone resorption by acting both directly and indirectly on osteoclasts [81].

The effects of LPS on OPG and RANKL expression in human periodontal ligament fibroblasts (HPLF) were reported. These suggest that LPS stimulates both OPG and RANKL expression in HPLF by up-regulating IL-1β and TNF-α [82].

All of these studies related to the dynamics of the inflammatory process allow a better understanding of the interaction of immunosenescence on cells periodontal. However, continuous research on this subject should be held.

5. Ageing as a risk factor for periodontal disease

The age-related changes in the periodontal tissues show that increasing age could potentially be a risk factor for periodontal disease [83]. Some moderate loss of periodontal attachment and alveolar bone is associated with age, but age alone in a healthy adult does not lead to a critical loss of periodontal support. Although moderate loss of alveolar bone and periodontal attachment is common in the elderly, severe periodontitis is not a natural consequence of ageing [3, 83]. Clinical attachment level and bone loss are irreversible measures of prior disease experience. Cross-sectional studies measuring disease experience demonstrated more attachment loss and alveolar bone loss among older age groups than other groups [3].

Longitudinal studies addressing potential relationships between age and attachment loss or bone loss showed statistically significant relationships between age and incidence of periodontal disease [84-86]. However, this age-associated increase in risk may not be linear, since some studies show no significant differences within age groups above 65 years [87-91].
The main issue related of this fact is the magnitude of any increase in risk. Studies that demonstrate statistically significant associations do not necessarily indicated that these will lead to severe clinical outcome for older adults [92]. A 28-year follow-up study reported an odds ratio of 10.4 for people aged 36-50 years compared with people aged 5-15 years. While this result is comparable in magnitude with other clinically important risk factors (smoking odds ratio in the same study was 14), it corresponds to a mean increase in clinical attachment level of only 1.34 mm over 28 years [85].
This level of increased risk probably is not sufficient, alone, to cause tooth loss. Consequently, periodontal disease may be considered as time-associated, and ageing itself appears to be responsible for some attachment and bone loss, it is of a magnitude that is unlikely to have a clinical significance [83, 92]. This fact is influenced by multiple factors that have been found to be associated with the prevalence and incidence of the periodontal disease [88].

6. Clinical Implications on ageing

Periodontal disease is not thought to be the major cause of tooth loss among adults, the loss of teeth in epidemiological studies usually induce an underestimate of periodontal disease incidence, since attachment loss tends to be greater in teeth that are extracted (whether or not the extraction is due to periodontal disease), and such teeth cannot be measured in follow-up studies [92].
Although longitudinal studies showed moderate levels of attachment loss in a high percentage of middle-aged and elderly subjects, severe loss is confined to a minority. Approximately one-fifth of older patients have experienced more generalized severe loss. The rate is higher in the oldest subjects [92]. The habitual observation in elderly populations is some loss of periodontal attachment and alveolar bone, but age alone in a healthy adult does not lead to a critical loss of periodontal support [3].
The most important clinical conclusion to draw from the longitudinal studies concerning the effects of aging is that increased age poses some increased risk for periodontal loss, but the amount of loss due to age alone is probably consistent with "successful aging" rather than accelerated pathological processes [92]. Really, it is probably appropriate to view the aging-periodontitis association as a rationale for redefining appropriate endpoints of periodontal therapy, such that the objective of treatment is to maintain a functioning dentition rather than a perfect level of periodontal attachment. Models for decision making regarding periodontal treatment needs in elderly have been proposed. Age-related thresholds could be used to decide on appropriate levels of therapy [92, 93].
Recognition of the dental needs of this special category of the population compels us to bear the responsibility of treating them now and in the future. One of the major criteria of successful ageing is to maintain a natural, healthy, functional dentition throughout life, including all the social and biological benefits, such as aesthetics and comfort, and the ability to chew, taste and speak. However, the oral health of elderly people is far from optimal. The demand for treatment is much lower than the need. In the future the elderly will retain their natural dentition and more teeth per individual will be present [94]. This fact can result in an increase in periodontal disease expectancy among the dentate elderly [2].

Certainly, in a short time, the trends for oral health care will be change. The new elderly populations will be more critical and more demanding for oral health care services than current elderly population. The dental profession must be aware of these trends which should be reflected in undergraduate and postgraduate dental education [94]. In worldwide, some countries recognized the Geriatric Dentistry as a new specialty into the dentistry [95] or included specific dental programs for elderly treatment and research [96]. If as an specific specialty or developed by a established specialty, such as the Periodontics, periodontal care services for elderly people must show proficient dental professionals, including knowledge about the ageing interactions on periodontal treatment.

7. Conclusions

In conclusion, ageing alone leads to no critical loss of the periodontal attachment in the healthy elderly. The effects of ageing human on periodontal tissues were based on biomolecular changes of the cells of periodontium that exacerbate bone loss in elderly patients with periodontitis [83].

These effects may be associated with: 1) alterations in differentiation and proliferation of osteoblasts and osteoclasts; 2) an increase in periodontal cell response to the oral microbiota and mechanical stress leading to the secretion of cytokines involved in bone loss; and 3) systemic endocrine alterations in the elderly [83].

8. References

[1] Sternberg SA, Gordon M. Who are older adults? Demographics and major health problems. Periodontol 2000. 1998; 16: 9-15.

[2] Ellen RP. Periodontal disease among older adults: what is the issue? Periodontol 2000. 1998; 16: 7-8.

[3] Burt BA. Periodontitis and ageing: reviewing recent evidence. J Am Dent Assoc. 1994; 125: 273-9.

[4] Mombelli A. Ageing and the periodontal and peri-implant microbiota. Periodontol 2000. 1998; 16: 44-52.

[5] Savitt ED, Kent RL. Distribution of Actinobacillus actinomycetemcomitans and Porphyromonas gingivalis by subject age. J Periodontol. 1991; 62: 490-494.

[6] Abiko Y, Shimizu N, Yamaguchi M, Suzuki H, Takiguchi H. Effect of ageing on functional changes of periodontal tissue cells. Ann Periodontol. 1998; 3: 350-369.

[7] Miura S, Yamaguchi M, Shimizu N, Abiko Y. Mechanical stress enhances expression and production of plasminogen activatorin ageing human periodontal ligament cells. Mech Ageing Dev. 2000; 112: 217-231.

[8] Beck JD, Koch G, Rozier RG, Tudor GE. Prevalence and risk indicators for periodontal attachment loss in a population of older community-dwelling blacks and whites. J Periodontol. 1990; 61: 521-528.

[9] Van der Velden U. Effect of age on the periodontium. J Clin Periodontol. 1984; 11: 281-294.

[10] Hou LT, Yaeger JA. Cloning and characterization of human gingival and periodontal ligament fibroblasts. J Periodontol. 1993; 64: 1209-1218.

[11] Dumas M, Chaudagne C, Bont F, Meybeck A. In vitro biosynthesis of type I and III collagens human dermal fibroblasts from donors of increasing age. Mech Ageing Dev. 1994; 73: 179-187.

[12] Lee W, McCulloch CA. Deregulation of collagen phagocytosis in ageing human fibroblasts: effects of integrin expression and cell cycle. Exp Cell Res. 1997; 237: 383-393.
[13] Takatsu M, Uyeno S, Komura J, Watanabe M, Ono T. Age-dependent alterations in mRNA level and promoter methylation of collagen alpha1(I) gene in human periodontal ligament. Mech Ageing Dev. 1999; 110: 37-48.
[14] Sismey-Durrant HJ, Hopps RM. Effect of lipopolysaccharide from Porphyromonas gingivalis on prostaglandin E2 and interleukin-1β release from rat periosteal and human gingival fibroblasts in vitro. Oral Microbiol Immunol. 1991; 6: 378-380.
[15] Johnson BD, Page RC, Narayanan AS, Pieters HP. Effects of donor age on protein and collagen synthesis in vitro by human diploid fibroblasts. Lab Invest. 1986; 55: 490-496.
[16] Bartold PM, Boyd RR, Page RC. Proteoglycans synthesized by gingival fibroblasts derived from human donors of different ages. Aust N Z J Med. 2000; 30: 209-214.
[17] Somerman MJ, Young MF, Foster RA, Moehring JM, Imm G, Sauk JJ. Characteristics of human periodontal ligament cells in vitro. Arch Oral Biol. 1990; 35: 241-247.
[18] Groessner-Schreiber B, Neubert A, Muller WD, Hopp M, Griepentroq M, Lang KP. Osteoclast recruitment in response to human bone matrix is age related. Mech Ageing Dev. 1992; 62: 143-154.
[19] Nishimura F, Terranova VP, Braithwaite M, Orman R, Ohyama H, Mineshiba J, et al. Comparison of in vitro proliferative capacity of human periodontal ligament cells in juvenile and aged donors. Oral Dis. 1997; 3: 162-166.
[20] Asahara Y, Nishimura1 F, Arai1 H, Kurihara H, Takashiba1 S, Murayama1Y. Chemotactic response of periodontal ligament cells decreases with donor age: association with reduced expression of c-fos. Oral Dis. 1999; 5: 337–343.
[21] Sawa Y, Phillips A, Hollard J, Yoshida S, Braithwaite MW. Impairment of osteocalcin production in senescent periodontal ligament fibroblasts. Tissue Cell. 2000; 32: 198-204.
[22] Tonna EA. Factors (ageing) affecting bone and cementum. J Periodontol 1976: 47: 267-280.
[23] Roholl PJM, Blauw E, Zurcher C, Dormans J, Theuns HM. Evidence for a diminished maturation of pre-osteoblasts into osteoblast during ageing in rats: an ultrastructural analysis. J Bone Miner Res. 1994; 9: 355-366.
[24] Sodek J, McKee MD. Molecular and cellular biology of alveolar bone. Periodontol 2000. 2000; 24: 99-126.
[25] Selkoe DJ. Deciphering Alzheimer's disease: the amyloid precursor protein yields new clues. Science 1990; 248: 1058-1060.
[26] McCord JM. Free radicals and inflammation: protection of synovial fluid by superoxide dismutase. Science 1974; 185: 529-531.
[27] Inderjeeth CA, Nicklason F, Al-Lahham Y, Greenaway TM, Jones G, Parameswaran VV, et al. Vitamin D deficiency and secondary hyperparathyroidism: clinical andbiochemical associations in older non-institutionalised Southern Tasmanians. Aust N Z J Med 2000; 30: 209-214.
[28] Freaney R, McBrinn Y, McKenna MJ. Secondary hyperparathyroidism in elderly people: combined effect of renal insufficiency and vitamin D deficiency. Am J Clin Nutr. 1993; 58: 187-91.

[29] Lips P. Vitamin D deficiency and secondary hyperparathyroidism in the elderly: consequences for bone loss and fractures and therapeutic implications. Endocr Rev 2001; 22: 477-501.

[30] Mohammad AR, Hooper DA, Vermilyea SG, Mariotti A, Preshaw PM. An investigation of the relationship between systemic bone density and clinical periodontal status in post-menopausal Asian-American women. Int Dent J. 2003; 53: 121-125.

[31] Yoshihara A, Seida Y, Hanada N, Miyazaki H. A longitudinal study of the relationship between periodontal disease and bone mineral density in community-dwelling older adults. J Clin Periodontol. 2004; 31: 680-684.

[32] Payne JB, Reinhardt RA, Nummikoski PV, Patil KD. Longitudinal alveolar bone loss in postmenopausal osteoporotic/osteopenic women. Osteoporos Int. 1999; 10: 34-40.

[33] Tezal M, Wactawski-Wende J, Grossi SG, Ho AW, Dunford R, Genco RJ. The relationship between bone mineral density and periodontitis in postmenopausal women. J Periodontol. 2000; 71: 1492-1498.

[34] Reinhardt RA, Payne JB, Maze CA, Patil KD, Gallagher SJ, Mattson JS. Influence of estrogen and osteopenia/osteoporosis on clinical periodontitis in postmenopausal women. J Periodontol 1999; 70: 823-828.

[35] Ronderos M, Jacobs DR, Himes JH, Pihlstrom BL. Associations of periodontal disease with femoral bone mineral density and estrogen replacement therapy: cross-sectional evaluation of US adults from NHANES III. J Clin Periodontol. 2000; 27: 778-786.

[36] Civitelli R, Pilgram TK, Dotson M, Muckerman J, Lewandowski N, Armamento-Villareal R, et al. Alveolar and postcranial bone density in postmenopausal women receiving hormone/estrogen replacement therapy: a randomized, double-blind, placebo-controlled trial. Arch Intern Med. 2002; 162: 1409-1415.

[37] Krall EA, Wehler C, Garcia RI, Harris SS, Dawson-Hughes B. Calcium and vitamin D supplements reduce tooth loss in the elderly. Am J Med. 2001; 111: 452-456.

[38] Biscup P. Risks and benefits of long-term hormone replacement therapy. Am J Health Syst Pharm. 2003; 60: 1419-1425.

[39] Franceschi C, Valensin S, Fagnoni F, Barbi C, Bonafè M. Biomarkers of immunosenescence within an evolutionary perspective: the challenge of heterogeneity and the role of antigenic load. Exp Gerontol. 1999; 34: 911–921.

[40] Malaguarnera L, Ferlito L, Imbesi RM, Gulizia GS, Di Mauro S, Maugeri D, Malaguarnera M, Messina A. Immunosenescence: a review. Arch Gerontol Geriatr 2001; 32:1–14.

[41] Aspinall R, Andrew D. Thymic involution in aging. J Clin Immunol 2000; 20:250–256.

[42] Tosi P, Kraft R, Luzi P, Cintorino M, Fankhauser G, Hess MW, et al. Involution patterns of the human thymus. I Size of the cortical area as a function of age. Clin Exp Immunol. 1982; 47: 497-504.

[43] Douek DC, Koup RA. Evidence for thymus function in the elderly. Vaccine 2000; 18: 1638–1641.

[44] Straub RH, Cutolo M, Zietz B, Scholmerich J. The process of aging change interplay of the immune, endocrine and nervous systems. Mech Ageing Dev. 2001; 122: 1591–1611.

[45] Gavazzi G, Krause KH. Aging and infection. Lancet Infect Dis. 2002; 2: 659-666.

[46] Caruso C, Di Lorenzo G, Modica MA, Candore G, Portelli MR, Crescimanno G, Ingrassia A, Sangiorgi GB, Salerno A. Soluble interleukin-2 receptor release defect in vitro in elderly Subjects. Mech Ageing Dev. 1991; 59: 27-35.

[47] McArthur WP. Effect of ageing on immunocompetent and inflammatory cells. Periodontol 2000. 1998; 16: 53-79.

[48] Rink L, Cakman I, Kirchner H. Altered cytokine production in the elderly. Mech Ageing Dev. 1998; 102: 199-209.

[49] Pawelec G, Barnett Y, Forsey R, Frasca D, Globerson A, McLeod J, et al. T cells and ageing. Front Biosci. 2002; 7: 1056-1183.

[50] Burns EA, Leventhal EA. Ageing, immunity, and cancer. Cancer Control. 2000; 7: 513.

[51] Fransson C, Berglundh T, Lindhe J. The effect of age on the development of gingivitis. Clinical, microbiologicaland histological findings. J Clin Periodontol. 1996; 23: 379-385.

[52] Fransson C, Mooney J, Kinane DF, Berglundh T. Differences in the inflammatory response in young and old human subjects during the course of experimental gingivitis. J Clin Periodontol. 1999; 26: 453-460.

[53] Mochizuki K, Yamaguchi M, Abiko Y. Enhancement of LPS-stimulated plasminogen activator production in aged gingival fibroblasts. J Periodontal Res. 1999; 34: 251-260.

[54] Okamura H, Yamaguchi M, Abiko Y. Enhancement of ipopolysaccharides-stimulated PGE2 and IL-1beta production in gingival fibroblast cells from old rats. Exp Gerontol. 1999; 34: 379-392.

[55] Ogura N, Matsuda U, Tanaka F, Shibata Y, Takiguchi H, Abiko Y. In vitro senescence enhances IL-6 production in human gingival fibroblasts induced by ipopolysaccharides from Campylobacter rectus. Mech Ageing Dev. 1996; 87: 47-59.

[56] Ogawa T, Uchida H, Amino K. Immunobiological activities of chemically defined lipid A from lipopolysaccharides of Porphyromonas gingivalis. Microbiology. 1994; 140: 1209-1216.

[57] Kinnby B. The plasminogen activating system in periodontal health and disease. Biol Chem. 2002; 383: 85-92.

[58] Schmid J, Cohen RL, Chambers DA. Plasminogen activator in human periodontal health and disease. Arch Oral Biol. 1991; 36: 245-50.

[59] Yin X, Bunn CL, Bartold PM. Detection of tissue plasminogen activator (t-PA) and plasminogen activator inhibitor 2(PAI-2) in gingival crevicular fluid from healthy, gingivitis and periodontitis patients. J Clin Periodontol. 2000; 27: 149-156.

[60] Shimizu N, Goseki T, Yamaguchi M, Iwasawa T, Takiguchi H, Abiko Y. In vitro cellular ageing stimulates interleukin-1 beta production in stretched human periodontal-ligament-derived cells. J Dent Res. 1997; 76: 1367-1375.

[61] Takiguchi H, Yamaguchi M, Mochizuki K, Abiko Y. Effect of in vitro ageing on Campylobacter rectus lipopolysaccharide-stimulated PGE2 release from human gingival fibroblasts. Oral Dis. 1996; 2: 202-209.

[62] Ohzeki K, Yamaguchi M, Shimizu N, Abiko Y. Effect of cellular ageing on the induction of cyclooxygenase-2 by mechanical stress in human periodontal ligament cells. Mech Ageing Dev. 1999; 108: 151-163.

[63] Lader CS, Flanagan AM. Prostaglandin E2, interleukin 1alpha, and tumor necrosis factor-alpha increase human osteoclast formation and bone resorption in vitro. Endocrinology. 1998; 139: 3157-3164.

[64] Nakashima K, Roehrich N, Cimasoni G. Gazi MI, Cox SW, Clark DT, et al. Characterization of protease activities in Capnocytophaga spp., Porphyromonas gingivalis, Prevotella spp., Treponema denticola and Actinobacillus actinomycetemcomitans. Oral Microbiol Immunol. 1997; 12: 240-248.
[65] Tsai CC, Hong YC, Chen CC, Wu YM. Measurement of prostaglandin E2 and leukotriene B4 in the gingival crevicular fluid. J Dent. 1998; 26: 97-103.
[66] Shimizu N, Yamaguchi M, Uesu K, Goseki T, Abiko Y. Stimulation of prostaglandin E2 and interleukin-1beta production from old rat periodontal ligament cells subjected to mechanical stress. J Gerontol A Biol Sci Med Sci. 2000; 55: B489-95
[67] Bertolini DR, Nedwin GE, Bringman TS, Smith DD, Mundy GR. Stimulation of bone resorption and inhibition of bone formation in vitro by human tumour necrosis factors. Nature. 1986; 319: 516-518.
[68] Faizuddin M, Bharathi SH, Rohini NV. Estimation of interleukin-1beta levels in the gingival crevicular fluid in health and in inflammatory periodontal disease. J Periodontol Res. 2003; 38: 111-114.
[69] Tsalikis L, Parapanisiou E, Bata-Kyrkou A, Polymenides Z, Konstantinidis A. Crevicular fluid levels of interleukin-1alpha and interleukin-1beta during experimental gingivitis in young and old adults. J Int Acad Periodontol. 2002; 4: 5-11.
[70] Payne JB, Reinhardt RA, Masada MP, DuBois LM, Allison AC. Gingival crevicular fluid IL-8: correlation with local IL-1 beta levels and patient estrogen status. J Periodontal Res. 1993; 28: 451-453
[71] Chien HH, Lin WL, Cho MI. Expression of TGF-beta isoforms and their receptors during mineralized nodule formation by rat periodontal ligament cells in vitro. J Periodontol Res. 1999; 34: 301–309.
[72] Wada N, Maeda H, Tanabe K, Tsuda E, Yano K, Nakamuta H, et al. Periodontal ligament cells secrete the factor that inhibits osteoclastic differentiation and function: the factor is osteoprotegerin/osteoclastogenesis inhibitory factor. J Periodontol Res. 2001; 36: 56 – 63.
[73] Kanzaki H, Chiba M, Shimizu Y, Mitani H. Dual regulation of osteoclast differentiation by periodontal ligament cells through RANKL stimulation and OPG inhibition. J Dent Res. 2001; 80: 887– 891.
[74] Lacey DL, Timms E, Tan H-L, Kelley MJ, Dunstan CR, Burgess T, et al. Osteoprotegerin ligand is a cytokine that regulates osteoclast differentiation and activation. Cell 1998; 93: 165–176.
[75] Nakagawa N, Kinosaki M, Yamaguchi K, Shima N, Yasuda H, Yano K, et al. RANK is the essential signaling receptor for osteoclast differentiation factor in osteoclastogenesis. Biochem Biophys Res Commun 1998; 253: 395– 400.
[76] Yasuda H, Shima N, Nakagawa N, Mochizuki S, Yano K, Fujise N, et al. Identity of osteoclastogenesis inhibitory factor (OCIF) and osteoprotegerin (OPG): a mechanism by which OPG/OCIF inhibits osteoclastogenesis in vitro. Endocrinology 1998; 139: 1329-1337.
[77] Park HJ, Park OJ, Shin J. Receptor activator of NF-kappaB ligand enhances the activity of macrophages as antigen presenting cells. Exp Mol Med. 2005; 37: 524-532.

[78] Takeuchi O, Hoshino K, Kawai T, Sanjo H, Takada H, Ogawa T, et al. Differential roles of TLR2 and TLR4 in recognition of Gram-negative and Gram-positive bacterial cell wall components. Immunity 1999; 11: 443–51.
[79] Hatakeyama J, Tamai R, Sugiyama A, Akashi S, Sugawara S, Takada H. Contrasting responses of human gingival and periodontal ligament fibroblasts to bacterial cell-surface components through the CD14/Toll-like receptor system. Oral Microbiol Immunol 2003; 18: 14–23.
[80] Miyauchi M, Sato S, Kitagawa S, Hiraoka M, Kudo Y, Ogawa I, et al. Cytokine expression in rat molar gingival periodontal tissues after topical application of lipopolysaccharide. Histochem Cell Biol 2001; 116: 57–62.
[81] Kobayashi K, Takahashi N, Jimi E, Udagawa N, Takami M, Kotake S, et al. Tumor necrosis factor alpha stimulates osteoclast differentiation by a mechanism independent of the ODF/RANKL-RANK interaction. J Exp Med 2000; 191: 275– 86.
[82] Wada N, Maeda H, Yoshimine Y, Akamine A. Lipopolysaccharide stimulates expression of osteoprotegerin and receptor activator of NF-kappa B ligand in periodontal ligament fibroblasts through the induction of interleukin-1 beta and tumor necrosis factor-alpha. Bone 2004; 35: 629-35.
[83] Huttner EA, Machado DC, de Oliveira RB, Antunes AG, Hebling E. Effects of human aging on periodontal tissues. Spec Care Dentist. 2009; 29:149-55.
[84] Papapanou PN; Wennström JL; Grondahl K. A 10-year retrospective study of periodontal disease progression. J Clin Periodontol 1989; 16: 403-411.
[85] Ismail AI; Morrison EC; Burt BA; Cafesse RG; Kavanagh MT. Natural history of periodontal disease in adults: findings from the Tecumseh Periodontal Study, 1959-87. J Dent Res 1990; 69: 430-435.
[86] Haffajee A; Socransky SS; Lindhe J; Kent RL; Okamoto H; Yoneyama T. Clinical risk indicators for periodontal attachment loss. J Clin Periodontol 1991; 18: 117-125.
[87] Albandar JM. A 6-year study on the pattern of periodontal disease progression. J Clin Periodontol 1990; 17: 467-471.
[88] Grbic JT; Lamster IB; Celenti RS; Fine JB. Risk indicators for future clinical attachment loss in adult periodontitis: patient variables. J Periodontol 1991; 62: 322-329.
[89] Brown LF; Beck JD; Rozier RG. Incidence of attachment loss in community-dwelling older adults. J Periodontol 1994; 65: 316-323.
[90] Beck JD; Koch GG. Incidence of attachment loss over 3 years in older adults – new and progressing lesions. Community Dent Oral Epidemiol 1995; 23: 291-296.
[91] Ship JA; Beck JD. Ten-year longitudinal study of periodontal attachment loss in healthy adults. Oral Surg Oral Med Oral Pathol Oral Radiol Endod 1996; 81: 281-290.
[92] Locker D, Slade GD, Murray H. Epidemiology of periodontal disease among older adults: a review. Periodontol 2000. 1998; 16: 16-33.
[93] Wennstrom JL, Papapanou PN, Grondahl K. A model for decision making regarding periodontal treatment needs. J Clin Periodontal 1990: 17: 217-222.
[94] Kalk W, de Baat C, Meeuwissen JH. Is there a need for gerodontology? Int Den J. 1992; 42: 209-16.
[95] Hebling E, Mugayar L, Dias PV. Geriatric dentistry: a new specialty in Brazil. Gerodontol. 2007; 24: 177-80.
[96] Ettinger RL. The development of geriatric dental education programs in Canada: an update. J Can Dent Assoc 2010; 76:a1.

17

Aging, Oral Health and Quality of Life

Vinicius Cappo Bianco and José Henrique Rubo
*Department of Prosthodontics, Bauru School of Dentistry,
University of São Paulo, Bauru, SP,
Brazil*

1. Introduction

The aging of populations is a global phenomenon that presents great challenges as humanity seeks to meet and promote the physical and mental wellbeing of the elderly (United Nations, 2002). As a population ages, a demographic and epidemiological transition occurs caused by the comparative increase of elderly individuals within the population. This is accompanied by a changing profile of disease as the incidence of chronic degenerative diseases, such as diabetes, arthritis, osteoarthritis, cardiovascular disease, rheumatism, depression and oral health problems increases, and the prevalence of infectious disease decreases.

The oral health of the elderly is, in part, precarious, as the majority use or require some form of dental prostheses. The average number of teeth in the oral cavity is typically minimal and the incidence of root caries and periodontal disease is high. This trend often directly influences the quality of life of the elderly, causing psychological, physical and social detriment to the patient (Correa da Silva and Fernandes, 2001). This demographic of the population also commonly experience xerostomia, temporomandibular joint problems and a reduction in taste sensation. Often, these physiological changes inhibit the maintenance of a proper diet as patients seek to mitigate the challenges associated with an inability to chew (Cassolato and Turnbull 2003, DeBoever et al. 1999, DeMarchi et al. 2008, Moynihan et al. 2009, Thonsom et al. 2006).

Decayed, Missing, Filled Teeth (DMFT) and Community Periodontal Index for Treatment Needs (CPITN) are instruments used to perform oral assessments of patients in populations. Using the data collected from these indexes, the oral health of populations can be evaluated in an objective manner. However, the simple assessment of the mouth does not answer a clinical question that has been a more recent concern of health research: What is the effect of poor oral conditions on quality of life?

Several rating systems have been proposed and subsequently used to answer this question, most prominently when considering those patients that are greater than 60 years of age. Certainly, the impact of health on quality of daily life is deeply conditioned by cultural, socioeconomic standards and the level of social interrelations.

2. Demographic and epidemiological transition

Aging is a biological, pathological, socioeconomic and psychosocial process. It varies from one individual to another according to patient health, culture and life expectancies (Kalk et al. 1992). Epidemiological aging is a result of the mortality rates in a population. As the

mortality rate decreases, there is an increase in the average life span of the population, bringing it to the biological limit of the species. This increase in life span is a natural aspiration of any society, but it is also important that the desire improve the quality of life for those who are elderly occurs in conjunction with this phenomenon (Ramos 1993).
The growth of the aging population is a global fact. The graphic below (Graphic 1, Graphic 2, Graphic 3) shows a representation of this growth along with projections of population increase for this demographic in the future (United Nations, 2010).

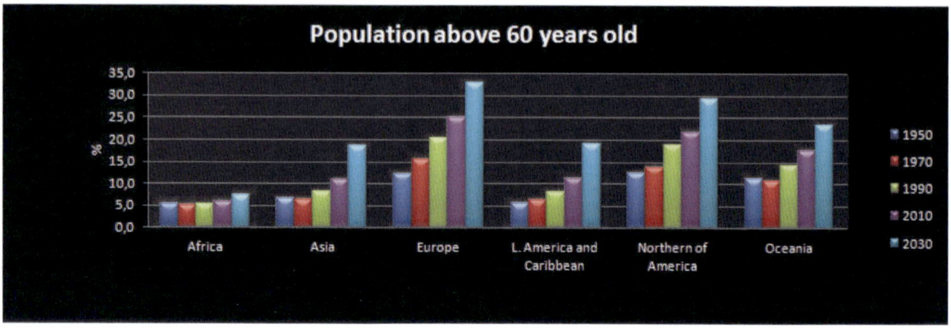

Source: United Nations 2010

Graphic 1.

A primary concern when considering demographic and epidemiological transition is how to prepare health care services to better suit the needs of this new segment of the population. This concern is most prominently raised in developing countries where public attention is urgently needed to address the lack of sufficient oral health care. As mentioned previously, a main feature in an aging population is the increase of chronic disease prevalence and the subsequent decrease of infectious disease.

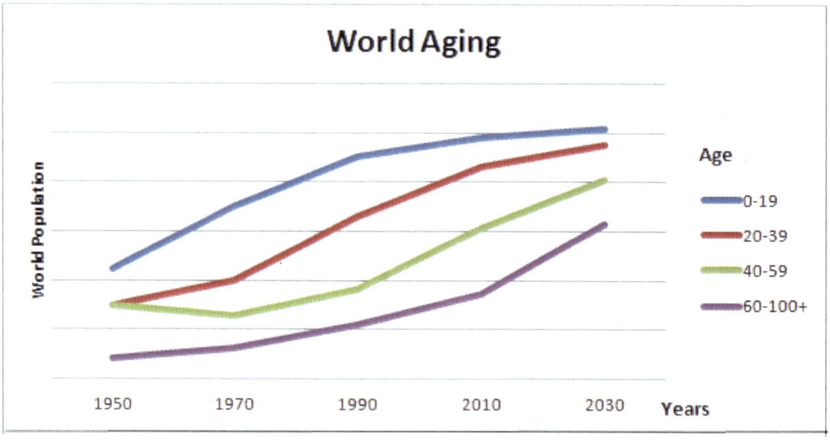

Source: United Nations 2010

Graphic 2.

This change results in an increased demand for continual treatment in an demographic of elderly individuals. Historically, treatment of the oral cavity was not prioritized to the elderly population. Consequently, the evaluation of oral health treatment requires attention as elderly individuals, who suffer more prominently from a high prevalence of caries and periodontal disease, become more numerous in modern populations (Moreira et al. 2005).

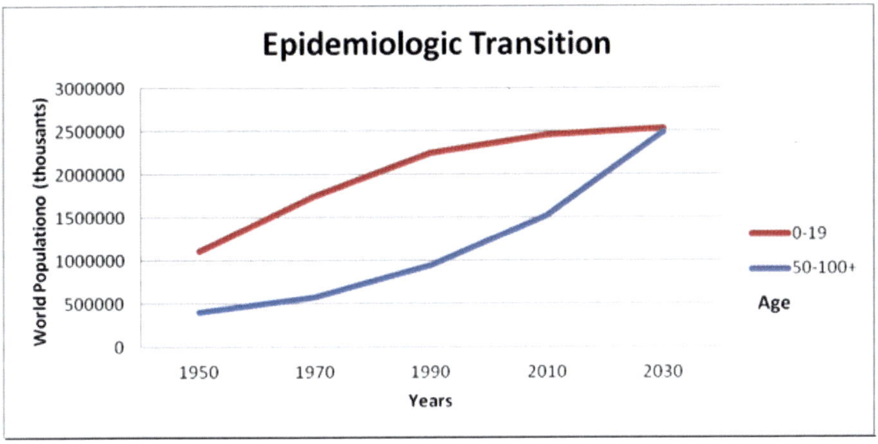

Source: United Nations 2010

Graphic 3.

3. Self perception of oral health and quality of life index

Epidemiological indicators such as the DMFT Index are used to analyze the amount of caries, restorations and missing teeth in a patient's oral cavity, while the CPITN Index can assess periodontal disease as well as the need for removable prostheses (WHO 1987). Since the 1990's there has been a growing recognition of the social and psychological impact that changes in oral health can have on the daily life of a patient. This impact on quality of life can be assessed through a variety of procedures that have been proposed in recent years and are primarily aimed at reaching the older generations of populations. These developments improve the understanding of oral health by adding a subjective component and revealing that oral abnormalities have significant social, psychological and economic consequences to overall quality of life.

3.1 Oral health impact profile (Slade and Spencer 1994)

The Oral Health Impact Profile (OHIP) is a self-perception measuring instrument that contains 49 questions divided into seven areas: functional limitation, physical pain, psychological discomfort, physical disability, psychological difficulty, social obstacle and social handicap. Questions are answered on a Likert scale from 0 to 4, with 0 = never, 1 = almost never, 2= sometimes, 3 = often and 4 = very often. The most significant advantage of this index is that it can represent both an individual as well as a group of individuals, while measuring the extent with which poor oral health can affect daily life. In more recent years, the Oral Health Impact Profile Short Form or OHIP-14 was developed. This index is a reduced form of the original, containing only 14 questions divided into the same seven domains (Slade 1997).

3.2 Dental impacts on daily living (Leao and Sheihan 1996)

The Dental Impacts on Daily Living (DIDL) index consists of 36 items divided into five scales or domains including comfort, appearance and pain. The responses to this questionnaire are scored within a range of +1 to -1, where +1 signifies a positive impact, 0 shows no impact, and -1 corresponds to a negative patient impact. The weight of each domain is represented by the sum of the patient responses to the questions within the domain being assessed.

3.3 Oral impacts on daily living (Adulyanon and Sheihan 1997)

The Oral Impacts of Daily Living (OIDP) Index was created to quantify the relative frequency of oral health problems impacting quality of life. This questionnaire pertains to the effects of oral health on such things as feeding and the utilization of food, the clear pronunciation of words, sleep and relaxation, the ability to show teeth without shame, the maintenance of a stable emotional state, and the willingness to go to work or social events. Responses to the test questions range from zero (no effect in the last six months) to five (often happening in the last six months).

3.4 General oral health assessment index (Atchison and Dolan 1990)

The General Oral Health Assessment Index (GOHAI) assesses the impact of oral health and oral disorders on the quality of life of individuals. It consists of 12 questions that can be answered with scores of zero to five.

4. Oral health and quality of life studies

It was found that data collected using the GOHAI Index differed from data found by clinical examination, with interviewees noting dental and gingival problems. When asked to evaluate their individual oral health, 42.7% of dentate patients considered their condition to be fair, while edentulous patients had the overall best self-assessment, with 55.8% of patients evaluating their overall oral health as good. In general, interviewees with a better self-evaluation (those with good or excellent) had, on average, more carious teeth than those who assessed their own oral health as fair, poor or very poor. Those patients with an oral environment that had been evaluated as poor or very poor had at least one tooth that was intended for extraction (Correa Silva and Fernandes 1999).

A study was conducted on the impact of oral health on quality of life by applying the OHIP-14 and comparing two techniques of denture fabrication. Sixty-five patients were selected, thirty-two of which had their dentures made in the conventional technique while the remaining thirty-three had the "copies of the edge" technique used. The OHIP-14 was applied before and after treatment. The results showed that there were no significant differences in impact on quality of life when comparing the denture fabrication techniques. However, in most cases, the patients reported an improvement with the use of their new prostheses (Scott Forgie and Davis 2006).

Two hundred and twenty-four patients were evaluated with the OHIP-49 before, during and after oral rehabilitation treatments with dental prostheses. After the completion of the treatment, another questionnaire was completed to measure patient satisfaction and evaluate subsequent improvements in oral health. It was observed that the results of the OHIP questionnaire performed before and during treatment were almost constant. However, the results changed after the completion of treatment, indicating a decrease in the effect of oral health on the quality of life. The vast majority of patients (59%) described an improvement in their oral health status after treatment, while 15.5% maintained that their oral hygiene remained stable, and 0.5% felt it was worse after treatment (John et al. 2009).

The OHIP-49 was used in a population of 224 patients aged 50 or older. By including patients between 50 and 60 years of age as well as those in the more elderly demographic, the "floor" effect, which occurs when a large number of zero scores affect an indexes ability to discriminate, is avoided (Locker and Allen 2002). In addition to the OHIP-49, clinical examinations were also conducted that included an assessment of patient dental status (DMFT Index), community periodontal index (CPITN), and periodontal attachment loss. As well, the use or need for use of full or partial dental prostheses was assessed according to the instructions of the WHO-Oral Health Surveys (Basic Methods 4th Edition 1987).

The index showed that the OHIP impacts of oral health on social domains are less severe than they are on the physical and psychological domains. Individual age was a significant factor in all areas. With the exception of the 'functional limitations' domain, age is inversely correlated with the amount of impact oral health has on quality of life (Graphic 4).

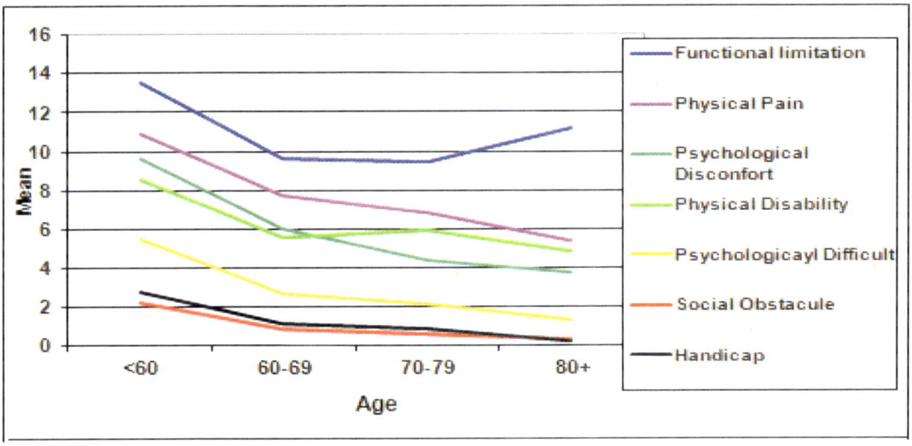

Graphic 4. OHIP outcomes from Bianco et al., 2010.

In the functional limitation domain, 90.63% of patients reported some sort of impact, while 83.48% described physical pain, and 73.22% experienced physical disability. In the psychological discomfort domain, the impact percentage was 70.54% and 53.57% in psychological incapacity. The impact experienced by patients in the social disability and social disadvantage domains was significantly less at 24.55% and 26.79% respectively. These results were similar to those in the original OHIP Slade and Spencer (1994) (Table 1). The Community Periodontal Index (CPI) emerged as significant in the functional limitation, physical pain, physical disability and disadvantage domains. The number of missing teeth had significant impact on functional limitation and disability.

Domains	Alfa (Bianco et al.2010)	(Slade and Spencer1994)
Functional limitation	0,67	0,70
Physical Pain	0,61	0,76
Psychological discomfort	0,80	0,77
Physical disability	0,71	0,82
Psychological difficulty	0,74	0,83
Social Obstacle	0,71	0,73
Handicap	0,65	0,37

Table 1. OHP Alfa Cronbach Coefficient comparison among Bianco et al. (2010) and Slade & Spencer (1994).

The interpretation of these indexes allows for the formation of a clinical profile of a population that can be correlated with the social and psychological aspects of oral health. This information can then be used to influence public policies for this age demographic and help to improve prevention programs and ensure adequate treatment opportunities (Bianco et al. 2010).

5. Oral health of the elderly

Oral health is inseparable from overall health. General characteristics of the individual and the environment affect the stomatognathic system, which makes an understanding of these interactions extremely important to the diagnosis of the needs and priorities of elderly patients (Shinkai 2000). An absence, or inability to adequately conduct the mechanical acts of oral hygiene, such as brushing and flossing, allows for the accumulation of plaque to such a degree that it can disrupt the balance of oral microbiota. The maintenance of the oral environment is the single most important preventative measure for the elderly, especially in reference to caries, periodontal problems, and opportunistic infections such as *Candida albicans*. The diagnosed conditions and risks of elderly patients must be assessed individually by the dental team in order for an effective treatment plan to be established. Using this evaluation, the proper course of oral hygiene, professional cleaning, fluoridation and antimicrobial use can be determined. Note that in older patients there is a higher occurrence rate of lesions on the oral mucosa, most predominantly in denture wearers. Chart 1 shows the main mucosal changes found in elderly patients.

These injuries are so common in the elderly due to the decreased elasticity of the mucosa, causing it to behave in a brittle fashion and be more susceptible to damage from irritants. Elderly patients are also more susceptible to injuries of the oral mucosa as a secondary result of a systemic problem, such as an inability to complete proper oral hygiene maintenance, reduction in oral flora due to prescription drugs, xerostomia, diabetes and leukemia (Rosa et al. 1999, Shay and Ship 1995, Smith and Sheiham 1979).

Amalgam tattoo	Denture stomatitis	Nicotinic stomatitis
Angular cheilitis	Erythroplakia	Nonspecific tumor
Burning mouth syndrome	Fissured tongue	Nonspecific ulcer
Cheek or lip biting	Geographic tongue	Pseudomembranous candidiasis
Cleft lip/palate	Homogeneous leukoplakia	Recurrent aphthous ulcers
Coated-hairy tongue	Macroglossia	

Source: Ship and Baum (1993), Avcu et al. (2005).

Chart 1. Most frequent mucosal lesions in elderly persons.

Another important consideration when dealing with the oral health of the elderly population is the nutrition status of patients who are partially edentulous or who use ill-fitting dentures. Many of these prostheses are no longer able to exercise proper function due to the wearing away of the artificial teeth. It is also fairly common for edentulous patients to use only an upper denture since adaptation to the lower prosthesis is more difficult due to its lack of stability (Bianco 2010). Typically, these patients tend to consume foods with a lower nutritional value in order to allow for ease of chewing. The maintenance of the teeth, gingiva and proper use of well fitted prostheses have a crucial role in the nutritional status of these patients (DeMarchi et al. 2008, Moynihan et al. 2009).

Temporomandibular joint problems are also commonly observed in this demographic of the population. Pops, crackles, pain and reduced mouth opening may be related to the systemic health of the patient. In general however, the clinical profile of temporomandibular dysfunction in the elderly does not differ from that of younger patients. Consequently, the same conservative treatments for these dysfunctions in younger patients can also be used for the elderly (DeBoever, DeBoever, Keersmaekers, 1999).

5.1 Edentulism

The most common causes of tooth loss are caries and periodontal disease. Often, edentulism occurs as a secondary result of systemic diseases that enhance periodontal disease, or as a result of iatrogenic effects, trauma, or damaging patient habits such as drug, alcohol or tobacco use. As well, patients who suffer from various congenital syndromes may exhibit an absence of some or all teeth (anodontia) (Dolan et al. 2001, Muller et al. 2007). Elderly patients also tend to exhibit a low demand for professional dental care, and are often non-compliant for both preventative and restorative dental treatments. It has been found that there is an adaptation of sorts to edentulism by elderly patients as they age. Typically, as age increases, the impact of oral health on the overall quality of life decreases. Graphic 5 shows the distribution of the use of denture according to their age (Bianco; 2010).

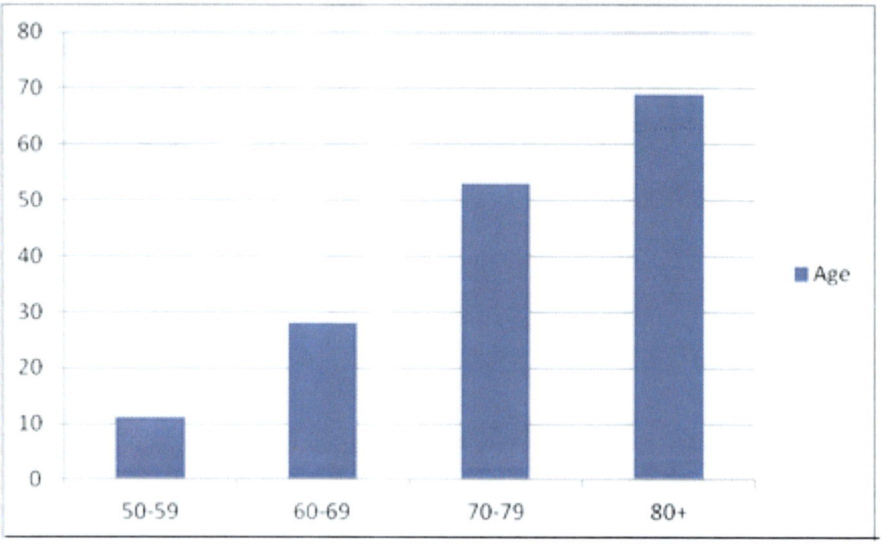

Graphic 5. Percentage of Dentures wearing according with age, Bianco et al. (2010).

Epidemiologically, edentulism is present in most studies involving the elderly population. One study examined 247 patients between the ages of 50 and 88 years old and discovered that among those examined, 25.9% were edentulous, 74.1% had at least one tooth present in the oral cavity, and the average number of teeth present in each individual was 17.9 (Locker et al. 1989).

In a survey of 303 individuals, those between the ages of 60 to 69 years old had a 58.3% prevalence of edentulism, while 65.9% of patients in the 70 to 79 year age group were edentulous. In patients older than 80 years, the number of edentulous patients reached 68% of the population (Bergman et al. 1991).

A longitudinal study was conducted between 1992 and 1994 that shows the prevalence of tooth loss in patients over 65 years of age. The first part of the survey was conducted with 1,667 subjects, and it revealed that 54.8% of this sample size was edentulous. In the second part of the survey, 1108 patients were assessed, and 56% were determined to be edentulous (Pucca Jr 1998).

In a study evaluating 201 elderly patients, the DMFT results lead to an average of 26.66, while each patient had an average of 11.42 teeth in the oral cavity. Root caries were detected in 37.8% of the dentate patients. As well, the need for and use of prosthetic appliances were also evaluated and it was determined that, clinically, most patients that did not use dental prostheses needed them. Of the edentulous patients, the majority used some form of dental prostheses. However, over 62.5% of these patients required the fabrication of a new prosthetic due to the clinical ineffectiveness of their current one (Correa da Silva and Fernandes 1999).

In a study of 224 patients, aged 50 or older, 117 participants (52%) were total upper denture wearers. Seventy-four of these patients also wore lower dentures (33% of the total sample size). Of the denture wearers, 54.7% needed the upper prosthetic replaced, while 59.7% of those who wore lower dentures required replacement as well. Three patients in the study wore only a lower full denture, and eight edentulous subjects wore no prostheses at all (Bianco et al. 2010).

A study of elderly individuals observed that the patients involved had an average of 17 teeth in the oral cavity, and as age increased, this average decreased. Patients aged 60 to 65 had an average of 20 teeth while older patients (80 years of age or older) had an average tooth count of only 12 (Varela 2011).

5.2 Periodontal disease

Periodontal disease is caused by the accumulation of plaque as it adheres to tooth surfaces, leading to the destruction of the surrounding periodontal tissues. Metabolic products synthesized by the bacteria in the accumulating plaque cause an inflammatory response in the gingival tissues surrounding the affected teeth. Consequently, the periodontal support is compromised and a loss of crestal bone results. Both horizontal and vertical alveolar bone resorption occurs, resulting in subsequent gingival recession, mobility and the potential for tooth loss. As a patient ages, unevenness on the surface of cementum and alveolar bone occurs, and there is an increased deposition of cementum at the apical region of the roots. Bone tissue begins to change as the amount of mineralized material in both cortical and trabecular bone decreases. This alteration leads to a reduced resilience in the bone structure, and an increased fragility. Typically, the amount of bone resorption increases while bone formation decreases, resulting in overall bone porosity (Gomes et al. 2010, Locker et al. 1998). In the gingival tissues, aging may result in a decrease in keratinized tissue that can indicate tissue permeability, and a decreased resistance to infection and trauma (Needleman 2004). As well, fibroblast formation and activity is also reduced in older patients, and as a result, there is a decrease in the production of organic matrix and vascularization, with a subsequent increase in elastic fibers (Johson et al. 1989, Needleman 2004, Severson et al. 1978, Zenobio et al. 2004).
The apical migration of the junctional epithelium (JE) is associated with aging, as well as with periodontal disease. However, the insertion loss that results as a consequence of age alone has been suggested to have no clinical significance (Locker et al. 1998). The progression of gingival recession can occur as a result of several factors, such as passive eruption caused by wearing away of tooth structure, anatomical factors and traumatic tooth brushing. It has been found that gingival recession is caused not only by aging, but by the progressive and cumulative effects of periodontal disease or trauma throughout life (Needleman 2004).
The presence of dental calculus, gingivitis and periodontal disease is a common finding in elderly patient populations. In a study of 120 elderly patients, gingivitis was found in 100% of those that were examined. Nineteen percent had pocket depths of 3-5mm and 5% had depths of 6mm or more (Mojon 1995). Another study conducted using the CPITN Index found that on average, 3.53 of the six sextants in the human dentition were excluded for elderly patients as a result of missing teeth. Of the 1.29 sextants with periodontal pockets, 43.7% of these were deep, 28.1% were shallow, and dental calculus was present in 26% of the valid sextants. Bleeding on probing was found for 8.2% of the applicable sextants, and areas of health were represented by only 3% (Correa da Silva and Fernandes 1999). In a study of elderly patients using the CPINT and Periodontal Attachment Loss (PAL) Indexes, edentulous patients were excluded, leaving only 57.6% of the sample to be assessed. For the CPINT and the PAL Index, a score of zero represents a healthly periodontal environment. A score of 1 signifies the presence of bleeding on probing for the CPINT Index, and an attachment loss of 4 to 5mm for the PAL Index. A score of 2 is characterized by the presence of calculus (CPINT) and attachment loss of 6 to 8mm (PAL Index). Lastly, an individual who receives a score of 3 will have pocket depths of 4 to 5mm (CPINT) and attachment loss of 9 to 11mm (PAL). In general, most of the subjects had zero scores for both indexes. However, when those subjects with scores of 1 or higher were summed, those individuals outnumbered the patients with scores of zero. Specifically, for the CPITN Index, 60.9% of

patients tested had a score of 1 or above, and the same was true for 55.8% of patients using the Periodontal Attachment Loss Index (Bianco 2010). Another study found that only 6% of patients had periodontal problems, while 26% experienced gingival bleeding, 57% had dental calculus, and 31% had some extent of periodontal attachment loss (Varela et al. 2011). It is evident that aging is not solely responsible for the occurrence of periodontal disease. Other influences such as the accumulation of plaque, along with environmental, systemic and economic factors, can also increase the risk of developing periodontal disease. This can be visualized in the schematic below (Schema 1).

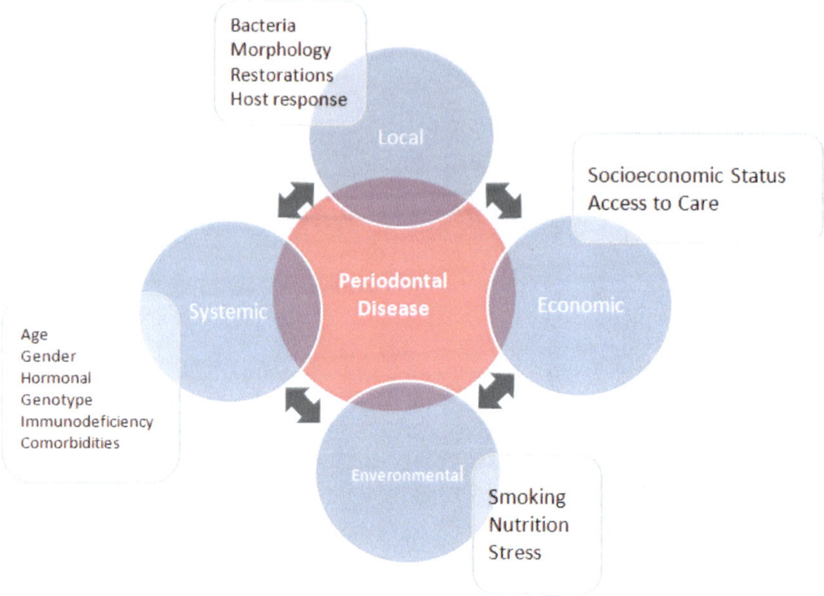

Schema 1. Risk model for periodontal disease. (*Based in* Novak 2008).

6. Concluding remarks

It has been proven that the elderly population is increasing in prominence worldwide, and the importance of preparing both private and public health services for this phenomenon is becoming increasingly apparent. Planning for health services accessibility and specialized prevention for this new demographic should be seriously assessed, most commonly in developing countries. It is imperative that health professionals work as a unit, both within the dental field and otherwise.

The assessment of the general health of the patient should be part of the dental treatment protocol, and should be completed well before beginning any procedure. As well, how treatment will affect the daily life of the patient must also be taken into consideration. A plan for appropriate treatment of elderly individuals must be cautious and allow for the development of treatment options that suit the needs of the patient. It is necessary for health professionals to develop preventative dental programs for future generations of adults who will, one day, be part of this elderly demographic. By doing so, dental professionals will be able to better provide oral care and quality of life to these patients.

7. References

[1] Adulyanon, S; Sheiham, A. Oral Impacts on Daily Performances. In: Slade GD. Measuring Oral Health and Quality of Life. Chapel Hill: University of North Carolina;1997.

[2] Atchison KA, Dolan TA. Development of the Geriatric Oral Health Assessment Index. J Dental Educ, v.54, p.680-7, 1990.

[3] Avcu, N; Ozbek, M; Kurtoglu, D; Kurtoglu, E; Kansu, O; Kansu, H. Oral findings and health status among hospitalized patients with physical disabilities, aged 60 or above .Archives of Gerontology and Geriatrics, v. 41, p.69–79, 2005.

[4] Bergman, JD; Wright, FAC; Hammond, RH. The Oral Health of Eldery in Melbourne. Aust. Dent. J.,v.36, p.280-285, 1991.

[5] Bianco, VC; Lopes, ES; Borgato, MH; Moura e Silva, P; Marta, SN. O impacto das condições bucais na qualidade de vida de pessoas com cinquenta ou mais anos de vida. Ciênc. saúde coletiva, v.15, p.2165-72, 2010.

[6] Cassolato, SF; Turnbull, RS. Xerostomia: clinical aspects and treatment. Gerodontology, v.20, p.4, 2003.

[7] Corrêa da Silva, SR; Fernandes, RAC. Auto Percepção das Condições de Saúde Bucal por Idosos. Revista Saúde Publica, v.35, p.349-55, 2001.

[8] DeBoever, VBL; DeBoever, AL; Keersmaekers, K. Comparison of clinical profiles and treatment outcomes of an elderly and ayounger temporomandibular patient group. J Prosthet Dent, v.81, p.312-7, 1999.

[9] DeMarchi, RJ; Hugo, FN; Hilgert, JB; Padilha, DMP. Association between oral health status and nutritional status in south Brazilian independent-living older people. Nutrition, v.24, p.546–553, 2008.

[10] Dolan, TA; Gilbert, GH; Duncan, RP; Foerster, U. Risk indicators of edentulism, partial tooth loss and prosthetic status among black and White middle-aged and older adults. Commun. Dent. Oral Epidemiol., v.29, p.329-40, 2001.

[11] Gomes, SGF; Meloto, CB; Custodio, W; Rizzatti-Barbosa, CM. Aging and the periodontium. Braz J Oral Sci., v. 9, p. 1-6, 2010.

[12] Johnson, BD; Mulligan, K; Kiyak, HA; Marder, M. Aging or disease? Periodontal changes and treatment considerations in the older dental patient. Gerontology, v. 8, p.109-18, 1989.

[13] Jonh, MT; Reibmann, DR; Szentpetery, A. Steele, J. An Approach to Define Clinical significance in prostohodontics. Jour. Prosth., v.18, p.455-460, 2009.

[14] Kalk, W; Boot, C; Meeuwissen, JH. Is there a need for Gerontology? Int. Dent., v.42, p.209-216, 1992.

[15] Leao, A; Sheiham, A. .The Development of socio - Dental Measure of Dental Impact of Daily Living. Community Dental Health, v.13, p.22-26, 1996.

[16] Locker D, Slade GD, Murray H. Epidemiology of periodontal disease among older adults: a review. Periodontol., 2000, v.16, p.16-33, 1998.

[17] Locker, D; Allen, PF. Developing Short Form Measures of Oral Health - Related Quality of Life. Journal of Public Health Dentistry, v.62, p.13-20, 2002.

[18] Locker, D; Miller, Y. Prevalence of and Factors Associated with Tooth Decay in Older Adults in Canada. Journal Dent. Res., v.68, p.765-772, 1989.

[19] Mojon, P; Rentsch, A; Budtz-Jorgensen, E. relationship Between Prosthodontic Status, Caries, and Periodontal Disease in a Geriatric Population. Int. J. Prosthodont, v.8, p.564-571, 1995.

[20] Moreira, RS; Nico, LS; Tomita, NE; Ruiz, T. A saúde bucal do idoso brasileiro: Revisão sistemática sobre o quadro epidemiológico e acesso aos serviços de saúde bucal. Cad. Saúde Pública, v.21, p.1665-1675, 2005.

[21] Moynihan, P; Thomason, M; Walls, A; Gray-Donald, K; Morais, JÁ; Ghanem, H; Wollin, S; Ellis, J; Steele, J; Lund, J; Feine, J. Researching the impact of oral health on diet and nutritional status: Methodological issues. Journal of Dentitry, v.37, p.237-49, 2009.

[22] Müller, F; Naharro, M; Carlsson, G E. What are the prevalence and incidence of tooth loss in the adult and elderly population in Europe? Clin. Oral Impl. Res. 18 (Suppl. 3), p.2-14, 2007.

[23] Needleman, I. Envelhecimento e o periodonto. In: Newman MG, Takei HH, Carranza FA. Periodontia clínica. 9.ed. Rio de Janeiro: Guanabara Koogan, p.51-5, 2004.

[24] Novak, KF. Periodontal disease and associated risck factors. In: Prevention in Clinical Oral Health Care. Mosby Elsevier, p. 56-67, 2008.

[25] Pucca Jr., GA. Saúde Bucal do Idoso: Aspectos Sociais e Preventivos. In. Gerontologia (M. Papaléo Neto, org.), São Paulo, Ed. Atheneu, p.297-310, 1996.

[26] Ramos, LR. A Explosão Demográfica da Terceira Idade no Brasil: Uma Questão de Saúde Pública. Revista de Gerontologia, v.1, 1993.

[27] Rosa, AGF; Fernandes, RAC; Pinto, VG, Ramos, LR. Condições de Saúde Bucal em Pessoas de 60 anos ou mais no Município de São Paulo (Brasil). Revista de Saúde Pública, n.26, p.155-166,1992.

[28] Scott, BJJ; Forgie, AH; Davis, DM. A Study to Compare the Oral Health Impact Profile and Satisfaction Before and After Having Replacement Complete Dentures Constructed by Either the Copy or the Conventional Technique. The gerontol. Assoc. and Blackwell Munksgaard, gerodontology, v.23, p.79-86, 2006.

[29] Severson, JA; Moffett, BC; Kokich, V; Selipsky, H. A histologic study of age changes in the adult human periodontal joint (ligament). J Periodontol., v.49, p.189-200, 1978.

[30] Shay, K; Ship, JA. The Importance of Oral Health in the Older Patient. J. Am. Geriatric. Soc., v.43, p.1414-1422, 1995.

[31] Shinkai, RSA; Cury, AADB. O Papel da Odontologia na Equipe Interdiciplinar: Contribuindo para Atenção Integral ao Idoso. Caderno de Saúde Publica, v.16, p.1099-109, 2000.

[32] Ship, JA; Baum, BJ. Old age in health and disease. Oral Surg Oral Med Oral Pathol, v.76, p.40-4, 1993.

[33] Slade, GD; Spencer, AJ. Development and Evaluation of the Oral Health Impact Profile. Community Dental Health, v.11, p.3-11, 1994.

[34] Slade, GD. Derivation and validation of a short form Oral Health impact Profile. Comm. Dent Oral Epidemiol, v.25, p.284-290, 1997.

[35] Thomson, WM; Chalmers, JM; Spencer, AJ; Slade, GD. A longitudinal study of medication exposure and xerostomia among older people. Gerodontology, v.23, p.205-13, 2006.

[36] United Nations. Web site: http://esa.un.org/unpd/wpp/ExcelData/population.htm. World Population Prospects, the 2010 Revision, 2011.

[37] Varela, MMS; Cabanell, PI; Clemente, NG; Garciia, JMR; Garcıa, MAN; Gonzalez, AL. Oral and dental health of non-institutionalized elderly people in Spain. Archives of Gerontology and Geriatrics, v.52, p.159–163, 2011.

[38] WHO. Oral Health Surveys Basic Method .4 th Edition,p.26-29,Geneva,1987.

[39] Zenóbio, EG; Toledo, BEC; Zuza. EP. Fisiologia, patologia e tratamento das doenças do periodonto do paciente geriátrico. In: Campostrini E. Odontogeriatria. Rio de Janeiro, Revinter, p.184-98, 2004.

Permissions

The contributors of this book come from diverse backgrounds, making this book a truly international effort. This book will bring forth new frontiers with its revolutionizing research information and detailed analysis of the nascent developments around the world.

We would like to thank Dr. Jane Manakil, for lending her expertise to make the book truly unique. She has played a crucial role in the development of this book. Without her invaluable contribution this book wouldn't have been possible. She has made vital efforts to compile up to date information on the varied aspects of this subject to make this book a valuable addition to the collection of many professionals and students.

This book was conceptualized with the vision of imparting up-to-date information and advanced data in this field. To ensure the same, a matchless editorial board was set up. Every individual on the board went through rigorous rounds of assessment to prove their worth. After which they invested a large part of their time researching and compiling the most relevant data for our readers. Conferences and sessions were held from time to time between the editorial board and the contributing authors to present the data in the most comprehensible form. The editorial team has worked tirelessly to provide valuable and valid information to help people across the globe.

Every chapter published in this book has been scrutinized by our experts. Their significance has been extensively debated. The topics covered herein carry significant findings which will fuel the growth of the discipline. They may even be implemented as practical applications or may be referred to as a beginning point for another development. Chapters in this book were first published by InTech; hereby published with permission under the Creative Commons Attribution License or equivalent.

The editorial board has been involved in producing this book since its inception. They have spent rigorous hours researching and exploring the diverse topics which have resulted in the successful publishing of this book. They have passed on their knowledge of decades through this book. To expedite this challenging task, the publisher supported the team at every step. A small team of assistant editors was also appointed to further simplify the editing procedure and attain best results for the readers.

Our editorial team has been hand-picked from every corner of the world. Their multi-ethnicity adds dynamic inputs to the discussions which result in innovative outcomes. These outcomes are then further discussed with the researchers and contributors who give their valuable feedback and opinion regarding the same. The feedback is then collaborated with the researches and they are edited in a comprehensive manner to aid the understanding of the subject.

Apart from the editorial board, the designing team has also invested a significant amount of their time in understanding the subject and creating the most relevant covers. They scrutinized every image to scout for the most suitable representation of the subject and create an appropriate cover for the book.

The publishing team has been involved in this book since its early stages. They were actively engaged in every process, be it collecting the data, connecting with the contributors or procuring relevant information. The team has been an ardent support to the editorial, designing and production team. Their endless efforts to recruit the best for this project, has resulted in the accomplishment of this book. They are a veteran in the field of academics and their pool of knowledge is as vast as their experience in printing. Their expertise and guidance has proved useful at every step. Their uncompromising quality standards have made this book an exceptional effort. Their encouragement from time to time has been an inspiration for everyone.

The publisher and the editorial board hope that this book will prove to be a valuable piece of knowledge for researchers, students, practitioners and scholars across the globe.

List of Contributors

Charlene W.J. Africa
University of the Western Cape, South Africa

Akihiro Yoshida and Toshihiro Ansai
Division of Community Oral Health Science, Kyushu Dental College, Japan

Vincent K. Tsiagbe
Department of Oral Biology, New Jersey Dental School, USA
Graduate School of Biomedical Science, USA
Department of Pathology and Laboratory Medicine, New Jersey Medical School, University of Medicine and Dentistry of New Jersey, Newark, NJ, USA

Daniel H. Fine
Department of Oral Biology, New Jersey Dental School, USA
Graduate School of Biomedical Science, USA

Whasun Oh Chung and Jonathan Y. An
University of Washington, Seattle, WA, USA

T. Hanioka
Fukuoka Dental College, Japan

M. Ojima
Graduate School of Dentistry, Osaka University, Japan

M. Nakamura
Osaka Medical Centre for Health Science and Promotion, Japan

R.S. Preethanath
Department of Periodontics and Community Dentistry, College of Dentistry, King Saud University, Riyadh, Saudi Arabia

S. V. Varma
Sri Sankara Dental College, Trivandrum, Kerala, India

P. S. Anand
People's College of Dental Sciences & Research Centre, Bhanpur, Bhopal, Madhya Pradesh, India

A. Al Farraj Aldosari
Department of Prosthetic Science, College of Dentistry, King Saud University, Riyadh, Saudi Arabia

S. Anil
Dental Implant and Osseointegration Research Chair, King Saud University, Riyadh, Saudi Arabia
Department of Periodontics and Community Dentistry, College of Dentistry, King Saud University, Riyadh, Saudi Arabia

Emil Kozarov and John Grbic
Columbia University College of Dental Medicine, Section of Oral and Diagnostic Sciences, New York, NY, USA

Ayse Basak Cinar
Faculty of Health Sciences, Dental Institute, University of Copenhagen, Denmark

Liliana Foia and Vasilica Toma
University of Medicine and Pharmacy "Gr. T. Popa" Iasi, Romania

Petra Surlin
University of Medicine and Pharmacy Craiova, Romania

Amin E. Hatem
Faculty of Dentistry, Tanta University, Egypt

Surajit Mistry and Debabrata Kundu
Department of Periodontics, Dr. R. Ahmed Dental College, Kolkata, India

Premananda Bharati
Biological Anthropology Unit, Indian Statistical Institute, Kolkata, India

Eleni Mamai-Homata, Vasileios Margaritis, Argy Polychronopoulou and Constantine Oulis
Dental School, National and Kapodistrian University of Athens, Greece

Vassiliki Topitsoglou
Dental School, Aristotle University of Thessaloniki, Greece

Hisashi Fujita
Department of Anthropology, Niigata College of Nursing, Japan

Juan Antonio García Núñez, Alicia Herrero Sánchez and Ana Isabel García Kass
Faculty of Odontology, Universidad Complutense of Madrid (UCM), Spain

Clara Gómez Hernández
Instituto Fisica-Quimica Rocasolano, Consejo Superior de Investigaciones Científicas (CSIC), Madrid, Spain

Renata S. Leite
Department of Stomatology, USA
Center for Oral Health Research, Medical University of South Carolina, Charleston, SC, USA

Keith L. Kirkwood
Craniofacial Biology, College of Dental Medicine, USA
Center for Oral Health Research, Medical University of South Carolina, Charleston, SC, USA

Eduardo Hebling
Department of Community Dentistry, Piracicaba Dental School, University of Campinas, Piracicaba, Brazil

Vinicius Cappo Bianco and José Henrique Rubo
Department of Prosthodontics, Bauru School of Dentistry, University of São Paulo, Bauru, SP, Brazil